C. Si
Antit
2nd e

Antibiotic Therapy
in Clinical Practice

Prof. Dr. C. Simon
University Children's Hospital, Kiel, Germany

Prof. Dr. W. Stille
University Centre for Internal Medicine,
Frankfurt am Main, Germany

Dr. P. J. Wilkinson
Microbiology and Public Health Laboratory,
Plymouth, England

Second, completely revised edition

With 65 Figures and 86 Tables

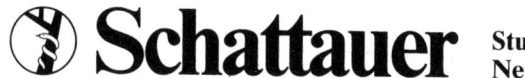 Schattauer Stuttgart –
New York 1993

The reproduction of general descriptive names, trade names, trade marks etc. in this publication, even when there is no special identification mark, is not to be taken as a sign that such names, as understood by the Trade Marks and Merchandise Marks Law, may be freely used.
For various reasons, the lists of antibiotics and chemotherapeutic agents in this book may not be complete. The omission of a commercially available preparation does not necessarily imply that it less suitable for therapy than the alternatives described.

Notice

Not all of the drugs mentioned in this book have been approved by FDA for use in infants or in children under the ages of 6 or 12. Such drugs should not be given in these age-groups if effective alternatives are available; they may be used if there is no alternative or if the known risk of toxicity of alternative drugs or of non-treatment is outweighed by the probable advantages of treatment. Any national regulations governing the consideration of clinical trial data must be complied with, particularly with respect to indications for antibiotic use that have not been specifically licensed by the appropriate regulatory authorities.
When prescribing new or unfamiliar drugs, our readers are urged to confirm the dosage in current appropriate references such as local or national formularies, or the manufacturer's data sheet or package insert.   The Authors

CIP-Kurztitelaufnahme der Deutschen Bibliothek

Simon, Claus:
Antibiotic therapy in clinical practice / C. Simon ; W. Stille ;
P. J. Wilkinson. – 2., completely rev. ed. – Stuttgart ; New York : Schattauer, 1993
   Einheitssacht.: Antibiotika-Therapie in Klinik und Praxis ‹engl.›
   ISBN 3-7945-1368-1

NE: Stille, Wolfgang; Wilkinson, Peter J.:

Authorized English edition, originally translated by Dr. F. MIELKE, Hamburg.

Completely revised, up-dated, and adapted version (1992) of the original German edition: C. SIMON, W. STILLE: Antibiotika-Therapie in Klinik und Praxis. 7th edition. Schattauer, Stuttgart – New York 1989.

All rights reserved. This book is protected by copyright. No part of it may be reproduced, stored in a retrieval system, or transmitted in any form or by any means, electronic, mechanical, photocopying, recording, or otherwise, without written permission from the publisher.

© 1985 and 1993 by F. K. Schattauer Verlagsgesellschaft mbH, Lenzhalde 3,
W-7000 Stuttgart 1, Germany. Printed in Germany

Composition, printing and binding: Mayr Miesbach, Druckerei und Verlag GmbH,
Am Windfeld 15, W-8160 Miesbach, Germany

ISBN 3-7945-1368-1

Foreword

This book attempts to give a clear, systematic and up-to-date presentation of the pharmacology and mode of action of antimicrobial agents, together with practical guidance in their use in the treatment of infectious disease. It should prove to be useful as a ready source of reference to answer specific questions that arise in the course of hospital and community practice. We believe it will be of value not only to the clinical specialist but also to general practitioners, doctors in training, pharmacologists, pharmacists, microbiologists and to all concerned with the diagnosis and management of infection.

A range of new antimicrobials has become available since the first edition was published in 1985. These include new penicillins (some in combination with β-lactamase inhibitors), new cephalosporins (both oral and parenteral), new macrolides (azithromycin, clarithromycin, roxithromycin), new glycopeptide alternatives to vancomycin (teicoplanin, daptomycin), and a succession of new quinolones. New approaches to the treatment of tuberculosis, mycoses and viral infections (particularly AIDS and its associated opportunistic infections) have necessitated substantial expansion of several chapters. To accommodate this, other chapters have been shortened and, after a brief introduction, the text has been rearranged into three principal sections which describe the properties of antimicrobial agents, the treatment of infections and infectious diseases, and general rules for antimicrobial chemotherapy.

First published in 1969 in Germany, this book has achieved seven editions in that language, as well as three in Hungarian, one in Spanish and one in Italian; a French edition is in preparation. Expert co-authors from each of these countries (D. Münnich, E. J. Perea and S. Guandalini) have collaborated closely in this project, and successive German and English editions have taken their contributions into account. The result is an evolution into a truly European text which should give useful guidance to prescribers of antibiotics in the single European market after 1993. This English edition should also provide for the needs of a wider international readership. The intention is to harmonise recommendations for antimicrobial treatment in European countries, to which end we have taken the recommendations of official bodies and of national professional organisations into account. We have paid particular attention, however, to recent scientific publications (especially within the last five years) and include these in the bibliography to each chapter, together with more general guidance for further reading.

The authors are very grateful to the staff of Schattauer Verlag, and in particular to Dr. med. Christine von Busch, for their help in the production of this book.

Autumn 1992   C. SIMON, W. STILLE and P. J. WILKINSON

Authors' Addresses

Prof. Dr. C. SIMON
　　Universitäts-Kinderklinik
　　Schwanenweg 20, W-2300 Kiel, FRG

Prof. Dr. W. STILLE
　　Zentrum der Inneren Medizin der Universität
　　Theodor-Stern-Kai 7, W-6000 Frankfurt/M., FRG

Dr. P. J. WILKINSON FRC Path.
　　Public Health Laboratory, Derriford Hospital
　　Derriford Road, Plymouth PL6 8DH, UK

Contents

A. Basic Concepts of Chemotherapy 1
  1. Classification of Antibiotics 3
  2. Antibacterial Activity 6
  3. Bacterial Resistance 8
  4. Pharmacokinetics 12

B. Properties of Antimicrobial Agents 17
    β-Lactam Antibiotics 19
  1. Penicillins 23
    a) Benzylpenicillin (Penicillin G) 26
    b) Phenoxypenicillins 33
    c) Isoxazolyl Penicillins (Anti-staphylococcal Penicillins) 36
    d) Aminopenicillins 39
        α) Ampicillin 39
        β) Amoxycillin 43
        γ) Pivampicillin 44
        δ) Bacampicillin 45
        ε) Talampicillin 47
    e) Carboxypenicillins 48
        α) Carbenicillin 48
        β) Carbenicillin Esters 48
        γ) Ticarcillin 50
        δ) Temocillin 52
    f) Acylaminopenicillins 53
        α) Azlocillin 53
        β) Mezlocillin 55
        γ) Piperacillin 57
        δ) Apalcillin 59
    g) Mecillinam 60
    h) Penicillin Combinations 62
  2. Cephalosporins 62
    a) Cefazolin Group (Basic Cephalosporins) 63
    b) Cefuroxime Group (Intermediate Cephalosporins) 66
    c) Cefoxitin Group (Cephamycins) 71
        α) Cefoxitin 71

β) Cefotetan 74
γ) Cefmetazole 75
δ) Latamoxef 76
ε) Flomoxef 78
d) Cefotaxime Group (Aminothiazole Cephalosporins) 80
e) Other Parenteral Cephalosporins 88
α) Cefsulodin 88
β) Cefoperazone 89
γ) Ceforanide 90
δ) Cefpirome 91
f) Older Oral Cephalosporins (Cephalexin Group) 92
g) Newer Oral Cephalosporins 95
α) Cefixime 95
β) Cefetamet.................................. 98
γ) Cefuroxime Axetil 99
δ) Cefpodoxime Proxetil 100
ε) Loracarbef 102
ζ) Cefotiam Hexetil 102
3. Other β-Lactam Antibiotics............................ 103
a) Imipenem/Cilastatin 103
b) Aztreonam 107
c) β-Lactamase Inhibitors 110
α) Co-amoxiclav (Amoxycillin/Clavulanic Acid) 110
β) Ticarcillin/Clavulanic Acid 113
γ) Sulbactam/Ampicillin 114
δ) Tazobactam 117
4. Tetracyclines 118
5. Chloramphenicol Group 126
a) Chloramphenicol 126
b) Thiamphenicol................................. 131
6. Aminoglycosides................................... 134
a) Gentamicin 135
b) Tobramycin 141
c) Sisomicin 142
d) Netilmicin 144
e) Amikacin 145
f) Spectinomycin 149
7. Macrolides 150
a) Erythromycin 150
b) Josamycin 159
c) Roxithromycin 160
d) Clarithromycin 161

| | | Contents | XI |

- e) Azithromycin 164
- f) Spiramycin 166
8. Lincosamides 168
    - a) Lincomycin 168
    - b) Clindamycin 171
9. Fusidic Acid 174
10. Glycopeptide Antibiotics 176
    - a) Vancomycin 176
    - b) Teicoplanin 180
    - c) Daptomycin 182
11. Fosfomycin 183
12. Topical Antibiotics 185
    - a) Bacitracin 186
    - b) Tyrothricin 186
    - c) Polymixins (Colistin and Polymixin B) 186
    - d) Kanamycin 188
    - e) Neomycin 188
    - f) Paromomycin 190
    - g) Mupirocin 190
    - h) Fusafungin 191
13. Antifungal Agents 191
    - a) Polyenes 191
        - α) Amphotericin B 191
        - β) Nystatin 195
        - γ) Natamycin (Pimaricin) 196
    - b) Azoles 196
        - α) Miconazole 197
        - β) Ketoconazole 199
        - γ) Itraconazole 202
        - δ) Fluconazole 204
    - c) Azoles for Topical Use 205
        - α) Clotrimazole 205
        - β) Econazole 206
        - γ) Isoconazole 208
        - δ) Oxiconazole 208
        - ε) Bifonazole 208
    - d) Flucytosine 209
    - e) Griseofulvin 211
    - f) Ciclopiroxolamine 213
    - g) Naftifin 214
    - h) Tolnaftate 214

14. Chemotherapeutic Agents 215
    a) Sulphonamides 215
    b) Co-trimoxazole 220
    c) Other Diaminopyrimidine-Sulphonamide Combinations 225
    d) Trimethoprim 226
    e) Nitrofurans 227
       α) Nitrofurantoin 227
       β) Nitrofurazone 231
    f) Quinolones 231
       α) Older Quinolones (Nalidixic Acid Group) 233
       β) Newer Quinolones (Fluoquinolones) 236
          (1) Norfloxacin 236
          (2) Ofloxacin 239
          (3) Ciprofloxacin 242
          (4) Enoxacin 246
          (5) Fleroxacin 248
          (6) Pefloxacin 250
          (7) Lomefloxacin 251
          (8) Temafloxacin 251
    g) Nitroimidazoles 252
15. Antimycobacterial Agents 258
    a) Isoniazid (INH) 258
    b) Rifampicin 261
    c) Ethambutol 265
    d) Streptomycin 267
    e) Thioamides (Ethionamide and Prothionamide) 270
    f) Pyrazinamide 272
    g) Capreomycin 273
    h) Dapsone 274
    i) Clofazimine 276
    j) Rifabutin 277
16. Antiviral Agents 278
    a) Acyclovir 278
    b) Ganciclovir 286
    c) Azidothymidine (Zidovudine, AZT) 288
    d) Vidarabine (Adenine Arabinoside) 292
    e) Tribavirin 293
    f) Idoxuridine 295
    g) Trifluridine 296
    h) Amantadine 297
    i) Interferons 298
    j) Immunoglobulins 302

C. Treatment of Infections and Infectious Diseases 305

1. Infections with Facultative Pathogenic Bacteria 307
   a) Infections Caused by Enterobacteriaceae 307
   b) Serratia marcescens Infections 312
   c) Pseudomonas Infections 313
   d) Haemophilus influenzae Infections 314
   e) Staphylococcal Infections 316
   f) Streptococcal and Pneumococcal Infections 319
   g) Anaerobic Infections 321
2. Septicaemia 325
   a) Initial Therapy (Pathogen Unknown) 330
   b) Directed Therapy (Pathogen Known) 335
3. Bacterial Endocarditis 342
4. Bacterial Pericarditis 349
5. CNS Infections 351
   a) Meningitis 351
      α) Initial Therapy (Pathogen Unknown) 356
      β) Directed Therapy (Pathogen Known) 357
   b) Cerebral Abscess 365
   c) Subdural Empyema 366
6. Respiratory Infections 367
   a) Rhinitis 368
   b) Tonsillitis, Pharyngitis 368
   c) Peritonsillar or Retropharyngeal Abscess, Ludwig's Angina 369
   d) Diphtheria 370
   e) Infectious Mononucleosis (Glandular Fever) 370
   f) Candida Stomatitis (Oral Thrush) 371
   g) Acute Necrotising Gingivitis 371
   h) Secondary Throat Infections 371
   i) Laryngitis and Acute Epiglottitis 372
   j) Acute Bronchitis 372
   k) Chronic Bronchitis 373
   l) Bronchiolitis 375
   m) Bronchiectasis 375
   n) Cystic Fibrosis (Mucoviscidosis) 376
   o) Pneumonia 376
      α) Best-guess Therapy 381
      β) Directed Therapy 384
   p) Legionellosis 388
   q) Lung Abscess 390
   r) Empyema 391

7. Infections of the Gastrointestinal Tract 393
   a) Gastritis and Peptic Ulcer 393
   b) Enteritis 395
   c) Appendicitis 410
   d) Peritonitis 411
   e) Pancreatitis 413
   f) Liver Abscess 413
   g) Infections of the Biliary Tract 414
8. Infections of the Urogenital Tract 417
   a) Treatment of Acute Urinary Infections 421
   b) Pyelonephritis 424
   c) Cystitis 426
   d) Urethritis 426
   e) Prostatitis, Epididymitis, Orchitis 428
9. Surgical Infections 430
   a) Wound Infections 430
   b) Infected Burns 433
   c) Hand Infections 434
   d) Postoperative Septicaemia 435
   e) Postoperative Pneumonia 436
   f) Infected Gangrene 436
10. Osteomyelitis and Septic Arthritis 437
    a) Osteomyelitis 437
    b) Acute Purulent Arthritis 440
11. Gynaecological Infections 441
    a) Bartholinitis 441
    b) Vulvitis 442
    c) Vulvovaginitis in Children 442
    d) Vaginitis in Adults 443
    e) Pelvic Inflammatory Disease 447
    f) Febrile Abortion 448
    g) Puerperal Fever 449
    h) Mastitis 450
    i) Pyrexia During Labour 451
    j) Pyelonephritis During Pregnancy 451
    k) Toxic Shock Syndrome 451
12. Eye Infections 453
    a) Lid Infections 458
    b) Conjunctival Infections 460
    c) Corneal Infections 463
13. Infections of the Ear, Nose and Throat 467

14. Skin Infections 475
    a) Acute Bacterial Infections 478
    b) Chronic Bacterial Infections 480
    c) Bacterial Infections Secondary to Viral Infections 481
    d) Viral Infections of the Skin 481
    e) Secondary Infections in Dermatoses 481
    f) Acne and Rosacea 482
    g) Fungal Infections of the Skin 482
15. Sexually Transmitted Diseases 484
    a) Syphilis 484
    b) Gonorrhoea 488
    c) Lymphogranuloma venereum 491
    d) Chancroid 491
    e) Granuloma inguinale (Donovanosis) 492
16. Rheumatic Fever 493
17. Scarlet Fever 495
18. Tetanus 496
19. Gas Gangrene 497
20. Anthrax 499
21. Erysipeloid 499
22. Listeriosis 500
23. Salmonella Infections 502
    a) Typhoid and Paratyphoid Fevers 502
    b) Gastrointestinal Salmonellosis 504
    c) Salmonella Excretors 505
       α) Persistent Excretors of Salmonella typhi and S. paratyphi 505
       β) Excretors of Other Salmonellae 505
24. Brucellosis 506
25. Tularaemia 508
26. Pertussis 509
27. Leptospirosis 510
28. Rickettsial and Coxiella Infections 511
29. Actinomycosis 512
30. Tuberculosis 513
    a) Principles of Antituberculous Chemotherapy 515
    b) Treatment of Tuberculosis and their Chemotherapy 523
31. Leprosy 526
32. Influenza 529
33. AIDS 530
    a) Pneumocystis carinii Pneumonia (PCP) 536
    b) Toxoplasmosis 538
    c) Cryptosporidial Infections 539

d) Candida Infections 540
e) Cryptococcal Meningitis 541
f) Aspergillus Infections 542
g) Mycobacterial Infections 543
h) Salmonella Septicaemia 544
i) Herpes 545
j) Varicella and Zoster 545
k) Cytomegalovirus 545
l) Papovaviruses 546
34. Fungal Infections 548
35. Toxoplasmosis 554
36. Malaria 559
37. Helminth Infections 565

D. General Rules for Antimicrobial Therapy 573
1. Choice of Antibiotic 575
   a) Preliminary Remarks 575
   b) Forms of Therapy 575
   c) Chemotherapy in Practice 581
      α) Parenteral Therapy 582
      β) Oral Therapy 582
2. Antibiotic Combinations 583
3. Route of Administration 585
4. Dosage 588
5. Side-effects 592
6. Cost of Treatment 596
7. Antibiotic Therapy in Renal Insufficiency 598
8. Antibiotic Therapy and Abnormal Liver Function 603
9. Antibiotic Therapy in Granulocytopenic Patients 605
10. Antibiotics in Pregnancy 610
11. Antibiotic Therapy in the Neonatal Period 612
12. Prophylaxis 613

Index 617

A. Basic Concepts of Chemotherapy

1. Classification of Antibiotics

Antibiotics are substances produced by fungi and bacteria, which in small quantities can inhibit the growth of microorganisms or even kill them. *Chemotherapeutic agents* are synthetic substances with antimicrobial activity and are not found in nature. Although most antiviral agents are synthetic, they can also be derived from fungi (e. g. vidarabine is obtained from the fermentation of Streptomyces antibioticus). There are no fundamental differences between antibiotics and chemotherapeutic agents. Synthetic antibiotics (e. g. chloramphenicol) and chemically modified (semisynthetic) antibiotics (e. g. ampicillin) occupy an intermediate position.

Table 1. Classification of the β-lactam antibiotics.

Group	Subgroup	Important derivatives
Penicillins (Penams)	Benzylpenicillin	Benzylpenicillin sodium Procaine penicillin Benzathine penicillin
	Phenoxypenicillins	Phenoxymethylpenicillin Propicillin Phenethicillin
	Amino-penicillins	Ampicillin Amoxycillin Pivampicillin Bacampicillin
	Acylamino-(Ureido-) penicillins	Azlocillin Mezlocillin Piperacillin Apalcillin
	Carboxy-penicillins	Carbenicillin Carfecillin Carindacillin Ticarcillin Temocillin
	Isoxazolyl penicillins	Oxacillin Cloxacillin Dicloxacillin Flucloxacillin

Table 1. (continued).

Group	Subgroup	Important derivatives
Penicillins	Amidino penicillins	Mecillinam
Cephalosporins	Cefazolin group	Cefazolin Cefazedone Cefonicid
	Cefuroxime group	Cefuroxime Cefamandole Cefotiam
	Cefoxitin group	Cefoxitin Cefotetan Latamoxef Cefmetazole Flomoxef
	Cefotaxime group	Cefotaxime Ceftriaxone Ceftizoxime Cefmenoxime Ceftazidime Cefpirome
	Other parenteral cephalosporins	Cefsulodin Cefoperazone Ceforanide
	Older oral cephalosporins	Cephalexin Cefaclor Cefadroxil Cephradine
	Newer oral cephalosporins	Cefixime Cefetamet Cefuroxime axetil Cefpodoxime proxetil Loracarbef Cefotiam hexetil
Carbapenems	–	Imipenem
Monobactams	–	Aztreonam
β-Lactamase inhibitors	–	Clavulanic acid Sulbactam Tazobactam

Antibiotics and chemotherapeutic agents of clinical importance may be classified on the basis of their chemical structure, their biological origin and their therapeutic use (Tables 1–3). Antibiotics of the same class have similar modes of action and spectra of activity; in general, they show partial cross-resistance and are similar in their toxicity.

Table 2. Classification of antibiotics other than β-lactams.

Group	Subgroup	Important derivatives
Aminoglycosides	Older aminoglycosides	Neomycin Paromomycin Kanamycin Spectinomycin
	Newer aminoglycosides	Gentamicin Sisomicin Tobramycin Netilmicin Amikacin
Other broad-spectrum antibiotics	Tetracyclines	Tetracycline Oxytetracycline Doxycycline Minocycline
	Chloramphenicol group	Chloramphenicol Thiamphenicol
Narrow-spectrum antibiotics	Macrolides	Erythromycin Roxythromycin Clarithromycin Azithromycin Josamycin Spiramycin
	Polymyxins	Polymyxin B Colistin
	Lincosamides	Lincomycin Clindamycin
	Glycopeptides	Vancomycin Teicoplanin

Table 3. Classification of the antibacterial chemotherapeutic agents.

Group	Derivatives
Sulphonamides	Short-acting sulphonamides Medium-acting sulphonamides Long-acting sulphonamides Ultra-long-acting sulphonamides
Sulphonamide-diaminopyrimidine combinations	Co-trimoxazole Co-trimetrole Co-trimazine Co-tetroxazine

Table 3. (continued).

Group	Derivatives
Nitrofurans	Nitrofurantoin Nitrofurazone
Older Quinolones	Nalidixic acid Pipemidic acid Cinoxacin Rosoxacin
Newer Quinolones	Norfloxacin Ciprofloxacin Ofloxacin Fleroxacin Pefloxacin Enoxacin Lomefloxacin Temafloxacin
Nitroimidazoles	Metronidazole Tinidazole

A few antibiotics, which act selectively on certain pathogens (e. g. staphylococci, pseudomonas or Mycobacterium tuberculosis) are called *narrow-spectrum antibiotics*. Broad-spectrum antibiotics are effective against a wider range of pathogens. A complete spectrum of activity cannot yet be achieved by a single drug, however, and a combination is always required for this purpose. Because of their toxicity, some antibiotics are restricted to local use (e. g. neomycin, kanamycin, bacitracin) and may be grouped as *topical antibiotics*.

2. Antibacterial Activity

Mode of action: The antibacterial activity of an antibiotic may be measured in vitro by determining its minimal inhibitory concentration (MIC).

For most antibiotics, there are concentrations below the MIC at which a degree of partial activity is shown. One measure of this subinhibitory activity is the minimal active concentration (MAC) of the antibiotic, i. e. the lowest concentration that will bring about a measurable reduction in the multiplication of a bacterial population.

While some antibiotics merely inhibit the multiplication of bacteria, that is, they are *bacteriostatic*, others actively kill microorganisms and so are *bactericidal*. The most important bactericidal antibiotics are the penicillins, the cephalosporins and the aminoglycosides.

2. Antibacterial Activity

Whether or not an antibiotic is bactericidal depends not only on the type of antibiotic, its mode of action and concentration at the site of action, but also on the bacterial species, the numbers of bacteria present (i.e. the inoculum size *in vitro*), the duration of action and the phase of growth of the micro-organism. Thus penicillins and cephalosporins are bactericidal only to actively proliferating microorganisms; polymyxin and the aminoglycosides, on the other hand, also act on bacteria in the resting phase.

The bactericidal effect is of greatest importance during the first 4–8 hours, and is only clinically relevant if a high percentage of the bacteria (>99%) are killed during this period. Bacteria can also die as part of their own aging process while under the influence of bacteriostatic drugs. A bactericidal effect is valuable in certain diseases in which the causative agent can only be eradicated with difficulty (e.g. bacterial endocarditis). Many aspects of the clinical importance of bactericidal activity are obscure. The existing bactericidal antibiotics are by no means instantly bactericidal; the bacteria generally die after a latent period. The superior clinical efficacy of chloramphenicol over ampicillin in typhoid fever shows that a bacteriostatic antibiotic can be better than a bactericidal one in intracellular infections.

Some **pathogenic organisms may persist** when β-lactam antibiotics act on resting bacteria, that is, small numbers of dormant, sensitive bacteria survive. The explanation is that autolytic bacterial enzymes necessary for cell division are inhibited by the antibiotic. These *persisters* are thus morphologically normal bacteria which have survived lethal concentrations of penicillin. The daughter cells, produced subsequently, remain fully sensitive when the effect of the antibiotic ceases. Because of this phenomenon, antibacterials may fail to sterilise the lesion in many infections, which explains in part the failures of treatment encountered in immune deficiency diseases and bone marrow suppression. In other words, despite satisfactory tissue concentrations, the bactericidal antibiotics currently available may be unable to eradicate the pathogens of infection without the aid of the body's defence mechanisms.

The **mechanism of action** of most antibiotics is well known and is generally similar in drugs of the same group, giving rise to a pattern of complete cross-resistance. For example, penicillins interfere with synthesis of the bacterial cell wall and activate cell wall autolysins; after penetrating the cell wall, they are bound by penicillin-binding proteins (PBP) in the cell membrane. Antibiotics act by inhibiting bacterial cell wall synthesis, inhibiting the synthesis of cytoplasmic components, damaging the cytoplasmic membrane or disrupting nucleic acid synthesis (Table 4). A knowledge of these mechanisms is important in understanding the basis of the combined action of antibiotics, since a synergistic (potentiated) effect only occurs when the partners in the combination have different sites of action.

Table 4. Sites of action of antibiotics.

Cell wall synthesis	Cytoplasmic membrane (permeability)	Synthesis of cytoplasmic components	Nucleic acid synthesis
β-Lactam antibiotics Vancomycin Teicoplanin Fosfomycin	Colistin Polymyxin B Amphotericin B Nystatin	Chloramphenicol Tetracycline Erythromycin Lincosamides Aminoglycosides	Rifampicin Griseofulvin Fusidic acid Quinolones

3. Bacterial Resistance

Sensitivity to antibiotics varies between different species of bacteria, between different strains of the same species and even within the same bacterial population. The antibiotic sensitivity pattern of some bacterial species such as Streptococcus pyogenes (group A) is largely predictable; other species such as staphylococci, gonococci, enterococci, Escherichia coli, klebsiella, Pseudomonas aeruginosa, proteus, etc. show considerable variation. The antibiotic susceptibility of these species should therefore be tested in vitro before antibiotic treatment is initiated.

Bacterial resistance is recognised when the bacteria multiply at an antibiotic concentration which can be achieved in the tissues. Resistance is due either to inherent insensitivity to the antibiotic or to inactivation by bacterial enzymes (Table 5).

Table 5. Examples of chromosomal and plasmid-mediated antibiotic resistance.

Mechanisms of antibiotic resistance	
Chromosomal mutation	**Plasmid transfer (extrachromosomal)**
Increased formation of an inactivating enzyme (e.g. by Escherichia coli against *ampicillin*).	Enzymatic hydrolysis of the β-lactam ring (by *penicillin* and *cephalosporin* β-lactamases).
Decreased permeability (e.g. to *benzylpenicillin* in gonococci).	Acetylation by bacterial acetyl transferases (e.g. of *chloramphenicol* by Haemophilus influenzae).
Reduced binding to bacterial ribosomes (e.g. of *streptomycin* in enterococci).	Enzymatic changes by phosphorylases (e.g. of *gentamicin* by gram-positive bacteria).
	Disruption of transport across the cell membrane *(tetracyclines)*.
	Metabolic by-pass by the formation of a new bacterial enzyme (e.g. of dihydrofolate reductase, which confers resistance to *trimethoprim*).

3. Bacterial Resistance

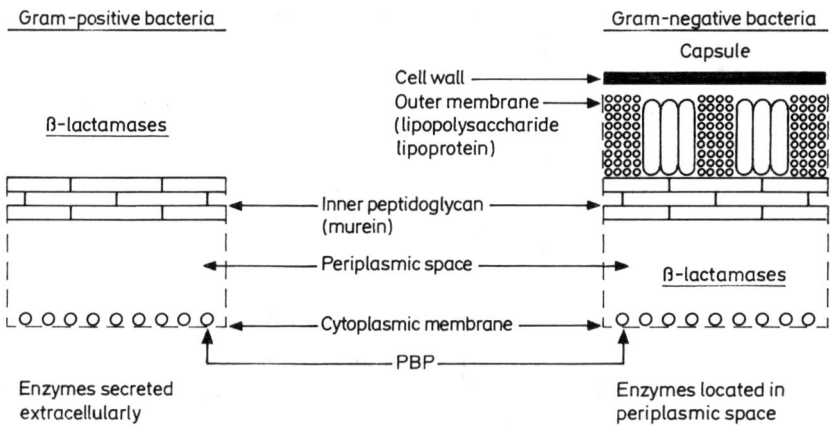

Fig. 1. Structure of capsule, cell wall and cell membrane of gram-positive and gram-negative bacteria. PBP = penicillin binding protein.

Certain penicillins and cephalosporins are inactivated by species-specific β-lactamases which hydrolyse the β-lactam ring of the antibiotic. The β-lactamases of gram-positive bacteria are secreted outside the cell, while those of gram-negative bacteria remain within the periplasmic space (Fig. 1). There are also β-lactamase inhibitors (e. g. clavulanic acid) which reduce the resistance of certain bacteria to penicillins. Aminoglycosides are also modified by bacterial enzymes (acetylase, phosphorylase, adenylase), which explains differences in the spectrum of activity of different members of this group. Chloramphenicol can be acetylated by the action of a bacterial acetyl transferase on the two free hydroxyl groups, which destroys its antibacterial activity. Other factors determining resistance to penicillins and cephalosporins are the ability of the antibiotic to penetrate the outer layers of the bacterial cell wall, and changes in the cell wall structure which can lead to antibiotic tolerance.

Resistance may be classified as follows:
1. **Natural resistance,** where the sensitivity of a bacterial species is permanent and genetically determined (e. g. the inactivity of benzylpenicillin against Pseudomonas aeruginosa). Such resistance is chromosomally mediated.
2. **Mutational resistance:** This is unrelated to previous antibiotic therapy. Individual members of a bacterial population which have become resistant to an antibiotic through mutation do not increase in relation to other members of that population until selected by exposure to that antibiotic.

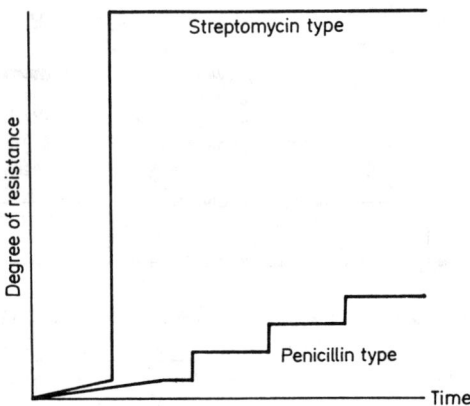

Fig. 2. One-step resistance (streptomycin type) and multiple-step resistance (penicillin type).

3. **Secondary resistance** does not develop until therapy has begun. Exposure to the antibiotic selects for resistant variants which appear in small numbers in larger bacterial populations and arise through mutation. Secondary resistance can develop at varying speeds according to the rate of mutation and transfer. Resistance develops rapidly with streptomycin *(one-step resistance)*, within a few days with erythromycin and fusidic acid, and much more slowly with polypeptide antibiotics and others *(multiple-step resistance)* (Fig. 2). This is why antibiotics to which resistance develops rapidly have a higher clinical failure rate. In such cases regular bacteriological cultures are recommended to detect any relapse or change in infecting organism promptly. In some strains of pseudomonas and enterobacteria, β-lactamase synthesis is induced by certain β-lactam antibiotics. Such strains appear sensitive *in vitro*, but therapy with a β-lactam antibiotic can fail. A similar situation obtains for so-called heterogeneous resistance of staphylococci to penicillinase-resistant penicillins (see p. 37).

4. **Transferable resistance** does not usually lead to secondary infections in humans or animals treated with antibiotics. As a rule, transferable resistance begins insidiously and occurs predominantly in gram-negative bacilli (Escherichia coli, klebsiella, salmonella, shigella, Pseudomonas aeruginosa, serratia, proteus, vibrio and yersinia). During the process of conjugation, plasmids (extrachromosomal genetic material) are transferred from one bacterial species to another; this process requires the mediation of a "resistance transfer". The multiple resistance of salmonellae or shigellae against sulphonamides, tetracycline, chloramphenicol or streptomycin can thus be transferred to a sensitive

3. Bacterial Resistance

strain of Escherichia coli. Other examples of transferable resistance include that to ampicillin and ticarcillin, kanamycin and gentamicin or trimethoprim. Resistance can also be transferred between bacteria of the same species. Extrachromosomal resistance transfer by plasmids has also been observed in staphylococci. The transfer of multiple resistance occurs not only *in vitro* but also *in vivo;* it has been demonstrated in the human intestine, on other mucous membranes and on the skin, and is often lost spontaneously later. Antibiotic additives to animal feedstuffs, which could play a part in the encouragement of such resistance, are nowadays restricted in most countries.

Genetics of antibiotic resistance: Bacteria can acquire resistance to antimicrobials either through chromosomal mutation or by plasmid transfer. Plasmids are extrachromosomal elements of bacterial DNA (including *R-factors*) which can, like the chromosome, carry genetic information about antibiotic resistance. Mutations mediating antibiotic resistance arise spontaneously with a frequency which is not affected by exposure to antibiotics. Plasmid-mediated resistance is generally of greater clinical importance than chromosomal, since bacteria which have undergone chromosomal mutation are usually metabolically impaired and less well able to multiply than non-mutant members of the population.

Plasmid-mediated resistance is usually based on the synthesis of proteins which either act as enzymes or change the cell wall in such a way that the antibiotic can no longer penetrate. R-(Resistance-)plasmids can be transferred from one bacterial cell to another by conjugation, transduction mediated by bacteriophages or by transformation (direct DNA transfer after the destruction of a cell). Conjugation is the main method of transfer for gram-negative organisms and bacteriophage transduction for gram-positive ones (e. g. staphylococci).

Another means of resistance transfer is by means of minute mobile elements of DNA *(transposons)* which are often found on plasmids and can move from plasmid to plasmid or to the chromosome. A transposon can mediate single or multiple resistance and can, after entering a bacterial cell, become incorporated in its plasmid or chromosome.

Chromosomal and plasmid-mediated resistance involve different mechanisms (Table 5). It is not uncommon for more than one resistance mechanism to be present in a single bacterial strain.

Clinical importance of resistance: Necessary antibiotics should not be withheld because of the fear of resistance, although patients at particular risk (e. g. with severe burns or leukaemia) should be carefully monitored for the development of secondary infections with resistant organisms during and after antibiotic treatment. The danger of resistance can be reduced by the use of combinations (e. g. in tuberculosis or agranulocytosis); the use of rifampicin or fusidic acid as single agents should be avoided since both can give rise to one-step mutational resistance. The prophylactic use of these drugs is also contraindicated.

When an antibiotic becomes ineffective against a proportion of cases of a certain infection in a hospital (e. g. benzylpenicillin against staphylococcal infection), an alternative antibiotic which is normally effective (e. g. flucloxacillin) should be used for the initial, "blind" therapy of severe infections such as osteomyelitis which are likely to be caused by those organisms.

In large hospitals it is sometimes worth monitoring systematically the pattern of resistance in clinical isolates as a basis for general recommendations for antibiotic use. Broad-spectrum antibiotics which favour the selection of resistant organisms in patients should then only be used for clear indications such as infections with many possible bacterial causes. In such situations, antibiotics which have been found to exert only a slight selection pressure, e. g. piperacillin, are preferable to agents such as ampicillin which select strongly. The uncritical use of antibiotics for general prophylaxis or in viral infections should always be avoided because of the risk of spread of resistant strains. Careful measures to minimise the risk of cross-infection will also help to control the dissemination of such bacteria in hospitals.

Cross-resistance (more precisely: *parallel resistance*) is the simultaneous resistance in a given bacterial strain to several antibiotics of the same group, that is, with generally similar chemical structures and the same or related modes of action. Two-way cross-resistance involving a single antibiotic is always related to resistance to another antibiotic of the same group; examples occur amongst the tetracyclines, between neomycin and kanamycin, and between polymyxin B and colistin. Cross-resistance can also be one-way where, for example, resistance to antibiotic A is linked with resistance to antibiotic B, but resistance primarily to antibiotic B may be associated with sensitivity to antibiotic A. An example of this is kanamycin resistance in mycobacteria which is linked with resistance to streptomycin; streptomycin-resistant strains are mostly sensitive to kanamycin, however. Differentiation between one-way and two-way cross-resistance is important in therapy because giving a closely related antibiotic will be unsuccessful where cross-resistance is two-way. There is no point in giving amoxycillin when ampicillin has failed.

4. Pharmacokinetics

Pharmacology must be taken into account when planning antibiotic treatment, particularly the choice of agent, route of administration and dosage. Antibiotics vary greatly in their absorption, blood concentrations, tissue diffusion, distribution in the body, metabolism, accumulation and excretion. Antibiotic pharmacokinetics also vary with the patient's age, disease and organ function. Another important factor is the galenic form of the preparation, which may differ considerably with different preparations of the same antibiotic.

The **absorption rate** after oral administration affects the blood concentration-time curve. Some antibiotics are well absorbed when taken by mouth, whereas others require parenteral administration. Rapid oral absorption leads to higher tissue concentrations than slow absorption in drugs which diffuse well and whose half-life is not too short. The rate of absorption after i. m. injection also varies, as between benzylpenicillin and procaine penicillin, and this is shown as variations in peak blood levels and the duration of adequate therapeutic concentrations, both of which are important for bactericidal activity at the site of infection. Bacteriostatic antibiotics need prolonged concentration at the site of infection in order to exceed the minimal inhibitory concentration of the infecting organism.

Tissue diffusion is very important in therapy, although the tissue concentration is unfortunately difficult to determine. Studies with radioactively labelled antibiotics in animals are also difficult to evaluate, since they fail to distinguish between the active agent and labelled metabolites. Intracellular antibiotic concentrations of agents such as rifampicin, chloramphenicol and tetracyclines are extremely difficult to measure. The extent to which an antibiotic penetrates tissues is reflected by its concentrations in lymph, synovial fluid, cerebrospinal fluid, saliva, tears and in artificially produced blisters; in animals it may be measured in subcutaneous fibrin implants or perforated synthetic capsules.

There is a general tendency towards an equilibrium between blood and tissue concentrations which requires a variable time to achieve since it depends on the capacity for diffusion of the antibiotic concerned. Maximal tissue concentrations therefore occur later than maximal blood concentrations and they also decline more slowly. The concentration in inflamed tissues is particularly important. Since this concentration is difficult to measure, it may be estimated as the serum concentration at the mid-point of the interval between two consecutive doses. Median concentrations are just as important as the serum peak and trough concentrations. The *trough* (or valley) *concentration* is the residual concentration just before the next dose.

Comparison of single tissue concentrations should be based on measurements made in the steady state, i.e. during constant i.v. infusion. The different composition and metabolism of different tissues can easily explain the variability of tissue kinetics in different organs. Glomerular filtration, tubular secretion and tubular reabsorption affect the concentration in the renal parenchyma, so blood and urine concentrations are both unsuitable indices of antibiotic concentrations in the kidney itself. The concentration in renal lymph, which is often regarded as an indicator of the interstitial antibiotic content, is the result of both tubular reabsorption and plasma transudation and is not, therefore, the same as the renal parenchymal concentration. Antibiotic concentrations in well perfused tissues such as lung and liver are usually higher than in poorly perfused ones such as eye or bone.

The **antibiotic concentrations in body fluids** (cerebrospinal fluid, bile, urine, amniotic fluid etc.) are important in the treatment of certain infections such as meningitis, cholangitis, urinary infections and chorioamnionitis. Note that the pharmacokinetics of an antibiotic in inflamed tissue or in systemic disease may differ greatly from those found in the healthy person. Thus cerebrospinal fluid concentrations of penicillin are higher in meningitis than when the meninges are not inflamed. Antibiotic concentrations in the bile, on the other hand, can be lower in obstructive jaundice. The concentration in bronchial secretions is affected by bronchiectasis, that in pleural effusion or empyema pus by pleurisy, and that in wound secretions by wound infection. The tissue diffusion, total clearance and renal clearance of antibiotics with a short half-life, such as the penicillins and cephalosporins, are impaired or delayed in elderly patients, who generally have higher blood and lower tissue concentrations than young adults.

Protein binding: It is generally accepted that only the unbound portion has antibacterial activity. However, the proportions of bound to unbound antibiotic depend on the plasma and tissue concentrations and are kept in an equilibrium defined by the adsorption isotherms (steady state). The degree of protein binding varies with different antibiotics and depends not only on the concentration but also on the pH, the protein content of the blood and inflamed tissue, the simultaneous administration of other drugs which can displace the first antibiotic, and the age (protein binding is less in the newborn). Many drugs are much less bound in chronic renal failure. There are also different physico-chemical mechanisms of protein binding (ionic bonds, hydrophobic interactions) and different types of protein (human, animal). Blood and tissue concentrations in animals are therefore not generally applicable to man.

The variation in published information about protein binding *in vitro* is partly due to differences of method and partly to the dependence of protein binding on drug concentration. Theoretical calculations of tissue ("free") concentrations based on the percentage protein binding do not relate to the true situation *in vivo*. Many questions about the clinical relevance of protein binding are still unanswered (e. g. protein binding to cell membranes and within cells). An important function is the transport of substances in the blood and their deposition in inflamed, protein-rich tissue. Free and bound antibiotics are concentrated in infected organs and tissues in relation to their degree of protein binding. Highly protein-bound drugs are less well bound in inflamed tissue with a low protein content in the blood, and their antibacterial activity at these sites is correspondingly greater. Highly protein-bound antibiotics can also achieve high total concentrations in inflamed tissues by virtue of their normal properties of diffusion, which depend on molecular size, lipophilia, ionic dissociation etc. Increased vascular permeability also increases the concentration of antibiotics at sites of inflammation. Protein binding cannot therefore be considered in isolation; it must always be related to other properties of the antibiotic such as solubility, tissue penetration, metabolism and excretion rate.

Most antibiotics are **metabolised** to varying extents and at different rates. The products of oxidation, reduction, hydrolysis and conjugation are usually antibacterially inactive or less active than the parent compound, and appear in the blood, urine, bile or faeces. This inactivation is usually associated with detoxification of the antibiotic, as happens to chloramphenicol through its conjugation with glucuronic acid. Occasionally, however, metabolic products can have enhanced toxicity, as in the acetylation of sulphonamides.

Most antibiotics are **eliminated** predominantly through the kidneys, by glomerular filtration and also, in some cases, by tubular secretion. A few antibiotics (e. g. rifampicin, fusidic acid, cefoperazone, ceftriaxone, apalcillin) are mainly excreted in the bile and faeces (partially through the intestinal wall). Intestinal reabsorption may occur; failure of reabsorption may result in excessively high intraluminal gut concentrations. Biliary elimination of an antibiotic tends to be a disadvantage. Renal insufficiency leads to the accumulation of antibiotics whose primary route of elimination is through the kidneys, and this may cause toxic side-effects. The plasma half-life of the agent is one index of its rate of elimination and is used to determine the optimal dose interval. The plasma half-life in premature babies, in the full-term neonate and in infants of up to one month may be prolonged because of immaturity of renal function. Antibiotics in this group of patients should usually be given at lower dosage or at extended dose intervals.

B. Properties of Antimicrobial Agents

β-Lactam Antibiotics

The penicillins and cephalosporins are the most important β-lactam antibiotics. They have a similar mechanism of action which is to inhibit peptidoglycan synthesis within the bacterial cell wall. The differences of activity between penicillins and cephalosporins are due to variations in their affinity for the binding proteins of the bacteria, their ability to penetrate the bacterial cell membrane *(crypticity)* and their stability to β-lactamase.

A number of new β-lactam antibiotics have been discovered in recent years, including ring-substituted cephalosporins such as latamoxef, and others which are neither penicillins nor cephalosporins (see Fig. 3). New possibilities for treatment are provided by the clavulanic acid derivatives, carbapenems and monobactams (monocyclic β-lactams).

Most β-lactam antibiotics in current use are semi-synthetic. The 6-aminopenicillanic acid or the 7-aminocephalosporanic acid rings can be substituted in a number of different ways. The apparently random nature of derivatives is in fact subject to fixed rules which have become clear as understanding of the structure-activity relationships of the β-lactam antibiotics has increased (Fig. 4). Thus acylamino derivatives are generally active against pseudomonas and the Enterobacteriaceae, and are concentrated well in the bile. Oxime thiazole cephalosporins have particularly good antibacterial activity and are very stable to the β-lactamases of the Enterobacteriaceae. Oxymethyl derivatives are also very stable to the β-lactamase of Bacteroides fragilis. Because the oxymethyl derivatives penetrate the bacterial cell poorly, they are generally less active. Tetrazolium derivatives have good pharmacokinetic qualities but cause intolerance to alcohol. There may be problems of inactivation with acetyl derivatives.

Group	Basic structure	Example
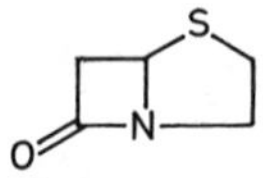 Penam	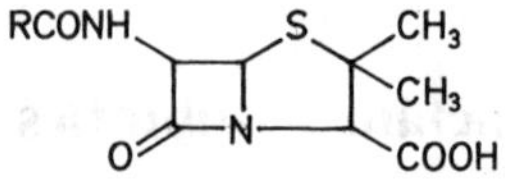 (structure with S, CH₃, CH₃, COOH, RCONH)	Penicillins (e.g. benzylpenicillin)
	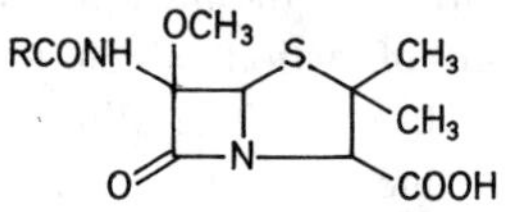 (structure with OCH₃, S, CH₃, CH₃, COOH, RCONH)	Oxymethyl penicillins (e.g. temocillin)
	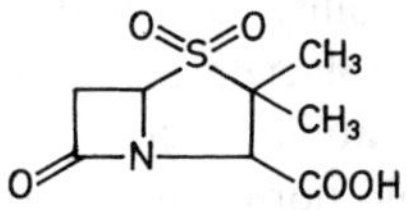 (sulfone structure with O=S=O, CH₃, CH₃, COOH)	Sulfone penicillins (e.g. sulbactam)
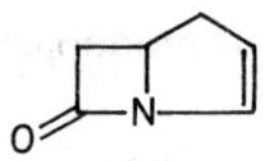 Carbapenem	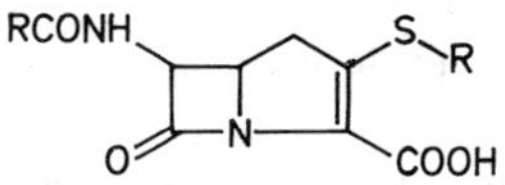 (structure with S–R, COOH, RCONH)	Thienamycins (e.g. imipenem)
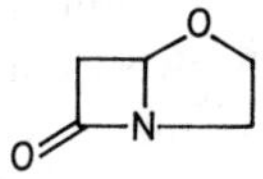 Clavam	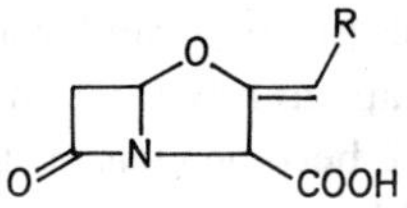 (structure with O, R, COOH)	e.g. clavulanic acid
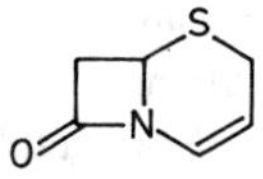 Cephem	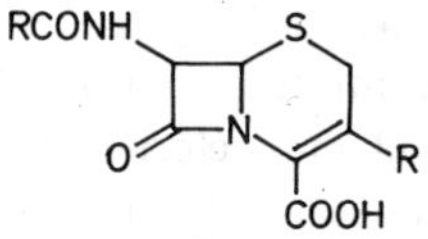 (structure with S, R, COOH, RCONH)	Cephalosporins (e.g. cephalothin)
	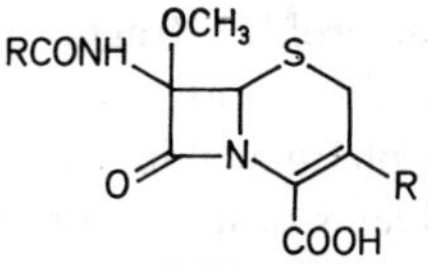 (structure with OCH₃, S, R, COOH, RCONH)	Oxymethyl cephalosporins (cephamycins) (e.g. cefoxitin)
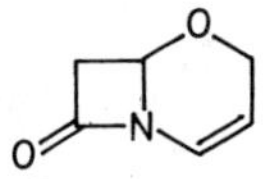 Oxacephem	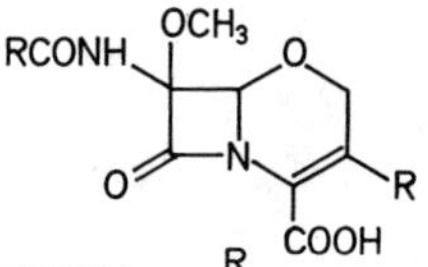 (structure with OCH₃, O, R, COOH, RCONH)	Oxa-cephalosporins (e.g. latamoxef)
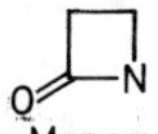 Monocyclic β-lactams	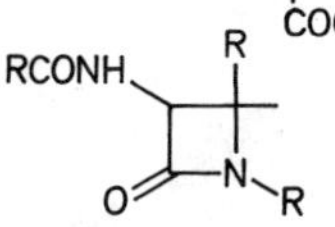 (structure with R, N–R, RCONH)	Monobactams (e.g. aztreonam)

Fig. 3. Structural formulae of the β-lactam antibiotics (penicillins, cephalosporins, carbapenems and monobactams).

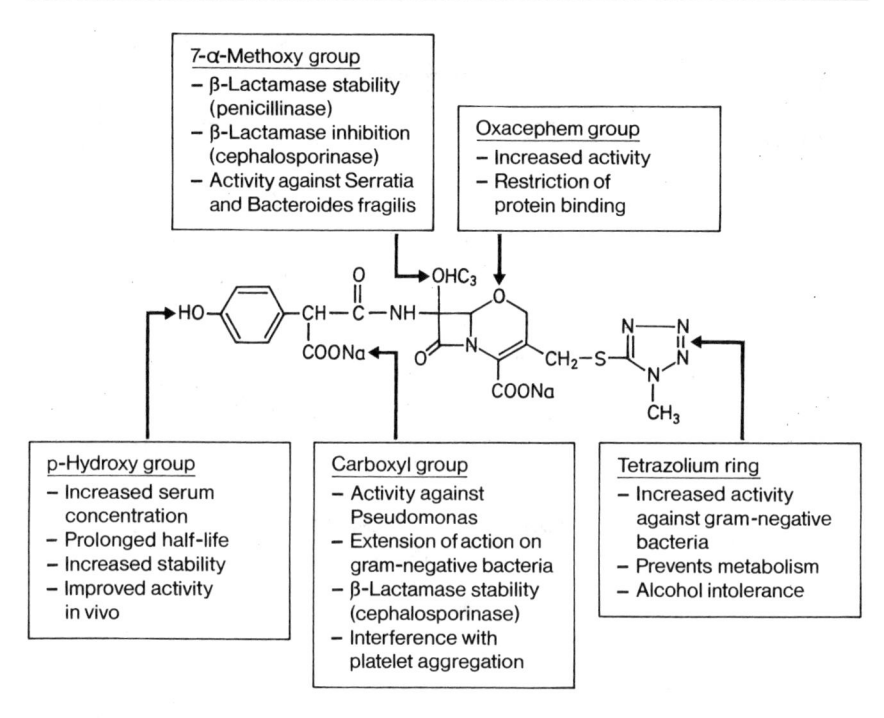

7-α-Methoxy group
− β-Lactamase stability (penicillinase)
− β-Lactamase inhibition (cephalosporinase)
− Activity against Serratia and Bacteroides fragilis

Oxacephem group
− Increased activity
− Restriction of protein binding

p-Hydroxy group
− Increased serum concentration
− Prolonged half-life
− Increased stability
− Improved activity in vivo

Carboxyl group
− Activity against Pseudomonas
− Extension of action on gram-negative bacteria
− β-Lactamase stability (cephalosporinase)
− Interference with platelet aggregation

Tetrazolium ring
− Increased activity against gram-negative bacteria
− Prevents metabolism
− Alcohol intolerance

Fig. 4. Structure-activity relationships in the β-lactam antibiotics, exemplified by latamoxef.

R=H: 6-Aminopenicillanic acid

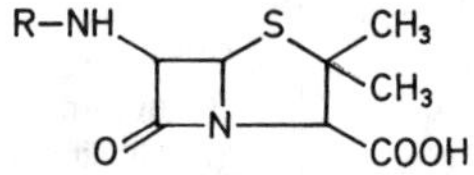

Category	Derivative	R
Penicillins with a narrow spectrum	Benzylpenicillin (Penicillin G)	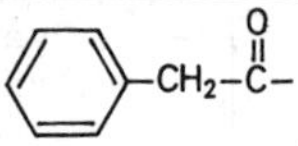 C₆H₅-CH₂-C(=O)-
	Phenoxymethyl penicillin (Penicillin V)	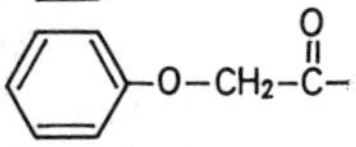 C₆H₅-O-CH₂-C(=O)-
Penicillins with a broader spectrum	Ampicillin	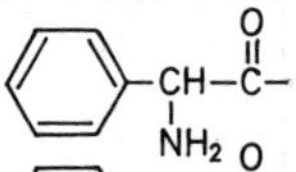 C₆H₅-CH(NH₂)-C(=O)-
	Amoxycillin	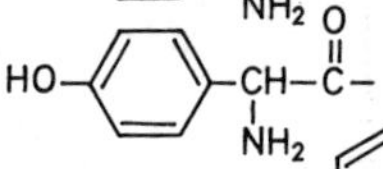 HO-C₆H₄-CH(NH₂)-C(=O)-
	Mezlocillin	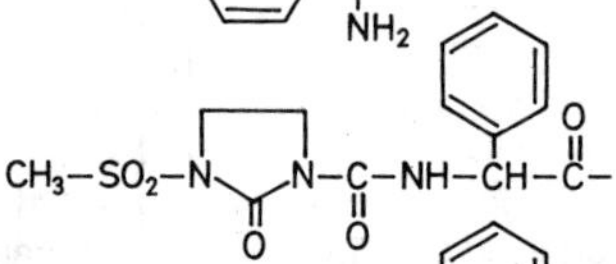 CH₃-SO₂-N(—)N-C(=O)-NH-CH(C₆H₅)-C(=O)-
	Azlocillin	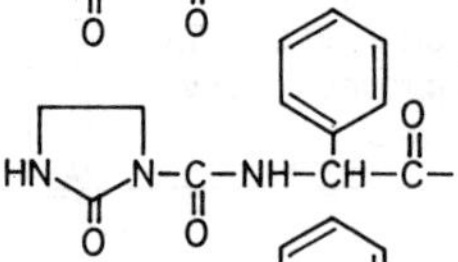 HN(—)N-C(=O)-NH-CH(C₆H₅)-C(=O)-
	Piperacillin	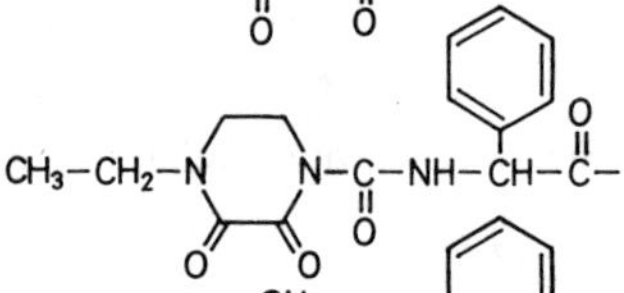 CH₃-CH₂-N(—)N-C(=O)-NH-CH(C₆H₅)-C(=O)-
	Apalcillin	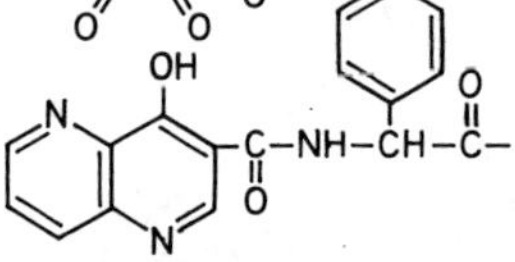 (naphthyridinyl-OH)-C(=O)-NH-CH(C₆H₅)-C(=O)-
Penicillinase-stable penicillins	Oxacillin	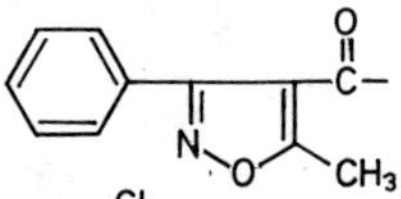 (phenyl-isoxazolyl-CH₃)-C(=O)-
	Dicloxacillin	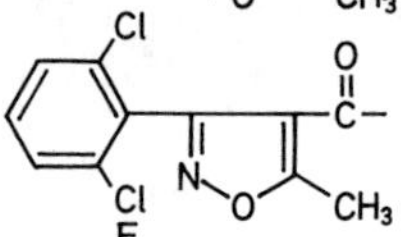 (2,6-dichlorophenyl-isoxazolyl-CH₃)-C(=O)-
	Flucloxacillin	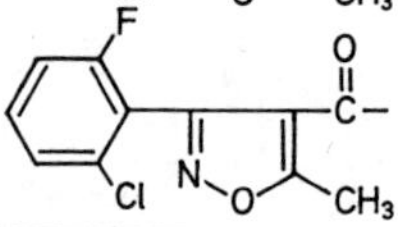 (2-fluoro-6-chlorophenyl-isoxazolyl-CH₃)-C(=O)-

Fig. 5. Chemical structure of the most important penicillins.

1. Penicillins

Classification: The penicillins are all derivatives of 6-aminopenicillanic acid. Acid radicals (R) can be attached to the amino group and determine the different types of penicillin (Fig. 5). The side-chain affects antibacterial activity. Penicillins in the form of weak acids are not very stable molecules. Neutral salts (particularly sodium salts) are more stable, as are esters, which are also more water-soluble. The penicillins may be classified according to their chemical structure as follows:

1. *Benzylpenicillin* (penicillin G) has the greatest activity against gram-positive bacteria but is inactivated through hydrolysis by bacterial β-lactamases.
2. The *phenoxypenicillins* (phenoxymethylpenicillin [penicillin V], propicillin, phenethicillin) have the same spectrum as benzylpenicillin but are relatively stable to gastric acidity and may therefore be used orally.
3. The *isoxazolyl penicillins* (oxa-, cloxa-, dicloxa- and flucloxacillin) are resistant to staphylococcal β-lactamase and so are often termed penicillinase-stable or anti-staphylococcal penicillins. They are less active than benzylpenicillin against other gram-positive bacteria and are inactive against gram-negative bacilli.
4. The *aminopenicillins* (ampicillin, amoxycillin) are resistant to the amidase formed by gram-negative bacilli, which catalyses the hydrolysis of the penicillin side-chain. Ampicillin and amoxycillin are therefore active against a number of species of gram-negative bacillus and thus are moderately broad-spectrum penicillins. Like benzylpenicillin, however, they are not stable to penicillinase and so are inactivated by staphylococcal β-lactamase.
5. The *acylaminopenicillins* (azlo-, mezlo-, pipera- and apalcillin) have a spectrum of activity similar to that of the aminopenicillins, but are generally more active against gram-negative bacilli, including Pseudomonas aeruginosa. They are not stable to penicillinase.
6. The *carboxypenicillins* (carbenicillin, ticarcillin, temocillin) are similar in their spectrum to the acylaminopenicillins and are also active against pseudomonas, though less so than azlocillin or piperacillin. Temocillin is more active in this respect than ticarcillin, but is inactive against gram-positive bacteria.
7. *Amidinopenicillins* (mecillinam, known as amdinocillin in the USA) is a derivative of amidino penicillanic acid. Its antibacterial action differs from that of other penicillins, in that it binds to penicillin-binding protein 2 and is thereby more active against gram-negative than against gram-positive bacteria. This different mechanism of action allows mecillinam to act synergistically with other penicillins.

Antibacterial activity and resistance: The differences in activity between individual penicillins are mainly due to differences in affinity for bacterial binding proteins, to variations in ability to penetrate the bacterial cell membrane (crypticity) and differences in β-lactamase stability. The availability of penicillin receptors, the peptidoglycan content of the bacterial cell wall (which is greater in gram-positive than in gram-negative bacteria) and the lipid content of the bacterial cell wall also play a part.

Resistance of bacteria to penicillins can be due to the following:
1. β-lactamase formation. At least 50 different β-lactamases have been described which can split the β-lactam ring. The β-lactamases produced by certain bacteria can be inhibited by β-lactamase inhibitors such as clavulanic acid, sulbactam and tazobactam (see p. 110, 114 and p. 117), thus extending the spectrum of a particular penicillin.
2. Lack of suitable receptors or poor penetration of the penicillin through the outer layer of the cell wall, so that the penicillin does not reach its receptors.
3. Failure of activation of autolytic bacterial enzymes in the cell wall, so that the bacteria are not killed. This phenomenon is known as bacterial tolerance.
4. Absence of a bacterial cell wall (e.g. mycoplasma) or of cell wall synthesis (as in the bacterial resting phase).

The **main indications** for the different penicillins are listed in Table 6. Benzylpenicillin is the drug of choice for streptococcal and pneumococcal infections as well as for infections with sensitive strains of staphylococci. Ampicillin is the first choice for infections with enterococci, haemophilus and Proteus mirabilis. Oxacillin, cloxacillin, dicloxacillin, flucloxacillin and nafcillin are used as penicillinase-stable antistaphylococcal penicillins. Azlocillin, ticarcillin and piperacillin are effective agents in infections with sensitive strains of Pseudomonas aeruginosa, although they are not stable to penicillinase. Ticarcillin and amoxycillin are available in combination with clavulanic acid as the proprietary combinations Timentin® and Augmentin®, respectively.

Parenteral penicillins are given at intervals corresponding to their pharmacokinetics. Treatment should be started with a loading dose. In acute and serious infections, benzylpenicillin is given parenterally as a short i.v. infusion or i.v. injection in a medium or high dosage (2.4–12 g).

After clinical signs of improvement, treatment may be continued with high doses of an oral penicillin (3 g), usually either phenoxymethylpenicillin or amoxycillin. Mild infections may be treated with oral penicillins from the outset. Depot penicillins give relatively low serum levels and are therefore only recommended for infections with very sensitive bacteria (streptococci, pneumococci, treponemes), as prophylaxis for rheumatic fever, and for patients who vomit when given penicillins by mouth. Topical and rectal administration of penicillins are not recommended because they are often ineffective and carry a considerable risk of allergy.

General evaluation *of the penicillins:*

Advantages: Bactericidal, well tolerated, large dose range, no or only slow development of resistance during therapy.

Disadvantages: Gaps in the spectrum of activity, instability towards the various β-lactamases, allergy and rapid excretion.

Table 6. Clinical efficacy of penicillins (principal indications shown thus: +++ or ++).

Drug	Staphylococci (without production of penicillinase)	Staphylococci (with production of penicillinase)	Str. pneumoniae, Str. pyogenes, gono-, meningococci, Treponema pallidum	Enterococci	Esch. coli	Klebsiella	Proteus mirabilis	Proteus vulgaris	Pseudomonas aeruginosa	Haemophilus	Serratia marcescens
Benzylpenicillin, phenoxymethyl penicillin	+++	∅	+++	+	∅	∅	∅	∅	∅	∅	∅
Ampicillin	++	∅	++	++	++	∅	++	∅	∅	++	∅
Mezlocillin	+	∅	++	++	++	++	++	++	+	++	++
Piperacillin	+	∅	++	++	++	++	++	++	++	++	++
Azlocillin	+	∅	+	++	++	∅	++	++	++	++	∅
Oxacillin, cloxacillin, flucloxacillin	++	++	+	∅	∅	∅	∅	∅	∅	∅	∅

a) Benzylpenicillin (Penicillin G)

Properties: Benzylpenicillin is used as its readily soluble sodium or potassium salt or as a poorly soluble depot penicillin (procaine penicillin, benzathine penicillin, clemizole penicillin). One international unit of sodium or potassium penicillin is equivalent to 0.6 µg (1 µg = 1.67 units). One megaunit is therefore 600 mg. One megaunit of procaine penicillin corresponds to 1 g, and 1 megaunit of benzathine penicillin corresponds to 750 mg of the pure substance.

Mode of action: Bactericidal on proliferating bacteria, by inhibition of cell wall synthesis by blocking bacterial transpeptidase.

Spectrum of activity:
Good or moderate sensitivity (minimal inhibitory concentration 0.001 to 0.25 mg/l) is shown by Streptococcus pyogenes, Lancefield group B streptococci, Streptococcus pneumoniae, viridans streptococci, anaerobic streptococci, gonococci, meningococci, corynebacteria, spirochaetes (treponemes, borrelia), Actinomyces israeli and Pasteurella multocida.

Variable sensitivity is shown by Staphylococcus aureus, S. epidermidis, Listeria monocytogenes, clostridia, Bacillus anthracis, and Campylobacter spp. Many gram-negative anaerobes (e.g. Bacteroides melaninogenicus, fusobacteria) are very sensitive. Most staphylococcal strains are resistant, but benzylpenicillin is very active against sensitive strains.

Weak sensitivity (or resistance) is shown by enterococci (Enterococcus faecalis, Enterococcus faecium), Proteus mirabilis, Brucella spp., Haemophilus influenzae and Bordetella pertussis.

Resistance (minimal inhibitory concentration greater than 4 mg/l) is shown by members of the Enterobacteriaceae, salmonellae, Bacteroides fragilis, Nocardia asteroides and Vibrio cholerae.

Resistance: The frequency of *primary resistance* amongst staphylococci differs from place to place (30–90%), and amongst pneumococci and gonococci is low but increasing. Multiresistant pneumococci are resistant not only to benzylpenicillin but also to tetracycline, chloramphenicol, erythromycin and clindamycin. Some strains are also resistant to rifampicin. Penicillin-resistant gonococci from East Asia are also mostly resistant to tetracycline, erythromycin and spectinomycin.

Secondary resistance is uncommon and develops slowly (multiple-step resistance) through mutation, the selection of resistant variants, or the induction of penicillinase in potential penicillinase producers under the prolonged influence of penicillin. The β-lactam ring of the penicillin is split hydrolytically by bacterial penicillinase, giving rise to antibacterially inactive penicilloyl compounds. *Penicillin-tolerant* strains of Staphylococcus aureus and Streptococcus sanguis are inhibited bacteriostatically, but they are only very slowly destroyed, if at all.

Penicillin-tolerant strains of Staphylococcus aureus may also be tolerant to cephalosporins and vancomycin, but not to gentamicin.

Cross-sensitivity to acylaminopenicillins is found in bacteria sensitive to benzylpenicillin.

Pharmacokinetics:

Oral administration is ineffective because the drug is not stable to gastric acid.

Absorption is rapid and complete after i.m. injection of the water-soluble benzylpenicillin, but is retarded with depot penicillins.

Serum concentrations after i.m. or i.v. administration depend on the dose and dose-interval, and differ between benzylpenicillin and the depot penicillins (Fig. 6).

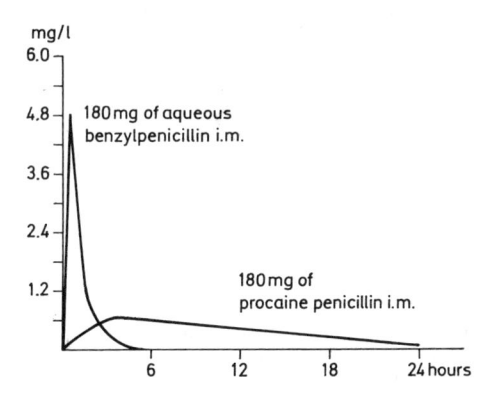

Fig. 6. Serum concentrations with benzylpenicillin and procaine penicillin.

The maximum serum level is 45 mg/l after an *i.v. bolus injection* of 0.6 g of benzylpenicillin; after an *i.v. infusion over one hour* it is 14.4 mg/l. The corresponding mean peak concentrations after 3 g are 236.4 mg/l and 80.4 mg/l. *Constant infusion* of 0.1 and 0.5 g/h (equivalent to a daily dose of 2.4 and 12 g) gives rise to mean serum concentrations of 3.5 and 13.3 mg/l respectively. Thus, as a rule of thumb, the mean serum concentrations in mg/l achieved with constant i.v. infusion correspond approximately to the daily dose in g. Because excretion is so rapid, the serum concentrations after i.v. bolus injection fall below those achieved through constant i.v. infusion within 1¼ h; concentrations after a short (1 h) i.v. infusion fall below those of constant infusion within 1¾ h (Fig. 7).

Mean serum concentrations of 1.7, 4.8, 12.0 and 42.0 mg/l are found 1 h after the *i.m. injection* of 0.12, 0.3, 0.6 and 3.0 g of benzylpenicillin sodium. Depot penicillins give a slower rise and fall with relatively low serum concentrations. The serum concentrations after 0.24 g of procaine penicillin are 0.36 mg/l at 1 and 2 h,

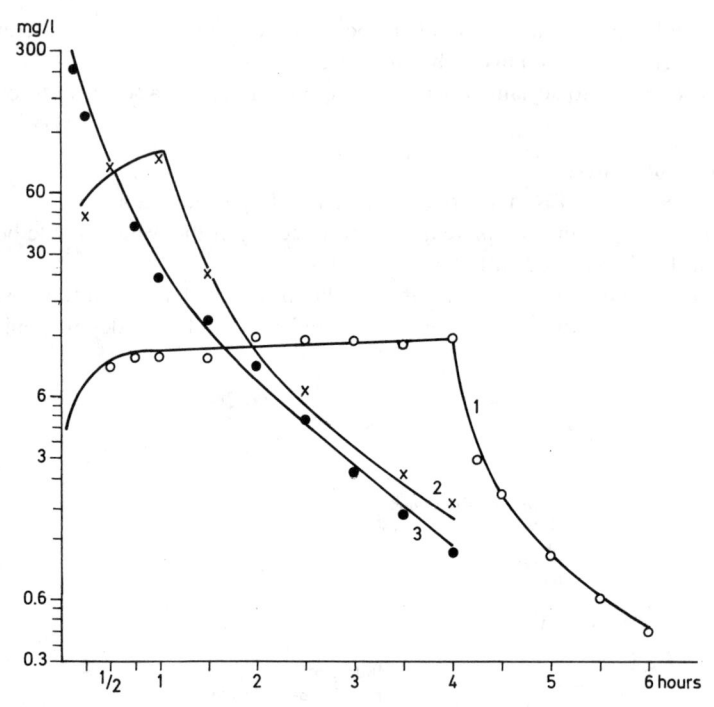

Fig. 7. Measured serum concentrations of benzylpenicillin (sodium salt) and curves calculated from them, after 4 hours of continuous infusion (0.3 g/h = 7.2 g/day, curve 1), after a short infusion of one hour (3 g, curve 2), and after a bolus intravenous injection (3 g, curve 3; own data).

0.3 mg/l at 6 h and 0.06 mg/l at 12 h; after 0.36 g of procaine penicillin they are 0.6 mg/l at 1 and 2 h, 0.54 mg/l at 6 h and 0.36 mg/l at 12 h.

Low serum concentrations of at least 0.018 mg/l for 3–4 weeks, which are useful in the long-term prophylaxis of rheumatic fever, are maintained *after benzathine penicillin* (0.72 g i.m.). 0.12 mg/l persist in the serum 2 weeks after 1.44 g of this preparation.

Half-life after parenteral benzylpenicillin: 40 min.

Plasma protein binding: ca. 50%.

CSF penetration is poor, but improved in the presence of meningeal inflammation. In purulent meningitis, large single doses of benzylpenicillin give cerebrospinal fluid concentrations which are high enough to kill pneumococci and meningococci (0.05–0.2 mg/l 1 h after 2.4 g i.v.).

Tissue concentrations: Good penetration of kidneys, lungs, liver, skin and mucous membranes.

Poor diffusion into muscle, bone, nervous tissue, brain and aqueous humor. Because of the failure to penetrate cells, there is no useful intracellular activity.

Concentrations in inflammatory, pleural, pericardial, peritoneal and synovial effusions reach 25–75% of the serum concentrations. About ¼ of the maternal serum concentration is found in the fetal circulation. High concentrations in amniotic fluid. 5–10% of serum concentration in breast milk.

Excretion: 85–95% excreted in the urine after parenteral administration with high urinary concentrations. Urinary recovery is reduced in renal insufficiency and with the simultaneous administration of probenecid.

Low biliary excretion; the concentrations in bile are similar to those in the blood.

Side-effects:
1. *Penicillin hypersensitivity* is the most frequent complication of penicillin therapy (0.5 – 2.0%). The allergens are the intact penicillin molecule and also antibacterially inactive metabolites of 6-aminopenicillanic acid, e.g. penicilloic acid. Since all penicillins are derived from 6-aminopenicillanic acid, they can all produce an allergic response in the hypersensitive individual.

Cross-allergy between the penicillins and cephalosporins is rare, so cephalosporins may still be considered as alternative agents in cases of penicillin allergy, though the patient should be carefully observed during therapy.

The occurrence of penicillin allergy depends on *several factors*, e.g.

a) the type of penicillin: skin reactions are commoner after ampicillin than after benzyl- or phenoxymethyl penicillin;

b) the functional state of the reticuloendothelial system: patients with infectious mononucleosis more frequently develop allergy after ampicillin;

c) the route of administration: topical application of penicillin on the skin or mucous membranes increases the likelihood of an allergic reaction.

If hypersensitivity has been present for some time, the allergic response may occur immediately after the first dose or develop within 8–14 days during treatment. A mild reaction may consist only of a morbilliform or scarlatiniform rash on the trunk and extremities which can disappear spontaneously during treatment. Such reactions following ampicillin are usually not allergic, but are due to a cumulative toxic effect of the ampicillin. Mild reactions are often expressed as drug fever, general uneasiness during the infusion, and eosinophilia. Urticarial or oedematous skin rashes with or without fever and sometimes accompanied by joint swelling, laryngeal oedema, cerebral oedema, conjunctivitis or other symptoms should be taken more seriously. The development of urticaria is a clear contraindication to any further penicillin therapy. *Anaphylactic shock* is fortunately rare but may be extremely serious, and lethal in 10% of cases. Affected patients suffer sudden vasomotor collapse, loss of consciousness, muscle cramps and respiratory distress. Rapid and intensive therapy (see below) may be lifesaving. Neutropenia, thrombocytopenia, haemolytic anemia and interstitial nephritis are uncommon allergic effects.

True penicillin allergy may be confused with the rare *allergy to procaine*. The non-allergic Hoigné syndrome, which follows the accidental intravascular injection of depot penicillin, is accompanied by severe general reactions, fear of imminent death, loss of consciousness without circulatory collapse, hallucinations, double vision, tinnitus, vertigo, paraesthesiae and tachycardia. These symptoms are not due to allergy and disappear completely within 15–30 min. They are caused by microemboli of the depot penicillin in capillaries.

Tests: No satisfactory method of testing for the presence of penicillin allergy has so far been developed. Specific serum IgE (RAST test) can be demonstrated in individuals who have never shown signs of allergy. A negative result, however, does not exclude allergy. When a patient gives a history, or for other reasons is suspected of penicillin allergy, the following *preliminary tests* may be useful if there is a need for further penicillin therapy:

Scratch test: A drop of penicillin solution (600–3000 mg/l) is applied to a fresh skin scratch. An immediate reaction with erythema and pruritus occurs within 15 min in allergic individuals.

Intradermal test with 0.02 ml of a solution of 600 mg/l. This test is dangerous and serious, even fatal, reactions have occurred. False positive and false negative reactions have been reported. When procaine allergy is suspected, 0.1 ml of a 1% solution of procaine may be injected, strictly intradermally. A wheal and flare reaction may result and there is a danger of shock. The value of skin testing, for which the scratch test is the best, is the recognition of patients in whom an immediate and severe reaction is likely to follow a further dose of a penicillin.

When the scratch and intradermal tests are negative, a careful *exposure test* may be performed. A solution of 0.12 g of benzylpenicillin in 500 ml of fluid is infused very slowly and stopped immediately at the first sign of an allergic reaction. Depot penicillins must never be given when penicillin allergy is suspected, because of the danger of a prolonged allergic response.

Treatment of penicillin allergy:
When rashes occur during treatment, discontinue penicillin. For allergic shock, which is often associated with pulmonary, laryngeal and cerebral oedema, inject 0.5–1 mg adrenaline i.m. or subcutaneously, followed, if necessary, by 0.5 mg slowly i.v.; repeat up to 3 times at intervals of 5–10 min. Continuous infusion of vasoconstrictors may be needed to maintain the blood pressure, together with 50–100 mg of prednisone i.v. For laryngeal oedema, intubate and ventilate mechanically. Injections of penicillinase and antihistamines are

ineffective. The patient should be observed carefully for a few hours after clinical improvement has been established, since symptoms can recur. When severe, protracted shock follows the injection of depot penicillins, particularly clemizole and benzathine penicillin, excision of the injection site may be necessary.
2. *Neurotoxicity* with convulsions is reported after intrathecal instillation and also in meningitis, epilepsy and uraemia after very high systemic doses of benzylpenicillin, in excess of 12 g. The potassium salt of benzylpenicillin can give rise to hyperkalaemia, muscle spasm, coma and cardiac arrest when given in excess and the sodium salt is preferable. 0.6 g of benzylpenicillin potassium contains 1.5 milliequivalents of potassium. In most high dose penicillin preparations, the sodium and potassium salts are mixed in a ratio intended to avoid electrolyte disturbances. A maximum daily dosage of 12–18 g of benzylpenicillin in adults, or of 7.2 g in children, should not generally be exceeded. Patients in severe renal failure (decompensated retention of uraemia) require only 50% of the normal dose of penicillin.
3. The *Herxheimer reaction* at the beginning of treatment of syphilis, particularly congenital and secondary syphilis, with penicillin consists of fever, chills, systemic and focal reactions. *Treatment:* 50–100 mg prednisone i. v.
4. Accidental intravascular injection of procaine or benzathine penicillin can result in *transverse myelitis* and paralysis, *gangrene* of the fingers, toes, or other extremities, and oedema or *necrosis* at the injection site. Injection in or near a nerve can give rise to permanent *neurological damage.*

Indications: Infections caused by streptococci, pneumococci, meningococci, penicillin-sensitive staphylococci; syphilis, gonorrhoea, diphtheria, scarlet fever, follicular tonsillitis, peridontitis, erysipelas, rheumatic fever, treatment and prophylaxis of infective endocarditis, erysipeloid, lobar pneumonia, meningitis due to sensitive pathogens, anthrax, animal bites infected with Pasteurella multocida, leptospirosis, actinomycosis, tetanus, gas gangrene, wound infections developed outside hospital. Benzylpenicillin is the antibiotic of choice in Lyme borreliosis, acrodermatitis atrophicans and other manifestations of borrelia infection. Depot penicillin gives lower blood concentrations than benzylpenicillin, which is rapidly absorbed after i. m. injection. Depot penicillins are indicated in patients who are prevented by vomiting from taking a penicillin by mouth, and also in infections with very sensitive bacteria such as spirochaetes and gonococci, where quite low concentrations are effective. Severe infections should be treated with high doses of an aqueous preparation i. v.

Inappropriate use: Benzylpenicillin *should not be used alone* in severe sepsis where the causative organism is unknown, since it is ineffective against penicillinase-producing strains, in urinary infections or in atypical pneumonia, where the pathogen is likely to be insensitive to penicillin.

Contra-indication: Penicillin allergy. Caution with doses greater than 6 g, in renal failure and in epilepsy (risk of neurotoxicity). Avoid the potassium salt in severe renal failure.

Route: Use a 5–10% solution for i.m. injection of benzylpenicillin sodium, and up to 20% for i.v. injection. Give frequently, either every 4–6 h in small doses, or by short i.v. infusion over ½–1 h for higher doses and in severe illness. In some cases, benzylpenicillin infusion can be given by day and i.m. depot penicillin at night. A depot injection of penicillin can be given at the start of outpatient therapy of infections with very sensitive organisms, followed by oral phenoxymethylpenicillin. Care must always be taken when injecting a penicillin preparation i.m. that the drug is not accidentally injected into a vein or artery. Always test the position of the needle by aspiration before injection. The vicinity of peripheral nerves must also be avoided, hence the preference for the upper, outer quadrant of the buttock in adults and the middle third of the outer aspect of the thigh in small children. Change infection sites regularly for repeated i.m. injection.

Dosage:
Adults: 0.6 g daily for sensitive pathogens, and 1.2–12 g i.m. or i.v. for less sensitive bacteria.
Small children: 24–36 mg/kg or 120–300 mg/kg i.m. or i.v. daily.
Infants: 24–60 mg/kg daily or 120–600 mg/kg i.m. or i.v. In *severe renal failure*, do not exceed a daily dose of 6 g of benzylpenicillin (adults) or 50% of the normal daily dose; depot penicillin should only be given every 2 (–6) days.

Dose interval: Every 4–6 hours with benzylpenicillin sodium and potassium and every 8 hours in the newborn and infants (delayed excretion because of renal immaturity); depot penicillins vary according to preparation and dose (generally every 12–24 h).

The administration of **probenecid** can inhibit the tubular secretion of benzylpenicillin, resulting in higher serum levels. Adults are given 0.5 g orally 4 times a day and children (2 years and above) 10 mg/kg 4 times a day. Contra-indicated in blood dyscrasia, renal failure, uric acid calculus, and gout. Probenecid used to be particularly recommended in severe sepsis and endocarditis in order to achieve higher blood and tissue concentrations, and is used in some countries in the single dose treatment of gonorrhoea with benzylpenicillin or ampicillin.

Instillation of benzylpenicillin is possible in principle, but has only a brief effect because of its rapid absorption and can no longer be recommended.

Preparations:
Benzylpenicillin: vials of 0.24, 0.6, 6 and 12 g.
Clemizole penicillin: vials of 0.6 g.
Procaine penicillin: vials of 0.36, 0.72 and 1.44 g.
Benzathine penicillin: vials of 0.72 g.

Benethamine penicillin 475 mg + procaine penicillin 250 mg + benzylpenicillin sodium 300 mg (Triplopen).
Clemizole penicillin: 0.24 g + benzylpenicillin 2.16 g.

Summary:
Advantages: Wide therapeutic range, maximum concentrations achieved by injection, more active against sensitive strains than other penicillins, depot effect with procaine, clemizole, and benzathine penicillins.
Disadvantages: Inactivation by penicillinase-producing bacteria. Oral administration not possible because of instability to acid and poor oral absorption. Hypersensitivity reactions complicating parenteral administration (particularly of depot preparations) are more dangerous than with the oral route.

References

MENDELSON, L. M. et al.: Routine elective penicillin allergy skin testing in children and adolescents: Study of sensitization. J. Allergy Clin. Immunol. *73:* 76 (1984).
REDELMEIER, D. A., H. C. Sox: The role of skin testing for penicillin allergy. Arch. Intern. Med. *150:* 1939–1945 (1990).
SOGN, D. D. et al.: Interim results of the NIAID collaborative clinical trial of skin testing with major and minor penicillin derivatives in hospitalized adults. J. Allergy Clin. Immunol. *71:* 147 (1983).

b) Phenoxypenicillins

Common proprietary names:
Phenoxymethylpenicillin: Apsin VK, Beromycin, Cliacil, Co-Caps, Crystapen V, Distaquaine VK, Econocil VK, Fenoxypen, Icipen, Isocillin, Megacillin oral, Pencompren, Penicillin VK, Ospen, Stabillin V-K, Star-Pen, Ticillin V-K, V-Tablopen, V-Cil-K.
Propicillin: Baycillin, Oricillin. Not available in Britain.
Phenethicillin: Broxil.
Azidocillin: Longatren, Nalpen, Syncillin. Not available in Britain.

Synonyms: Acid-resistant penicillins, oral penicillins.

Properties: Phenoxymethylpenicillin (penicillin V) is a biosynthetic product; propicillin (phenoxypropyl penicillin), phenethicillin (phenoxyethyl penicillin) and azidocillin (α-azidobenzyl penicillin) are semi-synthetic products. The potassium salts of phenoxymethylpenicillin, phenethicillin, propicillin and azidocillin are readily soluble in water, while the phenoxymethylpenicillin free acid is only poorly water-soluble. Acid-stability is quite good with all the phenoxy penicillins. In some countries (e.g. Germany), phenoxypenicillins are still dosed in units. 1 megaunit of phenoxymethyl penicillin, phenethicillin and azidocillin correspond approximately to 600 mg (1 g contains approx. 1.6 megaunits). For propicillin, 1 megaunit corresponds to 700 mg (1 g = 1.42 megaunits).

Mechanism and spectrum of action: All the phenoxypenicillins act like benzylpenicillin. Propicillin is a little more stable to penicillinase than the others, but it is quite inadequate in infections caused by penicillinase-producing staphylococci.

Antibacterial activity: Propicillin and phenethicillin are 2–4 times less active than benzylpenicillin, phenoxymethylpenicillin and azidocillin against sensitive gram-positive bacteria. Azidocillin has some activity against Haemophilus influenzae, Bordetella pertussis and enterococci.

Resistance: Uncommon and slow to develop (like benzylpenicillin). Cross-resistance to penicillinase-producing bacteria occurs between the phenoxypenicillins, benzylpenicillin and ampicillin.

Pharmacokinetics:
Maximal serum concentrations in mg/l (Fig. 8) after oral administration of
propicillin 700 mg   10.1 (after 2.50 h),
phenoxymethylpenicillin potassium 600 mg   6.4 (after 0.75 h),
phenethicillin 600 mg   5.7 (after 0.75 h),
azidocillin 600 mg   8.8 (after 0.50 h).

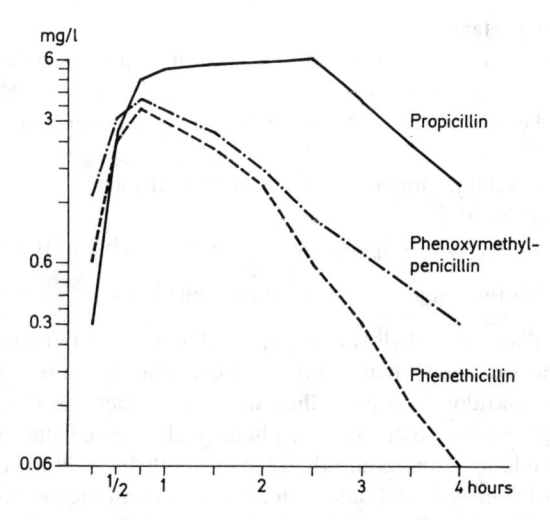

Fig. 8. Mean serum concentration-time curves in healthy adults after oral administration of propicillin 700 mg, phenoxymethylpenicillin and phenethicillin 600 mg (own data).

The rates of absorption of propicillin and phenoxymethylpenicillin are about the same (approx. 50%), as shown by comparisons of the areas under the blood concentration-time curves for intravenous and oral administration. The blood concentration of propicillin is twice as high as that of phenoxymethylpenicillin, which may be explained by the fact that propicillin is metabolised more slowly than phenoxymethylpenicillin. With azidocillin, at least 75% of the oral dose is absorbed and blood levels after oral and i.m. administration are comparable. Phenoxymethylpenicillin and phenethicillin are absorbed less well after meals than fasting. Half-life of phenoxymethylpenicillin, propicillin and azidocillin: 30 min; of phenethicillin: 20 min.

Plasma protein binding: Phenoxymethylpenicillin: 60%, propicillin: 80–85%, phenethicillin: 80%, and azidocillin: 84%.

Tissue diffusion and *CSF penetration* are similar to benzylpenicillin.

Excretion: Phenoxymethylpenicillin is 30–50% excreted in the urine, propicillin 50%, phenethicillin 20–30% and azidocillin 60%. More inactive metabolites (penicilloic acid) are excreted with phenoxymethylpenicillin than with propicillin. 5% of the dose of azidocillin is excreted in the urine as ampicillin, which is formed from azidocillin in the body.

Side-effects: The risk of sensitisation is smaller than with benzylpenicillin, which is given parenterally. Neurotoxicity does not occur.

Main indications: Mild infections caused by penicillin-sensitive bacteria, e.g. sore throat, erysipelas, periodontal infections, scarlet fever, borrelia infections, prevention of rheumatic fever and scarlet fever.

Inappropriate use: Meningitis, septicaemia, endocarditis, infections caused by less sensitive bacteria which require large i.v. doses.

Contra-indication: Penicillin allergy.

Administration and dosage: Can only be given by mouth. The unpleasant taste of certain preparations causes difficulties in dosing children. The minimum recommended doses are:
Adults and children aged 13 or over: 500 mg 3 times a day;
Children aged 6–12 years: 250 mg 3 times a day;
Children aged 1–5 years: 125 mg 3 times a day;
Newborn and infants up to 1 year: 62.5 mg 2–3 times a day.
Azidocillin: 1.5–2 g a day for adults, 750 mg a day for children (2–10 years); 60 mg/kg a day for children under 2 years. Give in 3 divided doses in each case.

Preparations: *Phenoxymethylpenicillin:* Capsules or tablets of 125 mg, 250 mg and 500 mg; syrup with 125 mg or 250 mg in 5 ml.
Propicillin: Tablets or coated tablets of 140, 280, 520 and 700 mg; syrup.
Azidocillin: Tablets of 750 mg, granules in sachets of 250 mg.

Summary: Despite differences in their antibacterial activity and pharmacokinetics, the different phenoxypenicillins have similar clinical activity when given for appropriate indications in sufficient dosage. Azidocillin has additional activity against Haemophilus influenzae and is therefore particularly suitable for the treatment of respiratory infections and otitis media.

References

BUCHANAN, G. R., J. D. SIEGEL, S. J. SMITH, B. M. DE PASSE: Oral penicillin prophylaxis in children with impaired splenic function: a study of compliance. Pediatrics *70:* 926 (1982).

c) Isoxazolyl Penicillins (Anti-staphylococcal Penicillins)

Common proprietary names:
Dicloxacillin: Dichlor-Stapenor, Diclocil, Dycill, Dynapen, Pathocil. Not marketed in Britain.
Flucloxacillin: Floxapen, Staphylex.
Oxacillin: Bactocill, Cryptocillin, Oxacillin, Prostaphlin, Stapenor. Not marketed in Britain.
Cloxacillin: Cloxapen, Orbenin. No longer marketed in Germany.
Methicillin: Celbenin, Staphcillin. No longer marketed in Britain or Germany.
Nafcillin: Nafcil, Unipen. Not marketed in Britain or Germany.

Properties: Methicillin was the first penicillinase-stable penicillin to be used in therapy. It could only be given parenterally, was relatively toxic and was less active *in vitro* on penicillinase-producing staphylococci than the newer penicillinase-stable isoxazolyl penicillins, oxacillin, nafcillin, cloxacillin, dicloxacillin and flucloxacillin, which have superceded methicillin in treatment. These penicillins are water-soluble, can be given by mouth and differ from each other in pharmacokinetic properties only, not in antibacterial activity.

Spectrum of activity: Effective against penicillinase-producing staphylococci. The isoxazolyl penicillins are generally only one tenth as active as benzylpenicillin against penicillin-sensitive staphylococci, streptococci, pneumococci and other gram-positive bacteria.

Resistance: Methicillin is traditionally used to test for resistance to all the penicillinase-stable penicillins. Methicillin-resistant Staphylococcus epidermidis has increased in recent years and now accounts for more than 50% of isolates in many hospitals. The incidence of methicillin-resistant Staphylococcus aureus (MRSA) shows wide local and regional variation; in addition to strains of low or moderate virulence, some hospitals now report outbreaks of severe infection with virulent, multiresistant epidemic strains (EMRSA), which may be susceptible to treatment with vancomycin or quinolone antibiotics only. Methicillin resistance is best detected *in vitro* either in culture media containing 5% NaCl or after overnight incubation at 30° C. Secondary resistance has not been observed during therapy. There is complete cross-resistance in staphylococci between all the penicillinase-stable penicillins and the cephalosporins. Penicillin-sensitive staphylococci are always sensitive to methicillin and the isoxazolyl penicillins.

Pharmacokinetics:
Oral absorption is best with dicloxacillin and flucloxacillin. Cloxacillin and oxacillin, which are less acid-stable than dicloxacillin, are less well absorbed. Absorption is better on an empty stomach (1 h before or 2–4 h after meals). Maximal blood concentrations occur after 1–2 h. Methicillin is not acid-stable and is virtually not absorbed after oral administration.

Serum concentrations (mg/l) after 500 mg by mouth 1 h after a meal (Fig. 9): flucloxacillin 7.6 and 2.3 (after 1½ and 4 h), dicloxacillin 5.9 and 2.0 (after 1½ and 4 h).

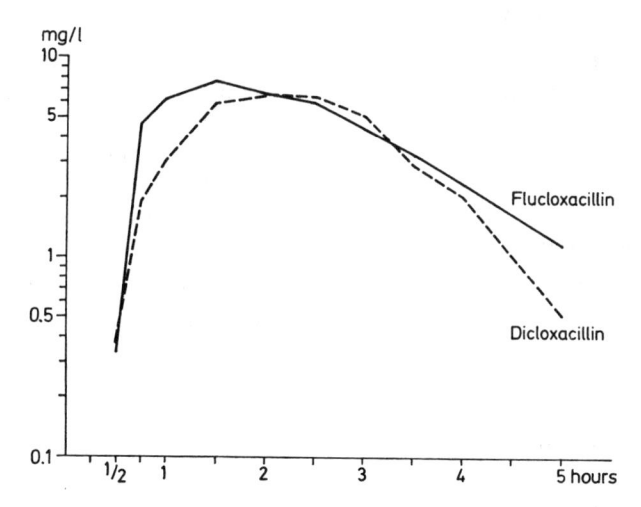

Fig. 9. Mean serum concentration-time curve in 10 healthy adults after a single oral dose of 500 mg of flucloxacillin or dicloxacillin, 1 h after a standard breakfast (own data).

Serum concentrations (mg/l) after i.v. injection of 500 mg: flucloxacillin 15.7 and 2.0 (after 1 and 4 h), oxacillin 1.7 and less than 0.1 (after 1 and 4 h).
Half-life of dicloxacillin and flucloxacillin: 45 min; oxacillin: 25 min.
Plasma protein binding: dicloxacillin 97%, flucloxacillin 95%, oxacillin 93%.
CSF penetration is poor, up to 10% of the serum concentration in meningitis. Passes into the fetal circulation.

Excretion in the urine after parenteral administration: dicloxacillin up to 65%, flucloxacillin up to 35% and oxacillin up to 25%. Oxacillin is more rapidly excreted than dicloxacillin and is more completely metabolised than either dicloxacillin or flucloxacillin. Excretion of inactive metabolites (penicilloic acid) is greatest with oxacillin, less with cloxacillin and flucloxacillin, and least with dicloxacillin.

Side-effects: Similar to benzylpenicillin. Methicillin has occasionally caused allergic bone marrow depression (granulocytopenia) and renal damage. Increased serum transaminases and neutropenia have been reported after oxacillin. Local irritation is frequently found with dicloxacillin, both i.m. (pain) and i.v. (phlebitis), but is uncommon with oxacillin and flucloxacillin.

Indication: Suspected or proven infections with penicillin-resistant staphylococci.

Inappropriate use: Infections with penicillin-sensitive or methicillin-resistant staphylococci, streptococci, pneumococci, gonococci or meningococci.

Contra-indication: Allergy to penicillin.

Administration: For oral administration (before meals), dicloxacillin and flucloxacillin are preferable because of their better absorption and higher, more persistent serum concentrations.

When given by injection, oxacillin, cloxacillin and flucloxacillin have better local tolerance than dicloxacillin. Oxacillin (1% solution) is preferable for local instillation. Intravenous injection should be given slowly to avoid venous irritation, and short i.v. infusions over 30 min are preferable.

Dosage: Daily doses lower than the following are inadvisable:
Oral administration of dicloxacillin and flucloxacillin (fasting) in 4 to 6 divided doses:
    Adults and children over 10 years: 2–4 g daily,
    children aged 2–10 years: 1–2 g daily (50 mg/kg),
    children under 2 years: 0.5–1 g daily (50 mg/kg).
I.m. or i.v. administration of flucloxacillin or cloxacillin in 4–6 hourly injections or short infusions:
    Adults and children over 10 years: 3–4 (–10) g daily,
    children aged 2–10 years: 2–3 (–6) g,
    children under 2 years: 1–2 (–4) g,
    newborn: 40 mg/kg daily.
Probenecid may be given in addition (500 mg 4 times a day for adults), which delays the renal excretion of the penicillinase-resistant penicillins and thus increases the serum concentration. It should not be given to children under 2 years.
Intralumbar instillation of oxacillin: 10–20 g (adults) and 5–10 mg (children).

Preparations:
Dicloxacillin: Capsules of 250 mg.
Flucloxacillin: Capsules of 250 and 500 mg, syrup (25 mg/ml and 50 mg/ml), vials of 250, 500 mg and 1 g.
Oxacillin: Capsules of 250 mg, vials of 500 mg and 1 g.
Cloxacillin: Capsules of 250 and 500 mg, vials of 0.25, 0.5 and 1 g.

Summary: Effective in infections with penicillinase-producing staphylococci. Severe staphylococcal infections are better treated with other antibiotics having better tissue penetration. Dicloxacillin or flucloxacillin are preferable for oral use, and flucloxacillin parenterally.

References

BRUCKSTEIN, A. H. A. A. ATTIA: Oxacillin hepatitis. Two patients with liver biopsy, and review of the literature. Amer. J. Med. *64:* 519 (1978).
FARRINGTON, M., A. FENN, I. PHILLIPS: Flucloxacillin concentration in serum and wound exudate during open heart surgery. J. Antimicrob. Chemother. *16:* 253 (1985).
SMITH, A. L., C. A. MEEKS, J. R. KOUP, K. E. OPHEIM, A. WEBER, D. T. VISHWANATHAN: Dicloxacillin absorption and elimination in children. Rev. Pharmacol. Ther. *14:* 35–44 (1990).
SPINO, M., R. P. CHAI, A. F. ISLES et al.: Cloxacillin absorption and disposition in cystic fibrosis. J. Pediatr. *105:* 829 (1984).
TURNER, I. B., R. P. ECKSTEIN, J. W. RILEY, M. R. LUNZER: Prolonged hepatic cholestasis after flucloxacillin therapy. Med. J. Aust. *151:* 701–705 (1989).

d) Aminopenicillins

The aminopenicillins in current use are ampicillin, bacampicillin, pivampicillin and talampicillin. They differ from ampicillin in their pharmacokinetic properties but not in their antibacterial activity.

α) Ampicillin

Proprietary names: Penbritin and many others.

Properties: A semisynthetic penicillin derivative (α-aminobenzylpenicillin) with an extended spectrum; relatively unstable in solution.

Mode of action: Bactericidal, by inhibition of peptidoglycan synthesis in the cell wall. Not stable to penicillinases from staphylococci, enterobacteria and bacteroides.

Spectrum of action: As benzylpenicillin, but with additional moderate or good activity (inhibitory concentration up to 5 mg/l) against enterococci, listeria, Haemophilus influenzae and Campylobacter fetus. Benzylpenicillin is 2–4 times more active against gram-positive bacteria. The frequency of ampicillin-resistant strains of haemophilus is increasing, but these are still reliably sensitive to cefuroxime, cefamandole, cefotaxime and cefaclor. Simultaneous resistance of haemophilus to ampicillin and chloramphenicol is rare. Resistance amongst enterococci has increased in some parts of the world.

Variable activity against salmonellae, shigellae, Escherichia coli (resistance rate up to 50%) and Proteus mirabilis (non-penicillinase-producing strains), klebsiella, enterobacter, citrobacter, Yersinia enterocolitica, Serratia marcescens, Bacteroides fragilis, Pseudomonas aeruginosa, Proteus vulgaris, Proteus rettgeri and Morganella morganii. When combined with a β-lactamase inhibitor such as clavulanic acid or sulbactam, there is synergistic action on β-lactamase-producing strains of Escherichia coli, klebsiella, Bacteroides fragilis and Staphylococcus aureus.

Resistance: Complete cross-resistance with amoxycillin. Penicillin-resistant strains of gonococci are also resistant to ampicillin. Some cross-resistance of aerobic gram-negative bacilli with azlocillin, mezlocillin, piperacillin, apalcillin, temocillin and the cephalosporins. Resistance rarely develops during therapy but is sometimes seen in haemophilus infections. Selection of primarily resistant bacteria may occur during therapy and should be distinguished from secondary resistance.

Pharmacokinetics:
Absorption by mouth is 30–40%.
Maximum serum concentrations after 500 mg by mouth (after meals): mean of 2 mg/l after 1½ hours; after 500 mg i.m.: 10 mg/l after ½ hour (Fig. 10). *Half-life:* 1 hour. *Plasma protein binding:* 18%.

Good *tissue diffusion; CSF penetration* poor, as with benzylpenicillin, but sufficient to treat meningitis when a large dose is given i.v. Concentrations in hepatic bile are as high as in serum, and higher in gall-bladder bile. Ampicillin crosses the placenta and passes into the fetal circulation and amniotic fluid.

Excretion: 20–30% of the oral dose and 60% of the i.v. dose are *excreted* in the urine after 24 hours; high urine concentrations (1000–2000 mg/l are found after 0.5–1 g.i.m.). Eliminated also in the bile and faeces. Biliary recovery after i.v. administration: 0.1%.

Side-effects: Toxicity is as low as benzylpenicillin. Typical allergy, as shown in urticaria or anaphylactic shock, is no more frequent than with benzylpenicillin. Macular rashes occur in 5–20% of patients during or after 8–14 days of treatment. The cause of the rash seems in part to be toxic, since it is more frequent at higher dosage and with degradation of ampicillin in the infusion. Other penicillins should be used subsequently with care, since cross-allergy may occur, although they are usually tolerated after a typical ampicillin rash. 5–20% of cases have gastrointesti-

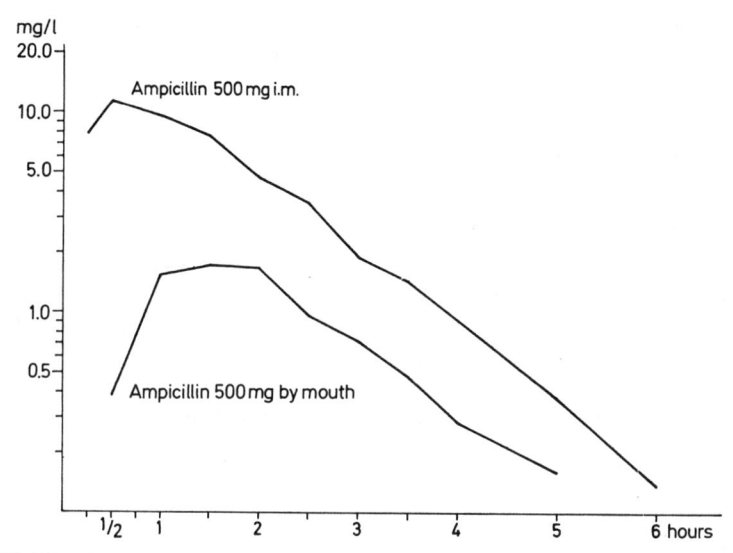

Fig. 10. Blood concentrations after 500 mg of ampicillin i.m. and orally (1 h after a meal; own data).

nal reactions (nausea, vomiting, diarrhoea) due in part to disturbance of the normal intestinal flora. Like clindamycin, ampicillin can cause pseudomembranous enterocolitis, which may become chronic and is related to the presence of toxin-producing strains of Clostridium difficile in the large bowel. This serious complication may be effectively treated with oral vancomycin (see p. 406). Urinary infection is often followed by a reinfection with resistant bacteria (klebsiella or enterobacter).

Main indications: Haemophilus meningitis and other haemophilus infections (where shown to be sensitive), enterococcal endocarditis and other severe enterococcal infections, salmonella endocarditis, osteomyelitis and meningitis, listeriosis.

Other indications: Acute and chronic urinary infections with sensitive pathogens, long-term treatment of chronic bronchitis, cholecystitis and cholangitis. For oral treatment, amoxycillin or the ampicillin esters, which are better absorbed, are preferable.

Inappropriate use: Typical or proven staphylococcal, streptococcal and pneumococcal infections, sore throat, fever of unknown origin, primary pneumonia, wound infections, topical or local application.

Contra-indications: Penicillin allergy, infectious mononucleosis and chronic lymphatic leukaemia (>50% of patients develop a rash).

Administration: In severe infections and in patients who are unable to swallow, give as a 10–20% solution i.m., slowly i.v., or if in large doses, by short i.v. infusion. Prepare a fresh solution every 6–8 hours if given by slow i.v. infusion because of progressive inactivation in vitro at room temperature; do not give other additives in the same infusion. Ampicillin is poorly absorbed by the oral route, so amoxycillin or an ampicillin absorption ester are preferable by mouth.

Dosage: Standard daily dosage in *adults* of 2–4 g by mouth and 1.5–2 g parenterally; this dosage may be increased to 10–20 g i.v. Reduce dosage in renal failure giving the normal single dose every 12 hours when the creatinine clearance is 10–50 ml/min, and every 24 hours at creatinine clearances below 10 ml/min. In *children:* 60–100 mg/kg (orally) and 100–200 mg/kg (parenterally); 200–400 mg/kg in meningitis. Divide daily dose into 3–4 single doses. For *intrathecal* use in adults, give 10–20 mg once a day only, and in children 5–10 mg.

Preparations: Capsules of 250 mg and tablets of 500 mg and 1 g, vials of 500 mg, 1, 2, and 5 g, syrup of 50 mg/ml.

Summary:
Advantages: Broader spectrum of activity than benzylpenicillin; good tissue penetration.
Disadvantages: Inactivity against klebsiella and enterobacter strains, incomplete absorption by mouth, frequent rashes. In many cases, better replaced by piperacillin or azlocillin for parenteral use, and by amoxycillin for oral use.

Referenes

MacMahon, P., J. Sills, E. Hall, T. Fitzgerald: Haemophilus influenzae type b resistant to both chloramphenicol and ampicillin in Britain. Brit. Med. J. *284:* 1229 (1982).
Mendelman, P. M., D. O. Chaffin, T. L. Stull et al.: Characterization of non-beta-lactamase-mediated ampicillin resistance in Haemophilus influenzae. Antimicrob. Ag. Chemother. *26:* 235 (1984).
Parr, T. R. Jr., L. E. Bryan: Mechanism of resistance of an ampicillin-resistant, beta-lactamase-negative clinical isolate of Haemophilus influenzae type b to beta-lactam antibiotics. Antimicrob. Ag. Chemother. *25:* 747 (1984).
Uchiyama, N., G. R. Greene, D. B. Kitts, L. D. Thrupp: Meningitis due to Haemophilus influenzae type b resistant to ampicillin and chloramphenicol. J. Pediatr. *97:* 421 (1980).
Walterspiel, J. N., S. L. Kaplan, M. J. Kessler, L. F. Reid: Ampicillin and chloramphenicol resistance in systemic Haemophilus influenzae disease. J. Am. Med. Assoc. *251:* 884 (1984).

β) Amoxycillin

Proprietary names: Amoxil etc.

Properties: Chemically α-amino-p-hydroxybenzylpenicillin (Fig. 5, p. 22) as the trihydrate, which is poorly soluble in water but dissolves better in phosphate buffer (pH 8.0). Relatively acid-stable, like ampicillin. Monosodium salt for injection is very water-soluble.

Antibacterial activity: Spectrum and *in vitro* activity similar to ampicillin. Rapidly bactericidal to gram-negative bacilli.

Pharmacokinetics: *Absorption* is almost complete after oral administration. Maximum blood concentrations after 2 hours are more than twice as high as after the same dose of ampicillin by mouth (Fig. 11). Absorption is unaffected by food intake. Mean serum concentrations of 20 mg/l (1 h) and 2 mg/l (4 h) follow the i.v. injection of 1 g. *Plasma protein binding:* 17%. *Urinary recovery* 60–70% in 6 hours after oral intake, and 70–80% after i.v. administration.

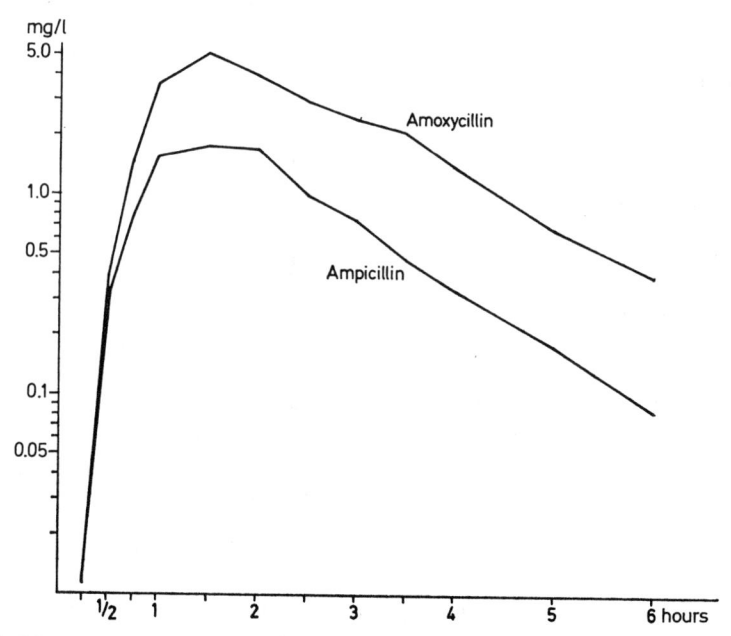

Fig. 11. Mean serum concentrations after the oral administration of 500 mg of amoxycillin and ampicillin (own data).

Indications: As for ampicillin.

Side-effects: As with ampicillin. Intestinal upset is less frequent because of the almost complete absorption after oral administration.

Administration and dosage: 1–1.5 (–3) g daily according to bacterial sensitivity; 50 (–100) mg/kg in small children, in 3 (–4) divided doses.

Larger doses may be given i.v. in severe infections. Intravenous injection or short infusion (1 g every 6–8 h) may also be given at the beginning of treatment and in patients with vomiting or unconsciousness.

Preparations: Tablets of 500 mg, 750 mg and 1 g, syrup containing 50 mg/ml and vials containing 500 mg, 1 g and 2 g.

Summary: Almost complete absorption after oral administration, hence smaller dosage possible than with ampicillin, with a lower risk of intestinal upset. Because of the high rate of resistance in many organisms, amoxycillin, like ampicillin, cannot be recommended as a single agent in the initial treatment of severe infections.

References

HILL, S. A., K. H. JONES, L. J. LEES: Pharmacokinetics of parenterally administered amoxycillin. J. Infect *2:* 320: (1980).

IRVINE, A. E., A. N. D. AGNEW, T. C. M. MORRIS: Amoxycillin induced pancytopenia. Brit. Med. J. *290:* 968 (1985).

γ) Pivampicillin

Proprietary name: Pondocillin.

Properties: Pivaloyl oxymethyl ester of ampicillin, marketed as the hydrochloride. Readily soluble in water, odourless, with a bitter taste. When taken by mouth, pivampicillin is rapidly and almost completely (99%) transformed by nonspecific esterases in the serum and intestinal wall into pivalinic acid (20%) and ampicillin-hydroxymethyl ester. The latter then breaks down spontaneously into ampicillin (70%) and formaldehyde (6%). 50% of the pivalinic acid (trimethyl acetic acid) produced in this way is excreted as the glucuronide in the urine. Formaldehyde breaks down rapidly in the body, particularly in the erythrocytes and the liver, into formic acid and then into CO_2 and H_2O.

Antibacterial action: Pivampicillin itself is almost completely inactive. The ampicillin released by its metabolism in the body has the characteristic spectrum and normal activity of ampicillin (see p. 39). The combination of pivampicillin with mecillinam (see p. 60) is synergistic against haemophilus and certain intestinal bacteria.

Pharmacokinetics: Rapid and almost complete (90%) *absorption* after oral administration. Maximal blood concentrations after 1–1½ h are proportional to the dose. The maximal *blood concentrations* are at least twice as high as those found after oral ampicillin, and of the same order as those found after i.m. ampicillin. The *urine recovery* is 65–75% (20–30% with ampicillin). The simultaneous intake of food considerably impairs the absorption of ampicillin but improves absorption and gastric tolerance of pivampicillin. Thus a much smaller dose of pivampicillin is needed to achieve the same blood concentration as oral ampicillin. The *half-life, plasma protein binding and excretion* are similar to those of ampicillin (p. 40). *Tissue concentrations* are related to blood concentrations.

Side-effects: As for oral ampicillin. Ingestion when fasting occasionally leads to heartburn, a sensation of epigastric distension, and vomiting; intestinal upset is less frequent than with ampicillin because the intestinal flora is less disturbed on account of the better absorption. Pivalinic acid is slightly toxic in animals.

Indications: As for ampicillin.

Administration and dosage: 1.4–2.8 g a day for *adults* (corresponding to 1.0 – 2.0 g of free ampicillin), 50 mg/kg for *small children* (corresponding to 35 mg/kg of free ampicillin), in 2 or 3 divided doses, preferably after meals.

Preparations: Tablets of 700 mg (equivalent to 500 mg ampicillin); suspension of 175 mg/5 ml; granules (175 mg/sachet).

Summary: Pivampicillin is preferable to ampicillin on account of its improved absorption; it can nevertheless give rise to dyspepsia and vomiting. The fixed combination with mecillinam is suboptimal.

References

LÖNNERHOLM, G., S. BENGTSSON, U. EWALD: Oral pivampicillin and amoxycillin in newborn infants. Scand. J. Infect. Dis. *14:* 127 (1982).
NERINGER, R., A. STRÖMBERG: A comparison of the side-effects of amoxycillin and pivampicillin. Scand. J. Infect. Dis *12:* 133 (1980).

δ) Bacampicillin

Proprietary name: Ambaxin.

Properties: An ampicillin ester (aminopenicillin) for oral use, which is almost completely absorbed from the gastrointestinal tract and very rapidly hydrolysed to ampicillin in the body. 800 mg of the ester correspond to 556 mg of free ampicillin. Bacampicillin hydrochloride is readily soluble in water and chloroform, and is acid-stable (Fig. 12).

Fig. 12. Structural formula of bacampicillin.

Mode and spectrum of activity: As ampicillin.

Pharmacokinetics: *Rapid absorption* of about 95% of the oral dose; maximal serum concentrations after 1 h (but after 2½ h with ampicillin).

Maximal serum concentrations after 800 mg orally are generally much higher than those after the equimolar dose of ampicillin (556 mg) (Fig. 13), with a mean maximum concentration of 15.9 mg/l, which declines after 4 h to 2.0 mg/l and after 6 h to 0.5 mg/l. After oral bacampicillin, the concentrations in blister fluid

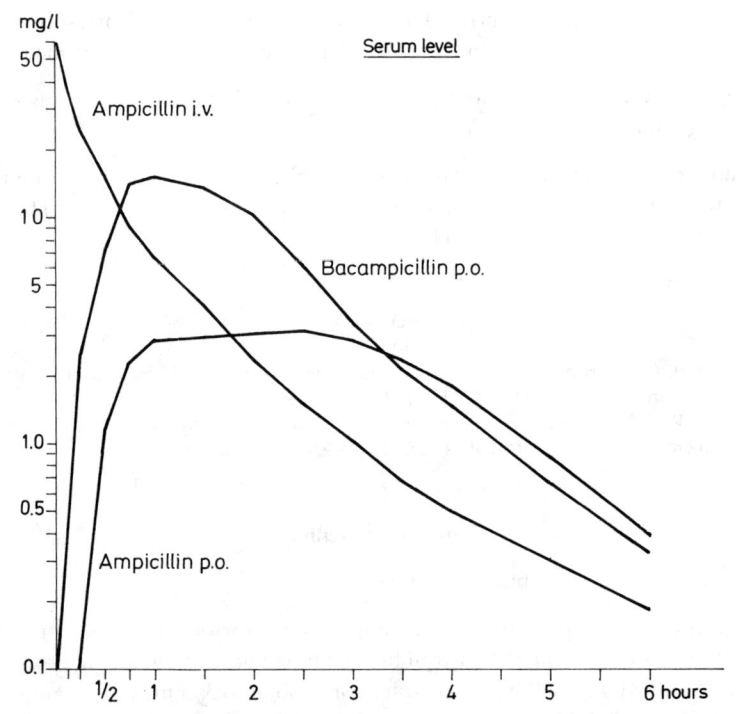

Fig. 13. Mean serum concentrations after 800 mg of bacampicillin by mouth, compared with 556 mg of ampicillin by mouth and i.v. (own data).

are four times higher, and in saliva and tears three times higher than those found after oral ampicillin at equimolar dosage. There is a dose-related increase in serum concentration when the dose is doubled from 400 to 800 mg. Food intake does not impair absorption.

Urine recoveries over the first 6 h with oral bacampicillin: 57%, with i.v. ampicillin: 60%, with oral ampicillin: 30%.

Side-effects as with oral ampicillin though loose stools and diarrhoea are less frequent because of the almost complete gastrointestinal absorption. Well tolerated by mouth.

Main indications: Respiratory and urinary infection by sensitive pathogens.

Contra-indications: as for benzylpenicillin and ampicillin.

Administration and dosage: 800 mg 2–3 times a day in tablet form (20 mg/kg 2–3 times a day for children).

Preparations: Film tablets of 400 and 800 mg.

Summary: Better than oral ampicillin because of its complete absorption and good gastrointestinal tolerance.

References

EDWARDS, L. D., T. GARTNER: Comparison between bacampicillin and amoxycillin in treating genital and extragenital infection with Neisseria gonorrhoeae and pharyngeal infection with Neisseria meningitidis. Brit. J. Vener. Dis. *60:* 380 (1984).
GINSBURG, C. M., G. H. MCCRACKEN Jr., J. C. CLAHSEN, T. C. ZWEIGHAFT: Comparative pharmacokinetics of bacampicillin and ampicillin suspensions in infants and children. Rev. Infect. Dis. *3:* 177 (1981).
NEU, H. C.: The pharmacokinetics of bacampicillin. Rev. Infect. Dis. *3:* 110 (1981).
SJÖVALL, J.: Tissue levels after administration of bacampicillin, a prodrug of ampicillin, and comparisons with other aminopenicillins: a review. J. Antimicrob. Chemother. *8 (Suppl. C):* 41 (1981).
SJÖVALL, J., L. MAGNI, E. VINNARS: Bioavailability of bacampicillin and talampicillin, two oral prodrugs of ampicillin. Antimicrob. Ag. Chemother. *20:* 837 (1981).
SUM, Z. M., A. M. SEFTON, A. P. JEPSON, J. D. WILLIAMS: Comparative pharmacokinetic study between lenampicillin, bacampicillin and amoxycillin. J. Antimicrob. Chemother. *23:* 861–868 (1989).

ε) Talampicillin

Proprietary name: Talpen.

Properties: The phthalidyl thiazolidine carboxylic ester of ampicillin which, like bacampicillin and pivampicillin, is rapidly and completely absorbed from the gastro-intestinal tract after oral dosage. Mucosal and erythrocytic esterases release free ampicillin into the circulation and the inactivated ester moiety is excreted through the liver and kidneys. 500 mg of the ester corresponds to 338 mg of free ampicillin.

Mode and spectrum of activity: As ampicillin.

Pharmacokinetics: Identical behaviour to that of pivampicillin and bacampicillin.

Side-effects: As with oral ampicillin, except that, as with pivampicillin and bacampicillin, gastro-intestinal intolerance is much reduced.

Main indications and contra-indication: As with the other ampicillin esters.

Administration and dosage: 500 mg 3–4 times a day in tablet form (10 mg/kg 3–4 times a day for children).

Summary: This was the first of the ampicillin esters to be marketed in Great Britain. A good form of delivery of ampicillin by the oral route.

References

LEIGH, D. A., D. S. REEVES, K. SIMMONS, A. L. THOMAS, P. J. WILKINSON: Talampicillin: a new derivative of ampicillin. Brit. med. J. *1:* 1378 (1976).

e) Carboxypenicillins

α) Carbenicillin

The first carboxybenzyl penicillin, which is still commercially available for the treatment of infections with pseudomonas and proteus but, because of its weak activity, has now been largely superceded by ticarcillin, azlocillin and piperacillin.

β) Carbenicillin Esters

Proprietary names: For *carindacillin:* Carindapen, Geocillin.
For *carfecillin:* Uticillin.

Description: Carindacillin is the indanyl ester and carfecillin the phenyl ester of carbenicillin. Both esters are acid-stable and absorbed after oral administration, by being rapidly hydrolysed into carbenicillin (Fig. 14) which passes into the bloodstream. The indanol or phenol released by hydrolysis is bound to glucuronic acid and excreted predominantly in the urine.

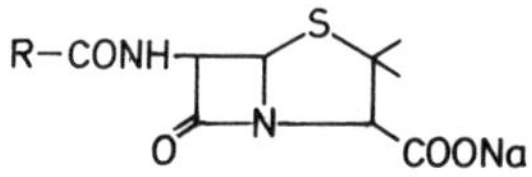

1. Penicillins

Generic Name	R
Carbenicillin	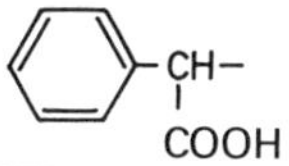 phenyl–CH(COOH)–
Carindacillin	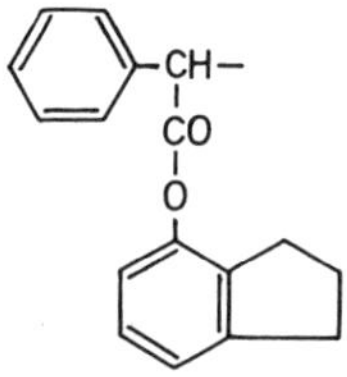 phenyl–CH(CO–O–indanyl)–
Carfecillin	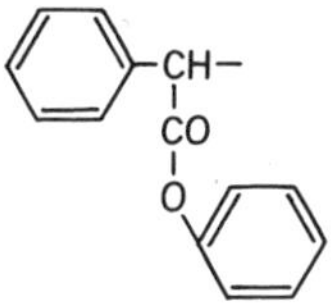 phenyl–CH(CO–O–phenyl)–

Fig. 14. Structural formulae of carbenicillin and its absorption esters.

Spectrum of activity: Sufficient carbenicillin for effective treatment of Pseudomonas aeruginosa and Proteus species is only present in the urine. Infections with pseudomonas at other sites must be treated with an alternative antibiotic.

Pharmacokinetics: Maximal serum concentrations average 10 mg/l after 1 g of carindacillin by mouth, and 8 mg/l after the same dose of carfecillin. *Urinary concentration* of carindacillin: 300–2000 mg/l; of carfecillin: 200–1000 mg/l. *Urinary recovery:* 30% and 20–25% respectively. The urinary concentrations are not sufficient for treatment in patients with *renal failure* (creatinine clearance less than 10 ml/min).

Side-effects: Relatively frequent diarrhoea, vomiting, nausea, disagreeable taste, all of which occur more frequently with carindacillin.

Indications: Oral continuation of the treatment of persistent or recurrent urinary infection with Pseudomonas aeruginosa, Proteus vulgaris and other indole-positive species (Morganella morganii and Proteus rettgeri).

Administration and dosage: 1 g 3–4 times a day by mouth as film tablets for 1–2 weeks; 20 mg/kg 3–4 times a day for children. Longer treatment is possible. 500 mg 3 times a day is often sufficient with carfecillin.

Preparations: Tablets of 500 mg.

Summary: When tolerated by the patient, a possible antibiotic treatment of chronic and recurrent urinary infections caused by Pseudomonas aeruginosa, Proteus vulgaris and related indole-positive species. Now largely superceded in adults by norfloxacin, ciprofloxacin or other new quinolones.

γ) Ticarcillin

Proprietary name: Tiear.

Properties: A carbenicillin derivative, α-carboxy-3-thienylmethyl penicillin, commercially available as the disodium salt, containing 5.2–6.5 mmol/g of sodium. It is water-soluble and the solution is colourless or slightly yellow. Solutions stored at 4° C should be discarded after 3 days.

Spectrum of activity: As carbenicillin, but 2–3 times more active *in vitro* against proteus and Pseudomonas aeruginosa. The frequency of resistant strains of Pseudomonas, which are inhibited at concentrations of 100 mg/l or more, is less than for carbenicillin. There is no difference in activity from carbenicillin on Escherichia coli and Proteus species (particularly the indole-positive strains). Most strains of Acinetobacter, Klebsiella, Citrobacter and Serratia are resistant as are all strains of Enterobacter species and the enterococci. Synergy with the aminoglycosides (tobramycin, gentamicin, amikacin) is found against Pseudomonas aeruginosa. Secondary resistance in Pseudomonas aeruginosa may develop rapidly.

Pharmacokinetics: Rapid *absorption* after intramuscular injection (maximal serum concentration after 30–45 min). Not absorbed by mouth.

Mean serum concentrations: 107 and 175 mg/l respectively, 1 h after i.v. injection of 3 g and 5 g, and 14 and 28 mg/l respectively after 4 h. 740 ± 56 mg/l after short i.v. infusion of 5 g over 30 min; 981 ± 53 mg/l after i.v. infusion of 10 g over 60 min. Serum concentration of 260 mg/l found with constant i.v. infusion of 1 g/h. *Half-life* 70 min. *Plasma protein binding* 45%.

Excretion almost entirely through the kidneys. *Urinary recovery* greater than 95%.

Side-effects: As for benzylpenicillin (allergy, neurotoxicity etc.). Hypernatraemia, hypokalaemia and thrombophlebitis are less frequent than with carbenicillin on account of the smaller dose. Daily sodium load 104 mmol with 20 g of ticarcillin daily. Bleeding disorders with prolongation of bleeding time are dose-related and are caused by impaired platelet function.

Interaction: Coagulation disorders and bleeding tendency are potentiated by acetyl salicylic acid.

Indications: Pseudomonas infections, which, when severe, should be treated in combination with an aminoglycoside such as gentamicin, tobramycin, amikacin or netilmicin.

Contra-indication: Penicillin allergy. Use with caution in patients receiving anticoagulants because of the possibility of an increased bleeding tendency.

Administration: Adequate dilution is necessary with the i.v. route (1 g in 10–20 ml of water for injection) to avoid local venous irritation. Short i.v. infusion is preferable. Dissolve in 1% lignocaine for i.m. injection (1 g in 2 ml) and do not exceed 2 g per injection. Do not mix with aminglycosides (gentamicin, tobramycin, netilmicin or amikacin) in the same solution for injection or infusion, because inactivation has been reported *in vitro*, though not *in vivo*.

Dosage: 15–20 g a day for *adults;* 300 mg/kg for *children* and *neonates*, in 4 (–6) i.v. injections or short infusions daily and preferably in combination with tobramycin or gentamicin (for dosage, see p. 138, 141). 2 g every 8 h are sufficient in severe renal failure (creatinine clearance 10–30 ml/min), or 2 g every 12 h (creatinine clearance less than 10 ml/min).

Preparations: Vials of 1 g, 2 g, 5 g and 10 g and of 1.6 g, 3.2 g and 5.2 g for paediatric use.

Summary: Less active than azlocillin and piperacillin against pseudomonas, enterococci and the Enterobacteriaceae. Dose-dependent side-effects.

References

DROUET, F. H., T. DAVIES, D. A. LEDERER, G. P. MCNICOL, U. K. LEEDS: The effect of ticarcillin on the haemostatic mechanism. J. Pharm. Pharmacol. *27:* 1964 (1975).

GASTINEAU, D., R. SPECTOR, D. PHILIPS: Severe neutropenia associated with ticarcillin therapy. Ann. Intern. Med. *94:* 711 (1981).

JOHNSON, G. J., H. R. GUNDU, J. G. WHITE: Platelet dysfunction induced by parenteral carbenicillin and ticarcillin. Am. J. Pathol. *91:* 85 (1978).

NELSON, J. D., S. SHELTON, H. KUSMIESZ: Clinical pharmacology of ticarcillin in the newborn infant: Relation to age, gestational age, and weight. J. Pediat. *87:* 474 (1975).

OHNING, B. L., M. D. REED, C. F. DOERSHUK, J. L. BLUMER: Ticarcillin-associated granulocytopenia. Amer. J. Dis. child. *136:* 645 (1982).

SOMANI, P., M. R. SMITH, A. GOHARA et al.: The effects of mezlocillin, ticarcillin and placebo on blood coagulation and bleeding time in normal volunteers. J. Antimicrob. Chemother. *11 (Suppl. C):* 33–41 (1983).

δ) Temocillin

Proprietary name: Temopen.

Properties: Temocillin was the first 6-methoxypenicillin to show stability to the β-lactamases produced by gram-negative bacteria. Like ticarcillin, temocillin has a free carboxylic acid group and a thienyl group, and may be designated 6-methoxyticarcillin (Fig. 15). It is available as the disodium salt.

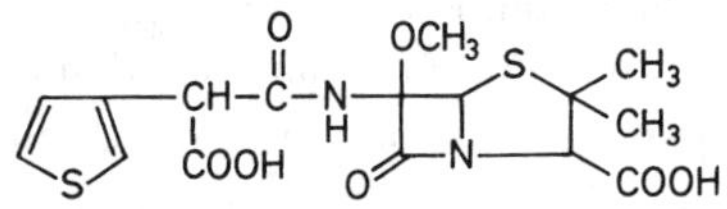

Fig. 15. Structural formula of temocillin.

Spectrum of activity: Temocillin is active against the majority of gram-negative bacteria including β-lactamase-producing strains of Haemophilus influenzae and Neisseria gonorrhoeae. Gram-positive bacteria, Pseudomonas aeruginosa, Acinetobacter species, Campylobacter jejuni and Bacteroides fragilis are resistant. Against sensitive gram-negative bacteria the in vitro activity is generally superior to that of other penicillins. Some strains of Enterobacter cloacae, Serratia marcescens and Providencia stuartii are resistant. There is partial cross-resistance with other penicillins and cephalosporins.

Pharmacokinetics: *Mean serum concentrations* 90 mg/l 1 h, 35 mg/l 4 h and 10 mg/l 12 h after i. v. injection of 1 g. Not absorbed by mouth. *Plasma protein binding:* 85%. *Half-life:* 4.5 h. *Urinary recovery:* 80%, mostly filtered by the glomeruli.

Side-effects: Similar to ticarcillin (see p. 50).

Indications: Urinary and gynaecological infections with known sensitive gram-negative rods.

Administration and dosage: Preferably as i. v. injection or short i. v. infusion. 2–4 g a day in 2 or 3 divided doses are usually adequate because of the relatively long half-life.

Preparations: Vials of 0.5 g, 1 g and 2 g.

Summary: Highly active against most gram-negative bacteria, but inactive against Pseudomonas species, Bacteroides fragilis and many gram-positive organisms. Should only be used for infections with known sensitive microorganisms. Relatively long half-life.

References

BASKER, M. J., R. A. EDMONDSON, S. J. KNOTT et al.: In vitro antibacterial properties of BRL 36650, a novel 6 alpha-substituted penicillin. Antimicrob. Ag. Chemother. *26:* 734 (1984).
BOELAERT, J., R. DANEELS, M. SCHURGERS et al.: The pharmacokinetics of temocillin in patients with normal and impaired renal function. J. Antimicrob. Chemother. *11:* 349 (1983).
BRÜCKNER, O., M. TRAUTMANN, K. BORNER: A study of the penetration of temocillin in the cerebrospinal fluid. Drugs *29 (Suppl. 5):* 162 (1985).
COCKBURN, A., G. MELLOWS, D. JACKSON, D. J. WHITE: Temocillin summary of safety studies. Drugs *29 (Suppl. 5):* 103 (1985).
EDMONDSON, R. A., C. READING: β-Lactamase stability of temocillin. Drugs *29 (Suppl. 5):* 64 (1985).
GUEST, E. A., R. HORTON, G. MELLOWS et al.: Human pharmacokinetics of temocillin (BRL 17421) side chain epimers. J. Antimicrob. Chemother. *15:* 327 (1985).
NUNN, B., A. BAIRD, P. D. CHAMBERLAIN: Effect of temocillin and moxalactam on platelet responsiveness and bleeding time in normal volunteers. Antimicrob. Ag. Chemother. *27:* 858 (1985).

f) Acylaminopenicillins

This is a group of ampicillin derivatives whose amino group is substituted by a modified ureido side-chain, hence the alternative term, "ureidopenicillin", for this group. The individual derivatives contain complex rings and are better designated acylaminopenicillins.

All members of this group have activity against Pseudomonas aeruginosa, enterobacteria and enterococci. They penetrate rapidly into the bacterial cell wall (good crypticity), but are not stable against β-lactamases from staphylococci or resistant strains of enterobacter, serratia and klebsiella.

α) Azlocillin

Proprietary name: Securopen.

Properties: An acylaminopenicillin (see Fig. 5, p. 22). The monosodium salt is readily soluble in water. The 10% solution can be stored at room temperature for at least 6 h without loss of activity. 5 g azlocillin contain 11 millimoles of sodium.

Spectrum of activity: Broader than carbenicillin because of its much greater activity against Pseudomonas aeruginosa (4–8-fold), enterococci (10-fold) and Bacteroides fragilis (2-fold). Ticarcillin and mezlocillin are only ⅓ as active as azlocillin against pseudomonas (Table 28, p. 309). Mezlocillin is more active than azlocillin against other gram-negative bacilli such as Escherichia coli, Proteus species, klebsiella, enterobacter, serratia etc. All penicillinase-producing staphylococci are resistant, as are the majority of enterobacters and serratias. There is synergy with the aminoglycosides against pseudomonas, klebsiella, serratia, proteus and enterococci.

Resistance: Incomplete cross-resistance with piperacillin, ticarcillin, mezlocillin, temocillin and ampicillin. Some strains of pseudomonas are resistant to ticarcillin but sensitive to azlocillin. Azlocillin-resistant gram-negative rods are sometimes sensitive to mezlocillin and piperacillin (e. g. Escherichia coli, klebsiella, serratia). Complete cross-resistance with benzylpenicillin against staphylococci, mycoplasmas etc., and with ampicillin against Haemophilus influenzae.

Pharmacokinetics: *Not absorbed* by mouth.
Mean serum concentrations after i. v. injection of 2 g: 47 mg/l at 1 h, and 7.4 mg/l at 4 h; after i. v. infusion of 3 g over 30 min: 68 mg/l 1 h after end of infusion and 10 mg/l 4 h later.
Half-life: 55–70 min, dependent on dose. *Plasma protein binding:* 30%.
Urinary excretion 60% at 6 h in the active from. The biliary concentration is some 15-fold higher than the corresponding serum concentration. An unknown amount is transformed by the body into inactive metabolites.

Side-effects: As for benzylpenicillin. Diarrhoea or loose stools, eosinophilia and a transient rise in serum alkaline phosphatase may all occur. False-positive non-enzymatic tests for urinary sugar and urobilinogen may occur during therapy. Skin rashes are less common than with ampicillin. Reversible leucopenia occurs rarely.

Indications: Pseudomonas infections such as ecthyma gangrenosum, pneumonia in patients on ventilators, infected burns, septicaemia in leukaemics, aspiration pneumonia etc. Best given in combination with an aminoglycoside. When the causative organism is unknown, azlocillin may be combined with one of the β-lactamase-stable cephalosporins such as cefotaxime. Combinations with other antibiotics such as clindamycin, metronidazole or a quinolone may also be useful.

Inappropriate use: Infections against which other penicillins such as benzylpenicillin, mezlocillin or piperacillin would be more active. Infections with penicillin-resistant staphylococci.

Contra-indication: Penicillin allergy.

Administration and dosage: Preferably as a slow i. v. injection or short i. v. infusion. Intramuscular injection is possible but sometimes painful. In severe or fulminating infections, give 5 g 3 times a day as a short i. v. infusion to adults and 80 mg/kg 3 times a day to children; otherwise give 2 g 3 times a day to adults and 30 mg/kg 3 times a day to children. The dose in the newborn (up to the 7th day of life) is 100 mg/kg twice daily. In renal failure (creatinine clearance less than 10 ml/

min) the single dose of 1.5–3.0 g should be given every 12 instead of every 8 h. The 1% aqueous solution may be used for local irrigation.

Preparation: Vials of 500 mg, 1 g, 2 g, 4 g, 5 g and 10 g.

Summary: An effective anti-pseudomonal penicillin which has completely supplanted carbenicillin. An important partner in combination with the β-lactamase-stable cephalosporins in initial therapy.

References

BEHRENS-BAUMANN, W., R. ANSORG: Azlocillin concentrations in human aqueous humor after intravenous and subconjunctival administration. Graefe's Arch. Clin. Exp. Ophthalmol. *220:* 292–293 (1983).
DELGADO, F. A., R. L. STOUT, A. WHELTON: Pharmacokinetics of azlocillin in normal renal function: single and repetitive dosing studies. J. Antimicrob. Chemother. *11 (Suppl. B):* 79 (1983).
KAFTEZIS, D. A., D. C. BRATER, J. E. FANOURGAKIS: Materno-fetal transfer of azlocillin. J. Antimicrob. Chemother. *12:* 157 (1983).
LANDER, R. D., R. P. HENDERSON, D. R. PYSZCZYNSKI: Pharmacokinetic comparison of 5 g of azlocillin every 8 h and 4 g every 6 h in healthy volunteers. Antimicrob. Agents Chemother. *33:* 710–713 (1989).

β) Mezlocillin

Proprietary name: Baypen.

Properties: An acylaminopenicillin. The sodium monohydrate is readily soluble in water. The 10% aqueous solution for i. v. injection is colourless or slightly yellow and remains stable for up to 24 h at room temperature. Approx. 9.3 millimoles of sodium are contained in 5 g.

Spectrum of activity: Broader than ampicillin, to include some of the indole-positive strains of proteus (Proteus vulgaris), providencia, serratia, klebsiella, enterobacter and Pseudomonas aeruginosa. Mezlocillin is 2–3 times more active than azlocillin against the Enterobacteriaceae, with the exception of Pseudomonas aeruginosa (mean MIC of mezlocillin 32 mg/l, and of azlocillin 8 mg/l). A variable number of strains are resistant to mezlocillin at concentrations of 64 mg/l or more, however, including providencia (60%), Klebsiella pneumoniae (40%), Serratia marcescens (40%), Enterobacter aerogenes (20–40%), Pseudomonas aeruginosa (10–40%) and Escherichia coli (10–30%). At concentrations of 32 mg/l or more, mezlocillin is active against most of the non-sporing anaerobes (Bacteroides species, including Bacteroides fragilis). All penicillinase-producing staphylococci are resistant, as are ampicillin-resistant strains of haemophilus. Synergy is found in combination with the aminoglycosides against pseudomonas, klebsiella, serratia and proteus.

Pharmacokinetics: *Not absorbed* by mouth.
Mean serum concentrations: 56 mg/l 1 h and 4.4 mg/l 4 h after the i. v. injection of 2 g. Mean concentrations after i. v. infusion of 3 g over 30 min were 426 mg/l at the end of the infusion, 178 mg/l 1 h later and 33 mg/l 4 h after the end of the infusion. *Half-life:* 50 min; *plasma protein binding:* 30%.
Excretion: 55–60% in active form in the urine, and up to 25% in the bile. An unknown proportion breaks down into antibacterially inactive metabolites.

Side-effects: As with benzylpenicillin. Loose stools or diarrhoea, skin reactions (erythema, rashes) and an unusual taste can all occur during administration. An increase in serum transaminases and alkaline phosphatase and an eosinophilia are occasionally observed. The urinary excretion of metabolites can lead to false positive non-enzymatic urinary tests for sugar and urobilinogen.

Rashes are no more frequent than with benzylpenicillin. As with other β-lactam antibiotics, a transient neutropenia sometimes occurs.

Indications: Infections of the genitourinary and biliary tract with sensitive gram-negative bacilli including Bacteroides species. Metronidazole still remains the best first-line antibacterial agent in Bacteroides fragilis infections, however. Severe systemic infections (septicaemia, endocarditis, meningitis etc.) in combination with an aminoglycoside or with an isoxazolyl penicillin (e. g. flucloxacillin). Combinations with metronidazole, a β-lactamase inhibitor or a quinolone may also be useful.

Inappropriate uses: Infections with organisms sensitive to benzylpenicillin. Staphylococcal infections.

Contra-indication: Penicillin allergy.

Administration and dosage: Preferably as a slow i. v. injection or short i. v. infusion over 30 to 60 min. Do not mix with other drugs in the syringe or infusion solution, particularly aminoglycosides. Dosage for severe systemic infections: 5 g 3 times a day or 10 g twice a day (200–300 mg/kg/day for children); for urinary infections and non-life-threatening infections with sensitive bacteria: 2 g 3 times a day (80–100 mg/kg/day for children. 75 mg/kg every 12 h in the newborn up to the 6th day of live. In renal failure (creatinine clearance <10 ml/min), give 2 g 8 hourly in adults.

Preparations: Vials of 500 mg, 1 g, 2 g, 3 g, 4 g, 5 g and 10 g.

Summary: A broad-spectrum penicillin which is superior to ampicillin in both activity and breadth of spectrum. It is recommended for infections with sensitive gram-negative bacilli, particularly biliary and abdominal infections.

References

BALLARD, J. O., S. G. BARNES, F. R. SATTLER: Comparison of the effects of mezlocillin, carbenicillin, and placebo on normal hemostasis. Antimicrob. Ag. Chemother. *25:* 153 (1984).
BEHRENS-BAUMANN, W., R. ANSORG: Mezlocillin concentrations in human aqueous humor after intravenous and subconjunctival administration. Chemotherapy *31:* 169–172 (1985).
COPELAN, E. A., R. K. KUSUMI, L. MILLER et al.: A comparison of the effects of mezlocillin and carbenicillin on haemostasis in volunteers. J. Antimicrob. Chemother. *11 (Suppl. C)* 43–49 (1983).
CUSHNER, H. M., J. B. COPLEY, J. BAUMAN, S. C. HILL: Acute interstitial nephritis associated with mezlocillin, nafcillin, and gentamicin treatment for Pseudomonas infection. Arch. Intern. *145:* 1204 (1985).
GUNDERT-REMY, U., D. FÖRSTER, P. SCHACHT, E. WEBER: Kinetics of mezlocillin in patients with biliary t-tube drainage. J. Antimicrob. Chemother. *9 (Suppl. A):* 65 (1982).
JANICKE, D. M., T. T. RUBIO, F. H. WIRTH Jr. et al.: Developmental pharmacokinetics of mezlocillin in newborn infants. J. Pediatr. *104:* 773 (1984).
MEHTA, P., D. LAWSON, S. GROSS, J. GRAHAM-POLE: Comparative effects of mezlocillin and carbenicillin on platelet function and thromboxane generation in patients with cancer. Am. J. Pediatr. Hematol. Oncol. *11:* 286–291 (1989).
ODIO, C., N. THRELKELD, M. L. THOMAS, G. H. MCCRACKEN Jr.: Pharmacokinetic properties of mezlocillin in newborn infants. Antimicrob. Ag. Chemother. *25:* 556 (1984).

γ) Piperacillin

Proprietary name: Pipril.

Properties: An acylaminopenicillin related to azlocillin and mezlocillin. The monosodium salt is readily soluble in water and is relatively stable (10% loss of activity after 24 hours at 25° C in a buffered solution). The 10% aqueous solution is isotonic with blood. 1 g of piperacillin sodium contains 2 millimoles of sodium.

Spectrum of activity: Like mezlocillin, piperacillin is active against most of the Enterobacteriacae and, like azlocillin, is anti-pseudomonal. Mezlocillin is slightly more active against enterococci. There are no essential differences between piperacillin and azlo- or mezlocillin against haemophilus or anaerobes (including Bacteroides fragilis). Like all acylaminopenicillins, piperacillin has no activity on penicillinase-producing staphylococci. There is synergy with aminoglycosides against gram-negative bacilli and enterococci.

Resistance: Incomplete cross-resistance with ticarcillin, azlo-, mezlo-, and ampicillin. Complete cross-resistance with benzylpenicillin against staphylococci and with ampicillin against haemophilus. Piperacillin is inactivated by β-lactamases produced by staphylococci and Bacteroides fragilis.

Pharmacokinetics: *Mean concentrations:* 40 mg/l (1 h), 3.6 mg/l (4 h) and 1 mg/l (6 h) after i.v. injection of 2 g. After an i.v. infusion of 4 g serum concentrations are 60 mg/l 1 h after end of infusion, 8 mg/l (4 h) and 2.5 mg/l

(6 h). A constant serum concentration of 15 mg/l is maintained during continuous i.v. infusion (0.33 g/h = 8 g/24 h). *Half-life:* 1 h. *Plasma protein binding:* 20%. *Urinary excretion* in active form: 60–70%. *Urinary concentrations* after 2 g i.v.: 4000–10000 mg/l during the first 3 hours. Biliary concentrations (hepatic bile): 200–2400 mg/l. A proportion is metabolised in the body. *Tissue diffusion* good but *CSF concentration* relatively low.

Side-effects: As with benzylpenicillin. Skin rashes are less frequent than with ampicillin. Gastrointestinal upset (nausea, diarrhoea), pain at the site of i.m. injection and thrombophlebitis with repeated i.v. injection can occur. A transient rise in liver enzymes has been observed in <3% of patients. As with other β-lactam antibiotics, transient neutropenia occasionally occurs.

Indications: Urinary, genital and biliary infections caused by sensitive gram-negative bacilli, and proven or suspected pseudomonas infections (preferably in combination with tobramycin), as well as severe systemic infections (septicaemia, meningitis, pneumonia etc.) in combination with an aminoglycoside or cephalosporin. Combination with metronidazole, a β-lactamase inhibitor or a 4-quinolone can be useful in extending the spectrum of activity.

Inappropriate use: As a single agent in life-threatening systemic bacterial infections of unknown origin, particularly where resistant organisms such as Staphylococcus aureus, enterobacter or Bacteroides fragilis are possible pathogens.

Contra-indication: Penicillin allergy.

Administration and dosage: Preferably as a slow i.v. injection or short i.v. infusion. Do not mix in the syringe or the infusion solution with other drugs or with an aminoglycoside.

Normal dosage: 2 g 3–4 times a day (30 mg/kg 3–4 times a day in children). The dose can be doubled in severe or life-threatening infections (4 g 3–4 times a day). In renal failure (creatinine clearance <20 ml/min), no more than 4 g should be given every 12 h. I.m. injection is only recommended for single doses of up to 2 g, and the substance may be dissolved in 0.5% lignocaine solution if necessary.

Preparations: Vials of 1 g, 2 g, 3 g, 4 g and 6 g.

Summary: A broad-spectrum penicillin which is particularly active against gram-negative organisms, including pseudomonas. Not active against most staphylococci. In the initial treatment of life-threatening infections, therefore, give only in combination with an aminoglycoside or cephalosporin.

References

DICKINSON, G. M., D. G. DROLLER, R. L. GREENMAN, T. A. HOFFMANN: Clinical evaluation of piperacillin with observation on penetrability into cerebrospinal fluid. Antimicrob. Ag. Chemother. *20:* 481 (1981).

GENTRY, L. O., J. G. JEMSEK, E. A. NATELSON: Effects of sodium piperacillin on platelet function in normal volunteers. Antimicrob. Ag. Chemother. *19:* 532 (1981).

KUCK, N. A., N. V. JACOBUS, P. J. PETERSEN, W. J. WEISS, R. T. TESTA: Comparative in vitro and in vivo activities of piperacillin combined with the beta-lactamase inhibitors tazobactam, clavulanic acid, and sulbactam. Antimicrob. Agents Chemother. *33:* 1964–1969 (1989).

THIRUMOORTHI, M. C., B. I. ASMAR, J. A. BUCKLEY et al.: Pharmacokinetics of intravenously administered piperacillin in preadolescent children. J. Pediatr. *102:* 941 (1983).

WELLING, P. G., W. A. CRAIG, R. W. BUNDTZEN et al.: Pharmacokinetics of piperacillin in subjects with various degrees of renal function. Antimicrob. Ag. Chemother. *23:* 881 (1983).

δ) Apalcillin

Proprietary name: Lumota.

Description: An acylaminopenicillin developed in Japan with a similar spectrum and activity to piperacillin (see p. 57).

Spectrum of activity: Apparently slightly greater activity against pseudomonas, but little or no action on Bacteroides fragilis, Serratia marcescens or penicillin-resistant staphylococci. Intrinsically resistant strains of Escherichia coli, Klebsiella pneumoniae and Proteus species occur.

Pharmacokinetics: *Maximal serum concentrations* of 140 and 190 mg/l are found 2 hours after an i.v. infusion of 2 g and 3 g respectively. *Plasma protein binding:* 96%. *Half-life:* 80 min. *Urinary recovery:* 20%. High *excretion* in the bile and some metabolism in the body (caution in liver disease). Pharmacokinetic properties are not, therefore, as favourable as with piperacillin.

Side-effects: Increase in serum transaminases and diarrhoea in 5–10%.

Dosage: 2–3 g 3 times a day, as i.v. infusion.

Preparations: Vials of 1 g and 3 g.

Summary: No advantages in comparison to piperacillin. The pharmacokinetics of apalcillin differ markedly from those of other penicillins, and there are more frequent side-effects.

References

Barry, A. L., R. N. Jones, L. W. Ayers et al.: In vitro activity of apalcillin compared with those of piperacillin and carbenicillin against 6797 bacterial isolates from four separate medical centers. Antimicrob. Ag. Chemother. 25: 669 (1984).
Bergogne-Berezin, E., J. Pierre, J. Chastre et al.: Pharmacokinetics of apalcillin in intensive-care patients: study of penetration into the respiratory tract. J. Antimicrob. Chemother. 14: 67 (1984).
Brogard, J.-M., J.-P. Arnaud, J. F. Blickle, J. Lavillaureix: Biliary elimination of apalcillin in humans. Antimicrob. Ag. Chemother. 26: 428 (1984).
Dusart, G., M. Simeon de Buochberg, M. Zuccarelli, M. A. Attisso, C. Willemin: Comparative effect of apalcillin and other betalactam antibiotics against the Bacteroides fragilis group. Pathol. Biol. Paris 37: 523–527 (1989).
Gentry, L. O., B. A. Wood, E. A. Natelson: Effects of apalcillin on platelet function in normal volunteers. Antimicrob. Ag. Chemother. 27: 683 (1985).
Raoult, D., H. Gallias, P. Casanova et al.: Meningeal penetration of apalcillin in man. J. Antimicrob. Chemother. 15: 123 (1985).

g) Mecillinam

Proprietary name: Selexid, Selexidin (Pivmecillinam). Combined with pivampicillin as Miraxid.

Synonyms: Amdinocillin, amidino penicillin.

Spectrum of activity: A broad-spectrum penicillin (the amidino derivative of 6-aminopenicillanic acid), active against gram-negative bacilli such as Escherichia coli, Proteus mirabilis, Proteus vulgaris, Klebsiella pneumoniae, Enterobacter cloacae, yersinia, citrobacter, salmonellae and shigellae. Little activity against gram-positive bacilli such as streptococci, pneumococci or penicillin-sensitive staphylococci. No activity against Pseudomonas aeruginosa, enterococci or penicillinase-producing staphylococci, or against most strains of Serratia marcescens or Haemophilus influenzae. Synergy with ampicillin against most strains of Escherichia coli and Klebsiella pneumoniae, as well as with cephalosporins, aminoglycosides and tetracyclines against other bacteria. The mode of action of mecillinam differs from that of other penicillins because it is active on only one binding protein, leading to a marked production of spheroblasts and a slower bacteriolysis.

Pharmacokinetics: Poorly absorbed by mouth, but well absorbed as the ester (pivmecillinam). Mean *serum concentrations* 1 h after the oral administration of 200 mg and 400 mg of pivmecillinam are 3 and 5 mg/l respectively, and peak serum concentrations up to 12 mg/l are found after i. m. injection of 0.4 g. *Half-life:* 1 h. *Plasma protein binding:* 10%. *Urinary recovery:* 50% (after oral administration).

Side-effects: Headaches, nausea, vomiting and diarrhoea (after oral administration) occur not infrequently. Other side-effects as for benzylpenicillin and ampicillin.

Indications: Mecillinam is suitable for the treatment of urinary infections with gram-negative bacilli and may be given parenterally or orally (as pivmecillinam). Few data are available for other indications.

Contra-indications: Penicillin allergy, infectious mononucleosis and chronic lymphatic leukaemia (skin rashes).

Dosage: 200–400 mg of pivmecillinam orally 3 times a day, 5–15 mg/kg (as tablets) 3 times a day for children below the age of 6. 5–10 mg/kg 3 times a day parenterally, as a slow i.v. injection or short i.v. infusion. I.m. injection is possible. The dose of the combined preparation of pivmecillinam with pivampicillin is 1–2 film-coated tablets twice daily (adults) taken with at least 50–100 ml of fluid during or after meals. This dose is recommended in the hope that synergy will occur, but is in our opinion too low. A combination of mecillinam with amoxycillin would be better.

Preparations: Vials of 0.4 g, tablets (pivmecillinam) of 0.2 g and tablets of 0.225 g and 0.45 g (0.1 g and 0.2 g of pivmecillinam + 0.125 g and 0.25 g of pivampicillin respectively).

Summary: Against gram-negative bacilli, mecillinam has a broader spectrum and greater activity than ampicillin, but it is inactive against haemophilus and enterococci, though the combination with pivampicillin closes this gap in the spectrum. Penicillinase-producing staphylococci are always resistant. The ester moieties often cause gastrointestinal upset.

References

HARES, M. M., A. HEGARTY, J. TOMKYNS et al.: A study of the biliary excretion of mecillinam in patients with biliary disease. J. Antimicrob. Chemother. *9:* 217 (1982).

IGESUND, A., L. VORLAND: A fixed combination of pivmecillinam and pivampicillin in complicated urinary tract infections. A double-blind comparison with pivmecillinam. Scand. J. Infect. Dis. *14:* 159 (1982).

JODAL, U., P. LARSSON, S. HANSSON, C. A. BAUER: Pivmecillinam in long-term prophylaxis to girls with recurrent urinary tract infection. Scand. J. Infect. Dis. *21:* 299–302 (1989).

MEYERS, B. R., J. JACOBSON, J. MASCI et al.: Pharmacokinetics of amdinocillin in healthy adults. Antimicrob. Ag. Chemother. *23:* 827 (1983).

PATEL, I. H., L. D. BORNEMANN, V. M. BROCKS et al.: Pharmacokinetics of intravenous amdinocillin in healthy subjects and patients with renal insufficiency. Antimicrob. Ag. Chemother. *28:* 46 (1985).

SVENUNGSSON, B., E. EKWALL, H. B. HANSSON: Efficacy of the combination pivampicillin/pivmecillinam compared to placebo. Infection *18:* 163–165 (1990).

h) Penicillin Combinations

Certain fixed combinations are commercially available, in which ampicillin or mezlocillin are combined with penicillinase-stable penicillins, such as oxa- and dicloxacillin. Because of the relatively high proportion of bacteria resistant to ampicillin and mezlocillin they are now becoming obsolete. The optimal derivatives never seem to be combined in an optimal dosage. Free combinations of anti-pseudomonal penicillins such as azlocillin or piperacillin with other β-lactam antibiotics (e. g. cefotaxime), which would extend the spectrum and increase activity, are potentially much more useful.

2. Cephalosporins

Classification: The cephalosporins are bicyclic β-lactam antibiotics which are made up of a dihydrothiazine (A) and a β-lactam (B) ring (Fig. 16, p. 64). These two rings form 7-aminocephalosporanic acid, the common nucleus of the cephalosporins. The cephamycins are broadly similar in properties to the cephalosporins but have a different nucleus (an oxacephem ring).

The basic molecule, 7-aminocephalosporanic acid, can be modified by R_1 substitution in position 7 (left side-chain), R_2 substitution in position 3 (right side-chain) and, in the cephamycins, by a third (α-methoxy) substitution in the β-lactam ring. Various substitutions enable a range of compounds to be produced which differ in their antibacterial activity and in their pharmacological properties. The structure-activity relationships are illustrated well by the example of latamoxef (Fig. 3, p. 20).

The cephalosporins may be classified into groups, each designated by a representative member, on the basis of their microbiological properties, as follows:
1. *Cefazolin group* (basic cephalosporins).
2. *Cefuroxime group* (intermediate cephalosporins).
3. *Cefoxitin group* (anti-anaerobic cephalosporins).
4. *Cefotaxime group* (broad-spectrum cephalosporins).
5. *Cefoperazone group* (other parenteral cephalosporins).
6. *Cephalexin group* (older oral cephalosporins).
7. *Cefixime group* (newer oral cephalosporins).

Earlier, historical classifications on the basis of "generations" may lead to confusion and are not used in this book.

The representatives of each group should be considered for particular indications because of their spectrum of action and pharmacokinetic properties.

In American usage the first syllable of the generic name of all cephalosporins is spelled "cef". The English convention, used in this book, is to retain the classical spelling "ceph" for compounds described before 1975.

a) Cefazolin Group (Basic Cephalosporins)

Proprietary names:
for *cefazolin:* Kefzol;
for *cefazedone:* Refosporin.

Mode of action: Like the penicillins, the cephalosporins inhibit bacterial cell wall synthesis and are bactericidal only during bacterial growth.

Spectrum of activity: A range of gram-positive and gram-negative organisms are sensitive to members of this group. Cefazolin and cefazedone are much more active than cephalothin against gram-negative bacilli, particularly Escherichia coli and Klebsiella pneumoniae, of which there is therefore a lower percentage of resistant organisms. Cefazolin has particularly good activity against staphylococci, including β-lactamase-producing strains. Cefazedone and the other cephalosporins are inactive against the enterococci (Enterococcus faecalis and E. faecium). Cefazedone is more active than cefazolin against the other streptococci of Lancefield Group D (S. bovis, S. equi and S. zymogenes). The following bacteria are *resistant:* Pseudomonas aeruginosa, Proteus rettgeri, Morganella morganii, enterococci (Enterococcus faecalis), most strains of Proteus vulgaris and Haemophilus influenzae, as well as providencia, serratia, citrobacter, edwardsiella, arizona, acinetobacter, Bacteroides fragilis, campylobacter, nocardia, mycoplasma, moraxella, brucella and most strains of enterobacter.

Cefonicid (marketed in the USA as Monocid) has a spectrum similar to cefazolin but is less active against staphylococci and streptococci. Cefonicid is 98% protein bound, and its in vitro activity against Staphylococcus aureus is reduced if 50% serum is added to the test system. Because of its prolonged half-life (4 h) it is used as a single injection of 1–2 g every 24 h.

Resistance: *Primary* resistance is fairly common in gram-negative bacteria but quite rare with gram-positive organisms. *Secondary* resistance during therapy is rare and arises slowly. *Cross-resistance* occurs with Staphylococcus aureus between cephalosporins and penicillinase-stable penicillins (e. g. flucloxacillin) but not with Staphylococcus epidermidis (i. e. methicillin-resistant strains of Staphylococcus epidermidis can be sensitive to cefazolin). Partial cross-resistance is found with ampicillin, the acylaminopenicillins and ticarcillin. No cross-resistance with benzylpenicillin.

Pharmacokinetics: *Not absorbed after* oral administration. *Rapid* absorption after i. m. injection. *Serum concentrations* of cefazolin and cefazedone are much higher, dose for dose, than those found with cephalothin. The mean serum concentrations after 1 g of *cefazolin* i. v. are 52 mg/l after 1 h, 33 mg/l after 2 h and 5.6 mg/l after 6 h. The mean serum concentrations after 1 g of *cefazedone* i. v. are 65 mg/l (1 h), 34 mg/l (2 h) and 6.4 mg/l (6 h).

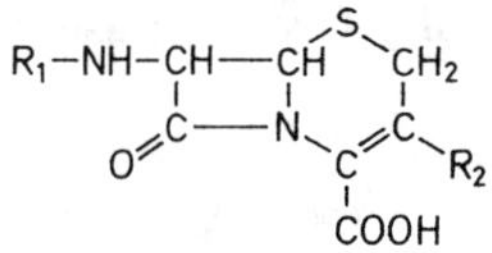

Compound	R₁	R₂
7-Aminocephalo-sporanic acid	H–	$-CH_2-O-C(=O)CH_3$
Cephalothin	(thienyl)$-CH_2-C(=O)-$	$-CH_2-O-C(=O)CH_3$
Cephaloridine	(thienyl)$-CH_2-C(=O)-$	$-CH_2-N^+$(pyridinium)
Cefazolin	(tetrazolyl)$N-CH_2-C(=O)-$	$-CH_2-S-$(thiadiazolyl)$-CH_3$
Cefamandole	(phenyl)$-CH(OCHO)-C(=O)-$	$-CH_2-S-$(tetrazolyl)$-CH_3$
Cefuroxime	(furyl)$-C(=N-O-CH_3)-C(=O)-$	$-CH_2-O-C(=O)-NH_2$
Cefsulodin	(phenyl)$-CH(SO_3Na)-CO-$	$-CH_2-N^+$(pyridinium)$-CONH_2$
Cefotiam	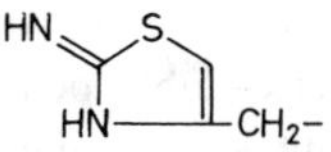 (aminothiazolyl)$-CH_2-$	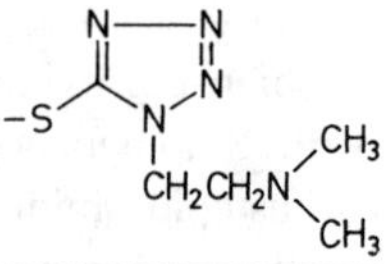 $-S-$(tetrazolyl)$-CH_2CH_2N(CH_3)_2$ · 2HCl

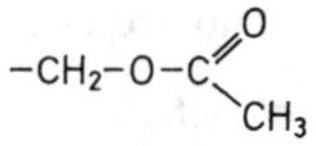

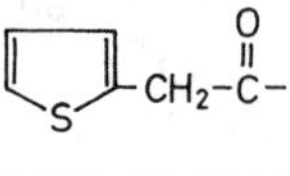

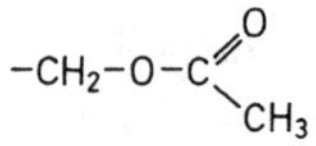

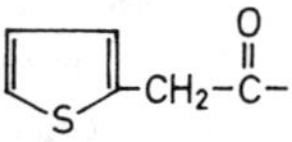

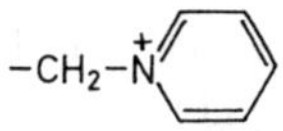

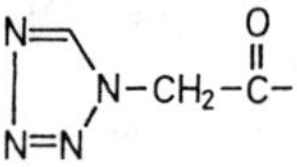

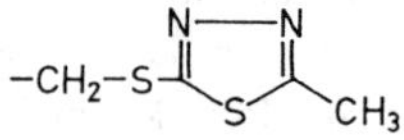

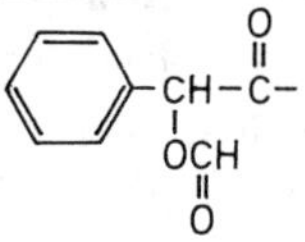

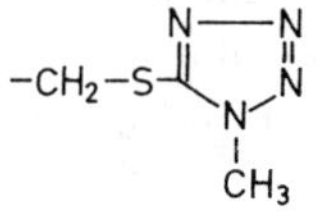

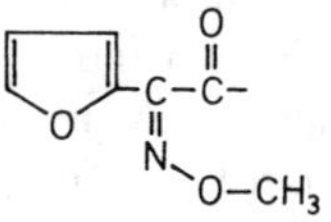

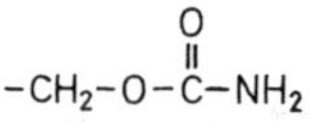

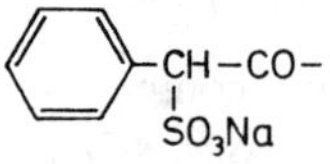

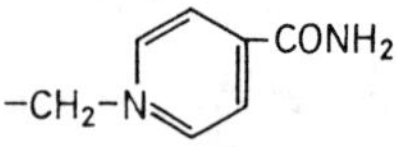

Fig. 16. Structural formulae of the cephalosporins.

Half-life of cefazolin 94 min, and of cefazedone 140 min. *Plasma protein binding* of cefazolin 84%, and of cefazedone 93%. *Urinary recovery* of cefazolin is 92%, and of cefazedone 95%. Biliary concentrations of both compounds are higher than that of cephalothin, and are therapeutically adequate.

Side-effects:
1. *Allergic reactions* (fever, rashes, urticaria etc.) in 1–4%. Anaphylactic shock is possible, but less common than with the penicillins. Cross-allergy with penicillins is not usually found. The great majority of patients with penicillin allergy tolerate cephalosporins because they do not release any penicilloyl compounds in the body.
2. *Allergic leukocytopenia*, rapidly reversible after cessation of therapy. Blood count should be checked after prolonged therapy or if allergic symptoms or fever occur during treatment.
3. *Renal tolerance* of all the newer cephalosporins, including the basic cephalosporins, is good. When renal function is severely impaired, cefazedone (and rarely cefazolin) very occasionally give rise to a bleeding tendency, but the clotting time rapidly returns to normal with vitamin K treatment. Transient rises in serum transaminases, alkaline phosphatase and bilirubin have been reported during cefazolin therapy.
4. The *direct Coombs test* can become *positive* during therapy with cephalosporins. The cephalosporins are assumed either to damage the surface of the red cells, allowing normal serum globulin to accumulate at this site, or to facilitate the deposition of a cephalosporin-globulin complex on the red cell surface which reacts with anti-human globulin. Haemolytic anaemia is nevertheless extremely rare during cephalosporin therapy.

Indications have become fewer with the introduction of the new β-lactamase-stable cephalosporins. Cefazolin and cefazedone are still useful in:
1. Primary pneumonia (community-acquired).
2. Wound infections (community-acquired).
3. Indications for benzylpenicillin in patients with penicillin allergy (cross-allergy with penicillin is very rare).
4. Perioperative prophylaxis.

Incorrect use: Methicillin-resistant Staphylococcus aureus infections (cross-resistance). Severe systemic infections (septicaemia), where multi-resistant enterobacteria may be involved.

Contra-indications: Cephalosporin allergy.

Dosage and administration: I. v. injection or short i. v. infusion. I. m. injection up to 1 g is possible but painful. Give 3–4(–6) g a day for adults, 60(–100) mg/kg for children, in 2–3 divided doses. In renal failure, reduce normal daily dose to 60% where creatinine clearance is 40–60 ml/min, to 25% where creatinine clearance is 20–40 ml/min and to 10% where creatinine clearance is 5–20 ml/min.

Preparations: Vials of 0.5 g, 1 g and 2 g. Lignocaine solution is provided for i. m. injection only.

Summary: These basic cephalosporins have good activity against staphylococci, a broad spectrum, and are well tolerated. Cefazolin and cefazedone are less active against gram-negative bacilli than cefotaxime, and are inactive against Pseudomonas. Cefazolin and cefazedone should not, therefore, be used alone in life-threatening infections of unknown cause.

References

ACTOR, P.: In vitro experience with cefonicid. Rev. Infect. Dis. *6* (Suppl. 4): S. 783, 1984.
BARRIERE, S. L., G. J. HATHEWAY, J. G. GAMBERTOGLIO, et al.: Pharmacokinetics of cefonicid, a new broad-spectrum cephalosporin. Antimicrob. Ag. Chemother; *21:* 935 (1982).
CONTE, J. E., Jr.: Clinical and economic impact of cefonicid: Overview and summary of the symposium. Rev. Infect. Dis. *6* (Suppl. 4): S. 777 (1984).
EL SEFI, T. A., H. M. EEL AWADY, M. I. SHEHATA, M. A. AAL-HINI: Systemic plus local metronidazole and cephazolin in complicated appendicitis: a prospective controlled trial. J. R. Coll. Surg. Edinb. *34:* 13–16 (1989).
MORGAN, S. I., R. E. PONTZER, L. M. CORTEZ et al.: Single-dose regimen of cefonicid for the treatment of uncomplicated infections of the lower urinary tract. Rev. Infect. Dis. *6* (Suppl. 4): 844 (1984).
MORRIS, D. L., J. A. JONES, J. D. HARRISON et al.: Randomised study of prophylactic parenteral sulbactam/ampicillin and cephalozolin in biliary surgery: significant benefit in jaundiced patients. J. Hosp. Infect. *13:* 261–266 (1989).
PABST, J., G. LEOPOLD, W. UNGETHÜM, E. DINGELDEIN: Clinical pharmacology phase I of cefazedone, a new cephalosporin, in healthy volunteers. II. Pharmacokinetics in comparison with cefazolin. Arzneimittel-Forsch. 29 *(I):* 437 (1979).
PHELPS, R. T., CONTE, J. E. Jr.: Multiple-dose pharmacokinetics of cefonicid in patients with impaired renal function. Antimicrob. Ag. Chemother. *29:* 913 (1986).
WALLACE, R. J. Jr., S. L. NIFFIELD, S. WATERS et al.: Comparative trial of cefonicid and cefamandole in the therapy of community-acquired pneumonia. Antimicrob. Ag. Chemother. *21:* 231 (1982).
WÜST, J. et al.: Comparative in Vitro Activity of Cefetamet and Fleroxacin against Anaerobic Bacteria. Eur. J. Clin. Microbiol. *6:* 688–690 (1987).
VAN MEIRHAEGHE, J., R. VERDONK, G. VERSCHRAEGEN et al.: Flucloxacillin compared with cefazolin in short-term prophylaxis for clean orthopedic surgery. Arch. Orthop. Trauma. Surg. *108:* 308–313 (1989).

b) Cefuroxime Group (Intermediate Cephalosporins)

Proprietary names: For *cefuroxime:* Zinacef; for *cefamandole:* Kefadol; for *cefotiam:* Halospor.

Properties: The intermediate cephalosporins include cefuroxime, cefamandole and cefotiam (for structural formula, see Fig. 16, p. 64). Cefuroxime has an oxime side-chain and cefotiam an aminothiazole side-chain, both of which increase antibacterial activity. The sodium salts of cefuroxime and cefamandole formiate are readily soluble in water, as is the dihydrochloride of cefotiam. The ampoules of cefamandole contain 63 mg of sodium carbonate per g of cefamandole. When dissolved in water, the ester is rapidly hydrolysed and CO_2 is released.

Spectrum of activity: Cefuroxime, cefamandole and cefotiam are largely stable to β-lactamases. β-lactamase resistance in these cephalosporins is due to the molecular grouping around the β-lactam ring which comprises the methyloxime group for cefuroxime and mandelamido and tetrazole groups for cefamandole. In contrast to cefazolin, the increase in activity is directed against almost all gram-negative bacilli and much less against the gram-positive cocci.

Table 7. Activity against 449 clinical bacterial isolates tested *in vitro* with cephalothin, cefuroxime, cefamandole, cefotiam and cefoxitin. n = number of strains examined. $MIC_{50\%}$ = minimal inhibitory concentration in ≤50% of the strains (own data).

Species	n	$MIC_{50\%}$ (mg/l)				
		Cepha-lothin	Cefur-oxime	Cefa-mandole	Cefo-tiam	Cefo-xitin
Escherichia coli	102	3.1	3.1	3.1	0.1	3.1
Proteus mirabilis	105	25.0	12.5	12.5	3.1	3.1
Proteus vulgaris	60	> 200.0	200.0	200.0	25.0	6.2
Klebsiella pneumoniae	65	6.2	3.1	6.2	0.2	3.1
Enterobacter aerogenes	102	> 200.0	12.5	0.8	0.4	50.0
Citrobacter freundii	15	50.0	12.5	25.0	25.0	50.0

Cefamandole, cefotiam and cefuroxime have reasonably good activity against staphyloccci. Cefuroxime and cefotiam are particularly active against streptococci of Lancefield groups A and B, gonococci including penicillinase-producing strains and meningococci. Cefamandole is quite active against Enterobacter species, salmonellae and staphylococci. Cefamandole, cefuroxime and cefotiam are all active against Haemophilus influenzae, mostly at concentrations of 0.4–1.6 mg/l, as well as against ampicillin-resistant strains. Table 7 shows the activity of cefamandole, cefuroxime and cefotiam against different enterobacteria. The following organisms are completely resistant: Pseudomonas aeruginosa, enterococci, mycoplasmas, chlamydiae and mycobacteria. Cefuroxime, cefamandole and cefotiam have little or no activity against Bacteroides fragilis, and cefuroxime and cefotiam have little or no activity against cephalothin-resistant staphylococci.

Resistance: A variable proportion of Enterobacteriaceae are resistant to cefuroxime, cefamandole and/or cefotiam (according to the organism involved, see Table 27, p. 308). There is incomplete cross-resistance between the old and the new (β-lactamase-stable) cephalosporins and incomplete cross-resistance between cefoxitin, cefuroxime, cefamandole and cefotiam, which should be taken into account in sensitivity testing.

Pharmacokinetics: *Not absorbed* by mouth. *Serum concentrations* after i.v. injection of 1 g (Fig. 17): 24.1 mg/l (1 h) and 3.7 mg/l (4 h) with cefuroxime; 16.5 mg/l (1 h) and 1.1 mg/l (4 h) with cefamandole; 19 mg/l (1 h) and 1.1 mg/l (4 h) with cefotiam. With a continuous i.v. infusion of 0.166 g/h (= 4 g/24 h), the *mean serum concentrations* are 12.0 mg/l with cefuroxime and 8.1 mg/l with cefamandole. *Half-life* of cefuroxime: 70 min, cefamandole: 50 min and cefotiam: 45 min. All penetrate tissues well but CSF poorly. Skin blister concentrations at equilibrium with cefuroxime are 8 times as high as with cephalothin and with cefamandole 3 times as high. *Plasma protein binding* of cefuroxime: 20%, cefamandole: 67%, cefotiam: 40%.

Urinary excretion of 90% of cefuroxime and cefamandole in active form within the first 6 h by glomerular filtration and active tubular secretion, and of 70% with cefotiam. A small amount is excreted with the bile. Little or no metabolism (except for cefotiam at approx. 20%). Probenecid retards renal excretion and doubles the half-life. Cefuroxime is almost completely removed and cefamandole partially removed by haemodialysis. Both are only partially removed by peritoneal dialysis.

Side-effects: Similar to cefazolin and cefazedone. Cefamandole may cause alcohol intolerance and hypoprothrombinaemia, which improves rapidly with vitamin K. This vitamin K antagonism is associated with the n-methyl-thiotetrazole side-chain, which cefmenoxime, cefoperazone and latamoxef also possess. The alcohol intolerance with cefamandole is also related to the methyl thiotetrazole ring and blockade of acetaldehyde dehydrogenase caused by the tetrazole side-chain. When the patient takes alcohol, the acetaldehyde concentration increases, leading to flushes, sweating, hypotension, tachycardia, vomiting, headache and dizziness. This effect can even occur 72 h after the last dose of antibiotic. This Antabuse (disulfiram)-like effect is best prevented by avoiding all alcohol (including alcohol-containing infusions) until 2–4 days after treatment. Cefuroxime, cefamandole and cefotiam occasionally give rise to a transient elevation of serum transaminases, alkaline phosphatase and bilirubin.

Indications: Initial therapy before culture and sensitivities are available of bacterial infections which could be due to staphylococci and/or resistant gram-negative rods. Indications of this sort are secondary pneumonia, postoperative urinary infections and severe wound and tissue infections. The gaps in the spectrum due to pseudomonas and enterococci can be covered by giving azlocillin or piperacillin at the same time. Combination with an aminoglycoside (gentamicin, tobramycin, amikacin or netilmicin) to enhance the antibacterial effect continues to be useful in severe infections with Enterobacteriaceae.

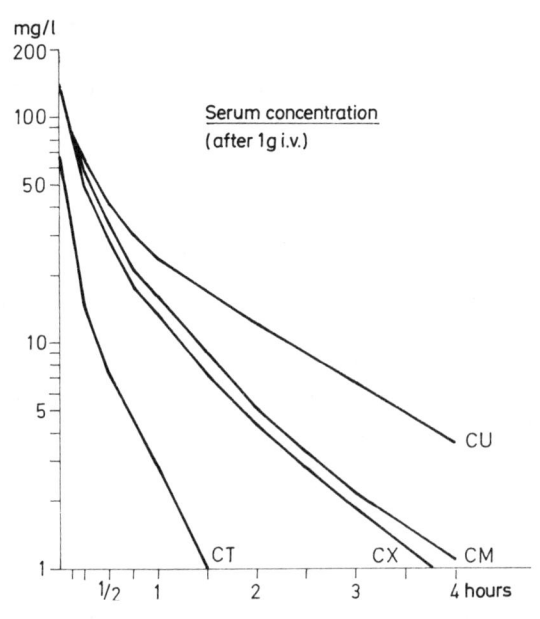

Fig. 17. Mean serum concentrations of cefuroxime (CU), cefamandole (CM), cefoxitin (CX) and cephalothin (CT) after i. v. injection of 1 g of each into 10 healthy adults, as a cross-over study (own data).

Cefuroxime, cefamandole and cefotiam are also indicated in infections with ampicillin-resistant strains of haemophilus and with organisms resistant to other antibiotics. Cefamandole and cefotiam are effective against infections with Enterobacter aerogenes and staphylococci, whereas cefuroxime and cefotiam are useful in infections with Klebsiella pneumoniae. A single dose of cefuroxime or cefotiam can also be used to treat gonorrhoea, even when the strain is penicillin-resistant. Cephalosporins of the intermediate group are also suitable for perioperative prophylaxis by virtue of their pharmacokinetics and spectrum of activity.

Contra-indications: Cephalosporin allergy.

Administration: Either by i. v. injection, short i. v. infusion (30 min) or continuous i. v. infusion. Cefamandole should not be added to solutions containing calcium or magnesium. Do not mix with other drugs (e. g. aminoglycosides) in the same solution. The i. m. injection of cefamandole can be painful and is better dissolved in 0.5% lignocaine.

Dosage: In *severe infections,* all members of this group should be given in the same dose, namely 2 g 3 times a day for adults (50 mg/kg 3 times a day for children). This can cause some difficulty with cefuroxime, whose ampoules contain 0.75 g and 1.5 g.

For *organ infections* (without severe systemic features): 1 g 3 times a day or 2 g twice daily for adults (25 mg/kg 3 times a day for children).

For *gonorrhoea:* Single dose of 1.5 g of cefuroxime i. m. divided between 2 separate injection sites and preferably combined with a single oral dose of 1 g probenecid.

For *perioperative prophylaxis,* adults receive 2 g i. v. 1–3 times for a maximum of 24 h, according to the operative circumstances.

The dosage interval should be prolonged in patients with *chronic renal failure* to 8 h when the creatinine clearance is 30–50 ml/min, to 12 h at 10–29 ml/min, to 24 h at 5–9 ml/min and to 48 h for less than 5 ml/min. The normal single dose, according to the severity of the infection, is then given at longer intervals. Do not give more than 0.75–1 g as a single dose when the creatinine clearance is less than 10 ml/min.

Preparations: *Cefuroxime:* vials of 250 mg, 750 mg, 1.5 g; *cefamandole:* vials of 500 mg, 1 g, 2 g; *cefotiam:* 500 mg, 1 g and 2 g.

Summary: Because of their broad spectrum and favourable pharmacokinetic properties, the intermediate group of cephalosporins has a useful role in the treatment of non-life-threatening infections such as pneumonia.

References

ARDITI, M., B. C. HEROLD, R. YOGEV: Cefuroxime treatment failure and Haemophilus influenzae meningitis: case report and review of literature. Pediatrics *84:* 132–135 (1989).
BROGARD, J. M., J. P. ARNAUD, J. F. BLICKLE et al.: Biliary elimination of cefotiam, an experimental and clinical study. Chemotherapy *32:* 222–235 (1986).
BROGARD, J. M., F. JEHL, B. WILLEMIN, A. M. LAMALLE, J. F. BLICKLE, H. MONTEIL: Clinical pharmacokinetics of cefotiam. Clin. Pharmacokinet. *17:* 163–174 (1989).
BURNS, G. P., T. A. STEIN, M. COHEN: Biliary and pancreatic excretion of cefamandole. Antimicrob. Ag. Chemother. *33:* 977–979 (1989).
DE LOS, A., M. DEL RIO, D. F. CHRANE et al.: Pharmacokinetics of cefuroxime in infants and children with bacterial meningitis. Antimicrob. Ag. Chemother. *22:* 990 (1982).
FREUNDT, K. J., E. SCHREINER, U. CHRISTMANN-KLEISS: Cefamandole – a competitive inhibitor of aldehyde dehydrogenase. Infection *13:* 91 (1985).
KONISHI, K., Y. OZAWA: Pharmacokinetics of cefotiam in patients with impaired renal function and in those undergoing hemodialysis. Antimicrob. Ag. Chemother. *26:* 647–651 (1984).
ROUAN, M.-C., J. B. LECAILLON, J. GUIBERT et al.: Pharmacokinetics of cefotiam in humans. Antimicrob. Ag. Chemother. *27:* 177 (1985).
UOTILA, L., J. W. SUTTIE: Inhibition of vitamin K-dependent carboxylase in vitro by cefamandole and its structural analogs. J. Infect. Dis. *148:* 571 (1983).

c) Cefoxitin Group (Cephamycins)

The cephamycins differ from the other cephalosporins by possessing a methoxy group in the 7-α position (Fig. 18). This group includes cefoxitin, cefotetan and cefmetazole. Latamoxef and flomoxef belong to a subsidiary group within the cephamycins, designated the oxacephems, in which one of the sulphur atoms in the cephem ring is substituted by oxygen. They are all very stable to β-lactamases, including those produced by Bacteroides fragilis. Except for latamoxef, however, they are not active against pseudomonas.

α) Cefoxitin

Proprietary name: Mefoxin.

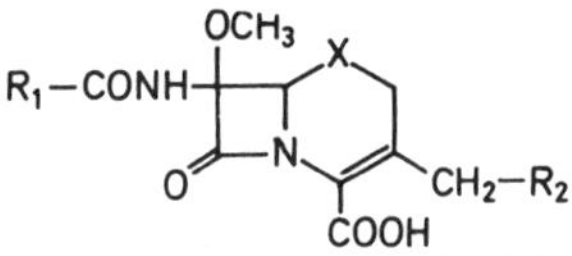

$$R_1-CONH-\underset{\underset{COOH}{|}}{\overset{OCH_3}{\text{[cephem ring with X]}}}-CH_2-R_2$$

Compound	R_1	R_2	X
Cefoxitin	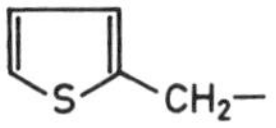 thiophene-CH_2-	$-OCONH_2$	S
Cefmetazole	$N\equiv C-CH_2-S-CH_2-$	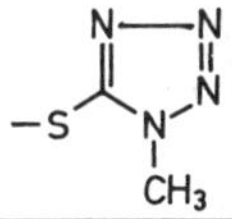 $-S-$(1-methyl-tetrazolyl)	S
Cefotetan	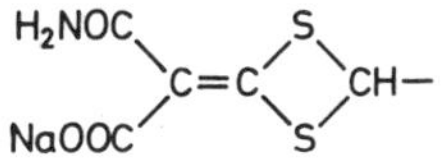 $H_2NOC\text{-}C(=C(S-CH-S-))\text{-}NaOOC$	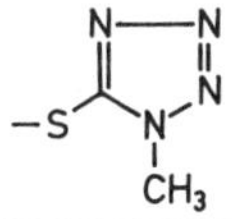 $-S-$(1-methyl-tetrazolyl)	S
Latamoxef	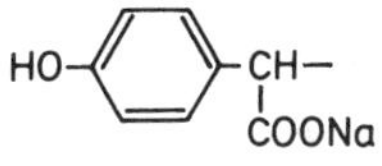 $HO-C_6H_4-CH(COONa)-$	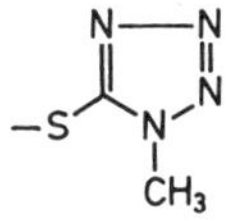 $-S-$(1-methyl-tetrazolyl)	O
Flomoxef	$F_2HC-S-CH_2-$	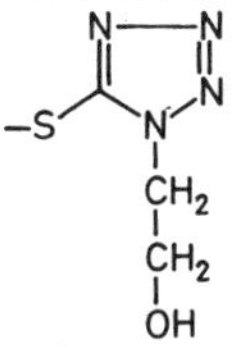 $-S-$(1-(2-hydroxyethyl)-tetrazolyl)	O

Fig. 18. Structural formula of the 7-methoxycephalosporins.

Mode of action: Highly resistant to almost all bacterial β-lactamases. Relatively poor penetration of the outer membrane of gram-negative bacteria.

Spectrum of activity: Cefoxitin is more active than cefazolin against gram-negative bacilli such as Escherichia coli and Proteus mirabilis by 1–2 or more geometric dilution steps. Moreover, cefoxitin inhibits the majority of cefazolin-resistant organisms (Proteus vulgaris, Proteus rettgeri, Morganella morganii, Klebsiella pneumoniae, Serratia marcescens, providencia and others). Cefoxitin is generally more active against Bacteroides species and is also stable to the β-lactamase of Bacteroides fragilis. Resistance to cefoxitin in Bacteroides fragilis is rare. Cefoxitin is also active against penicillin-resistant gonococci. Activity against staphylococci and streptococci of Lancefield groups A and B is less than with cefazolin, and the activity against haemophilus is less than that of cefuroxime, cefamandole, cefotiam and the cephalosporins of the cefotaxime group. The following bacteria are resistant: Pseudomonas aeruginosa, enterococci, methicillin-resistant staphylococci, some enterobacteria, all mycoplasmas, chlamydiae and mycobacteria.

Resistance: Primary resistance is rare amongst the Enterobacteriaceae with the exceptions of Citrobacter freundii and Enterobacter cloacae. Resistance does not arise during therapy. Some cross-resistance is found with other cephalosporins, so bacterial sensitivity to these agents should always be specifically tested. Cefoxitin may induce β-lactamase of Pseudomonas aeruginosa in vitro but there is no evidence that this is of clinical relevance.

Pharmacokinetics: *Not absorbed* by mouth.

Serum concentrations after *injection* of 1 g i.v.: 13.2 mg/l (1 h) and 0.9 mg/l (4 h). During continuous i.v. *infusion* of 0.166 g/h (= 4 g/24 h), the mean serum concentrations are 7.5 mg/l (3 times higher than with cephalothin).

Concentrations in blister fluid are also 3 times higher (80% of serum level). Penetrates *tissues* well but CSF poorly.

Half-life: 45 min. *Plasma protein binding:* 50%.

Excretion is predominantly renal, with 90% appearing in active form in the urine within 6 h. A small amount is secreted in the bile and some is also metabolised and excreted in the urine as decarbamoyl cefoxitin. Probenecid delays renal excretion and doubles the serum concentrations and half-life.

Side-effects: Similar to all cephalosporins. Usually no cross-allergy with penicillins, and administration in penicillin allergy is justifiable if the patient is under careful observation.

Indications:
1. *Initial therapy* of bacterial infections in which gram-positive cocci, resistant gram-negative bacilli and Bacteroides fragilis are considered as possible causes, e.g. secondary pneumonia, gynaecological infections and severe wound and

tissue infections. Because of its effectiveness against anaerobes, cefoxitin may be used in the treatment of mixed infections with anaerobes such as gangrene, tonsillar abscess and lung abscess. Combination with an aminoglycoside may potentiate the antibacterial effect.

2. Therapy of infections with *known sensitive organisms,* particularly where otherwise resistant pathogens are sensitive to cefoxitin (e.g. Klebsiella, Serratia, Proteus rettgeri).

Contra-indications: Allergy to cephalosporins.

Administration: Preferably by i.v. injection or short i.v. infusion (30 min). Continuous i.v. infusion and i.m. injection are also possible but, because i.m. injection is painful, dissolve in 0.5% lignocaine. Do not mix with other drugs, particularly aminoglycosides (risk of precipitation).

Dosage: For *severe infections:* 2 g 3–4 times a day (50 mg/kg 3–4 times a day for children); for *less severe infections* 1 g 3 times a day (25 mg/kg 3 times a day for children).

Prolong the dose-interval for patients with *chronic renal failure* to 8 h when the creatinine clearance is 30–50 ml/min, to 12 h when 10–29 ml/min, to 24 h when 5–9 ml/min and to 48 h when less than 5 ml/min. The normal single dose is then given at extended intervals, according to the severity of the infection. Only when the creatinine clearance is less than 10 ml/min should the single dose of 750 mg not be exceeded.

Cefoxitin is dialysable. Give 2 g at the end of each haemodialysis.

Preparations: Injection bottles of 1 g and 2 g.

Summary: A β-lactamase-stable, broad-spectrum antibiotic with good activity against anaerobes. Ineffective against Pseudomonas species, Enterobacter species, enterococci and methicillin-resistant staphylococci.

References

DASCHNER, F. D., E. E. PETERSEN et al.: Antibiotic prophylaxis in gynecology: Cefoxitin concentrations in serum, myometrium, endometrium and salpinges. Infection *10:* 341 (1982).

FELDMAN, W. E., S. MOFFITT, N. SPROW: Clinical and pharmacokinetic evaluation of parenteral cefoxitin in infants and children. Antimicrob. Ag. Chemother. *17:* 669 (1980).

FELDMANN, W. E., S. MOFFITT, N. S. MANNING: Penetration of cefoxitin into cerebrospinal fluid of infants and children with bacterial meningitis. Antimicrob. Ag. Chemother. *21:* 468 (1982).

GREAVES, W. L., J. H. KREEFT, R. I. OGILVIE, G. K. RICHARDS: Cefoxitin disposition during peritoneal dialysis. Antimicrob. Ag. Chemother. *19:* 253 (1981).

KAMPF, D., R. SCHURIG, I. KORSUKEWITZ, O. BRÜCKNER: Cefoxitin pharmacokinetics: relation to three different renal clearance studies in patients with various degree of renal insufficiency. Antimicrob. Ag. Chemother. *20:* 741 (1981).

PEREA, E. J., M. C. GARCIA-IGLESIAS, J. AYARRA, J. LOSCERTALES: Comparative concentrations of cefoxitin in human lungs and sera. Antimicrob. Ag. Chemother. *23:* 323 (1983).
SANDERS, C. C., W. E. SANDERS JR., R. V. GOERING: In vitro antagonism of betalactam antibiotics by cefoxitin. Antimicrob. Ag. Chemother. *21:* 968 (1982).
TALLY, F. P. et al.: Susceptibility of anaerobes to cefoxitin and other cephalosporins. Antimicrob. Ag. Chemother. *7:* 128 (1975).

β) Cefotetan

Proprietary name: Apatef.

Spectrum of activity: More active than cefoxitin against gram-negative rods but less effective against staphylococci. Activity against Bacteroides fragilis and other anaerobes is about the same as that of cefoxitin. Pseudomonas aeruginosa, Acinetobacter, enterococci (Enterococcus faecalis), Clostridium difficile and Bacteroides thetaiotaomicron are always resistant. Cefotetan is very stable against bacterial β-lactamase.

Pharmacokinetics: Mean serum concentrations after i. v. injection of 1 g and 2 g are 103 and 135 mg/l respectively after 1 h, and 9 and 12 mg/l respectively after 12 h. Relatively long *half-life* of 3–4 h. *Plasma protein binding:* 90%. 70% *excreted* unchanged in the urine, 15% in a tautomeric form with similar antibacterial activity. Partially excreted through the bile.

Side-effects as for other cephalosporins. The methylthiotetrazole side-chain is the reason for the observed prolongation of prothrombin time (bleeding tendency) and for alcohol intolerance (see p. 68).

Indications: As for cefoxitin (see p. 72).

Contra-indications: Cephalosporin allergy.

Administration and dosage: 1–2 g twice daily by i. v. or i. m. injection. When the creatinine clearance is 10–30 ml/min, the normal single dose is given every 24 h, and when less than 10 ml/min, every 48 h.

Preparations: Vials of 1 g and 2 g.

Summary: Cefotetan is more active than cefoxitin against gram-negative bacilli. As with latamoxef, disorders of blood coagulation can occur.

References

BROWNING, M. J., H. A. HOLT, L. O. WHITE et al.: Pharmacokinetics of cefotetan in patients with end-stage renal failure on maintenance dialysis. J. Antimicrob. Chemother. *18:* 103 (1986).
CONJURA, A., W. BELL, J. J. LIPSKY: Cefotetan and hypoprothrombinemia. Ann. Intern. Med. *108:* 643 (1988).

JONES, R. N. Cefotetan: A review of the microbiologic properties and antimicrobial spectrum. Am. J. Surg. *155* (5A): 16 (1988).
JUST, H.-M., E. E. PETERSEN, M. BASSLER, U. FRANK, F. D. DASCHNER: Penetration of cefotetan into serum, myometrium, endometrium and salpinges. Chemotherapy *30:* 305–307 (1984).
KLINE, S. S. et al.: Cefotetan-induced disulfiram-type reactions and hypoprothrombinemia. Antimicrob. Agents Chemother. *31:* 1328, 1987.
MARTENS, M., S. FARO: Cefotetan and the lack of associated bleeding (letter). Am J. Obstet. Gynecol. *163:* 251–252 (1990).
SMITH, B. R., J. L. LE FROCK, P. T. THYRUM et al.: Cefotetan pharmacokinetics in volunteers with various degrees of renal function. Antimicrob. Ag. Chemother. *29:* 887 (1986).
WARD, A., D. M. RICHARDS: Cefotetan: a review of its antibacterial activity, pharmacokinetic properties and therapeutic use. Drugs *30:* 382 (1985).
WATT, B., F. V. BROWN: The comparative in-vitro activity of cefotetan against anaerobic bacteria. J. Antimicrob. Chemother. *15:* 671 (1985).

γ) Cefmetazole

Proprietary name: Zefazone.

Spectrum of activity: A 7-methoxycephalosporin with better activity than cefoxitin, which is used in Japan and the U.S.A. Activity against staphylococci is greater than that of other cephalosporins of the cefoxitin and cefotaxime groups. More active (1–2 dilution steps) than cefoxitin against Enterobacteriaceae. Similar in activity against Bacteroides fragilis. Pseudomonas, Enterobacter spp. and enterococci are resistant. Cefmetazole is very stable to bacterial β-lactamases.

Pharmacokinetics: After i.v. infusion of 1 g and 2 g over 60 minutes mean serum concentrations are 31 mg/l and 70 mg/l respectively (1 h after the end of the infusion) and 3 mg/l and 6 mg/l respectively (5 h after the end of the infusion). *Half-life:* 60 min. *Plasma protein binding:* 85%. About 85% of the dose is excreted in the active form in the urine. Relatively high biliary concentrations.

Side-effects: Diarrhoea occurs occasionally; allergic reactions and other side-effects are rare. Laboratory changes include an increased glucose, decreased serum albumin, decreased total serum protein and fall in prothrombin activity. A disulfiram-like reaction has been reported after the ingestion of alcohol.

Indications: Urinary tract, lower respiratory tract and intra-abdominal infections caused by anaerobes and other susceptible bacteria (including staphylococci). Also used for the prophylaxis of postoperative infections (e.g. caesarean section, hysterectomy, colorectal surgery).

Administration and dosage: I. v. infusion over 10 to 60 minutes or i. v. injection over 5 minutes.

Daily dosage: 4 g (urinary infection), 6 g (other sites) and 8 g (severe infections), in 2, 3 or 4 divided doses respectively.

Summary: A broad spectrum of activity comparable to cefoxitin. Cefmetazole is a further development of cefoxitin and is of interest because of its good antistaphylococcal activity, even though it contains a tetrazole side-chain which can give rise to alcohol intolerance and hypoprothrombinaemia.

References

FINCH, R., R. C. MOELLERING, JR., and D. SPELLER. Cefmetazole: A clinical appraisal. J. Antimicrob. Chemother. *23* (Suppl. D): 1 (1989).
GRIFFITH, D. L., E. NOVAK, C. A. GREENWALD: Clinical experience with cefmetazole sodium in the United States: an overview. J. Antimicrob. Chemother. *23:* 21–33 (1989).
JONES, R. N.: Review of the in-vitro spectrum and characteristics of cefmetazole (CS-1170). J. Antimicrob. Chemother. *23:* 1–12 (1989).
KO, H., E. NOVAK, G. R. PETERS, W. M. BOTHWELL, J. D. HOSLEY, S. K. CLOSSON, W. J. ADAMS: Pharmacokinetics of single-dose cefmetazole following intramuscular administration of cefmetazole sodium to healthy male volunteers. Antimicrob. Ag. Chemother. *33:* 508–512 (1989).
Medical Letter. Cefmetazole sodium (Zefazone). Med. Lett. Drugs Ther. *32:* 65 (1990).
PETERS, G. R., C. M. METZLER: The effects of cefmetazole and latamoxef on platelet function in healthy human volunteers. J. Antimicrob. Chemother. *23 (Suppl. D):* 119–123 (1989).
SHIMADA, J., Y. HAYASHI, K. NAKAMURA: Cefmetazole: clinical evaluation of efficacy and safety in Japan. Drugs Exp. Clin. Res. *11:* 181 (1989).
TAN, J. S., S. J. SALSTROM, S. A. SIGNS, H. E. HOFFMAN, T. M. FILE: Pharmacokinetics of intravenous cefmetazole with emphasis on comparison between predicted theoretical levels in tissue and actual skin window fluid levels. Antimicrob. Ag. Chemother. *33:* 924–927 (1989).
YANGCO, B. C., V. S. KENYON, K. D. HALKIAS: Comparative evaluation of safety and efficacy of cefmetazole and cefoxitin in lower respiratory tract infections. J. Antimicrob. Chemother. *23:* 39–46 (1989).

δ) Latamoxef

Proprietary name: Moxalactam.

Synonym: Lamoxactam.

Properties: Latamoxef is an oxa-β-lactam compound, i.e., the sulphur atom has been substituted by oxygen.

Spectrum of activity is similar to cefotaxime. Latamoxef is more active than cefotaxime against Bacteroides fragilis, Enterobacter cloacae and Citrobacter freundii, but less active against Staphylococcus aureus, Staphylococcus epidermidis and Streptococcus viridans (Table 9, p. 82). Some strains of Pseudomonas aeruginosa are resistant to latamoxef but nearly all strains are sensitive to ceftazidime.

Pharmacokinetics: *Serum concentrations* (after 1 g i.v.): Table 11, p. 83. *Half-life:* 2 h. *Plasma protein binding:* 40%. *Urinary recovery:* 75%. The amount of latamoxef excreted in the bile is not known exactly but high concentrations of microbiologically active drug appear in the faeces and cause major changes in the stool concentration of certain bacteria (Escherichia coli, other enterobacteria and anaerobes).

Side-effects: As with other cephalosporins. Because of the presence of the methyltetrazole group, haemorrhages can occur, caused by hypoprothrombinaemia and/or disorders of platelet function. Such bleeding is uncommon with short courses of treatment, and can always be controlled. Before giving latamoxef, the prophylactic administration of vitamin K (10 mg per week) is recommended. The prothrombin time should be measured every second day during therapy. The risk of bleeding disorders is increased in patients with renal insufficiency, disturbed liver function, gastrointestinal disorders or during total parenteral nutrition. In such cases, other tests should also be performed (bleeding time, platelet count and platelet aggregation). When bleeding occurs, treatment with latamoxef should be discontinued; fresh frozen plasma, prothrombin complex or platelet concentrate may be given. Latamoxef may cause alcohol intolerance (see p. 68).

Interactions: The concurrent administration of heparin, oral anticoagulants, salicylates and other drugs which affect coagulation increases the risk of bleeding diatheses.

Indications: Use should be restricted to severe infections due to agents resistant to other, better tolerated antibiotics. Suitable for intra-abdominal and gynaecological bacterial infections of unknown origin, lung abscesses and aspiration pneumonia, which are often mixed infections with gram-positive or gram-negative bacteria, including fusobacteria and bacteroides. Latamoxef has been used in clinical trials for the treatment of meningitis caused by gram-negative bacilli (enterobacteria).

Daily dose: 2–4 g for adults, 50–100 mg/kg for children. Where the creatinine clearance is 5–25 ml/min, no more than 1.25 g should be given every 12 h; for a creatinine clearance less than 5 ml/min, give 1 g every 24 h.

Preparations: Vials of 1 g and 2 g.

Summary: Because of the particular risk of bleeding, other suitable cephalosporins are usually preferable to latamoxef.

References

Baxter, J. G., D. A. Marble, L. R. Whitfield et al.: Clinical risk factors for prolonged PT/PTT in abdominal sepsis patients treated with moxalactam or tobramycin plus clindamycin. Ann. Surg. *201:* 96 (1984).
Joehl, R., D. Rasbach, J. Ballard et al.: Moxalactam: Evaluation of clinical bleeding in patients with abdominal infection. Arch. Surg. *118:* 1259–1261 (1983).
Keyserling, H., W. E. Feldman, S. Moffitt et al.: Clinical and pharmacokinetic evaluation of parenteral moxalactam in infants and children. Antimicrob. Ag. Chemother. *21:* 898 (1982).
Lee, S., S. Spira, E. P. Gabor: Coagulopathy associated with moxalactam. JAMA *249:* 2019 (1983).
Lipsky, J. J., J. C. Lewis, W. J. Novick Jr.: Production of hypoprothrombinemia by moxalactam and 1-methyl-5-thiotetrazole in rats. Antimicrob. Ag. Chemother. *25:* 380 (1984).
Manthey, K. F., U. Ullmann: Studies on lamoxactam penetration into the aqueous humor of the human eye. Infection *11:* 210–211 (1983).
Pakter, R., T. Russell, H. Mielke et al.: Coagulopathy associated with the use of moxalactam. JAMA *248:* 1100 (1982).
Panwalker, A. P., J. Rosenfeld: Hemorrhage, diarrhea and superinfection associated with the use of moxalactam. J. Infect. Dis. *147:* 171 (1983).
Peters, G. R., C. M. Metzler: The effects of cefmetazole and latamoxef on platelet function in healthy human volunteers. J. Antimicrob. Chemother. *23 (Suppl. D):* 119–123 (1989).
Smith, Cr., J. Lipsky: Hypoprothrombinemia and platelet dysfunction caused by cephalosporin and oxalactam antibiotics. J. Antimicrob. Chemother. *11:* 496–499 (1983).
Whitekamp, M. R., G. M. Caputo, H. A. B. Al-Mondhiry, R. C. Aber: The effects of latamoxef, cefotaxime, and cefoperazone on platelet function and coagulation in normal volunteers. J. Antimicrob. Chemother. *16:* 95 (1985).
Whitekamp, M. R., R. C. Aber: Prolonged bleeding time and bleeding diathesis associated with moxalactam administration. JAMA *249:* 69–71 (1983).

ε) Flomoxef

Properties: Flomoxef differs from the other α-methoxy cephalosporins (cephamycins) by the introduction of a difluoromethyl-thioacetamide group in the 7-β position. Flomoxef has, like latamoxef, an oxygen atom in place of the sulphur atom in the cephem nucleus.

The **spectrum of activity** is almost identical with that of latamoxef. Flomoxef is as active as latamoxef, and much more active than cefoxitin and cefotetan, against Bacteroides fragilis (Table 8). Flomoxef is more active than the other cephamycins against other anaerobes and is effective as a single agent against Clostridium difficile (at concentrations of 6.2 mg/l). Like cefazolin, flomoxef has good antistaphylococcal activity. Like latamoxef, flomoxef is active against Branhamella catarrhalis and Bordetella pertussis at lower concentrations than other cephalosporins. Activity against intestinal gram-negative bacteria is good, but less than that of cefotaxime.

Table 8. Mean minimal inhibitory concentrations (MIC) of flomoxef (FL), cefoxitin (CX), cefotetan (CT) and latamoxef (LT) in anaerobes. After SIMON C. et al., Infection 16: 13 (1988)

Species	MIC 50% (mg/l)			
	FL	CX	CT	LT
Clostridium perfringens	0.8	1.6	1.6	0.2
Clostridium difficile	6.2	>100.0	25.0	50.0
Fusobacterium necrophorum	0.02	0.1	0.01	0.04
Fusobacterium fusiforme (nucleatum)	0.2	0.4	0.2	0.4
Eubacterium lentum	3.1	25.0	25.0	25.0
Peptostreptococcus asaccharolyticus	0.05	0.1	0.4	0.2
Peptostreptococcus anaerobius	0.2	0.8	3.1	1.6
Bacteroides fragilis	0.8	12.5	6.2	0.8
Bacteroides thetaiotaomicron	0.4	50.0	50.0	6.2
Bacteroides vulgatus	6.2	25.0	50.0	6.2
Bacteroides ovatus	6.2	50.0	100.0	50.0
Bacteroides eggerthii	1.6	3.1	25.0	0.8
Bacteroides bivius	>100.0	50.0	100.0	>100.0
Veillonella parvula	0.01	0.4	0.1	1.6

Pharmacokinetics: Mean serum concentrations of 40 mg/l are found after a short i.v. infusion of 1 g in 60 min. *Half-life:* 1 h. *Urinary recovery:* 90% (unchanged).

Side-effects are as for other cephalosporins (skin reactions etc.). No bleeding or coagulation disorders. No alcohol intolerance.

Use: Flomoxef has been the subject of numerous clinical trials in which it was clinically effective in 85% of patients with endometritis, Bartholin's abscess, adnexitis, pelvic peritonitis and pyometra, and in 65% of complicated urinary infections. An 80% cure rate was found in postoperative wound infections. Flomoxef has the advantages of latamoxef without the frequent side-effects. It is not licensed in Britain at present.

References

MATSUDA, S., M. SUZUKI: 6315-S (flomoxef) in obstetrics and gynecology. Chemotherapy 35: 1189–1195 (1987).
MATSUMOTO, T., S. KITADA: Clinical experience with 6315-S (flomoxef) in urinary tract infection. Chemotherapy 35: 1102–1120 (1987).

Neu, H. C., N.-X. Chin: In vitro activity and β-lactamase stability of a new difluoro oxacephem, 6315-S. Antimicrobial Ag. Chemother. *30:* 638–644 (1986).
Sagawa, T., K. Mure: 6315-S (flomoxef) in obstetrics and gynecology. Chemotherapy *30:* 1164–1171 (1987).
Simon, C., M. Simon, C. Plieth: In vitro activity of flomoxef in comparison to other cephalosporins. Infection *16:* 131 (1988).

d) Cefotaxime Group (Aminothiazole Cephalosporins)

Proprietary names:
for *cefotaxime:* Claforan;
for *ceftriaxone:* Rocephin;
for *ceftizoxime:* Cefizox, Ceftiz;
for *cefmenoxime:* Bestcall, Tacef;
for *ceftazidime:* Fortum.

Properties: The aminothiazole cephalosporins have an extended spectrum, excellent activity against enterobacteria and variable activity against Pseudomonas aeruginosa. This improvement has been achieved by coupling the aminothiazole side-chain of cefotiam with the oxime side-chain of cefuroxime. *Cefotaxime* is the parent compound of the group.

Ceftriaxone, ceftizoxime and *cefmenoxime* are chemical analogues of cefotaxime with substitution at position R_2 (Fig. 19) which gives different pharmacokinetics but the same activity. Ccftizoxime is the non-substituted derivative of cefotaxime. *Cefmenoxime* has the same methyltetrazole side-chain as cefamandole and cefoperazone. *Ceftazidime* has a carboxypropioimino group.

Mode of action: There are certain differences in β-lactamase stability, in the ability to penetrate the bacterial cell wall and in affinity for the so-called penicillin binding proteins (PBP) within this group, which are related to differences in structural formula.

Spectrum of activity: Very similar within the cefotaxime group and much broader than that of the other cephalosporins. Unlike the other cephalosporins, all agents in the cefotaxime group are effective even at very low concentrations against Haemophilus influenzae (ampicillin-sensitive and -resistant strains).

The **activity** varies according to the species of bacteria (Table 9). Of these cephalosporins, *cefotaxime* and analogous antibiotics are most active against Klebsiella pneumoniae and Proteus vulgaris. Ceftazidime is also relatively more active against Enterobacter cloacae. All cefotaxime derivatives are less active than

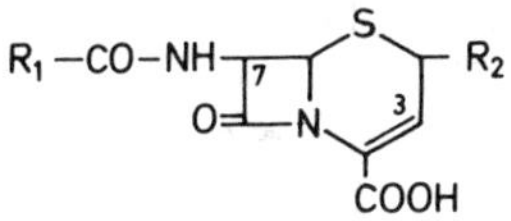

2. Cephalosporins

R₁—CO—NH— [β-lactam core with S, N, COOH] —R₂

Generic Name	R_1	R_2
Cefotaxime	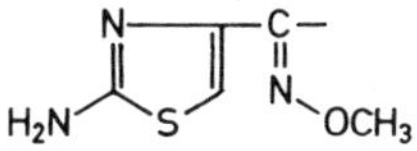 2-aminothiazol-4-yl with =N-OCH₃ (H₂N–thiazole–C(=N-OCH₃)–)	$-CH_2-OCOCH_3$
Ceftizoxime	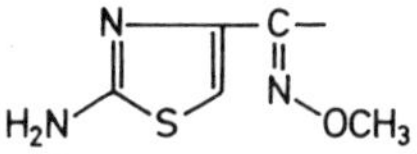 2-aminothiazol-4-yl with =N-OCH₃	$-H$
Cefmenoxime	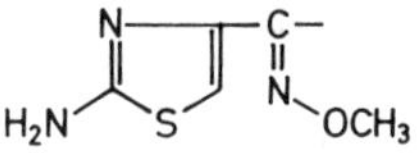 2-aminothiazol-4-yl with =N-OCH₃	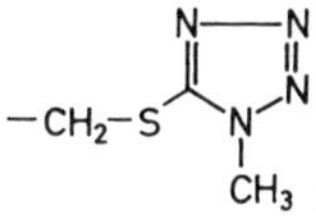 $-CH_2-S-$ (1-methyltetrazol-5-yl)
Ceftriaxone	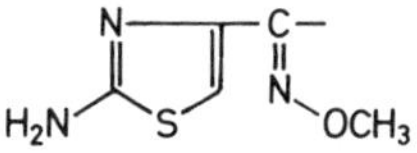 2-aminothiazol-4-yl with =N-OCH₃	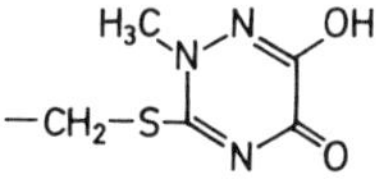 $-CH_2-S-$ (2-methyl-5,6-dioxo-1,2,4-triazin-3-yl with OH)
Ceftazidime	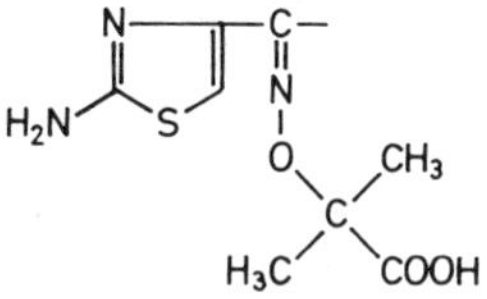 2-aminothiazol-4-yl with =N-O-C(CH₃)(CH₃)-COOH	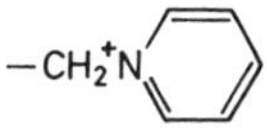 $-CH_2\overset{+}{N}$(pyridinium)
Cefoperazone	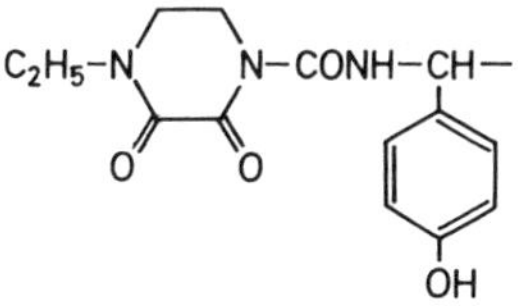 C_2H_5–N(piperazine-2,3-dione)–N–CONH–CH–(4-hydroxyphenyl)–	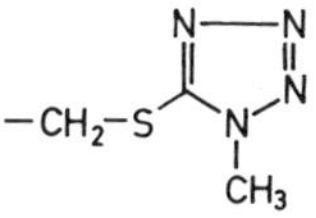 $-CH_2-S-$ (1-methyltetrazol-5-yl)

Fig. 19. Structural formulae of the newer cephalosporins.

Table 9. Differences of *in vitro* activity in members of the cefotaxime group in comparison with other cephalosporins. E. = Enterobacter, Staph. = Staphylococcus, Strept. = Streptococcus.

Agent	*In vitro* activity	
	relatively good	relatively poor
Cefotaxime Ceftriaxone Ceftizoxime Cefmenoxime	Klebsiella Proteus vulgaris	Pseudomonas Acinetobacter
Ceftazidime	Pseudomonas Acinetobacter E. cloacae Proteus vulgaris	Staph. aureus
Latamoxef	Bacteroides fragilis E. cloacae Citrobacter	Pseudomonas Staph. aureus Strept. viridans
Cefazolin Cefazedone	Staph. aureus Staph. epidermidis	Enterobacteriaceae

Table 10. Activity against Staphylococcus aureus of cephalosporins of the cefotaxime group in comparison with latamoxef, cefoperazone and cephalothin. GM = geometrical mean of minimal inhibitory concentrations (mg/l), MIC_{50} and MIC_{90} = minimal inhibitory concentrations at ≤50% or ≤90% of the strains examined.

Antibiotic	GM	MIC_{50}	MIC_{90}
Cefotaxime	2.0	1.6	3.1
Ceftriaxone	4.1	3.1	6.2
Ceftazidime	6.8	4.0	8.0
Ceftizoxime	2.0	1.5	3.1
Cefmenoxime	2.0	1.6	3.1
Latamoxef	10.0	8.0	16.0
Cefoperazone	3.8	3.1	6.2
Cephalothin	0.2	0.1	0.4

cephalothin against staphylococci (Table 10), and are inactive against oxacillin- and cephalothin-resistant staphylococci. Ceftizoxime is only slightly active against pseudomonas. Ceftazidime (p. 313) is the most active of the cephalosporins against Pseudomonas aeruginosa and acinetobacter. The differences of clinical relevance are also listed in Tables 27 and 28 (p. 308), which include the minimal inhibitory concentrations for 50% and 90% of the strains examined. As the percentage of resistant strains for each drug is continually changing, a combination should be used to cover gaps in the spectrum.

Combinations with an aminoglycoside (gentamicin, tobramycin) are often synergistic against sensitive bacteria. Combinations with an acylaminopenicillin are either synergistic or additive.

Resistance: Primary resistance is seen in enterococci, listeria, campylobacter, Clostridium difficile, Legionella pneumophila, mycoplasma and chlamydiae. Secondary resistance is uncommon (except against ceftazidime in pseudomonas strains). Partial cross-resistance occurs between the basic and intermediate groups of cephalosporins in gram-negative bacilli. Complete cross-resistance is found with methicillin-resistant strains of Staphylococcus aureus. Ampicillin-resistant strains of Haemophilus spp. and penicillin-resistant gonococci are sensitive to all the cephalosporins of the cefotaxime group (but not to cephalothin).

Pharmacokinetics: *Not absorbed* by mouth. After i.v. injection of 1 g (Table 11 and Fig. 20), the *serum levels* after 1 h are highest with ceftriaxone and lower with ceftazidime, ceftizoxime, cefmenoxime and cefotaxime. The *concentrations* are still relatively high after 6 h with ceftriaxone, while they decline to 5 mg/l, 2 mg/l, 1 mg/l and 0.3 mg/l with ceftazidime, ceftizoxime, cefmenoxime and cefotaxime, respectively. After 12 h the *serum concentrations* of ceftriaxone are 30 mg/l, whereas ceftizoxime, cefmenoxime and cefotaxime are undetectable. There are corresponding differences in concentration between the individual antibiotics in short i.v. infusion, continuous i.v. infusion and i.m. injection.

The *half-life* is 7–8 h with ceftriaxone, 110 min with ceftazidime, 70 min with ceftizoxime and cefmenoxime and 60 min with cefotaxime (Table 12). *Plasma protein binding* is 97% with ceftriaxone (in concentrations up to 150 mg/l), 60%

Table 11. Mean serum concentrations of aminothiazole cephalosporins in comparison with other cephalosporins after i.v. injection of 1 g.

Antibiotic	Serum concentration (mg/l) after			
	1 h	4 h	6 h	12 h
Cefotaxime	12	1.1	0.3	0
Ceftriaxone	120	65	50	30
Ceftazidime	40	10	5	0.6
Ceftizoxime	30	5	2	0
Cefmenoxime	25	4	1	0
Latamoxef	65	16	9	0.9
Cefoperazone	58	14	7	1.0

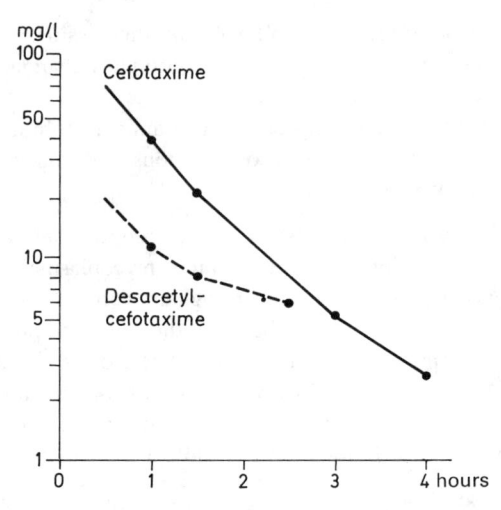

Fig. 20. Mean serum level of cefotaxime and desacetyl cefotaxime after i. v. injection of 2 g in 10 healthy adult volunteers (own data).

with cefmenoxime and less than 50% with the other members of this group. All members of this group diffuse quite well into tissues, but poorly into the CSF when the meninges are not inflamed. Therapeutically effective CSF concentrations for purulent meningitis are achievable, particularly with cefotaxime.

Urinary output of active agent in the first 24 h: 50% with cefotaxime, 40–60% with ceftriaxone, 70–80% with ceftizoxime and cefmenoxime and 80–90% with ceftazidime. The biliary concentrations are generally higer than the serum levels.

Table 12. Pharmacokinetic data for aminothiazole cephalosporins in comparison with other cephalosporins.

Antibiotic	Half-life (min)	Plasma protein binding (%)	Urinary recovery (%)	Tubular secretion	Biliary excretion
Cefotaxime	60	40	50	+	(+)
Ceftriaxone	385–480	97	40–60	∅	++
Ceftazidime	110	10	80	∅	(+)
Ceftizoxime	70	30	80	∅	(+)
Cefmenoxime	70	60	80	∅	(+)
Latamoxef	130	40	75	∅	(+)
Cefoperazone	110	90	25	(?)	++

Ceftriaxone is excreted through the biliary tract into the intestine to a much greater extent than the other members of the group. Approximately ⅓ of the dose of cefotaxime is metabolised in the body, which explains the relatively low serum concentrations. The metabolites detected have been desacetyl cefotaxime, which has reduced antibacterial activity, and 2 inactive lactones. Small quantities of metabolites have also been detected with ceftriaxone and ceftizoxime in animals. The renal excretion of cefotaxime is also by tubular secretion, so probenecid increases the serum concentrations. Excretion of the other members of this group is predominantly by glomerular filtration. In *renal failure,* the half-life of ceftriaxone and cefotaxime is less prolonged than that of the other antibiotics of this group.

Side-effects: Similar to the other parenteral cephalosporins. Good renal tolerance. Disorders of coagulation with prolongation of the prothrombin time have occasionally been reported with cefmenoxime, so the bleeding time should be checked every 2–3 days in patients with a bleeding tendency. With ceftriaxone, changes in density are occasionally seen on ultrasonography of the gall bladder, which resolve when the antibiotic is discontinued (pseudocholelithiasis). If pain develops symptomatic measures are recommended.

Interactions: When cefmenoxime is given at the same time as high-dose heparin or oral anticoagulants, bleeding and coagulation indices should be frequently and regularly checked. This also applies to the simultaneous administration of substances which can interfere with platelet function.

Alcohol intake after a dose of cefmenoxime can give rise to increased acetaldehyde concentrations, resulting in skin flushes, sweating, hypotension, tachycardia, vomiting, headache and giddiness. This can also occur as a late reaction up to 72 h after the antibiotic dose. To avoid this Antabuse- (disulfiram-) like effect, alcohol should be avoided for at least 2–4 days after treatment. Beware of infusion solutions containing alcohol.

Indications:
1. *Initial therapy* of severe, life-threatening infections (sepsis, pneumonia, osteomyelitis, wound and tissue infections), particularly when defences are impaired by severe underlying disease or when multi-resistant gram-negative bacilli may be present. May be used for the initial therapy of urinary infections in urological surgery, where multi-resistant bacteria occur more often. If Bacteroides fragilis is suspected, combine with metronidazole. Always combine these agents in severe systemic infections, either with an aminoglycoside or with an acylaminopenicillin.
2. Treatment of severe generalised or local infections (pneumonia, pyelonephritis, cholangitis) *due to cefazolin-resistant bacteria,* which are also insensitive to the acylaminopenicillins.

3. Severe infections in patients with *penicillin allergy* (cross-sensitivity should be excluded prior to therapy).
4. Other indications are typhoid fever, salmonella septicaemia, meningitis, neuroborreliosis.
5. Infections with Pseudomonas aeruginosa (use ceftazidime).

Inappropriate uses: Less severe bacterial infections and those which would be expected to respond to benzylpenicillin, amoxycillin, cefazolin, cefazedone or cefuroxime.

Contra-indication: Allergy to cephalosporins.

Administration and dosage: Preferably 2–3 times a day as a short i.v. infusion (20–30 min) or slow i.v. injection (5 min). Continuous i.v. infusion is also possible. I.m. injection may be painful; if necessary, dissolve in 0.5% lignocaine solution and do not exceed a dose of 1 g. Daily dose according to severity of infection: 2–4 g (50–100 mg/kg for children). Highest dose (e.g. for meningitis): 6 g a day for adults, 200 mg/kg for children. With *ceftriaxone*, 2 g every 24 h may be sufficient.

When renal function is severely impaired (creatinine clearance <5 ml/min), 0.5 g of cefotaxime is given every 12 h. With *ceftazidime,* the patient should receive 1 g every 12 h for a creatinine clearance of 31–50 ml/min, 1 g every 24 h for a creatinine clearance of 16–30 ml/min, and for creatinine clearance of 6–15 and <5, 0.5 g every 24 h or 48 h respectively. With ceftriaxone, normal dosage is possible.

Preparations: Ampoules of 500 mg, 1 g and 2 g.

Summary: This group of cephalosporins has been a major advance in therapy because of their considerably improved activity and extension of their spectrum.

Anti-pseudomonal activity is incomplete with most members of this group and the activity against staphylococci is generally less than with cephalothin. For life-threatening infections with unknown organisms, the remaining gaps in the spectrum (anaerobes, enterococci, Pseudomonas etc.) should be covered with another antibiotic.

Cefotaxime and ceftriaxone are preferable for blind therapy of life-threatening infections because of their good clinical efficacy and tolerance. Ceftazidime should be reserved for proven or suspected pseudomonas infections.

References

ASMAR, B. I., M. C. THIRUMOORTHI, J. A. BUCKLEY et al.: Cefotaxime diffusion into cerebrospinal fluid of children with meningitis. Antimicrob. Ag. Chemother. *28:* 138 (1985).

BILLSTEIN, S. A., T. E. SUDOL: Ceftriaxone-associated neutropenia (letter). Am. J. Med. *88:* 701–702 (1990).

BLACK, A. S., J. COHEN: Multiple beta-lactam resistance in Enterobacter cloacae following ceftazidime monotherapy. Lancet *2:* 331 (1985).

DAGAN, R. et al.: Outpatient treatment of serious community-acquired pediatric infections using once-daily intramuscular ceftriaxone. Pediatr. Infect. Dis. J. *6:* 1080 (1987).

FRENKEL, L. D., and the Multicenter Ceftriaxone Pediatric Study Group. Once-daily administration of ceftriaxone for the treatment of selected serious bacterial infections in children. Pediatrics *82:* 486 (1988).

DRUSANO, G. L., J. JOSHI, A. FORREST et al.: Pharmacokinetics of ceftazidime, alone or in combination with piperacillin or tobramycin, in the sera of cancer patients. Antimicrob. Ag. Chemother. *27:* 605 (1985).

GAMBERTOGLIO, J. G., D. P. ALEXANDER, S. L. BARRIERE: Cefmenoxime pharmacokinetics in healthy volunteers and subjects with renal insufficiency and on hemodialysis. Antimicrob. Ag. Chemother. *26:* 845 (1984).

GOLD, T. et al.: Controlled trial of ceftazidime vs. ticarcillin and tobramycin in the treatment of acute respiratory exacerbations in patients with cystic fibrosis. Pediatr. Infect. Dis. *4:* 172 (1985).

GUNDERT-REMY, U. G., R. HILDEBRANDT, A. STIEHL, P. SCHLEGEL: Pharmacokinetics of ceftizoxime. Eur. J. Clin. Pharmacol. *28:* 463 (1985).

HIGHAM, M., F. M. CUNNINGHAM, D. W. TEELE: Ceftriaxone administered once or twice a day for treatment of bacterial infections of childhood. Pediatr. Infect. Dis. *4:* 22 (1985).

HOOGKAMP-KORSTANJE, J. A. A.: Activity of cefotaxime and ceftriaxone alone and in combination with penicillin, ampicillin and piperacillin against neonatal meningitis pathogens. J. Antimicrob. Chemother. *16:* 327 (1985).

HÖFFKEN, G., H. LODE, P. KOEPPE, M. RUHNKE, K. BORNER: Pharmacokinetics of cefotaxime and desacetyl-cefotaxime in cirrhosis of the liver. Chemotherapy *30:* 7 (1984).

HUDSON, S. J., H. R. INGHAM: Ceftazidime for Pseudomonas meningitis. Lancet *1:* 464 (1985).

JACOBS, R. F.: Ceftriaxone-associated cholecystitis. Pediatr. Infect. Dis. J. *7:* 434 (1988).

KARACHALIOS, G. N., A. N. GEORGIOPOULOS, S. KANATAKIS: Treatment of various infections in an outpatient practice by intramuscular ceftriaxone: home parenteral therapy. Chemotherapy *35:* 389–392 (1989).

KEARNS, G. L., R. E. JACOBS, B. R. THOMAS, T. L. DARVILLE, J. M. TRANG: Cefotaxime and desacetylcefotaxime pharmacokinetics in very low birth weight neonates. J. Pediatr. *114:* 461–468 (1989).

LJUNGBERG, B., I. NILSSON-EHLE: Advancing age and acute infection influence the kinetics of ceftazidime. Scand. J. Infect. Dis. *21:* 327–332 (1989).

LJUNGBERG, B., I. NILSSON-EHLE: Pharmacokinetics of ceftazidime in elderly patients and young volunteers. Scand. J. Infect. Dis. *16:* 325 (1984).

MOSKOVITZ, B. L.: Clinical adverse effects during ceftriaxone therapy. Am. J. Med. *77 (4C):* 84 (1984).

MULHALL, A., J. DE LOUVOIS: The pharmacokinetics and safety of ceftazidime in the neonate. J. Antimicrob. Chemother. *15:* 97 (1985).

NAHATA, M. C., M. A. MILLER: Diarrhoea associated with ceftriaxone and its implications in paediatric patients. J. Clin. Pharm. Ther. *14:* 305–307 (1989).

NAQVI, S. H., M. A. MAXWELL, L. M. DUNKLE: Cefotaxime therapy of neonatal Gram-negative bacillary meningitis. Ped. Infect. Dis. *4:* 499 (1985).

PATEL, I. H., S. A. KAPLAN: Pharmacokinetic profile of ceftriaxone in man. Am. J. Med. *77 (4C):* 17 (1984).

QUENTIN, C. D., R. ANSORG: Penetration of cefotaxime into the aqueous humor of the human eye after intravenous application. Graefe's Arch. clin. exp. Ophthalmol. *220:* 245 (1983).
RICHARDS, D. M., R. N. BROGDEN: Ceftazidime: a review of its antibacterial activity, pharmacokinetic properties and therapeutic use. Drugs *29:* 105 (1985).
RODRIGUEZ, W. J. et al: Treatment of Pseudomonas meningitis with ceftazidime with or without concurrent therapy. Pediatr. Infect. Dis. J. *9:* 83 (1990).
SIMON, C.: In vitro activity of ceftazidime combined with other antibiotics. Infection *13:* 58 (1985).
SPRITZER, R., H. J. V. D. KAMP, G. DZOLJIC, P. J. SAUER: Five years of cefotaxime use in a neonatal intensive care unit. Pediatr. Infect. Dis. J. *9:* 92–96 (1990).
TANSINO, G. F., M. R. HAMMERSCHLAG, B. L. CONGENI et al.: Clinical efficacy and safety of cefmenoxime in children. Antimicrob. Ag. Chemother. *28:* 508 (1985).
TRANG, J. M., R. F. JACOBS, G. L. KEARNS et al.: Cefotaxime and desacetylcefotaxime pharmacokinetics in infants and children with meningitis. Antimicrob. Ag. Chemother. *28:* 791 (1985).

e) Other Parenteral Cephalosporins

α) Cefsulodin

Proprietary name: Monaspor.

Properties: A semi-synthetic cephalosporin (carbamoyl-cephalosporin, Fig. 16, p. 64). Readily water-soluble as the sodium salt.

Antibacterial activity: Greatest against Pseudomonas aeruginosa, including ticarcillin- and gentamicin-resistant strains. *Resistance* to pseudomonas occurs in 1–3% only. Synergy in combination with aminoglycosides is frequently found, as is additive activity in combination with an anti-pseudomonal β-lactam antibiotic.

Staphylococci, pneumococci and gonococci are inhibited at concentrations between 0.5 and 4 mg/l but most gram-negative bacilli other than pseudomonas are insensitive.

Pharmacokinetics: After i.v. injection of 500 mg, 1 g and 2 g, the mean serum concentrations are 20, 40 and 60 mg/l (1 h). *A serum concentration* of 100 mg/l is achieved after a short i.v. infusion of 2 g (30 min). *Half-life:* 1½ h. *Plasma protein binding:* 30%. *Urine recovery:* 90%. *Tissue diffusion* good.

Side-effects: Similar to other parenteral cephalosporins. Renal function should be closely monitored, particularly when cefsulodin is combined with an aminoglycoside.

Indications: Proven pseudomonas infections of the respiratory and urinary tracts, skin and bone, preferably in combination with an aminoglycoside. Combination with another cephalosporin or a penicillin without risk of antagonism is possible.

Administration and dosage: Preferably by short i.v. infusion over 30 min. Slow i.v. injection is also possible. Dissolve in 0.5% lignocaine solution for i.m. injection. 2–3(–6) g a day for *adults*, 50(–100) mg/kg for *children*, in 2–3 divided doses. Do not exceed a *maximum dose* of 6 g a day.

Preparations: Vials of 500 mg, 1 g and 2 g.

Summary: A highly effective antibiotic for infections with Pseudomonas aeruginosa, but with no activity against other gram-negative bacilli. For specific treatment, combine with an aminoglycoside.

References

CABEZUDO, I., R. L. THOMPSON, R. F. SELDEN et al.: Cefsulodin sodium therapy in cystic fibrosis patients. Antimicrob. Ag. Chemother. *25:* 4 (1984).
FURUSAWA, T., T. UETE, T. KAWADA et al.: Resistance to cefsulodin and gentamicin in Pseudomonas aeruginosa strains in five areas of Japan between 1980 and 1983. J. Antimicrob. Chemother. *17:* 755 (1986).
GIBSON, T. P. et al.: Kinetics of cefsulodin in patients with renal impairment. Rev. Infect. Dis. *6:* 689 (1984).
MATZKE, G. R., W. F. KEANE: Cefsulodin pharmacokinetics in patients with various degrees of renal function. Antimicrob. Ag. Chemother. *23:* 369 (1983).
POTTAGE, J. C. Jr., P. H. KARAKUSIS, G. M. TRENHOLME: Cefsulodin therapy for osteomyelitis due to Pseudomonas aeruginosa. Rev. Infect. Dis. *6 (Suppl. 3):* 728 (1984).

β) Cefoperazone

Proprietary name: Cefobid.

Activity: An acylamino-cephalosporin (Fig. 19, p. 81) with better activity against Pseudomonas aeruginosa than cefotaxime but less activity than ceftazidime. Spectrum of activity similar to cefotaxime. Cefoperazone has little activity against Acinetobacter calcoaceticus and Enterobacter cloacae.

Pharmacokinetics are less favourable than for the cefotaxime group. Urinary excretion of active agent is only 20–25%.

Serum concentrations (after 1 g i.v.): Table 11, p. 83. *Half-life:* 110 min; *plasma protein binding:* 90%. Excretion is predominantly biliary, into the intestinal tract.

When liver function is severely impaired, the half-life is prolonged 3–4 times, the extrarenal clearance reduced to ⅛, and urinary excretion is three times as great.

Side-effects: As for other cephalosporins but diarrhoea has been reported in 20–30% of cases and bleeding diatheses (caused by hypoprothrombinaemia and/or disorders of platelet function) are relatively frequent. Because of these side-effects and lower intrinsic activity, cefoperazone is inferior to the broad-spectrum aminothiazole cephalosporins such as cefotaxime, and may cause alcohol intolerance (see also p. 68).

Daily dose: 2–4 g for adults, 50–100 mg/kg for children.

Preparations: Vials of 500 mg, 1 g and 2 g.

References

ANDRIOLE, V. T., W. M. M. KIRBY: Overview/introduction: Cefoperazone. Am. J. Med. *85* (Suppl. 1A): 1 (1988).
CABLE, D., G. OVERTURF, G. EDRALIN: Concentrations of cefoperazone in cerebrospinal fluid during bacterial meningitis. Antimicrob. Ag. Chemother. *23:* 688 (1983).
CARLBERG, H., K. ALESTIG, C. E. NORD, B. TROLLFORS: Intestinal side-effects of cefoperazone. J. Antimicrob. Chemother. *10:* 483 (1982).
GREENFIELD, R. A., A. U. GERBER, W. A. CRAIG: Pharmacokinetics of cefoperazone in patients with normal and impaired hepatic and renal function. Rev. Infect. Dis. *5 (Suppl. 1):* 127 (1983).
LEUNG, J. W., R. C. CHAN, S. W. CHEUNG, J. Y. SUNG, S. C. CHUNG, G. L. FRENCH: The effect of obstruction on the biliary excretion of cefoperazone and ceftazidime. J. Antimicrob. Chemother. *25:* 399–406 (1990).
ROSENFELD, W. N., H. E. EVANS, R. BATHEJA et al.: Pharmacokinetics of cefoperazone in full-term and premature neonates. Antimicrob. Ag. Chemother. *23:* 866 (1983).

γ) Ceforanide

Proprietary name: Precef (not marketed in UK or Germany).

Spectrum of activity: Similar to that of cefamandole. In vitro less active than cefamandole and cefuroxime against staphylococci and Haemophilus influenzae and less active than cefoxitin against anaerobes.

Pharmacokinetics: Half-life 3 h (prolonged in renal insufficiency). Mainly excreted by the kidneys (unchanged).

Indications and dosage: Effective in community-acquired pneumonia and urinary tract infection. Daily dosage 2 g (in two divided doses), in children 40 mg/kg.

Summary: Ceforanide is less active than many other cephalosporins and unreliable in haemophilus infection.

References

BARRY, A. L., R. N. JONES, R. R. PACKER: Antistaphylococcal activity of ceforanide and cefonicid in the presence of human serum. Antimicrob. Ag. Chemother; *29:* 147 (1986).
Medical Letter. Ceforanide (Precef). Med. Lett. Drugs Ther. *26:* 91 (1984).

δ) Cefpirome

Cefpirome (Fig. 21) is a cefotaxime derivative with increased activity against Pseudomonas aeruginosa, Enterobacter cloacae, acinetobacter, Citrobacter species and staphylococci. It is also active against Enterococcus faecalis and E. faecium, but is inactive against Xanthomonas maltophilia and some Bacteroides species. Gram-positive anaerobes are generally susceptible, as are fusobacteria. Cefpirome is still under evaluation. The clinical position is not yet decided.

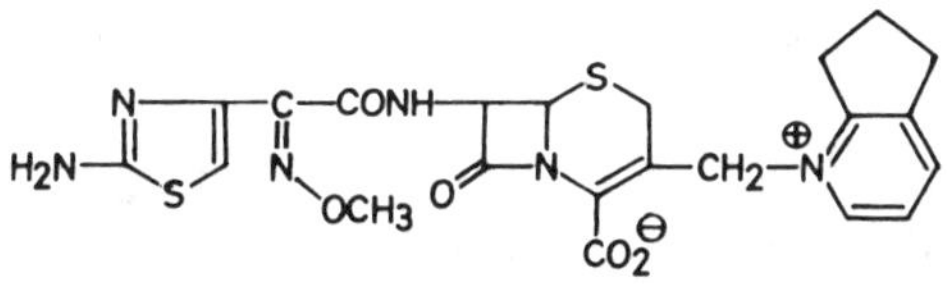

Fig. 21. Structural formula of cefpirome.

References

ENG, R. H. K., C. E. CHERUBIN, S. M. SMITH: In-vitro and in-vivo activity of cefpirome (HR 810) against methicillin-susceptible and -resistant Staphylococcus aureus and Streptococcus faecalis. J. Antimicrob. Chemother. 23: 373–381 (1989).
GOLDSTEIN, E. J. C., D. M. CITRON: Comparative in vitro inhibitory and killing activity of cefpirome, ceftazidime and cefotaxime against Pseudomonas aeruginosa, enterococci, Staphylococcus epidermidis, and methicillin-susceptible and -resistant and tolerant and nontolerant Staphylococcus aureus. Antimicrob. Ag. Chemother. 28: 160 (1985).
JONES, R. N., E. H. GERLACH: Antimicrobial activity of HR 810 against 419 strict anaerobic bacteria. Antimicrob. Ag. Chemother. 27: 413 (1985).
KAVI, J., J. M. ANDREWS, J. P. ASHBY, G. HILLMANN, R. WISE: Pharmacokinetics and tissue penetration of cefpirome, a new cephalosporin. J. Antimicrob. Chemother. 22: 11–916 (1988).
MAASS, L., V. MALERCZYK, M. VERHO: Pharmacokinetics of cefpirome (HR 810), a new cephalosporin derivative administered intramuscularly and intravenously to healthy volunteers. Infection 15: 207 (1987).
ROLSTON, K., M. E. ALVAREZ, J. F. HOY, B. LE BLANC, D. H. HO, G. P. BODEY: Comparative in vitro activity of cefpirome and other antimicrobial agents against isolates from cancer patients. Chemotherapy 32: 344–351 (1986).
VERHO, M., L. MAASS, V. MALERCZYK, H. GRÖTSCH: Renal tolerance of cefpirome (HR 810), a new cephalosporin antibotic. Infection 15: 215 (1987).

f) Older Oral Cephalosporins (Cephalexin Group)

Proprietary names:
for *cephalexin:* Ceporex, Ceporexin, Keflex;
for *cefadroxil:* Duracef, Ultracef, Baxan;
for *cefaclor:* Distaclor;
for *cephradine:* Velosef.

Properties: The chemical structure of cefadroxil differs from cephalexin solely by the addition of a para-hydroxyl group to the aromatic ring, and that of cephadrine by saturation of one of the double bonds in the aromatic ring (Fig. 22). Cefaclor is also very similar to cephalexin, but a methyl group has been replaced by chlorine. All compounds are readily soluble in water and relatively stable; only cefaclor is less stable than cephalexin in aqueous solution.

Spectrum of activity: Largely identical with cefazolin (see p. 63), but less active against some organisms, particularly gram-negative rods. Some strains of Escherichia coli, klebsiella and proteus are resistant. Not active against Enterobacter aerogenes, Serratia marcescens, Pseudomonas aeruginosa, Bacteroides fragilis or enterococci. Little activity against Bordetella pertussis and Haemophilus influenzae. Cefaclor is 4–8 times as active as the other oral

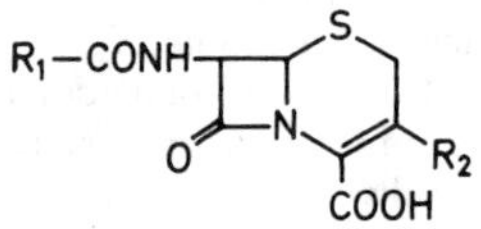

Generic Name	R_1	R_2
Cephalexin	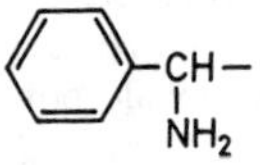 (phenyl)–CH(NH$_2$)–	–CH$_3$
Cephradine	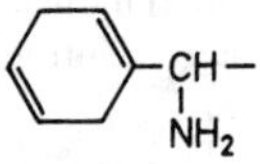 (cyclohexenyl)–CH(NH$_2$)–	–CH$_3$
Cefadroxil	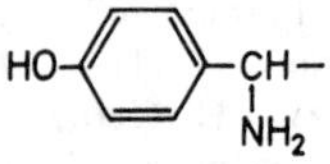 HO–(phenyl)–CH(NH$_2$)–	–CH$_3$
Cefaclor	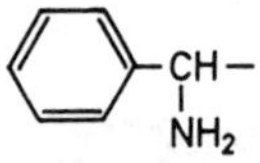 (phenyl)–CH(NH$_2$)–	–Cl

Fig. 22 Structural formulae of the older oral cephalosporins.

cephalosporins against streptococci, pneumococci and sensitive gram-negative bacilli (Escherichia coli, Klebsiella pneumoniae, Proteus mirabilis) and inhibits Haemophilus influenzae (ampicillin-sensitive) at concentrations of 1.6–3.2 mg/l and ampicillin-resistant strains at 3.2–6.4 mg/l. Resistance does not develop rapidly *in vitro* or *in vivo*.

Pharmacokinetics (Fig. 23): With **cephalexin** and **cephradine:** Absorption is largely complete after oral administration with maximal blood concentrations after 1½ hours (cephalexin) and 1 hour (cephradine). *Mean maximal serum concentration* is 24.7 mg/l after 1 g of cephalexin, and 7.5 mg/l after 4 h; after 1 g of cephradine orally, the maximum is 23 mg/l, and the concentration after 4 h 1.5 mg/l. *Half-life* of cephalexin: 60 min; of cephradine: 32 min. *Plasma protein binding:* 12% with cephalexin, 13% with cephradine. *Penetration* of cephalexin and cephradine into purulent bronchial secretions and amniotic fluid is good. At least 90% is excreted unchanged through the kidneys, and some is excreted in the bile.

Maximal serum concentrations after 1 g of **cefadroxil** by mouth are higher (28 mg/l) than after 1 g of cephalexin. Because of the longer half-life (1½ h), the serum concentrations decline more slowly than with cephalexin and the concentra-

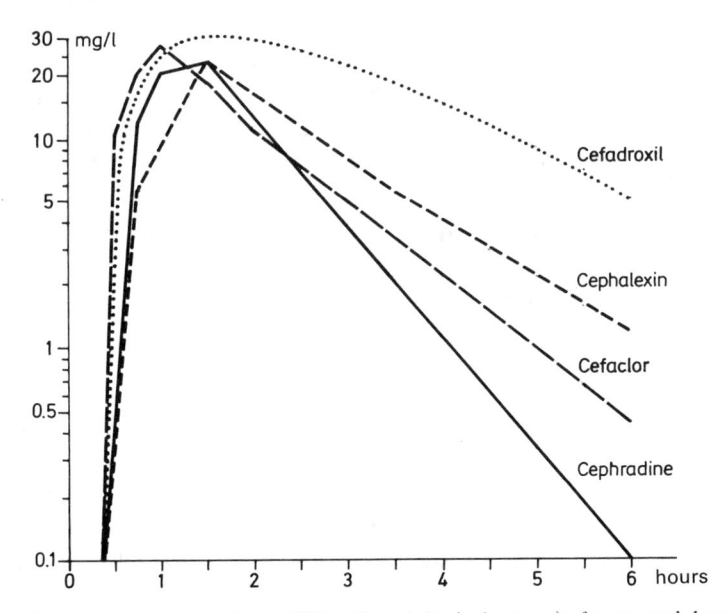

Fig. 23. Mean serum concentration in 10 healthy adults (volunteers) after an oral dose of 1 g cefadroxil (· · · ·), cephalexin (----), cefaclor (---) and cephradine (—), each given 1 h after a standardised breakfast (own data).

tion is 4 times as high after 6 h. *Plasma protein binding:* 20%. *Urinary recovery:* 85%.

Mean serum concentrations of **cefaclor** are 17 mg/l (1 h) and 3.1 mg/l (3 h) after 0.5 g, and 27 mg/l (1 h) and 5.1 mg/l (3 h) after 1 g. *Half-life:* 1 h. *Plasma protein binding:* 50%. *Urinary recovery* (over 8 h): 60%. Partially metabolised in the body.

Side-effects: As with parenteral cephalosporins, and also gastro-intestinal upset (vomiting, diarrhoea) in 1–3%. Transient elevation of serum ALT, AST and alkaline phosphatase can occur with cephalexin, cephradine and cefaclor, but cholestatic jaundice is uncommon.

Indications: Infections of the respiratory and urinary tracts and skin with sensitive bacteria, particularly staphylococci, as well as many strains of Escherichia coli, klebsiella and proteus. Cefaclor is also useful in infections with haemophilus. Prophylaxis of ascending urinary infections.

Inappropriate usage: Severe systemic infections where β-lactamase-stable cephalosporins (e.g. cefotaxime) would be more effective.

Contra-indications: Allergy to cephalosporins.

Administration and dosage: 0.5 (–1) g 3 times a day, 50 (–100) mg/kg for children; with cefadroxil: 1 g twice a day for adults, 50–100 mg/kg twice a day for children. In renal impairment, give the normal adult dose of 1 g at extended intervals, that is, every 24 h for creatinine clearances of 10–25 ml/min, and every 36 h when <10 ml/min. No dose reduction is necessary for cefaclor, because of the relatively small renal excretion.

Preparations:
Cephalexin: Capsules of 250 mg, tablets of 500 mg and 1 g, suspension (50 mg/ml), syrup (50 mg/ml) and drops (100 mg/ml).
Cefadroxil: Capsules of 500 mg, tablets of 1 g, syrup (50 mg/ml) and syrup forte (100 mg/ml).
Cefaclor: Capsules of 250 mg and 500 mg, syrup (25 mg/ml and 50 mg/ml) and drops (50 mg/ml).
Cephradine: Capsules of 500 mg, tablets of 1 g, suspension (50 mg/ml), ampoules of 1 g and 2 g.

Summary: Oral cephalosporins are frequently used and well tolerated in children but they are considerably less active than the β-lactamase-stable parenteral cephalosporins. Cefaclor is distinguished from the other oral cephalosporins by its effectiveness against haemophilus.

References

GINSBURG, C. M.: Comparative pharmacokinetics of cefadroxil, cefaclor, cephalexin and cephradine in infants and children. J. Antimicrob. Chemother. *10 (Suppl. B):* 27 (1982).

LA ROSA, F., S. RIPA, M. PRENNA et al.: Pharmacokinetics of cefadroxil after oral administration in humans. Antimicrob. Ag. Chemother. *21:* 320 (1982).

LEVIN, R. M., P. H. AZIMI, M. G. DUNPHY: Susceptibility of Haemophilus influenzae type b to cefaclor and influence of inoculum size. Antimicrob. Agents Chemother. *22:* 923–925 (1982).

OBERLIN, J. A., D. L. HYSLOP: Cefaclor treatment of upper and lower respiratory tract infections caused by Moraxella catarrhalis. Pediatr. Infect. Dis. J. *9:* 41–44 (1990).

ROTSCHAFER, J. C., K. B. CROSSLEY, T. S. LESAR et al.: Cefaclor pharmacokinetic parameters: serum concentrations determined by a new high-performance liquid chromatographic technique. Antimicrob. Ag. Chemother. *21:* 170 (1982).

SPYKER, D. A., L. L. GOBER, W. M. SCHEID et al.: Pharmacokinetics of cefaclor in renal failure: effects of multiple doses and hemodialysis. Antimicrob. Ag. Chemother. *21:* 278 (1982).

g) Newer Oral Cephalosporins

The older oral cephalosporins are variants of cephalexin, that is, aminocephalosporins with similarities in structure and spectrum of activity and good activity against gram-positive but relatively poor activity against gram-negative organisms. Most have favourable pharmacokinetic properties with little metabolism and a high urinary recovery. The only further development in this group is the carbacephem analogue of cefaclor, loracarbef.

Since 1982, new oral cephalosporins have been found which have much greater activity against gram-negative bacilli. They are generally less active against staphylococci, however, and are incompletely absorbed. Two lines of development have been followed, namely

1. Oral oxime cephalosporins (cefotaxime derivatives), the prototype of which is cefixime. Absorption in this group is also enhanced by the use of a better absorbed ester (e.g. cefetamet).
2. Absorption esters of existing parenteral cephalosporins provide another means of improving oral cephalosporins. The best-developed of these to date are cefuroxime axetil, cefpodoxime proxetil and cefotiam hexetil.

α) Cefixime

Proprietary name: Cephoral, Suprax.

Properties: New oral oxime cephalosporin (cefotaxime derivative, Fig. 24) that is soluble in methanol, ethanol and 0.1 N phosphate buffer (pH 7.0).

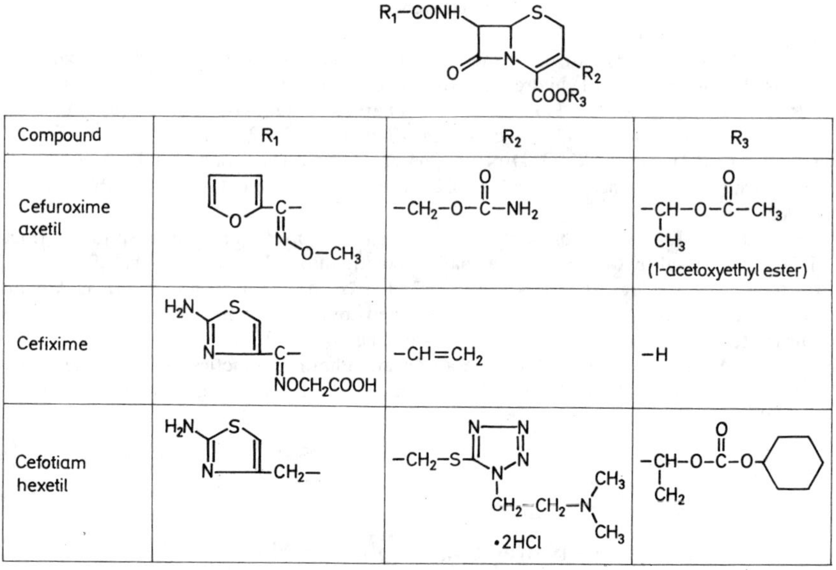

Compound	R₁	R₂	R₃
Cefuroxime axetil	(furan)-C(=NOCH₃)-	$-CH_2-O-\overset{O}{\overset{\|}{C}}-NH_2$	$-CH(CH_3)-O-\overset{O}{\overset{\|}{C}}-CH_3$ (1-acetoxyethyl ester)
Cefixime	H₂N-(thiazole)-C(=NOCH₂COOH)-	$-CH=CH_2$	$-H$
Cefotiam hexetil	H₂N-(thiazole)-CH₂-	$-CH_2-S-$(tetrazole-N)-$CH_2CH_2-N(CH_3)_2$ ·2HCl	$-CH(CH_2)-O-\overset{O}{\overset{\|}{C}}-O-$(cyclohexyl)

Fig. 24. Structural formulae of the newer oral cephalosporins.

Spectrum of activity: Like cefalexin and cefaclor, but much more effective *in vitro* against a variety of species. Cefixime is 6 times more active than cefaclor against Haemophilus influenzae (Tab. 13), 10 times more active against Streptococcus pyogenes (group A streptococci), 30 times more active against Klebsiella pneumoniae and 130 times more active against Proteus mirabilis (Tab. 14).

Table 13. Comparison of the *in-vitro* activities of the older and newer oral cephalosporins as well as of cefuroxime and cefotaxime against Haemophilus influenzae (own data). $MIC_{50\%}$ and $MIC_{90\%}$ = minimal inhibitory concentration for ≤50% and 90% of the strains, respectively.

Drug	Haemophilus influenzae	
	$MIC_{50\%}$	$MIC_{90\%}$
Cephalexin	25	100
Cefaclor	3.1	12.5
Cefixime	0.05	0.4
Cefetamet	0.25	0.5
Cefuroxime	0.8	0.8
Cefotaxime	0.02	0.02

Tab. 14. Comparison of the *in-vitro* activity of older and newer oral cephalosporins with that of cefuroxime and cefotaxime against various gram-negative species. n = number of strains, $MIC_{50\%}$ = minimal inhibitory concentrations for ≤50% of strains.

Species	n	$MIC_{50\%}$			
		Cefixime	Cefetamet	Cefaclor	Cephalexin
E. coli	102	0.1	0.2	0.8	6.2
Enterobacter aerogenes	54	0.2	0.4	1.6	6.2
Enterobacter cloacae	16	1.6	1.6	>100.0	>100.0
Klebsiella pneumoniae	48	0.05	0.2	1.6	6.2
Proteus mirabilis	48	<0.006	0.05	0.8	12.5
Proteus vulgaris	10	0.006	0.1	50.0	50.0
Yersinia enterocolitica	26	0.2	0.4	3.1	6.2
Bordetella pertussis	38	3.1	50.0	25.0	100.0
Branhamella catarrhalis	50	0.05	0.8	0.4	3.1

Cefixime is effective against Proteus vulgaris, Morganella morganii and Enterobacter cloacae, whereas cefaclor and cephalexin are not. The activity against pneumococci is equally good, but that against staphylococci weaker. There is some cross-resistance between older and newer oral cephalosporins.

Pharmacokinetics: Cefixime is incompletely absorbed (about 40%). Serum concentrations 4–5 h after oral intake of 0.1 g, 0.2 g and 0.4 g were 1.3, 2.7 and 3.7 mg/l, falling to 0.4, 0.7 and 1.1 mg/l respectively after 12 h. The half-life is 2.5 h, plasma protein binding 63% and urinary recovery 20%. Bile concentrations are fairly high. Mild gastrointestinal upset (nausea, vomiting, diarrhoea) has been occasionally reported.

Indications: Respiratory and urinary tract infections caused by susceptible organisms, especially in children. The broader spectrum and greater effectivity make cefixime superior to older cephalosporins in initial therapy.

Dosage: 0.2 g daily (adults) and 8 mg/kg daily (children) once a day or in 2 divided doses.

Preparations: Tablets of 0.2 g, suspension (0.1 g in 5 ml).

Summary: Because of its broad spectrum and greater efficacy, cefixime is superior to the older oral cephalosporins in infections of the urinary and respiratory tracts.

References

Carenfelt, C., I. Melen, L. Odkvist et al.: Treatment of sinus empyema in adults. A coordinated Nordic multicenter trial of cefixime vs. cefaclor. Acta Otolaryngol. Stockh. *110:* 128–135 (1990).
Chardon, H., O. Bellon, E. Lagier, E. Giraud: Activite in vitro du cefixime sur 200 souches de Branhamella catarrhalis. Comparison au cefotaxime. Presse Médicale *18:* 1556–1559 (1989).
Dorow, P.: Safety and efficacy of cefixime versus cefaclor in respiratory tract infections. J. Chemother. *1:* 257–260 (1989).
Kuhlwein, A., B. A. Nies: Efficacy and safety of a single 400 mg oral dose of cefixime in the treatment of uncomplicated gonorrhea. Eur. J. Clin. Microb. Inf. Dis. *8:* 261–262 (1989).
Mortenson, J. E., S. L. Himes: Comparative in vitro activity of cefixime against isolates of Haemophilus influenzae from pediatric patients including amipicillin resistant, non-β-lactamase producing isolates. Antimicrob. Ag. Chemother. *34:* 1456–1458 (1990).
Singlas, E., D. Lebrec, C. Gaudin, G. Montay, G. Roche: Influence de l'insuffisance hépatique sur la pharmacocinetique du cefixime. Presse Médicale *18:* 1587–1588 (1989).
Stone, J. W., G. Linong, J. M. Andrews, R. Wise: Cefixime, in vitro activity, pharmacokinetics and tissue penetration. J. Antimicrob. Chemother. *23:* 221–228 (1989).
Verghese, A., D. Roberson, J. H. Kalbleisch, F. Sarubbi: Randomized comparative study of cefixime versus cephalexin in acute bacterial exacerbations of chronic bronchitis. Antimicrob. Agents Chemother. *34:* 1041–1044 (1990).

β) Cefetamet

Proprietary name: not yet known (Roche).

Properties: A new oral oxime cephalosporin (cefotaxime derivative) which is given as the pivaloyl oxymethyl ester to enhance oral absorption. The pivaloyl group is split from the cephalosporin ring in the intestinal wall, and the active free acid appears in the blood.

Spectrum of activity is in part identical with that of cefaclor and cephalexin. Cefetamet is active in addition against Enterobacter cloacae and Proteus vulgaris, but not against staphylococci. Cefetamet is 10 times more active than cefaclor against Streptococcus pyogenes (Lancefield Group A) and 12 times more active against Haemophilus influenzae (Tab. 13). The activity against Escherichia coli, Klebsiella pneumoniae and yersinia is 8 times greater.

Pharmacokinetics: Peak serum concentrations after an oral dose of 0.5 g are between 4 and 5 mg/l after 3.5 h. *Half-life* 4 h. *Urinary recovery* 70%.

Clinical trials are still in progress.

References

Angehrn, P., P. Hohl, R. Then: In vitro antibacterial properties of cefetamet and in vivo activity of its orally absorbable ester derivative, cefetamet pivoxil. Eur. J. Clin. Microbiol. Infect. Dis. *8:* 536–543 (1989).
Blouin, R. A., J. Kneer, K. Stoeckel: Pharmacokinetics of intravenous cefetamet (Ro 15-8074) and oral cefetamet pivoxil (Ro 15-8075) in young and elderly subjects. Antimicrob. Agents Chemother. *33:* 291–296 (1989).
Hayton, W. L., J. Kneer, R. A. Blouin, K. Stoeckel: Pharmacokinetics of intravenous cefetamet and oral cefetamet pivoxil in patients with hepatic cirrhosis. Antimicrob. Agents Chemother. *34:* 1318–1322 (1990).
Kneer, J., Y. K. Tam, R. A. Blouin, F. J. Frey, E. Keller, C. Stathakis, B. Luginbuehl, K. Stoeckel: Pharmacokinetics of intravenous cefetamet and oral cefetamet pivoxil in patients with renal insufficiency. Antimicrob. Agents Chemother. *33:* 1952–1957 (1989).
Stoeckel, K., Y. Tam, J. Kneer: Pharmacokinetics of oral cefetamet pivoxil (Ro 15–8075) and intravenous cefetamet (Ro 15-8074) in humans: a review. Curr. Med. Res. Opin. *11:* 432–441 (1989).
Simon, C.: In vitro activity of Ro 15-8074 and Ro 19-5247 in comparison to cefaclor and cefalexin. Infection *15:* 2, 122–124 (1987).
Tam, Y. K., J. Kneer, U. C. Dubach, K. Stoeckel: Pharmacokinetics of cefetamet pivoxil (Ro 15-8075) with ascending oral doses in normal healthy volunteers. Antimicrob. Agents Chemother. *33:* 957–959 (1989).
Tam, Y. K., J. Kneer, U. C. Dubach, K. Stoeckel: Effects of timing of food and fluid volume on cefetamet pivoxil absorption in healthy normal volunteers. Antimicrob. Agents Chemother. *34:* 1556–1559 (1990).

γ) Cefuroxime Axetil

Proprietary name: Zinnat.

Properties: Acetoxyethyl ester of cefuroxime (Fig. 24, p. 96) which is hydrolysed in the intestinal wall to release acetaldehyde and acetic acid. After absorption, free cefuroxime is released into the bloodstream.

Spectrum of activity: Cefuroxime (see p. 66) has good stability to β-lactamases and is also active against ampicillin-resistant strains of haemophilus and penicillin-resistant gonococci. Cefuroxime is more active than cephalexin or cefaclor against Escherichia coli, Proteus mirabilis and Klebsiella pneumoniae. Cefuroxime is, however, inactive against pseudomonas, Enterobacter species, Proteus vulgaris and cephalothin-resistant staphylococci.

Pharmacokinetics: Incomplete oral absorption with relatively large individual variation. The mean peak serum concentrations after 0.5 g by mouth are 8.6 ml/l, with a range of 4.5 to 12.8 mg/l. Absorption is better with food than fasting. *Half-life* 1.2 h. *Urinary recovery* 33–40%. Loose stools and diarrhoea occur relatively frequently.

Preparations: Tablets of 125 mg, 250 mg and 500 mg, suspension (150 mg in 5 ml).

Dosage: 0.25–0.5 g twice a day by mouth and 0.125 g twice a day in uncomplicated urinary tract infection (adults); 15 mg/kg twice a day (children).

References

ADAMS, D. H., M. J. WOOD, I. D. FARREL et al.: Oral cefuroxime axetil: clinical pharmacology and comparative dose studies in urinary tract infection. J. Antimicrob. Chemother. *16:* 359 (1985).
FONG, I. W., W. LINTON, M. SIMBUL, N. A. HINTON: Comparative clinical efficacy of single oral doses of cefuroxime axetil and amoxicillin in uncomplicated gonococcal infections. Antimicrob. Ag. Chemother. *30:* 321–322 (1986).
GINSBURG, C. M., G. H. MCCRACKEN Jr., M. PETRUSKA, K. OLSON: Pharmacokinetics and bactericidal activity of cefuroxime axetil. Antimicrob. Ag. Chemother. *28:* 504 (1985).
HARDING, S. M., P. E. O. WILLIAMS, J. AYRTON: Pharmacology of cefuroxime as the 1-acetoxyethyl ester in volunteers. Antimicrob. Ag. Chemother. *25:* 78–82 (1984).
SCHLEUPNER, C. J., W. C. ANTHONY, J. TAN: Blinded comparisons of cefuroxime to cefaclor for lower respiratory tract infections. Arch. Intern. Med. *148:* 343–348 (1988).
SOMMERS, D., M. VAN WYK, P. E. O. WILLIAMS, S. M. HARDING: Pharmacokinetics and tolerance of cefuroxime axetil in volunteers during repeated doses. Antimicrob. Ag. Chemother. *25:* 344 (1984).
SYDNOR, A. J., JR., et al.: Comparative evaluation of cefuroxime axetil and cefaclor for treatment of acute bacterial maxillary sinusitis. Arch. Otolaryngol. Head Neck Surg. *115:* 1430 (1989).
WILLIAMS, P. E. O., S. M. HARDING: The absolute bioavailability of cefuroxime axetil in male and female volunteers after fasting and after food. J. Antimicrob. Chemother. *13:* 191 (1984).
WISE, R., S. A. BENNETT, J. DENT: The pharmacokinetics of orally absorbed cefuroxime compared with amoxycillin clavulanic acid. J. Antimicrob. Chemother. *132:* 603–610 (1984).

δ) Cefpodoxime Proxetil

Proprietary name: Orelox.

Properties: Cefpodoxime proxetil is the prodrug ester of the 3-methoxy-methyl derivative of ceftizoxime (see p. 8) which is hydrolysed in the intestine to its active compound cefpodoxime. No unchanged ester is detected in the blood. A small amount of two inactive metabolites of proxetil are excreted by the kidneys and the liver. The chemical structure of cefpodoxime proxetil is shown in figure 25.

Spectrum of activity: Similar to cefixime (see p. 96). Cefpodoxime is 10- to 20-fold more active than cefaclor, against Streptococcus pyogenes and Streptococcus pneumoniae and 30-fold more active against Haemophilus influenzae. Methicillin-sensitive staphylococci and Branhamella catarrhalis have similar sensitivity to

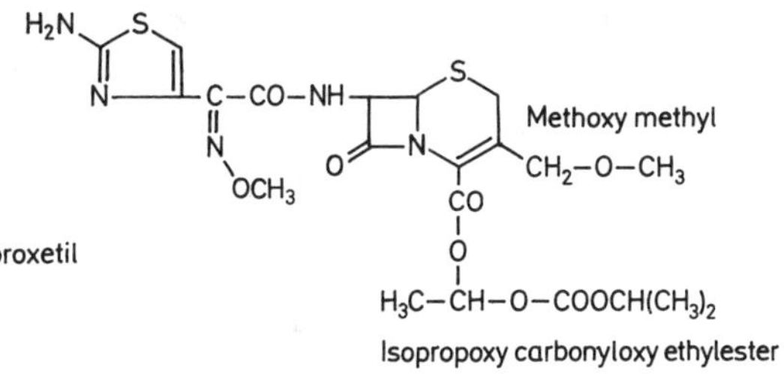

Fig. 25. Chemical structure of cefpodoxime proxetil.

cefpodoxime and cefaclor. Cefpodoxime has much greater activity than cefaclor against many gram-negative bacteria and is the only member of this group to have activity against most strains of Citrobacter freundii. Pseudomonas aeruginosa, Serratia marcescens, Bacteroides spp., enterococci and methicillin-resistant staphylococci are always resistant to cefpodoxime. There is incomplete cross-resistance between the newer oral cephalosporins.

Pharmacokinetics: Cefpodoxime is incompletely absorbed (better when given with food). Peak serum concentrations 2–3 h after oral intake of 0.2 g (fasting) are 2.0–2.4 mg/l, falling to about 0.1 mg/l after 12 h. The half-life is 2.3 h, plasma protein binding 40% and urinary recovery 30–40%. Bile concentrations are 3–4 mg/l (after 4–8 h). Inactive metabolites are found in the urine and faeces.

Side-effects: Diarrhoea, loose stools and allergic symptoms (rash and eruptions) occur occasionally.

Indications: Respiratory and urinary tract infections caused by susceptible organisms.

Dosage: 0.2 (–0.4) g daily by mouth (divided in 2 doses).

Summary: Because of its broad spectrum and greater efficacy, cefpodoxime proxetil is superior to the older oral cephalosporins in respiratory and urinary tract infections.

References

Borin, M. T., G. S. Hughes, C. R. Spillers, R. K. Patel: Pharmacokinetics of cefopodixime in plasma and skin blister fluid following oral dosing of cefpodoxime proxetil. Antimicrob. Ag. Chemother. *34:* 1094–1099 (1990).

Hoffler, D., P. Koeppe, M. Corcilius, A. Przyklinik: Cefpodoxime proxetil in patients with endstage renal failure on hemodialysis. Infection *18:* 157–162 (1990).

O'Neill, P., K. Nye, G. Douce, J. Andrews, R. Wise: Pharmacokinetics and inflammatory fluid penetration of cefpodoxime proxetil in volunteers. Antimicrob. Ag. Chemother. *34:* 232–234 (1990).

SCHAADT, R. D., B. H. YAGI, G. E. ZURENKO: In vitro activity of cefpodoxime proxetil (U-76,252; CS-807) against Neisseria gonorrhoeae. Antimicrob. Ag. Chemother. *34:* 371–372 (1990).
STOBBERINGH, E. E., A. W. HOUBEN, J. H. PHILIPS: In vitro activity of cefpodoxime, a new oral cephalosporin. Eur. J. Clin. Microbiol. Infect. Dis. *8:* 656–658 (1989).

ε) Loracarbef

Properties: A new carbacephem analogue of cefaclor (Lilly) which, unlike cefaclor, is very stable *in vitro*. The spectrum of activity and in vitro activity are similar those of cefaclor, whereas cephalexin is less active. Loracarbef is also active against ampicillin-resistant strains of haemophilus and branhamella, but not active against enterococci, pseudomonas, serratia or Enterobacter species.

Pharmacokinetics: Loracarbef is almost completely absorbed when taken by mouth. The peak serum concentrations 1 h after an oral dose of 0.1 g, 0.25 g and 0.5 g are 4, 10 and 16 mg/l respectively. *Half-life* 1.1 h. *Urinary recovery* 90% (unchanged).

Dosage: Because of its good absorption, daily doses of 400–800 mg are sufficient to treat most susceptible infections. The drug appears to be well tolerated.

References

JONES, R. N., A. L. BARRY: Beta-lactamase hydrolysis and inhibition studies of the new 1-carbacephem LY163892. Eur. J. clin. microbiol. *6/5:* 570–571 (1987).
KNAPP, C. C., J. A. WASHINGTON: II. In vitro activities of LY 163892. Antimicrob. Ag. Chemother. *32/1:* 131–133 (1988).
SHELTON, S., J. D. NELSON: In vitro susceptibilities of common pediatric pathogens to LY 163892. Antimicrob. Ag. Chemother. *32/2:* 268–270 (1988).

ς) Cefotiam Hexetil

Properties: Absorption ester of cefotiam (Fig. 24, p. 96). The ester is hydrolysed in the intestinal wall and absorbed as cefotiam.

Spectrum of action and activity of cefotiam are described on p. 67. *Peak serum concentrations* 1.5 h after an oral dose of 0.2 g are 2.3 mg/l. *Half-life* 40 min. *Urinary recovery:* 30%. Clinical testing is still in progress.

References

NISHIMURA, T., Y. YOSHIMURA, A. MIYAKE, M. YAMAOKA: Orally active 1-(cyclohexyloxycarbonyloxy)alkyl ester prodrugs of cefotiam. J. Antibiotics *40:* 81–90 (1987).

3. Other β-Lactam Antibiotics

a) Imipenem/Cilastatin

Proprietary name: Primaxin.

Properties: *Imipenem* (N-formimidoyl thienamycin) is an amidino derivative of thienamycin and has been found to be 5–10 times more stable than naturally occurring thienamycin; its antibacterial activity is equal or slightly superior to that of thienamycin. Imipenem is the first carbapenem in clinical use (Fig. 26).

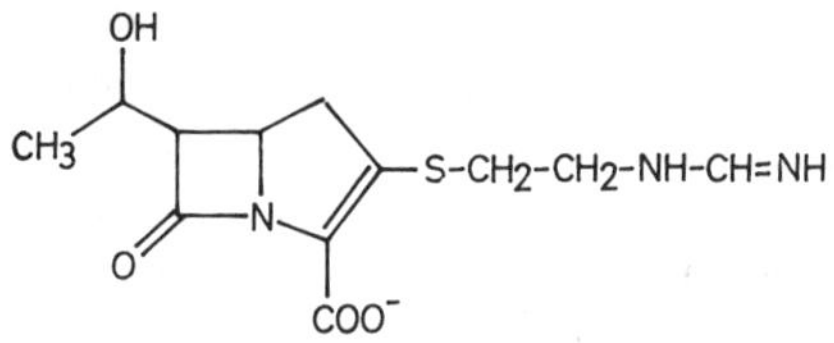

Fig. 26. Structural formula of imipenem.

The substitution of the sulphur atom by a methyl (CH_2) group potentiates the bactericidal effect of imipenem. Attachment of a hydroxyethyl side-chain to the β-lactam ring in transorientation is responsible for its exceptional stability to β-lactamases. Imipenem cannot be given alone because it is rapidly degraded in the kidneys by the tissue enzyme, dehydropeptidase I. It must therefore be combined with cilastatin (see below).

Cilastatin is a competitive reversible inhibitor of dehydropeptidase I, a renal enzyme which metabolises and inactivates imipenem. Cilastatin is a derivative of heptene carbonic acid (Fig. 27).

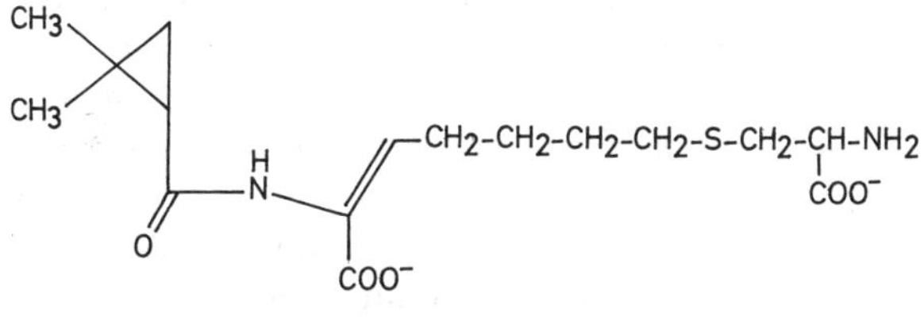

Fig. 27. Structural formula of cilastatin.

Cilastatin has two functions. Firstly, it reduces hydrolysis of imipenem in the kidneys and increases urinary concentrations of the active antibiotic; secondly, it inhibits nephrotoxicity of imipenem at a higher dosage (demonstrable in animals). Cilastatin has no effect on other human metallodipeptidases or on bacteria. Imipenem and cilastatin sodium are present in the proprietary preparation in a 1:1 ratio. The amount of cilastatin is not usually taken into account when calculating dosage.

Spectrum of activity: Imipenem inhibits bacterial cell wall synthesis and is highly bactericidal. It has an exceptionally broad spectrum of activity which encompasses practically all gram-positive bacteria, including enterococci, Listeria monocytogenes, nocardia, Mycobacterium avium-intracellulare, and virtually all gram-negative bacteria, including Pseudomonas aeruginosa, citrobacter, serratia, acinetobacter and enterobacter species. Imipenem also inhibits β-lactamase-producing strains of Haemophilus influenzae, Streptococcus pneumoniae and Neisseria gonorrhoeae. It is more active than clindamycin and metronidazole against Bacteroides fragilis and most other anaerobes (clostridia, peptococcus, peptostreptococcus, actinomyces, Fusobacterium species etc.). The activity of imipenem against Proteus vulgaris and Proteus mirabilis is somewhat less than against the other enterobacteria. Imipenem is inactive against Pseudomonas cepacia and Xanthomonas maltophilia, some strains of Enterococcus faecium and some methicillin-resistant staphylococci. There is very occasional partial cross-resistance with penicillins and cephalosporins. Secondary resistance in Pseudomonas aeruginosa can develop during therapy.

Pharmacokinetics: After i.v. infusion of 250 mg, 500 mg and 1 g of *imipenem* over 20 min, *peak serum concentrations* range from 14–24 mg/l to 20–60 mg/l. *Half-life:* 60 min. *Protein binding:* 25%. *Urinary recovery:* 15–20%. Poor *cerebrospinal fluid penetration.*

Cilastatin gives *peak serum levels* after i.v. infusion of 250 mg, 500 mg and 1 g over 20 min between 15–25 mg/l and 30–50 mg/l. *Half-life:* 45 min. *Protein binding:* 25%. *Urinary recovery:* 55% as the parent drug and ca. 15% as the N-acetyl metabolite (which has the same inhibitory activity as the parent substance). Renal dehydropeptidase I activity rapidly returns to normal after elimination of cilastatin from the bloodstream.

Concomitant administration of imipenem and cilastatin increases the serum levels of imipenem only slightly (Fig. 28); the half-life and protein binding are almost the same as when used singly but *urine concentrations* of imipenem are higher and exceed 10 mg/l for up to 8 hours after 500 mg imipenem +500 mg cilastatin i.v. *Urinary recovery* of imipenem (after combined treatment): 70% (the remainder is recovered as antibacterially inactive metabolites). Imipenem is only excreted in small quantities in the bile and hence into the faeces. No accumulation of imipenem in plasma or urine was found after repeated administration of the combination. Both imipenem and cilastatin are dialysable.

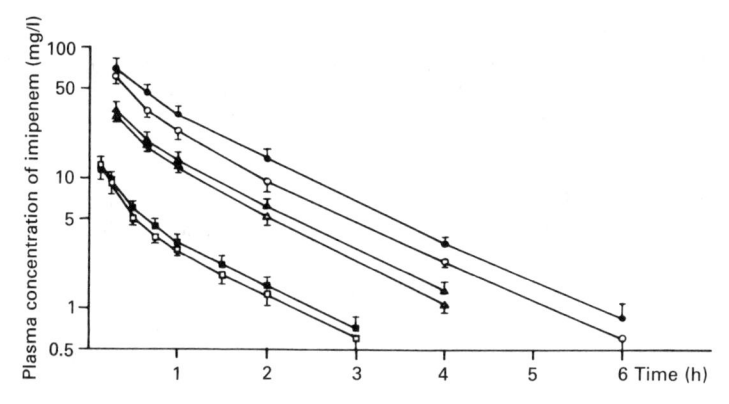

Fig. 28. Mean plasma concentration of imipenem after i. v. doses of 150 mg (□), 500 mg (△), or 1 g (○) alone (open symbols) or combined with equal doses of dehydropeptidase inhibitor (closed symbols). After: S. R. NORRBY et al.: Antimicrob. Ag. Chemother. *23:* 300 (1983).

Side-effects: Serious side effects are rare. 5–20% experience gastrointestinal upset (nausea, vomiting and diarrhoea), ≤5% local reactions (thrombophlebitis) and <3% allergic reactions (rashes). 1–2% suffer central-nervous side-effects (spasms, focal tremor, myoclonus, confusion, psychic disorders, giddiness, drowsiness), particularly at higher dosage or with impaired renal function or prior CNS damage. Haematological reactions are more frequently seen as eosinophilia and less commonly as leucocytopenia, thrombocytopenia and a fall in haemoglobin. The direct Coombs test can become positive. Transient prolongation of the prothrombin time occurs in <2% of cases. Disorders of renal function (oliguria, elevated serum urea or creatinine) are uncommon. Slight enhancement of serum transaminases, bilirubin and/or alkaline phosphatase are occasionally seen. Circulatory reactions can follow rapid i. v. injection, so imipenem should always be infused.

Indications: Mixed infections and initial treatment of severe infections, particularly in the presence of impaired immunity, septicaemia or intra-abdominal, gynecological, bone or joint infections. It can be life-saving when previous therapy with other broad-spectrum antibiotics has failed. Imipenem may be used with caution if the patient is allergic to penicillins and cephalosporins. In severe pseudomonas infections, always combine with an aminoglycoside. This combination is usually well tolerated. Combination therapy should also be considered for peritonitis and endocarditis. Imipenem is often started when other antibiotics have failed and any remaining gaps in the spectrum can usually be filled by combination with other antibiotics.

Contra-indications: Hypersensitivity to either component of the drug. In cases of proven penicillin allergy, the very uncommon cross-allergy to imipenem should be ruled out. There are no controlled studies in pregnancy, so imipenem should only be given in pregnancy when the benefits outweigh the possible risk to the fetus.

Administration and dosage: The intravenous preparation should be dissolved in an appropriate volume of compatible, lactate-free diluent and infused over 30 min. The daily dosage is 1.5–2 g given by short i.v. infusion in 3 or 4 divided doses. The maximum daily dose is 4 g or 50 mg/kg body weight. The single dose of 1 g should be infused over 60 min. Children aged 4 months and over should receive 30–60 mg/kg/day in 4 divided doses. Optimal dosage and indications in the neonate have not yet been determined.

In patients with renal impairment with a creatinine clearance of 20–30 ml/min, give 500 mg every 12 h, and when creatinine clearance is <5 ml/min, 250 mg every 12 h. A daily maximum of 1 g or 12.5 mg/kg should not be exceeded. Give an additional 500 mg after each haemodialysis.

Preparations: Vials containing 500 mg imipenem + 500 mg cilastatin.

Summary: Imipenem is the first of a new class of β-lactam antibiotics with a very broad spectrum of activity against almost all aerobic and anaerobic bacteria. It has a high antibacterial activity and therefore provides an alternative to a wide range of broad-spectrum combinations used previously for initial therapy in severe bacterial infections including mixed infections. To avoid metabolic degradation in the kidneys and to attain sufficient urinary concentrations, imipenem is combined with cilastatin which inhibits a renal dipeptidase that destroys imipenem and increases the renal tolerance of the drug.

References

AHONKHAI, V. I., G. M. CYHAN, S. E. WILSON, K. R. BROWN: Imipenem-cilastatin in pediatric patients: an overview of safety and efficacy in studies conducted in the United States. Pediatr. Infect. Dis. J. 8: 740–744 (1989).

ALARABI, A. A., O. CARS, B. G. DANIELSON, T. SALMONSON, B. WIKSTROM: Pharmacokinetics of intravenous imipenem/cilastatin during intermittent haemofiltration. J. Antimicrob. Chemother. 26: 91–98 (1990).

CALANDRA, G. B.: Review of adverse experiences and tolerability in the first 2,516 patients treated with imipenem/cilastatin. Am. J. Med. 78 (6A): 73 (1985).

D'AMATO, C., M. A. ROSCI, G. VISCO: The efficacy and safety of imipenem/cilastatin in the treatment of severe bacterial infections. J. Chemother. 2: 100–107 (1990).

DRUSANO, G. L., H. C. STANDIFORD: Pharmacokinetic profile of imipenem/cilastatin in normal volunteers. Am. J. Med. 78 (6A): 47 (1985).

ERON, L. J.: Imipenem/cilastatin therapy of bacteremia. Amer. J. Med. 78 (6A): 95 (1985).

FREIJ, B. J., G. H. MCCRACKEN Jr., K. D. OLSEN, N. THRELKELD: Pharmacokinetics of imipenem-cilastatin in neonates. Antimicrob. Ag. Chemother. 27: 431 (1985).

GIBSON, T. P. , J. L. DEMETRIADES, J. A. BLAND: Imipenem/cilastatin: pharmacokinetic profile in renal insufficiency. Amer. J. Med. *78 (6A):* 54 (1985).
GRUBER, W. C., M. A. RENCH, J. A. GARCIA-PRATS et al.: Single-dose pharmacokinetics of imipenem-cilastatin in neonates. Antimicrob. Ag. Chemother. *27:* 511 (1985).
KAGER, L., C. E. NORD: Imipenem/cilastatin in the treatment of intraabdominal infections: A review of worldwide experience. Rev. Infect. Dis. *7 (Suppl. 3):* 518 (1985).
KESADO, T., K. WATANABE, Y. ASAHI, M. ISONO, K. UENO: Susceptibilities of anaerobic bacteria to N-formimidoyl thienamycin (MK 0787) and to other antibiotics. Antimicrob. Ag. Chemother. *21:* 1016–1022 (1982).
MACGREGOR, R. R., G. A. GIBSON, J. A. BLAND: Imipenem pharmacokinetics and body fluid concentrations in patients receiving high-dose treatment for serious infections. Antimicrob. Ag. Chemother. *29:* 188 (1985).
OVERTURF, G. D.: Use of imipenem-cilastatin in pediatrics. Pediatr. Infect. Dis. J. *8:* 792 (1989).
PEDERSEN, S. S., T. PRESSLER, N. HIBY et al.: Imipenem/cilastatin treatment of multiresistant Pseudomonas aeruginosa lung infection in cystic fibrosis. J. Antimicrob. Chemother. *16:* 629 (1985).
QUINN, J. P., E. J. DUDEK, C. A. DI VICENZO et al.: Emergence of resistance to imipenem during therapy for Ps. aeruginosa infections. J. Infect. Dis. *154:* 289 (1986).
REED, M. D., R. C. STERN, C. A. O'BRIEN et al.: Pharmacokinetics of imipenem and cilastatin in patients with cystic fibrosis. Antimicrob. Ag. Chemother. *27:* 583 (1985).
REED, M. D., R. M. KLIEGMAN, T. S. YAMASHITA, C. M. MYERS, J. L. BLUMER: Clinical pharmacology of imipenem and cilastatin in premature infants during the first week of life. Antimicrob. Agents Chemother. *34:* 1172–1177 (1990).
SOBEL, J. D.: Imipenem and aztreonam. Infect. Dis. Clin. North Am. *3:* 613 (1989).
TAUSK, F., M. E. EVANS, L. S. PATTERSON, C. F. FEDERSPIEL, C. W. STRATTON: Imipenem-induced resistance to antipseudomonal β-lactams in Pseudomonas aeruginosa. Antimicrob. Ag. Chemother. *28:* 41 (1985).
VERPOOTEN, G. A., L. VERBIST, A. P. BUNTINX et al.: The pharmacokinetics of imipenem (thienamycin formamidine) and the renal dehydropeptidase inhibitor cilastatin sodium in normal subjects and patients with renal failure. Br. J. Clin. Pharmacol. *18:* 183 (1984).
WONG, V. K., H. T. WRIGHT, L. A. ROSS: Imipenem/cilastatin treatment of bacterial meningitis in children. Pediatr. Infect. Dis. J. *10:* 122–125 (1991).
ZAJAC, B. A., M. A. FISHER, G. A. GIBSON, R. R. MAC GREGOR: Safety and efficacy of high-dose treatment with imipenem-cilastatin in seriously ill patients. Antimicrob. Ag. Chemother. *27:* 745 (1985).

b) Aztreonam

Proprietary name: Azactam.

Properties: Aztreonam is the first monobactam to be used clinically. It is a monocyclic β-lactam antibiotic with an α-methyl-3-amino-monobactamic acid nucleus linked to the typical side-chain of ceftazidime (Fig. 29).

Mode of action: Aztreonam inhibits bacterial cell wall synthesis. Its strong affinity for penicillin-binding protein 3 explains its activity against gram-negative bacteria. It is very stable to the β-lactamases of gram-negative bacteria.

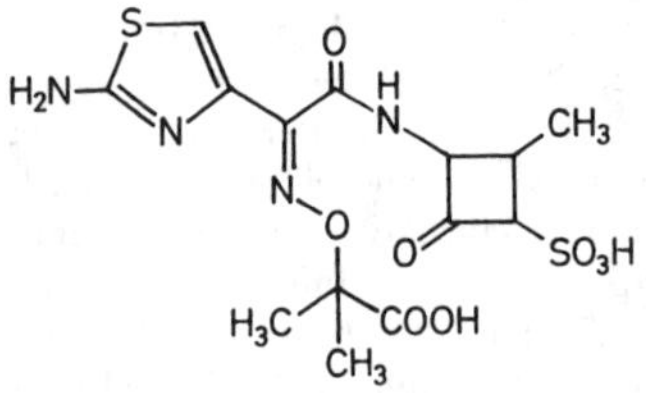

Fig. 29. Structural formula of aztreonam.

Spectrum of activity: Aztreonam is active against almost all aerobic gram-negative bacilli including Pseudomonas aeruginosa, Serratia marcescens, enterobacter and citrobacter, but is not active against anaerobes (Bacteroides species etc.), acinetobacter and Alcaligenes species. Like temocillin but unlike other penicillins and cephalosporins, aztreonam has no activity against gram-positive bacteria. The anti-pseudomonal activity is approximately similar to that of cefsulodin. Azetreonam acts synergistically with gentamicin against Pseudomonas aeruginosa and Klebsiella pneumoniae.

Pharmacokinetics: Mean serum concentrations of 54, 90 and 204 mg/l are attained after i.v. infusion (in 30 min) of 0.5, 1 and 2 g respectively. After i.v. injection of 1 g and 2 g, the initial serum concentrations of 125 and 242 mg/l fall after 8 h to 1.3 and 6 mg/l respectively. *Half-life:* 1.7 h. *Plasma protein binding:* 56%. *Urinary recovery:* 70% (a small proportion is also excreted as an inactive metabolite in the urine). *Biliary excretion* is slight, and *CSF penetration* poor.

Side-effects are similar to those reported for other β-lactam antibiotics, i.e., gastrointestinal upset, skin reactions. There is usually no cross-allergy with other β-lactam antibiotics. A transient rise in prothrombin and partial thromboplastin times may occur, but anaemia and thrombocytopenia are rare. Thrombophlebitis occasionally complicates repeated i.v. administration.

Indications: *Complicated urinary infections* with otherwise resistant organisms (also as an alternative to gentamicin). Use with metronidazole in *intra-abdominal infections,* and with clindamycin in *gynaecological infections* (aztreonam is also active against penicillin-resistant gonococci). Useful in *cystic fibrosis* in rotation with other antipseudomonal agents. Single-dose therapy of gonorrhoea (1 g i.m.).

Inappropriate use: Single-agent initial therapy of infections whose cause is not yet established.

Contra-indications: Use with caution in pregnant women and neonates until more experience has been gained.

Administration and dosage: I.v. injection or short i.v. infusion; i.m. injection is also possible. Daily dosage in adults is 3–6 (–8) g, and in children 45–90 (–100) mg/kg, in 3–4 divided doses. In *impaired renal function*, reduce the dose to ½ if creatinine clearance is 10–30 ml/min, and to ¼ if it is below 10 ml/min. Give ⅛ of a normal divided dose after each haemodialysis.

Preparations: Ampoules of 0.5 g, 1 g and 2 g.

Summary: Useful in suspected or proven infections by gram-negative bacteria (broad spectrum). Ineffective against anaerobic and gram-positive pathogens. Although this antibiotic is of great theoretical interest, its clinical value is limited. Aztreonam may be considered in patients allergic to penicillin (after a test dose).

References

BIROLINI, D., M. F. MORAES, O. S. DE SOUZA: Aztreonam plus clindamycin vs. tobramycin plus clindamycin for the treatment of intraabdominal infections. Rev. Infect. Dis. *7 (Suppl. 4):* 724 (1985).

CHANDRASEKAR, P. H., B. R. SMITH, J. L. LE FROCK, B. CARR: Enterococcal superinfection and colonization with aztreonam therapy. Antimicrob. Ag. Chemother. *26:* 280 (1984).

FERIS, J., N. MOLEDINA, W. J. RODRIGUEZ et al.: Aztreonam in the treatment of gram-negative meningitis and other gramnegative infections. Chemother. *35,* Suppl. *1:* 31–8 (1989).

GREENMAN, R. L., S. M. ARCEY, G. M. DICKINSON et al.: Penetration of aztreonam into cerebrospinal fluid in the presence of meningeal inflammation. J. Antimicrob. Chemother. *15:* 637 (1985).

JONES, P., K. ROLSTON, V. FAINSTEIN et al.: Aztreonam plus vancomycin (plus amikacin) vs. moxalactam plus ticarcillin for the empiric treatment of febrile episodes in neutropenic cancer patients. Rev. Infect. Dis. 7 (Suppl. 4): 741 (1985).

McLEOD, C. M., E. A. BARTLEY, J. A. PAYNE: Effects of cirrhosis on kinetics of aztreonam. Antimicrob. Ag. Chemother. *26:* 493 (1984).

MIHINGU, J. C. L., W. M. SCHELD, N. D. BOLTON et al.: Pharmacokinetics of aztreonam in patients with varying degrees of renal dysfunction. Antimicrob. Ag. Chemother. *24:* 252 (1983).

NEU, H. C. (ed.): Aztreonam's role in the treatment of gram-negative infections. Am. J. Med. *88* (3C): 1–43 (1990).

NEU, H. C.: Aztreonam activity, pharmacology, and clinical uses. Am. J. Med. *88* (Suppl. 3C): 2 (1990).

NEWMAN, T. J., G. R. DRESLINSKI, S. S. TADROS: Safety profile of aztreonam in clinical trials. Rev. Infect. Dis. 7 (Suppl. 4): 648 (1985).

SAXON, A., A. HASSNER, E. A. SWABB et al.: Lack of cross reactivity between the monobactam aztreonam and penicillin in penicillin allergic subjects. J. Infect. Dis. *149:* 16 (1984).

SHIBL, A. M., A. H. ISHAG, S. M. DURGHAM: Comparative in vitro antibacterial activity of aztreonam against clinical isolates of gram negative bacteria. Chemotherapy *35* Suppl. 1: 72–76 (1989).

STUTMAN, H. R., M. I. MARKS, E. A. SWABB: Single-dose pharmacokinetics of aztreonam in pediatric patients. Antimicrob. Ag. Chemother. *26:* 196 (1984).

c) β-Lactamase Inhibitors

β-lactamase inhibition is of great theoretical interest. Blockade of β-lactamases enables the spectrum of activity of a penicillin to be considerably extended. However, practical limitations soon become apparent. Not all β-lactamases are inactivated by β-lactamase inhibitors. Other forms of resistance, e. g., in methicillin-resistant staphylococci, are not mediated by β-lactamases. Some β-lactamases are tolerated only in small doses. β-lactamase inhibitors can themselves induce β-lactamases, thus interfering with the activity of penicillins.

As in other types of combined therapy, combination with a β-lactamase inhibitor involves variable ratios of the two components in different organs. The commercially available preparations are not optimum combinations of an optimum penicillin with a β-lactamase inhibitor in optimum dosage. At best, the effects are as good as those of basic cephalosporins. Combinations with inferior or obsolete penicillins serve to discredit β-lactamase inhibitors. Acylaminopenicillins, which penetrate very well, and benzylpenicillin are better suited for combination with a β-lactamase inhibitor. The β-lactamase inhibitors sulbactam is now available in some countries as a single agent and may be prescribed with any β-lactam agent.

α) Co-amoxiclav (Amoxycillin/Clavulanic Acid)

Proprietary name: Augmentin.

Properties: Clavulanic acid is obtained by the fermentation of Streptomyces clavuligerus and is structurally similar to the penicillin nucleus but has no acylamino side-chain and contains oxygen instead of sulphur at position 1 (Fig. 30).

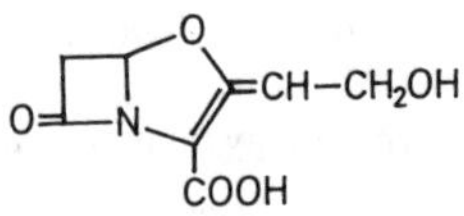

Fig. 30. Structural formula of clavulanic acid.

Activity: It has only weak antibacterial activity and would not be therapeutically effective if administered alone. Clavulanic acid is, however, a strong and irreversible β-lactamase inhibitor, especially of types II, III, IV and V. Clavulanic acid acts only against β-lactamases of type I if they are produced by Bacteroides fragilis. Amoxycillin-resistant (β-lactamase-producing) strains of Staphylococcus aureus and epidermidis, Haemophilus influenzae, Branhamella catarrhalis, gonococci, Escherichia coli, Klebsiella pneumoniae, Proteus mirabilis, Proteus vulgaris and Bacteroides fragilis are generally as sensitive in the presence of clavulanic acid as amoxycillin-sensitive strains. Clavulanic acid does not protect amoxycillin from inactivation by the β-lactamases of Pseudomonas aeruginosa, Serratia marcescens, Enterobacter species, Morganella morganii or Proteus rettgeri. Some strains of Escherichia coli, Staphylococcus epidermidis and Klebsiella are not rendered sensitive to amoxycillin by clavulanic acid because they produce a different type of β-lactamase. Enterobacteriaceae should therefore be tested *in vitro* for sensitivity to co-amoxiclav. Amoxycillin trihydrate for oral use and clavulanic acid as the potassium salt are combined in tablets in various ratios because the clavulanic acid component is limited by its tolerability.

For parenteral use the mixture is also variable, according to the amoxycillin content of the ampoule.

Pharmacokinetics: Clavulanic acid is well absorbed orally as the potassium salt. 125 mg of clavulanic acid by mouth give a maximal serum concentration after 1.5 h of 3 mg/l and 0.6 mg/l after 4 h. 9.2 mg/l are detected 1 h after 200 mg i. v., and 0.9 mg/l after 4 h. *Plasma protein binding:* 20%. *Half-life:* 60 min. Poor *CNS penetration. Urinary recovery:* 40% (after oral administration).

Amoxycillin has similar pharmacokinetics after oral and i. v. administration but the percentage urinary recovery is higher (see p. 43).

Side-effects: 10% of patients suffer nausea, abdominal cramps, vomiting, and diarrhoea, predominantly due to the clavulanic acid. The recommended oral dose of clavulanic acid should not, therefore, be exceeded.

Interactions: Skin rashes frequently occur when allopurinol is given simultaneously. Concurrent administration of disulfiram is poorly tolerated.

Indications: Infections with amoxycillin-resistant bacteria, the β-lactamases of which are inhibited by clavulanic acid. These include milder respiratory infections (sinusitis, otitis media and suppurative bronchitis with β-lactamase-producing strains of haemophilus and branhamella), urinary infections with ampicillin-resistant strains of Escherichia coli and with klebsiella, and skin and soft-tissue infections with penicillin-resistant staphylococci.

Inappropriate use: As a single agent in life-threatening infections (efficacy unreliable). Streptococcal, pneumococcal and clostridial infections (because penicillin or amoxycillin alone would be fully active).

Contra-indications: Infectious mononucleosis and lymphatic leukaemia (rashes), pregnancy, neonatal period.

Administration and dosage: by mouth, expressed as amoxycillin, 250–500 mg (adults) or 15 mg/kg (children), every 8 h, preferably after meals. By i. v. injection or infusion, expressed as amoxycillin, 1 g (adults) or 25 mg/kg (children) every 8 h, increased to every 6 h in serious infections, but every 12 h in premature and fullterm neonates.

This dose is reduced in renal failure as follows: Where the creatinine clearance is 10–30 ml/min, give the normal dose every 12 h, and where the creatinine clearance is <10 ml/min, give half the normal dose every 12 h, or the normal dose every 24 h.

Preparations: Tablets and dispersible tablets of 250/125 mg, junior suspension of 125/62 mg in 5 ml, paediatric suspensions of 125/31 mg in 5 ml, injections of 0.5/0.1 g and 1.0/0.2 g, all expressed as amoxycillin/clavulanate.

Summary: Clavulanic acid in combination with amoxycillin (called co-amoxiclav) is a valuable addition to the range of oral antibiotics. It extends the spectrum of activity of amoxycillin against certain β-lactamase-producing bacteria (staphylococci, haemophilus, gonococci, Escherichia coli, Klebsiella pneumoniae and Bacteroides fragilis). This combination is an alternative to oral cephalosporins. When administered parenterally, it is as effective as the basic cephalosporins.

References

Bush, L. M., J. Calmon, and C. C. Johnson: Newer penicillins and beta-lactamase inhibitors. Infect. Dis. Clin. North Am. *3:* 571 (1989).

Engelhard, D., D. Cohen, N. Strauss, T. G. Sacks, L. Jorczak-Sarni, M. Shapiro: Randomised study of myringotomy, amoxycillin/clavulanate, or both for acute otitis media in infants. Lancet 2 *(8655):* 141–143 (1989).

Grange, J. D., A. Gouyette, L. Gutmann, X. Amiot, M. D. Kitzis, S. Islam, J. F. Acar, P. Jaillon: Pharmacokinetics of amoxycillin/clavulanic acid in serum and ascitic fluid in cirrhotic patients. J. Antimicrob. Chemother. *23:* 605–611 (1989).

Lapointe, J. R., C. Lavallée: Antibiotic interaction of amoxycillin and clavulanic acid against 132 β-lactamase positive haemophilus isolates: a comparison with some other oral agents. J. Antimicrob. Chemother. *19:* 49–58 (1987).

Nilsson-Ehle, I., H. Fellner, S.-Å. Hedström et al.: Pharmacokinetics of clavulanic acid, given in combination with amoxycillin in volunteers. J. Antimicrob. Chemother. *16:* 491 (1985).

Odio, C. M., H. Kusmiesz, S. Shelton, J. D. Nelson: Comparative treatment trial of Augmentin versus cefaclor for acute otitis media with effusion. Pediatrics *75:* 819 (1985).

Todd, P. A., F. Benfield: Amoxicillin/clavulanic acid. An update of the antibacterial activity, pharmacokinetic properties and therapeutic use. Drugs *39:* 264–307 (1990).

Williams, M. E., D. Thomas, C. P. Harman et al.: Positive direct antiglobulin tests due to clavulanic acid. Antimicrob. Ag. Chemother. *27:* 125 (1985).

β) Ticarcillin/Clavulanic Acid

Proprietary names: Betabactyl, Timentin.

Properties: Injectable combined preparation consisting of a β-lactamase inhibitor, clavulanic acid (p. 110), and ticarcillin (p. 50). Clavulanic acid protects ticarcillin from inactivation by certain bacterial β-lactamases (particularly types II, III, IV and V), but not those produced by Pseudomonas aeruginosa and other pseudomonas, serratia, enterobacter, Morganella morganii or Proteus rettgeri. The combination is also ineffective against Enterococcus faecalis (enterococci), but is more active against other species of proteus. Ticarcillin/clavulanic acid inhibits most strains of pseudomonas, provided they do not produce β-lactamase. Since ticarcillin is less active against pseudomonas than azlocillin or piperacillin, and ticarcillin is used to combat pseudomonas infections, the combination of ticarcillin with clavulanic acid has no major advantages, despite superior efficacy against staphylococci, klebsiella and Bacteroides fragilis.

Pharmacokinetics: Mean serum levels 1 h after a 30-min i.v. infusion of 0.1 g and 0.2 g of clavulanic acid are 1.8 and 3.4 mg/l, respectively. If 1.5 g or 5 g ticarcillin is given at the same time, mean ticarcillin concentrations are 60 and 193 mg/l, respectively. Both substances have a *half-life* of about 1 h. *Urinary recovery* of clavulanic acid is 70% after parenteral administration, and that of ticarcillin >95%.

Side-effects are rare when clavulanic acid is given parenterally, although allergic reactions are possible. Ticarcillin is known to cause hypernatremia, thrombophlebitis and a bleeding tendency (see p. 50).

Interactions: Concurrent administration of anticoagulants may enhance the bleeding tendency.

Indications: Infections whose bacterial cause is not established, particularly where pseudomonas is suspected, but other species may also be involved (in which case, combination with an aminoglycoside is advisable).

Contra-indications: Penicillin allergy, pregnancy.

Administration and dosage: For adults, 3.2 g 3–4 times a day, either in 30-min i.v. infusions or slow i.v. injections (5 min); give children 80 mg/kg 3–4 times a day.

In adult patients with *impaired renal function:* 3.2 g every 8 h (creatinine clearance 31–60 ml/min), every 12 h (creatinine clearance 10–30 ml/min), and 1.6 g every 12 h (creatinine clearance 10 ml/min);
Children are given 80 mg/kg every 8, 12 or 24 h.

Preparations: Injection of 1.6 g and 3.2 g containing 1.5 g and 3 g of ticarcillin and 0.1 g and 0.2 g of clavulanic acid, respectively.

Summary: The combination with clavulanic acid does not enhance the activity of ticarcillin against pseudomonas. The necessity for high dosage imposes a considerable metabolic burden.

References

BENNETT, S., R. WISE, D. WESTON, J. DENT: Pharmacokinetics and tissue penetration of ticarcillin combined with clavulanic acid. Antimicrob. Ag. Chemother. *23:* 831 (1983).
FRICKE, G., M. DOERCK, D. HAFNER, R. HORTON, M. KRESKEN: The pharmacokinetics of ticarcillin/clavulanate acid in neonates. J. Antimicrob. Chemother. *24:* 111–120 (1989).
FUCHS, P. C., A. L. BARRY, C. THORNSBERRY, R. N. JONES: In vitro activity of ticarcillin plus clavulanic acid against 632 clinical isolates. Antimicrob. Ag. Chemother. *25:* 392 (1984).

γ) Sulbactam/Ampicillin

Proprietary name: Unacid.

Properties: An injectable combined preparation of sulbactam (a β-lactamase inhibitor) and ampicillin (see p. 39). Sulbactam is a penicillanic acid sulphone (Fig. 31) and is also available without ampicillin (Combactam) for combination with mezlocillin, piperacillin or cefotaxime.

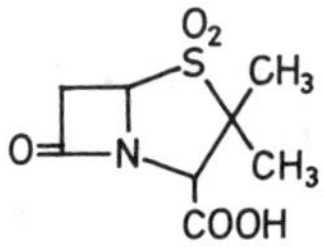

Fig. 31: Structural formula of sulbactam

Sulbactam itself has little intrinsic antibacterial activity but extends the spectrum of ampicillin by inhibition of certain β-lactamase (of types II, III, IV, and V) on a proportion of the ampicillin-resistant strains of Staphylococcus aureus, Staph. epidermidis, E. coli, Klebsiella pneumoniae, Proteus mirabilis, Proteus vulgaris and Bacteroides fragilis. β-lactamase-producing strains of gonococci, haemophilus and branhamella are also inhibited by the combination. Species and strains that are intrinsically resistant to ampicillin (e. g. pseudomonas, serratia, enterobacter, a proportion of methicillin-resistant staphylococci and all the enterobacteria that produce β-lactamase of type I) are also resistant to sulbactam/ampicillin.

In-vitro testing of isolates, particularly of Enterobacteriaceae, is therefore advisable. The activity of the combination is similar to that of the basic cephalosporins (cefazolin group).

Pharmacokinetics: One hour after the end of a 30-minute i. v. infusion of 1.5 g of the combination of sulbactam 0.5 g and ampicillin 1 g, the *mean serum concentration* of sulbactam is 7 mg/l and of ampicillin 17 mg/l. After a 15-minute i. v. infusion of 3 g of the combination (sulbactam 1 g + ampicillin 2 g), the mean serum concentrations are sulbactam 16 mg/l and ampicillin 35 mg/l, 1 h after the end of the infusion. *Half-life* of both substances is 1 h. *CSF penetration* is low. *Urinary recovery* of sulbactam is 75% and of ampicillin 60%. The ratio of the two components may vary considerably in different organs.

Side-effects: Anaemia, thrombocytopenia, eosinophilia and leucocytopenia occur rarely and are reversible after cessation of therapy. Occasional transient rises of liver enzymes have been reported, as have nausea, vomiting and diarrhoea; severe, persistent diarrhoea should alert one to pseudomembranous enterocolitis (see p. 406). Rashes, itching and other skin manifestations have occasionally been reported.

Pain at the i. m. injection site and phlebitis after i. v. use may occur. Very high serum concentrations can cause fits; allergic reactions and anaphylactic shock can all occur as with other penicillins.

Interactions: Concurrent intake of allopurinol enhances the risk of allergic skin reactions.

Indications: Mild infections with ampicillin-resistant bacteria whose β-lactamases are inhibited by sulbactam. Such infections include mild respiratory infections (sinusitis, otitis media and suppurative bronchitis due to β-lactamase producing strains of haemophilus and branhamella), urinary infections with ampicillin-resistant E. coli and klebsiella, and skin and soft tissue infections with penicillin- and ampicillin-resistant staphylococci.

Inappropriate use: As a single agent in life-threatening infection (activity unreliable). Infections with streptococci, pneumococci and clostridia (where benzylpenicillin or ampicillin alone are fully active).

Contra-indications: Infectious mononucleosis and lymphatic leukaemia (rashes), pregnancy, first year of life.

Administration and dosage: For adults, 1–3 g 3–4 times daily as a short i. v. infusion; children over the age of 1 year should receive 15–45 mg/kg 3–4 times a day. Since the i. m. injection can be painful, the solution for injection should be made up with 0.5% lignocaine. The daily dose should be reduced in renal impairment by giving the normal single dose every 12 h for creatinine clearances of 15–30 ml/min, every 24 h for creatinine clearances of 5–14 ml/min, and every 48 h for creatinine clearances less than 5 ml/min.

When sulbactam is prescribed as a single agent with e. g. mezlocillin, piperacillin or cefotaxime, the single dose of sulbactam for adults is 0.5–1 g every

6, 8 or 12 h (up to a maximum of 4 g daily), and for children 15 mg/kg (up to a maximum of 80 mg/kg daily).

Preparations: Vials of 0.75 g, 1.5 g and 3 g (containing ⅓ sulbactam and ⅔ ampicillin) and vials of 1 g (sulbactam alone).

Summary: For parenteral use only at present. The combination with sulbactam extends the spectrum of the ampicillin to include β-lactamase-producing strains of staphylococci, haemophilus, branhamella, gonococci, Esch. coli, klebsiella and other species. Since mechanisms of resistance other than β-lactamases can occur, the sensitivities of the causative organism should always be tested.

References

ALDRIDGE, K. E. et al.: Variation in the potentation of β-lactam antibiotic activity by clavulanic acid and sulbactam against multiple antibiotic-resistant bacteria. J. Antimicrob. Chemoth. *17:* 463–469 (1986).

CROMBLEHOLME, W. R., M. OHM-SMITH, M. O. ROBBIE et al.: Ampicillin/sulbactam versus metronidazole-gentamicin in the treatment of soft tissue pelvic infections. Am. J. Obstet. Gynecol. *156:* 507–512 (1987).

FRANK, U.: In Vitro Activity of Sulbactam Plus Ampicillin Against Hospital Isolates of Coagulase-negative Staphylococci and Acinetobacter Species. Infection *17:* 272–274 (1989).

FRANK, U.: Concentrations of Sulbactam/Ampicillin in Serum and Lung Tissue. Infection *18:* 307–309 (1990).

JACOBY, G. A.: Pseudomonas cepacia Susceptibility to Sulbactam. Antimicrob. Agents Chemoth. *33:* 583–584 (1989).

KIM, J. H., K.-H. CHOI: Treatment of multi-resistant N. gonorrhoeae infection with sulbactam/ampicillin. Rev. Infect. Dis. *8 (Suppl. 5):* 599–603 (1986).

KULHANJIAN, J., M. G. DUNPHY, S. HAMSTRA, K. LEVERNIER, M. RANKIN, A. PETRU, P. AZIMI: Randomized comparative study of ampicillin/sulbactam vs. ceftriaxone for treatment of soft tissue and skeletal infections in children. Pediatr. Infect. Dis. J. *8:* 605–610 (1989).

OLIVENCIA-YURVATI, A. H., S. P. SANDERS: Sulbactam induced hyperpyrexia. Arch. Intern. Med. *150:* 1961 (1990).

RIPA, S., L. FERRANTE, M. PRENNA: Pharmacokinetics of sulbactam/ampicillin in humans after intravenous and intramuscular injection. Chemotherapy *36:* 185–192 (1990).

SCHAAD, U. B.: Pharmacokinetics of sulbactam in pediatric patients. Rev. Infect. Dis. *8 (Suppl. 5):* 512–517 (1986).

WEXLER, H. M. et al.: In vitro efficacy of sulbactam combined with ampicillin against anaerobic bacteria. Ant. Ag. Chemoth. *Vol. 27, No. 5:* 876–878 (1985).

WRIGHT, N., R. WISE: The elimination of sulbactam alone and combined with ampicillin in patients with renal dysfunction. J. Antimicrob. Chemother. *11:* 583–587 (1983).

δ) Tazobactam

Properties: Tazobactam is an irreversible β-lactamase inhibitor (a derivative of penicillanic acid sulphone) with a triazolyl methyl ring in the 2β position. The compound has, in comparison with sulbactam and clavulanic acid, an improved range of inhibitory activity, particularly with gram-negative organisms.

Spectrum of activity: Tazobactam inhibits the majority of plasmid-mediated β-lactamases and many of the chromosomally coded cephalosporinases of groups II–IV. The inhibition of group I cephalosporinases is an advance, since these have not been susceptible to the other β-lactamase inhibitors available to date. Tazobactam has no antibacterial effect of its own, except against Acinetobacter calcoaceticus. Tazobactam has been developed for use in combination with piperacillin, and includes all β-lactamase-producing piperacillin-resistant strains of Staphylococcus aureus and most strains of Esch. coli, serratia, Klebsiella pneumoniae, Enterobacter cloacae, Citrobacter freundii, proteus and β-lactamase-producing Pseudomonas aeruginosa. The combination is ineffective against strains of pseudomonas whose resistance is due to lack of penetration of the bacterial cell. Tazobactam abolishes the β-lactamase-mediated resistance of anaerobes, particularly Bacteroides fragilis, to piperacillin.

The **pharmacokinetics** of tazobactam are very similar to those of piperacillin. Protein binding (about 20%) is comparable to that of piperacillin. The mode of elimination of each component of the combination is almost identical. About 80% of the inhibitor is excreted through the kidneys and a smaller proportion through the hepatobiliary tree.

The combination of tazobactam and piperacillin is currently undergoing clinical trials. It is a potent β-lactamase-stable penicillin preparation whose spectrum of action includes most gram-positive and gram-negative aerobes and anaerobes. Unlike other β-lactamase inhibitors available to date, tazobactam also inhibits most cephalosporinases.

References

HIGASHITANI, F., A. HYODO, N. ISHIDA, M. INOUE, S. MITSUHASHI: Inhibition of beta-lactamases by tazobactam and in-vitro antibacterial activity of tazobactam combined with piperacillin. J. Antimicrob. Chemother. *25:* 567–574 (1990).

JONES, R. N., M. A. PFALLER, P. C. FUCHS, K. ALDRIDGE, S. D. ALLEN, E. H. GERLACH: Piperacillin/tazobactam (YTR 830) combination. Comparative antimicrobial activity against 5889 recent aerobic clinical isolates and 60 Bacteroides fragilis group strains. Diagn. Microbiol. Infect. Dis. *12:* 489–494 (1989).

4. Tetracyclines

Common proprietary names:
Tetracycline: Achromycin, Hostacyclin etc. Deteclo contains tetracycline, chlortetracycline and demeclocycline.
Oxytetracycline: Terramycin etc.
Demeclocycline: Ledermycin.
Rolitetracycline: Reverin.
Doxycycline: Vibramycin.
Minocycline: Minocin.

Properties: A group of closely related broad-spectrum antibiotics with a naphthacene ring system. Tetracycline, oxytetracycline, rolitetracycline, minocycline and doxycycline differ from each other in the composition of their side-chains (Fig. 32), but they have an identical spectrum of action with the exception of minocycline, which retains activity against strains of staphylococci resistant to the other tetracyclines. There are various differences in activity and pharmacokinetic properties (absorption, blood concentrations, plasma protein binding, excretion) between the different tetracyclines, on the basis of which doxycycline and minocycline, which have sustained activity, can be separated from the other tetracyclines, whose half-lives are shorter.

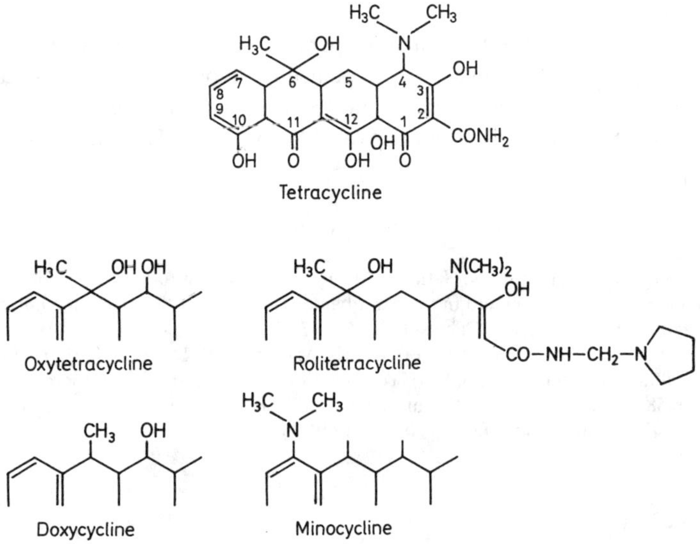

Fig. 32. Chemical structure of the tetracyclines.

Mode of action: The bacteriostatic activity of the tetracyclines is based on the inhibition of protein synthesis in the bacterial cell by prevention of acylation of amino acids as they enter the ribosome on the growing peptide chain. This action affects both extracellular and intracellular bacteria. The activity of the tetracyclines is very medium-dependent, and much activity is lost in certain body fluids (e. g. bile).

Spectrum of activity:
Moderate or good sensitivity: Streptococci, pneumococci, gonococci, meningococci, listeria, actinomycetes, Pasteurella multocida, yersinia, haemophilus, brucella, Pseudomonas mallei and pseudomallei, Vibrio cholerae and Vibrio parahaemolyticus, Campylobacter jejuni, Treponema pallidum, leptospira, Francisella tularensis and Bordetella pertussis. Good activity also against mycoplasmas, chlamydiae (ornithosis, trachoma, lymphogranuloma inguinale), Coxiella burnetii (Q fever) and rickettsiae (typhus).

Variable sensitivity: Enterococci, staphylococci, Escherichia coli, klebsiella, enterobacter, acinetobacter, salmonellae, shigellae, Bacteroides species, clostridia, corynebacteria, nocardia, Bacillus anthracis.

Little activity against mycobacteria.

Inactive against Pseudomonas aeruginosa, Proteus vulgaris, Serratia marcescens.

Resistance: There is little tendency for resistance to arise during therapy. The proportion of resistant strains of staphylococci varies from place to place (10–30%). Resistant strains of haemolytic streptococci, pneumococci, gonococci, clostridia and Haemophilus influenzae also occur (10–35% of Lancefield Group A streptococci, 2–30% of pneumococci and 3% of Haemophilus influenzae are resistant). Only 40–60% of strains of Bacteroides fragilis are sensitive to tetracyclines. Penicillin-resistant strains of gonococci are generally resistant to tetracyclines as well. There is cross-resistance between all the tetracyclines except minocycline against staphylococci, but no cross-resistance with other antibiotics.

Pharmacokinetics:
Absorption after oral administration is variable and depends on the individual preparation. Tetracycline and oxytetracycline are less completely absorbed than demeclocycline. Comparative studies of i. v. and oral administration show doxycycline to be 75% and minocycline to be almost completely absorbed. The absorption of tetracycline is impaired by food, particularly milk and certain drugs (aluminium hydroxide, sodium bicarbonate, potassium and magnesium salts, ferrous sulphate, activated charcoal and cholestyramine). Increasing the oral dose of tetracycline beyond 250 mg, which achieves maximum absorption, does not usually increase the blood level proportionally, but simply results in greater loss in the faeces. Blood concentrations of doxycycline (Fig. 33) and minocycline, on the

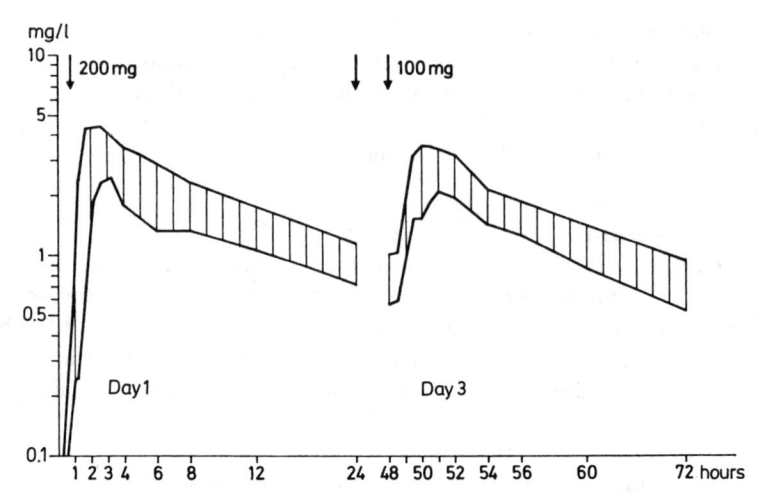

Fig. 33. Serum concentration in 8 adults after a single dose of 200 mg doxycycline (left) and after repeated oral doses of 100 mg doxycycline every 24 hours on day 3 (right) (own data).

other hand, are doubled by increasing the dose from 100 to 200 mg, and doubled again from 200 to 400 mg. Maximal blood concentrations after oral administration are achieved after 2–3 hours.

Mean serum concentrations with regular oral administration of 250 mg tetracycline or oxytetracycline are between 1 and 3 mg/l. Maximal serum concentrations of 3 mg/l are found after a single daily dose of 100 mg of doxycycline or 200 mg of minocycline. Unlike minocycline, doxycycline shows some non-toxic accumulation, so a maintenance dose of 100 mg following an initial dose of 200 mg is sufficient. Minocycline requires a maintenance dose of 200 mg.

Mean serum concentrations after a single i. v. injection of 250 mg of an injectable tetracycline (e. g. oxy- or rolitetracycline) are 3–5 mg/l after 3–4 h, 2–3 mg/l after 6 h and 1–2 mg/l after 12 h; for those after 200 mg doxycycline, see Fig. 34. 3.6 mg/l are achieved in the serum after an i. v. infusion of 200 mg of doxycycline for 1 hour, and 2.5 mg/l with 100 mg. After an i. v. infusion of doxycycline 200 mg over 1 h, 3.6 mg/l are found in the serum, and 2.5 mg/l after 100 mg.

After 200 mg of minocycline i. v. over 60 min, the serum concentration falls from 3.5 mg/l at the end of the infusion to 1 mg/l after 12 h and 0.6 mg/l after 24 h. *Half-lives* of tetracycline, oxytetracycline and rolitetracycline: 8–9 h; doxycycline and minocycline: 15 h. The half-life of doxycycline is reduced to 7 h when phenytoin or barbiturate are given at the same time, due to enzyme induction in the liver.

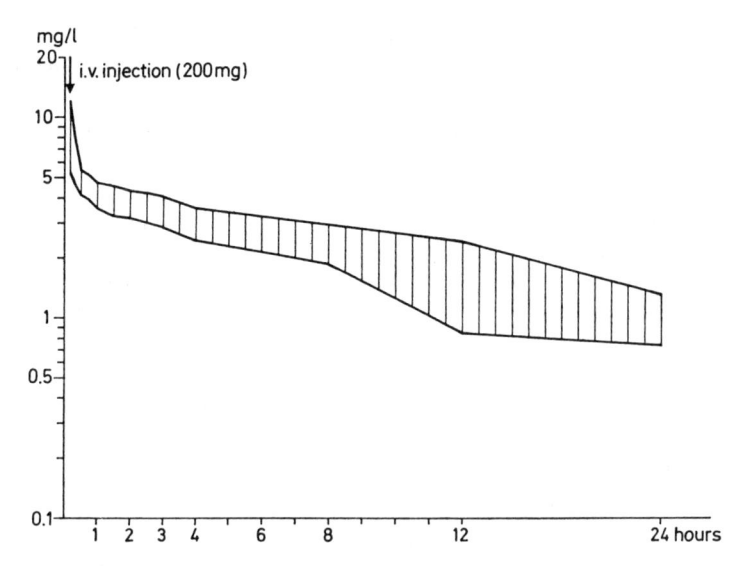

Fig. 34. Serum concentrations in 8 adults after 200 mg of doxycycline i. v. (own data).

Protein binding of tetracycline and oxytetracycline in the serum: 40%; rolitetracycline: 50%; doxycycline: 96%; minocycline: 75%.

Good *tissue diffusion* in the liver, kidneys, spleen, bones, lungs and genital tract. High biliary concentration. 50–75% of the maternal serum concentration is found in the cord blood, 20% in the amniotic fluid and 50–100% in the breast milk. Effective tetracycline concentrations are achieved in the pleural, pericardial, peritoneal and synovial fluids.

CSF penetration: Poor (at 1–10% of serum concentrations), but 20–40% with minocycline and improved penetration with meningeal inflammation.

Excretion of tetracycline and oxytetracycline is predominantly renal, mainly by glomerular filtration, at 10–25% after oral and 50–70% after i. v. administration. High urinary concentrations (50–300 mg/l). Delayed excretion of doxycycline and minocycline. *Urinary recovery* of doxycycline: 70% and 40% after i. v. and oral administration respectively; of minocycline: 5.9% and 5.5%. Urinary concentrations of doxycycline after 200 mg i. v. and orally: 60–200 mg/l; of minocycline after 200 mg orally: 4–25 mg/l. Because about 35% of absorbed minocycline is excreted into the intestines through the bile, more than 40% of the ingested antibiotic may be assumed to be metabolised in the body. The other tetracyclines are also excreted at high concentration in the bile when liver function is normal and the extrahepatic biliary tree is patent. They are then partly reabsorbed in the intestinal tract and partly metabolised in the body. After oral administration, the concentrations of tetracycline and oxytetracycline are particularly high in the faeces due to the incomplete absorption (200–2000 µg/g), while the better absorbed preparations (doxycycline and minocycline) are lost to a much lesser extent in the stools. Gastro-intestinal upset is therefore less common with these preparations, and they can be given in smaller doses.

Apart from doxycycline and minocycline, tetracyclines accumulate in *renal failure*. This can lead to liver damage and so require a reduction in dosage (see below). The half-life of doxycycline is prolonged to 15–24 hours depending on the severity of renal failure, but repeated administration of the normal dose does not result in accumulation. The half-life of minocycline is prolonged in chronic renal failure.

Side-effects:
1. *Gastrointestinal* upset with vomiting and diarrhoea due to irritation of the intestinal mucosa or disturbance of the gut flora. Stomatitis, glossitis, oesophagitis, proctitis, and vaginitis also occur. Pseudomembranous enterocolitis (caused by Clostridium difficile) is a rare but severe complication of tetracycline therapy and can develop after i. v. administration as well. It is doubtful whether the increased growth of candida in the intestines is the cause of gastrointestinal disturbances during tetracycline treatment. The prophylactic value of adding nystatin or amphotericin B to tetracycline preparations has not been established in comparative studies.
2. *Severe liver damage* can follow overdosage, particularly after parenteral administration in the third trimester of pregnancy or following the accumulation of tetracyclines in renal failure. The daily parenteral dose should not therefore exceed 750 mg (–1 g) of oxytetracycline or rolitetracycline, and 200 (–300) mg of doxycycline and minocycline. The combination of tetracyclines with other potentially hepatotoxic drugs such as chlorpromazine, phenylhydantoin and phenylbutazone derivatives should be avoided.
3. *Photosensitivity* occurs particularly after demeclocycline which should therefore no longer be used. It may also occur with other tetracyclines but is rare with minocycline. Erythema and oedema are found on exposed areas of the body. Regression is slow, requiring 2–4 weeks, and residual pigmentation and detachment of the nails may persist. Exposure to the sun should therefore be avoided in patients receiving tetracycline therapy.
4. *Allergies* (rashes, anaphylactic shock) have only been observed rarely. There is cross-allergy between all the tetracyclines.
5. *Reversible leucocytopenia* due to allergic bone marrow depression is rare.
6. *The teeth of small children* can be stained yellow irreversibly, often with associated enamel defects and an increased incidence of caries. The tetracycline is deposited in the teeth, bones and nails as tetracycline calcium phosphate. Both deciduous and permanent teeth may be affected, depending

on the phase of odontogenesis in which the tetracycline has been given between the 4th month of pregnancy and the end of the 7th year. Tetracycline should therefore be avoided between the 1st and 7th year. Infants should only be given tetracycline where alternative drugs have failed and there are very clear indications for treatment. In such cases, the yellow discoloration of the teeth may have to be accepted. A temporary and completely reversible delay of bone growth in premature infants has only been observed when overdosage was considerable.
7. Tetracycline therapy can give rise to a reversible increase in *intracranial pressure*, shown in the newborn as bulging of the fontanelle and as papilloedema in older children and adults, with visual disturbance and severe headache.
8. *Various types of renal damage* can occur, expressed either as deterioration of a pre-existing renal functional impairment and shown by an increase of serum creatinine and urea, or as renal damage associated with acute fatty change in the liver, also caused by tetracycline. A partially reversible *nephrogenic diabetes insipidus* which is resistant to vasopressin is occasionally caused by demeclocycline.
9. *Pseudoglycosuria:* Reduction tests in the urine may be falsely positive at high tetracycline concentrations, simulating glycosuria.
10. Because of their magnesium content, some tetracycline derivatives for intravenous injection may cause cardiac arrhythmias in digitalised patients. This can be avoided by injecting slowly over the recommended minimum period of 2 min. Injectable rolitetracycline, doxycycline and oxytetracycline are contra-indicated in myasthenia gravis on account of their magnesium content.
11. *Local irritation and phlebitis* sometimes complicate i. v. administration, and rapid injection can give rise to general symptoms such as dizziness, sweating, and circulatory collapse. Pain at the injection site commonly follows i. m. injection. *Ulceration of the oesophageal mucosa* has occasionally been reported after doxycycline and tetracycline capsules, but not tablets. This is mostly seen in patients with hiatus hernia.
12. Minocycline frequently causes *transient dizziness* at the onset of treatment, particularly in women, which is sometimes associated with drowsiness and nausea and may impair driving ability. It is probably due to central nervous system disturbance, and in some cases treatment has had to be stopped.

Interactions: Since tetracyclines can reduce plasma prothrombin activity, concurrent anticoagulant dosage should be reduced. The concurrent administration of oral antidiabetic agents (sulphonylureas) can potentiate the reduction in blood sugar. Simultaneous doxycycline and cyclosporin A may enhance the toxicity of cyclosporin A. Interactions have also been reported with methoxyflurane (increased nephrotoxicity), mineral antacids (impaired absorption of tetracyclines), amethopterin (enhanced amethopterin toxicity) and digoxin (increased plasma concentrations of digoxin).

Indications: Infections with sensitive gram-negative rods (Escherichia coli, haemophilus, bacteroides). Long-term treatment of chronic bronchitis, e. g. with one dose of doxycycline a day, which is well tolerated. Treatment of interstitial pneumonia with features suggestive of mycoplasma, Chlamydia pneumoniae, ornithosis or Q fever. Non-gonorrhoeal urethritis, due to Chlamydia trachomatis or Ureaplasma urealyticum. Infectious diseases such as brucellosis, yersinia infections, tularaemia, plague, leptospirosis, lymphogranuloma inguinale, trachoma, rickettsiosis (typhus etc.), listeriosis, melioidosis (caused by Pseudomonas pseudomallei), syphilis and gonorrhoea in patients with penicillin allergy, acne and rosacea, Whipple's disease.

Inappropriate usage: Clinically typical or bacteriologically proven infections with staphylococci, streptococci, pneumococci (which are often resistant) or Pseudomonas aeruginosa (commonly resistant).

Caution is advised in patients with severe liver disease (risk of further hepatotoxicity), especially in acute hepatitis, as well as in renal failure.

Contra-indications: Pregnancy. Children up to the age of 7 (yellow dental staining). Use in younger children only when there is no satisfactory alternative (e. g. doxycycline in ornithosis). Myasthenia gravis (applies to all intravenous tetracyclines on account of their magnesium content).

Administration: Generally as coated tablets, film tablets or capsules after meals, and as syrup in children. 3–4 divided doses are advised. 1–2 single i. v. doses a day may be given to seriously ill patients and to those who cannot take the antibiotic by mouth. Continuous infusion of tetracycline hydrochloride is not recommended because of the high incidence of phlebitis; it has been superceded by other injectable tetracyclines.

Dosage:
Oral: Doxycycline: 200 mg (4 mg/kg) on day 1, later reduced to 100 mg (2 mg/kg). Long-term treatment in doses up to 200 mg a day (4 mg/kg) in severe infections.

Minocycline 200 mg (4 mg/kg for children initially), then 100 mg every 12 h (or 2 mg/kg for children).

Tetracycline and oxytetracycline: 1–1.5 (–2) g, 20–30 mg/kg for children, in 2–4 divided doses 1 h before or 2 h after meals.

Intravenous: Doxycycline: 200 mg once a day initially followed by a maintenance dose of 100 (–200) mg as a slow i. v. injection; 2–4 mg/kg once a day for children. Minocycline: 200 mg a day for adults, 4 mg/kg for children, in 1 or 2 short i. v. infusions.

Rolitetracycline and oxytetracycline: 0.25–0.5 (–0.75) g a day in 2 (–3) divided doses, 10 mg/kg for children under 12 years (maximum single dose 100 mg). Because the preparations contain solubilisers and magnesium, injection must be slow (250 mg over at least 3 minutes). Do not mix with other drugs.

Preparations:
Tetracycline: Coated tablets, capsules and tablets of 50 mg, 250 mg and 500 mg.
Oxytetracycline: Capsules and tablets of 250 mg and 500 mg.
Doxycycline and *minocycline:* Capsules and tablets of 100 mg and 200 mg.
Demeclocycline: Tablets of 150 mg and 300 mg.
For children: Drops or syrup. For i. v. injection: Vials of 100 mg, 250 mg and 275 mg. For i. v. infusion: Vials of 250 and 500 mg.
There are also many topical preparations which contain tetracycline.

Summary:
Advantages: Effective against haemophilus and many intracellular infections (caused e. g. by mycoplasmas, chlamydiae and rickettsiae), good tissue diffusion, long-term therapy possible. Allergy very rare.
Disadvantages: Increasing resistance amongst the gram-negative bacilli, and only bacteriostatic at therapeutically attainable concentrations.

Doxycycline is preferred because it is well absorbed and tolerated and relatively little metabolised. I. v. preparations are nowadays only used in exceptional cases and for very few indications.

References

AMENDOLA, M. A., T. D. SPERA: Doxycycline-induced esophagitis. JAMA *253:* 1009 (1985).
FANNING, W. L., D. W. GUMP, R. A. SOFFERMAN: Side effects of minocycline: a double-blind study. Antimicrob. Ag. Chemother. *11:* 712 (1977).
PEARSON, M. G., S. M. LITTLEWOOD, A. N. BOWDEN: Tetracycline and benign intracranial hypertension. Brit. Med. J. *282:* 568 (1981).
ROGERS, H. J., F. R. HOUSE, P. J. MORRISON, I. D. BRADBOOK: Interaction of cimetidine with tetracycline absorption. Lancet *2:* 694 (1980).
SIMPSON, M. B.: Hemolytic anemia after tetracycline therapy. N. Engl. J. Med. *312:* 840 (1985).
WHO: Neisseria gonorrhoeae. Emergence of plasmid-mediated tetracycline-resistant strains. Wkly Epidem. Rec. *36:* 277 (1986).

5. Chloramphenicol Group

a) Chloramphenicol

Properties: *p*-Nitrophenyl-dichloroacetyl-aminopropanediol, a derivative of phenylalanine (Fig. 35). Unrelated to other antibiotics except for thiamphenicol. Chloramphenicol is very bitter, very stable, insoluble in water but readily soluble in lipids. Esterification of the alcohol group with certain higher fatty acids gives rise to esters such as the stearoyl glycolate and palmitate (available as granules) and the succinate (injectable). The esters possess no intrinsic antibacterial activity, and active chloramphenicol is released by the body's own esterases and lipases. Unlike free chloramphenicol, the succinate is readily soluble in water and is therefore suitable for parenteral use. *In-vitro* testing shows apparent resistance on account of the presence in many cultural media of the anatagonist, phenylalanine.

Mode of action: Bacteriostatic, with inhibition of bacterial protein synthesis by blocking the transfer of soluble ribonucleic acid to ribosomes.

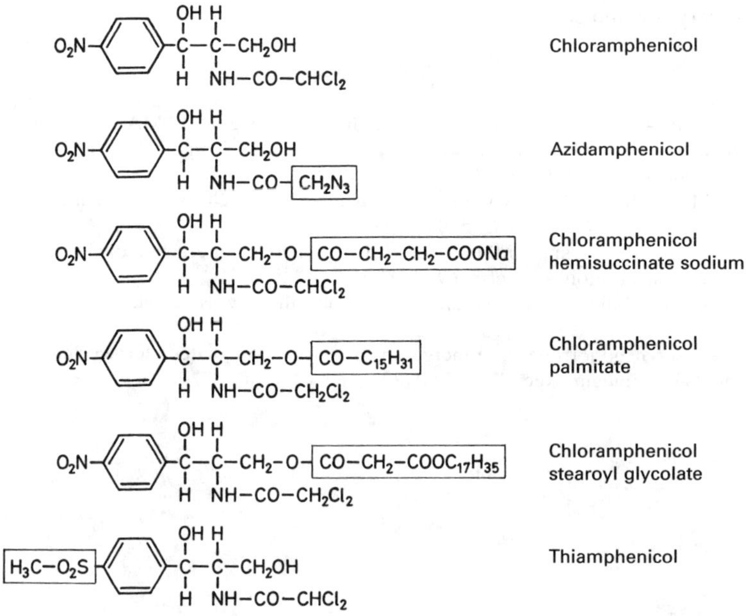

Fig. 35. Structural formulae of chloramphenicol, azidamphenicol and thiamphenicol.

Spectrum of activity: Activity against most gram-positive and gram-negative bacteria as well as against rickettsiae (typhus), spirochaetes, chlamydiae, mycoplasmas, leptospiras, and most non-sporing anaerobes (Bacteroides spp., fusobacteria, peptococci and peptostreptococci). Chloramphenicol is also active against salmonellae, rickettsiae (spotted fever), chlamydiae, mycoplasmas and leptospires. Mycobacteria, nocardia, fungi, protozoa and viruses are always resistant, as are most strains of Pseudomonas aeruginosa.

Resistance to chloramphenicol is increasingly emerging amongst salmonellae and shigellae; the former are also often resistant to ampicillin. Resistance is, however, seldom seen in Haemophilus influenzae, meningococci, pneumococci or other streptococci. The proportion of resistant gram-negative intestinal bacteria shows local variation, but some 20% of E. coli, 30% of Proteus, 50% of Klebsiella/Enterobacter and 20–40% of Serratia marcescens strains will typically be resistant. Chloramphenicol-resistant strains of Haemophilus influenzae may also be ampicillin-resistant. Resistance is usually due to bacterial production of acetyl transferase which inactivates chloramphenicol.

Staphylococci are less frequently resistant to chloramphenicol than to tetracycline. Streptococci can also be resistant to chloramphenicol. Enterococcus faecalis and other enterococci are usually sensitive, as are gonococci. Resistance of occasional strains of Bacteroides fragilis has been reported. There is a small risk of resistance development during therapy. Cross-resistance with other antibiotics (except thiamphenicol) is not generally found.

Pharmacokinetics: Rapid and almost complete *absorption* (90%) after oral administration which depends on particle size. Blood concentrations are 2–4 times higher with small particles. Maximal serum concentrations are reached after 2–4 hours. Chloramphenicol is available as two antibacterially inactive esters, the palmitate (a suspension) and the stearoyl glycolate (granules). They are hydrolysed in the gastrointestinal tract by esterases and lipases prior to absorption, and active chloramphenicol is released. Non-esterified chloramphenicol is preferable in patients with difficulties in digestion or enzyme deficiencies. After parenteral administration, the antibacterially inactive chloramphenicol monosuccinate sodium is transformed into free chloramphenicol by hydrolysis in the liver.

Serum concentrations after repeated oral doses of 500 mg: 4–6 mg/l; after repeated doses of 1 g: 10–16 mg/l. Values between 5–9 mg/l (after 1–2 h) are obtained after i.v. injection of 500 mg; 4–6 mg/l (after 3–4 h), 3–4 mg/l (after 5–7 h) and 3 mg/l (after 8–10 h). *Half-life:* 3 hours. Concurrent administration of phenobarbitone reduces the half-life due to induction of hepatic enzymes. *Binding to serum protein:* approx. 50%.

Chloramphenicol is mostly present in the active form in the blood. It is partially inactivated in the body by binding to glucuronic acid (10% in serum, 90% in urine), and also by hydrolysis and reduction of the nitro compound to amine.

Good tissue diffusion occurs in all organs and in cells. 50% of the serum concentrations are found in the CSF as well as in the pleural, peritoneal and synovial fluids. In meningitis, the CSF concentration can increase to the level of the serum concentrations. Therapeutically effective concentrations are also found in the aqueous and vitreous humors. 30–80% of the maternal serum values are found in the cord blood and amniotic fluid, and about 50% in the breast milk.

Excretion: Predominantly through the kidneys (up to 90%) by glomerular filtration of free chloramphenicol (5–12%) and tubular secretion of the inactive glucuronide (about 90%). Urinary free chloramphenicol concentrations are between 70 and 150 mg/l when 500 mg are given every 6 hours. Inactive metabolites accumulate in renal failure, but the serum concentrations of free chloramphenicol do not rise markedly. In patients with severe liver damage, the half-life of free chloramphenicol is prolonged up to 6 hours because of the reduced binding to glucuronic acid.

A small amount is excreted through the bile (concentrations of active chloramphenicol are about 20–50% of serum concentrations); only very small amounts pass out with the faeces.

Side-effects: *Aplastic blood dyscrasias* are the most dangerous side-effects of chloramphenicol. They almost always occur as irreversible pancytopenia or aplastic anaemia, leukopenia or thrombocytopenia, or a combination of these disorders. They mostly occur after a latent period of 2–8 weeks and are fatal in more than 50% of cases.

It is difficult to obtain reliable information about the frequency of aplastic chloramphenicol blood dyscrasias. The published figures range between 1:10,000 and 1:40,000. The frequency increases with increasing total dosage, but blood disorders have also followed short courses of treatment. Minor disorders also occur, such as reversible depression of erythropoiesis (hyporegeneratory anaemia), accompanied by a fall in the reticulocyte count and haemoglobin, vacuolisation of proerythroblasts and granulocyte precursors and neutropenia. The reduced utilisation of iron in haemoglobin synthesis causes the serum iron to rise. The cause of these toxic disturbances is the inhibition of protein synthesis by the action of chloramphenicol on messenger RNA, and they appear regularly when serum concentrations exceed 25 mg/l.

Mild gastrointestinal symptoms such as flatulence and loose stools are quite common but not dangerous.

Allergies occur only rarely.

"Grey baby" syndrome: Newborn babies and premature infants treated with doses of more than 25 mg/kg may react with vomiting, meteorism, hypothermia, respiratory problems, grey skin coloration and uncontrolled circulatory collapse. These symptoms are often fatal within a few hours and result from the toxic accumulation of chloramphenicol which is not adequately conjugated to

glucuronic acid in the immature liver for excretion in the urine. In such cases, the half-life is 6–7 times longer than usual.

Optic neuritis and peripheral neuritis: Very rare side-effects, found particularly after long-term treatment of children with chloramphenicol for recurrent pulmonary infection in cystic fibrosis; vision sometimes returns after discontinuation of the antibiotic and treatment with large doses of vitamin B complex.

Interactions: The combination of chloramphenicol with potentially haematotoxic drugs may precipitate blood dyscrasias. Chloramphenicol can potentiate the effects of sulphonylureas, coumarin and phenytoin drugs. The simultaneous administration of chloramphenicol and methotrexate can intensify methotrexate toxicity, and when chloramphenicol and paracetamol are given together the half-life of chloramphenicol may be prolonged.

Indications: Severe salmonella infections (typhoid, paratyphoid, salmonella septicaemia and meningitis) and life- or vision-threatening intraocular infections with chloramphenicol-susceptible organisms against which safer antibiotics are inactive or contraindicated. Chloramphenicol may also be necessary for brain abscesses, purulent meningitis and rickettsiosis, and continues to be used for the local treatment of skin and eye infections. In typical countries, chloramphenicol, which is cheap and very stable, remains an important antimicrobial.

Inappropriate use: Infections against which other, less dangerous antibiotics are also effective; infections where bactericidal therapy is important (endocarditis, osteomyelitis, salmonella carriage); topical instillation of inactive chloramphenicol succinate, which is only activated after i. v. administration when it is hydrolysed in the liver.

Contra-indications: Blood diseases like aplastic anaemia or pancytopenia; severe liver failure with jaundice. Combination with other potentially haematotoxic preparations (e. g. cytotoxic drugs, sulphonamides, phenothiazine, phenylbutazone, hydantoin etc.). The dose should be reduced in premature and full-term neonates. Because of the risk of cytotoxicity, chloramphenicol should not be given during pregnancy or lactation.

Administration: Usually oral, as a syrup for children. I. v. for unconscious and seriously ill patients, as 10–20% chloramphenicol succinate solution. Topical administration of free chloramphenicol for infections of the skin, eyes and ears. Intramuscular and rectal administration is not recommended (absorption unreliable).

Dosage: *Adults:* 1.5–3 g daily in 3–4 divided doses. Do not give less than the minimum dose of 1.5 g. The same dose is used orally and parenterally, because chloramphenicol is almost completely absorbed. *Children and infants:* 50 (–80) mg/kg daily, usually as a syrup or parenterally. *Neonates:* in 1st–2nd week:

25 mg/kg/day, in 3rd–4th week: 50 mg/kg/day. Serum concentrations should be measured at least once a week to ensure that peak concentrations are in the range 20–30 mg/l, and trough concentrations remain less than 15 mg/l. Serum concentrations should be measured even more frequently in patients treated concurrently with a barbiturate, diphenylhydantoin or paracetamol. Since the half-life is prolonged in patients with impaired liver function and serum and tissue levels are higher than in patients with normal liver function, the daily dose should be reduced in accordance with blood levels of chloramphenicol, whose peaks should not exceed 20 mg/l. The daily dose need not be reduced in severe renal failure, although there is some risk of side-effects due to increased concentrations of certain metabolites.

The total dose should generally be limited to 25–30 g for adults and 700 mg/kg for children, and should be exceeded only in life-threatening disease. Treatment with chloramphenicol should not, therefore, normally last longer than 14 days. If the total dose is exceeded, the blood count, platelet and reticulocyte counts should be checked frequently. Regular tests are also advisable to detect any fall in haematocrit or increase in serum iron, so that treatment can be stopped immediately at the first sign of incipient blood disease. Bone-marrow depression, which usually develops only after a latent period, is not preventable. The dosage and length of treatment are not restricted in topical therapy with eye drops, ear drops or skin ointments.

Preparations: For *oral administration:* capsules of 250 mg and 500 mg and a paediatric syrup of 25 mg/ml chloramphenicol as the palmitate or stearoyl glycolate.

Parenteral administration: as chloramphenicol succinate in 10–20% solution for slow i. v. injection but not i. v. infusion.

Topical chloramphenicol as a skin (2%) and ophthalmic (1%) ointment and as ear drops (5%) may be used without restriction.

Summary: No longer considered for routine clinical use because of its rare but irreversible bone marrow toxicity. It is malpractice to give chloramphenicol systemically without clear indications of a potentially life-threatening condition, but this antibiotic is still very valuable in such circumstances. The total dose of 25–30 g in adults should not be exceeded.

References

ADAMS, G. R., H. A. PEARSON: Chloramphenicol-responsive chronic neutropenia. New Engl. J. Med. *309:* 1039 (1983).
BURCKART, G. J.: Chloramphenicol dosage and pharmacokinetics in infants and children. J. Clin. Pharmacol. *23:* 106–112 (1983).
BURNS, J. L., P. M. MENDELMAN, J. LEVY et al.: A permeability barrier as a mechanism of chloramphenicol resistance in Haemophilus influenzae. Antimicrob. Ag. Chemother. *27:* 46 (1985).

CATRY, M. A., M. V. VAZ PATO: Haemophilus influenzae type b resistant to ampicillin and chloramphenicol. Brit. Med. J. *287:* 1471 (1983).
EKBLAD, H., O. RUUSKANEN, R. LINDBERG, E. IISALO: The monitoring of serum chloramphenicol levels in children with severe infection. J. Antimicrob. Chemother. *15:* 489 (1985).
GARVEY, R. J. P., G. P. MCMULLIN: Meningitis due to beta-lactamase-producing type b Haemophilus influenzae resistant to chloramphenicol. Brit. Med. J. *287:* 1183 (1983).
GOH, K.-O.: Chloramphenicol and chromosomal morphology. J. Med. *10:* 159–166 (1979).
KESSLER, D. L., A. L. SMITH, D. E. WOODRUM: Chloramphenicol toxicity in a neonate treated with exchange transfusion. J. Pediatr. *96:* 140 (1980).
KRASINSKI, K., H. KUSMIESZ, J. D. NELSON: Pharmacologic interactions among chloramphenicol, phenytoin and phenobarbital. Pediatr. Infect. Dis. *1:* 232 (1982).
LING, J., P. CHAU: Plasmids mediating resistance to chloramphenicol, trimethoprim and ampicillin in Salmonella typhi strains isolated in South-east Asian region. J. Infect. Dis. *149:* 652 (1984).
MACMAHON, P., J. SILLS, E. HALL, T. FITZGERALD: Haemophilus influenzae type b resistant to both chloramphenicol and ampicillin in Britain. Brit. Med. J. *284:* 1229 (1982).
MULHALL, A.: The pharmacokinetics of chloramphenicol in the neonate and young infant. J. Antimicrob. Chemother. *12:* 629–639 (1983).
MULHALL, A., J. DE LOUVOIS, R. HURLEY: Chloramphenicol toxicity in neonates: its incidence and prevention. Brit. Med. J. *287:* 1424 (1983).
PLAUT, M. E., W. R. BEST: Aplastic anemia after parenteral chloramphenicol: Warning renewed. N. Engl. J. Med. *306:* 1486 (1982).
ROBIN, E., M. BERMAN, N. BHOOPALAM, H. COHEN, W. FRIED: Induction of lymphomas in mice by busulfan and chloramphenicol. Cancer Res. *41:* 3478–3482 (1981).
SHALIT, J., M. J. MARKS: Choramphenicol in the 1980's (Leading Article). Drugs *23:* 281–291 (1984).
SHANKARAN, S., R. E. KAUFFMAN: Use of chloramphenicol palmitate in neonates. J. Pediatr. *105:* 113 (1984).
SHANN, F., V. LINNEMANN, A. MACKENZIE et al.: Absorption of chloramphenicol sodium succinate after intramuscular administration in children. New Engl. J. Med. *313:* 410 (1985).
SILLS, J. A., P. MCMAHON, E. HALL, T. FITZGERALD: Haemophilus influenzae type b resistant to chloramphenicol and ampicillin. Brit. Med. J. *286:* 722 (1983).
SKOLIMOWSKI, I. M.: Molecular basis of chloramphenicol and thiamphenicol toxicity to DNA in vitro. J. Antimicrob. Chemother. *12:* 535–542 (1983).
UCHIYAMA, N., G. R. GREENE, D. B. KITTS, L. D. THRUPP: Meningitis due to Haemophilus influenzae type b resistant to ampicillin and chloramphenicol. J. Pediatr. *97:* 421 (1980).

b) Thiamphenicol

Proprietary names: Fluimucil Antibiotic, Urfamycine.

Properties: Thiamphenicol (methylsulphonylamphenicol) is an analogue of chloramphenicol (Fig. 35, p. 126). It is a bitter, odourless, crystalline powder which is insoluble in water but readily soluble in organic solvents. The glycinate is water-soluble and suitable for parenteral use. Thiamphenicol is also available commercially as the acetate (ampoules and film tablets).

Mode of action: Thiamphenicol is bacteriostatic to intra- and extracellular bacteria by inhibition of bacterial protein synthesis.

Spectrum of activity: Similar to that of chloramphenicol, with *in-vitro* activity usually less.

Resistance: There is complete cross-resistance between thiamphenicol and chloramphenicol. It may be assumed that a number of strains of Esch. coli, Klebsiella, Enterobacter, Proteus, staphylococci and streptococci will be resistant to both chloramphenicol and thiamphenicol, though publications on this point are lacking. Salmonellae, shigellae, Haemophilus influenzae, meningococci, pneumococci and Bacteroides fragilis can all be resistant. Gonococci which are susceptible to penicillin are generally inhibited by thiamphenicol in concentrations less than 0.5 mg/l, whereas gonococci that are only moderately susceptible to penicillin require between 4 and 8 mg/l. Resistance does not usually develop during treatment.

Pharmacokinetics: An oral dose of 500 mg of thiamphenicol results in peak serum concentrations of 3–6 mg/l after 2 h. The half-life is 3 h. Thiamphenicol is not glucuronidated in the liver, and 70% is excreted in the active, unchanged form in the urine after oral dosage. The half-life is doubled in anuria. Thiamphenicol is not dialysable. Tissue diffusion, including penetration of bronchial secretions, is good.

Side-effects: Thiamphenicol can impair haemopoiesis and haemoglobin synthesis even in therapeutic doses. The danger is increased in the elderly and in patients with impaired renal function. This acute, dose-related toxicity is greater than that of chloramphenicol, but is always reversible. It may be demonstrated by sensitive methods in almost all patients who receive the drug. Irreversible bone marrow depression has not been reported to date. Gastrointestinal upsets such as nausea, vomiting and diarrhoea are relatively frequent, but allergic reactions are rare.

Interactions: Possible interactions with other drugs include potentiation of the haematotoxicity of other potentially haematotoxic substances (e. g. sulphonamides, phenothiazine, phenylbutazone and hydantoin) and potentiation of the methotrexate toxicity in combination with that substance. The pharmacological effects of the sulphonylureas, coumarin derivatives and phenytoin may be potentiated by concurrent thiamphenicol.

Indications: Because of its acute haematotoxicity, thiamphenicol should only be used where other, better tolerated antimicrobials are ineffective. Thiamphenicol may be used to treat typhoid fever, paratyphoid A and B, salmonella septicaemia and meningitis, haemophilus meningitis and intraocular bacterial infections. Thiamphenicol in combination with acetylcysteine (as thiamphenicol acetylcysteinate) may be used to treat chest infections resistant to other antibiotics. Thiamphenicol is frequently used in the tropics as a single-dose treatment of gonorrhoea.

Contra-indications: Blood disorders such as aplastic anaemia and pancytopenia, as well as pregnancy and lactation.

Administration and dosage: The dosage is the same by the oral and the parenteral route. Adults should receive 1.5 g daily in 3–4 divided doses, and small children 25 mg/kg/d, generally for a maximum of 10 days. Typhoid fever and meningitis may be treated with up to 3 g daily in the first week (and up to 100 mg/kg in small children), after which the dose should be reduced to 1.5 g or 25 mg/kg respectively.

In patients *aged over 65*, 500 mg of thiamphenicol should be given twice daily.

In patients with *impaired renal function*, the dose should be adjusted according to the severity of the renal impairment (Table 15).

Table 15. Dosage of thiamphenicol in renal failure.

Creatinine clearance (ml/min)	Serum creatinine (mg/dl)	Dose interval at 500 mg	750 mg (10 mg/kg in children)
>75	<1.5	8 h	12 h
50–75	1.5–2	12 h	18 h
25–50	2–2.5	18 h	24 h
20	2.5–3	24 h	36 h
10	3–4	48 h	72 h
0	>4	96 h	144 h

For the single-dose treatment of *gonorrhoea*, one dose of 2.5 g of thiamphenicol (= 5 capsules of 0.5 g) or a single i.m. or i.v. injection of 1.5 g thiamphenicol is recommended. In females a second dose of 2 g thiamphenicol (= 4 capsules) should be taken on the second day.

Thiamphenicol acetylcysteinate is available for i.m. use but can only be recommended for endobronchial instillation (1 ampoule of 250 mg thiamphenicol 1–2 times daily) or for inhalation (1 ampoule of 250 mg thiamphenicol twice daily).

Preparations: Capsules of 0.5 g. Vials of 0.5 g and 0.75 g, and in combination with acetylcysteine in vials of 0.25 g.

Summary: Spectrum of activity similar to chloramphenicol; pharmacokinetics superior, but *in-vitro* activity reduced and acute haematotoxicity considerably worse. Thiamphenicol is, like chloramphenicol, now rapidly being superceded by other antibiotics.

References

BOGAERTS, J., W. M. TELLO, L. VERBIST, P. PIOT, J. VANDEPITTE: Norfloxacin versus thiamphenicol for treatment of uncomplicated gonorrhea in Rwanda. Antimicrob. Ag. Chemother. *31:* 434–437 (1987).
LATIF, A. S.: Thiamphenicol in the treatment of chancroid in men. Br. J. Vener. Dis. *58:* 54–55 (1982).
TUPASI, T. E., L. B. CRISOLOGO, C. A. TORRES, O. V. CALUBIRAN, I. DE JESUS: Cefuroxime, thiamphenicol, spectinomycin, and penicillin G in uncomplicated infections due to penicillinase-producing strains of Neisseria gonorrhoeae. Br. J. Vener. Dis. *59:* 172–175 (1983).

6. Aminoglycosides

Chemical structure: The common component of the aminoglycosides is streptamine or a similar cyclic amino alcohol, joined to two amino sugars through glycosidic bonds. Aminoglycosides are therefore also designated *aminocyclitols*. The structural formula of tobramycin (Fig. 36) is given as an example of a typical aminoglycoside. The aminoglycoside group includes streptomycin, kanamycin, neomycin, paromomycin, spectinomycin, gentamicin, tobramycin, sisomicin, netilmicin and amikacin. The individual compounds are distinguished by the number and type of amino sugars.

The nomenclature of the aminoglycosides is not logical. Aminoglycosides formed by Streptomyces species are named with *"mycin"* as a suffix, whereas those produced by Micromonospora species are designated *"micin"*.

Mode of action: The principal effect of the aminoglycosides is to inhibit ribosomal protein synthesis in the bacterial cell. There are, however, several mechanisms of action. The most important **mechanism of resistance** results from the activity of bacterial enzymes which inactivate aminoglycosides. Some bacteria possess acetylases, others phosphorylases or adenylases. Amikacin is the least susceptible to enzymatic inactivation and can only be attacked at one site on the molecule. Amikacin is therefore effective against bacteria which are resistant to gentamicin and tobramycin.

Spectrum of action: Aminoglycosides are particularly active against the Enterobacteriaceae and staphylococci, and the newer ones are also active against pseudomonas. They generally have little activity against streptococci, Haemophilus influenzae or anaerobes (e. g. Bacteroides species, clostridia). The antibacterial activity of the older aminoglycosides such as streptomycin, neomycin, and kanamycin is much poorer than that of newer aminoglycosides such as gentamicin, tobramycin, and amikacin. Unlike β-lactam antibiotics, all the aminoglycosides are active against bacteria in both the proliferating and resting phase. Aminoglycosides in combination with certain β-lactam antibiotics have marked synergistic activity against some bacterial species (pseudomonas, Enterobacteriaceae, enterococci).

6. Aminoglycosides

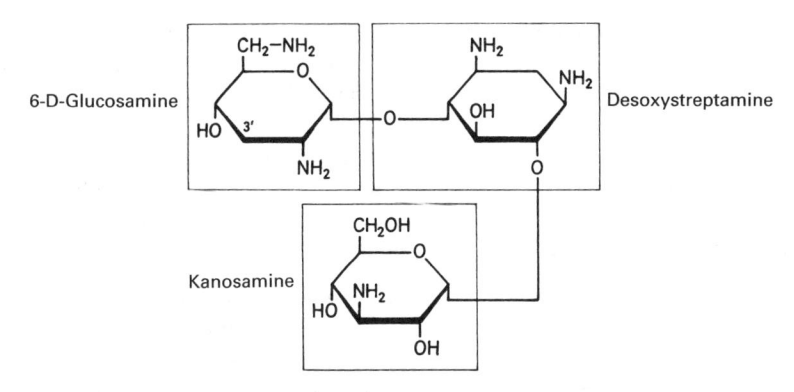

Fig. 36. Structural formula of tobramycin, a typical aminoglycoside.

Pharmacokinetics: Aminoglycosides all have similar pharmacokinetic properties; they are virtually not absorbed after oral administration and generally have a half-life of two hours. There are substantial differences between their antibacterial activities and tolerance. All aminoglycosides are freely water-soluble but are not soluble in lipids. They are very stable and can even be autoclaved.

Use: The first aminoglycoside to be used clinically, streptomycin, still plays a part in the treatment of tuberculosis. The other older aminoglycosides are, on account of their toxicity, no longer used systemically, but are exclusively for topical use. The newer aminoglycosides are almost indispensable in the treatment of severe infections, particularly in patients with immunological impairment.

a) Gentamicin

Proprietary names: Cidomycin, Garamycin, Genticin etc.

Description: Gentamicin (sometimes mis-spelled gentamycin) is an alkaline aminoglycoside complex of various fractions, the principal ones of which are C_1, C_{1a} and C_2. They are all-water-soluble, poorly lipid-soluble and stable.

Mode of action: Bactericidal activity in both the log and the lag phases of bacterial growth. Gentamicin potentiates *in vitro* the bactericidal activity of penicillins and cephalosporins even at low concentrations.

Spectrum of activity: Good activity against most strains of Pseudomonas aeruginosa, staphylococci, Enterobacter aerogenes, Klebsiella pneumoniae, Escherichia coli, Proteus vulgaris, uncommon species of Enterobacteriaceae, serratia, yersinia, pasteurellae, brucellae and Campylobacter fetus; moderate activity on gonococci, listeria, Haemophilus influenzae, Proteus mirabilis and salmonellae. Group A streptococci, pneumococci, enterococci, meningococci, clostridia, Bacteroides species, Nocardia asteroides, Pseudomonas cepacia, Xanthomonas maltophilia and Pseudomonas pseudomallei are all relatively resistant. Marked synergistic activity is found with azlo- and piperacillin against pseudomonas, with ampicillin against enterococci and with cephalosporins against klebsiella.

Resistance: Primary resistance in gram-negative bacilli is rare but has become more frequent recently, especially in hospitals, where outbreaks of infection with gentamicin-resistant staphylococci, klebsiella, acinetobacter, enterobacter, proteus, Serratia marcescens and Pseudomonas aeruginosa have been observed. Development of resistance during therapy is extremely rare. Partial cross-resistance is found with tobramycin, sisomicin, netilmicin, neomycin, kanamycin, amikacin, streptomycin and paromomycin. Gentamicin-resistant strains of pseudomonas are often still sensitive to amikacin.

Pharmacokinetics: Little *absorption* after oral and topical administration (up to 2% in gastro-enteritis); rapid absorption after i.m. administration. Maximal blood concentrations after 1 hour.

Serum concentrations (Fig. 37): Maxima of 2.8 mg/l after 40 mg i.m. (0.5 mg/l after 6 h); and of 5.1 mg/l after 80 mg i.m. (0.6 mg/l after 6 h).

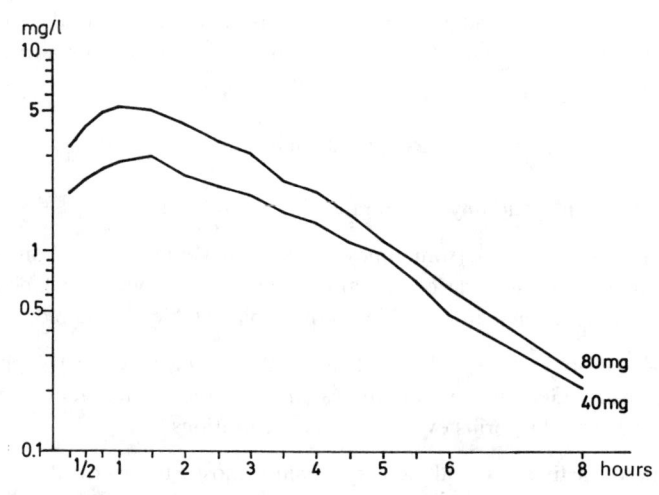

Fig. 37. Mean serum concentration-time curve in adults after 40 and 80 mg of gentamicin i.m. (own data).

Continuous i. v. infusion of 6.6 mg/h (i. e. 160 mg/24 h) gives a *blood concentration* of 1 mg/l. *Half-life:* 1½ h. No *plasma protein binding. Cerebrospinal fluid penetration* is very poor. Gentamicin diffuses into bronchial secretions and some passes into the fetal circulation. 30–50% of serum concentrations are found in pleural, peritoneal and synovial fluids. Very low concentrations are found in breast milk. Penetration into the eye and bone is poor.

Excretion: 85–95% in active form through the kidneys within 24 hours, predominantly by glomerular filtration. Urine concentrations in the first 3 hours are 60–115 mg/l after 40 mg i. m. and 90–500 mg/l after 80 mg i. m. As with other aminoglycosides, gentamicin is excreted in low concentrations in the urine for up to 1 month after the end of treatment (renal storage). A small amount passes out with the bile, but biliary concentrations are lower than the corresponding serum concentrations.

Side-effects:
1. *Vestibular damage* (dizziness, tinnitus, spontaneous or provocation nystagmus, Menière's disease) and *lesions of the acoustic nerves* can occur when renal function is impaired (peak serum concentrations in excess of 12 mg/l or trough concentrations above 2 mg/l) or dosage is high (above 0.45 g/d). Caloric tests show little or no excitability, and audiometry shows loss of hearing at high frequencies, although speech is heard normally until very late.
2. *Nephrotoxicity* is detected by oliguria and the presence of casts, protein and enzymes in the urine, and increased concentrations of creatinine and uric acid in the blood. It is commoner at persistent high dosage and where there is pre-existent renal disease. Deposits in the renal cortex can lead at very high dosage to acute tubular necrosis. Combination with large doses of cephalothin and cephaloridine can be acutely nephrotoxic under certain circumstances such as shock or the simultaneous administration of powerful diuretics such as frusemide. Other parenteral cephalosporins seem not to potentiate the nephrotoxicity of gentamicin to the same extent.
3. *Allergic reactions,* such as rashes, urticaria and laryngeal oedema, are uncommon. Cross-resistance with other aminoglycosides (e. g. neomycin) is found.
4. Paraesthesiae, tetany and muscle weakness (as a result of hypocalcaemia, hypomagnesaemia and hypokalaemia) occasionally occur.
5. Rapid i. v. injection of a large dose of gentamicin may lead to neuromuscular blockade with respiratory arrest, particularly when anaesthetics or muscle relaxants are given simultaneously or during transfusion of large quantities of citrated blood. Calcium gluconate is the antidote, and mechanical ventilation is sometimes required.
6. Some preparations for parenteral use contain sodium disulphite which can evoke allergic reactions.

Indications: Specific and non-specific treatment of severe bacterial infections (septicaemia, endocarditis etc.), preferably in combination with a second active agent such as an acylaminopenicillin or a cephalosporin.

Gentamicin may be used alone in urinary infections by resistant organisms and in combined therapy of severe infections, in endocarditis, and for topical application to bacterial eye infections, infected wounds, circumscribed burns etc.

Inappropriate use: Parenteral use in infections which should respond readily to less toxic antibiotics. Gentamicin should not be used alone in life-threatening infections, but should be combined as above.

Contra-indications: *Pregnancy* is a contra-indication. Do not combine with other potentially nephrotoxic antibiotics such as other aminoglycosides or, where avoidable, with rapidly acting diuretics such as frusemide or ethacrynic acid, since these potentiate the neurotoxicity. Use with caution in patients with myasthenia gravis and Parkinson's disease, since the curare-like action may potentiate their symptoms. Calcium gluconate is the antidote.

Administration and dosage: Rapid i.v. injection results in brief but high peak concentrations which may enhance toxicity. Slow intravenous injection, short i.v. infusion or i.m. injection are therefore preferred. Where the infection is caused by a very sensitive organism, doses of 80 mg (approximately 1 mg/kg) every 12 hours may suffice, but should be given every 8 hours for less sensitive infections (normally 2–3 mg/kg/day for 7–10 days). In severe or life-threatening infections, give up to 6 mg/kg/day in 3–4 divided doses. The use of higher doses has been reported but carries an increased risk of ototoxicity, and lower doses may suffice when synergistic combinations with β-lactam antibiotics are used. In obese patients one should base the dose on the ideal weight plus 40% of the excess weight. No dose reduction is necessary in the newborn or premature infant, whose volume of distribution is relatively greater.

Renal, auditory and vestibular function should be regularly checked when high doses are used for long periods.

In *renal failure,* the single dose of 1 mg/kg (generally 80 mg in adults) should be given at longer intervals in relation to the severity of the renal impairment (Table 16).

Whenever gentamicin or another aminoglycoside is used, serum concentrations should be assayed regularly to ensure that the maximal concentrations (peaks) lie within the therapeutic range (5–12 mg/l) and the troughs immediately prior to a dose are less than 2 mg/l, and preferably less than 1 mg/l. Peaks higher than 12 mg/l are in themselves less important associations with oto- or nephrotoxicity than high or progressively increasing troughs, which indicate accumulation. When renal function is impaired, care must also be taken with topical gentamicin (e.g. by inhalation or endotracheal instillation) when given at the same time as by a

Table 16. Gentamicin dosage in renal failure.

Creatinine clearance (ml/min)	Serum creatinine (µmol/l)	Serum urea (µmol/l)	Dose interval (h)	Single dose
>70	<125	<3	8	
35–70	125–170	3–5	12	
24–34	171–250	5–6.5	18	
16–23	251–330	6.5–8	24	1 mg/kg
10–15	331–470	8–12.5	36	
5–9	471–640	12.5–17.0	48	

systemic route. Gentamicin is dialysable and can be given in a dose of 1 mg/kg at the end of each dialysis when two haemodialyses are performed each week.

Intraperitoneal administration carries the risk of neuromuscular blockade with respiratory arrest.

Intrathecal instillation must be slow and should only be used in exceptional circumstances. Dosage: 5 mg for adults and 0.5–1 mg for the newborn and infants, of a preparation specifically for intrathecal administration which is free of the usual solvents.

A solution of 5 mg/ml of gentamicin can be instilled *intratracheally* after each tracheal aspiration in patients on long-term ventilation (30 mg 2–3 times daily in adults or 15 mg 2–3 times a day in children, each in 2 ml of physiological saline).

Subconjunctival injection for pseudomonas infections of the eye is also possible (10–20 mg). Gentamicin should not be mixed *in vitro* with other preparations, e. g. azlocillin, heparin, vitamins, because of the danger of mutual inactivation.

Gentamicin-PMMA-beads with a diameter of 7 mm can be used for the *topical treatment of bone and soft-tissue infections*. They consist of tissue-compatible PMMA (polymethylmethacrylate) and the x-ray contrast medium zirconium dioxide (Septopal). The beads, which are implanted into the bone or soft-tissue defect, each contain 7.5 mg of gentamicin sulphate which is slowly released in bactericidal concentrations by diffusion. The beads are wired together as a chain which is inserted into the bone cavity. The last bead protrudes from the wound which has been closed by a suture. A tube drain without suction allows any exudate to escape. The beads can be removed without an anaesthetic during the first 2 weeks. In some cases, the beads can be implanted permanently within the bone as treatment of chronic and post-traumatic osteomyelitis and of infected osteosynthesis. The beads, which are available either loose or as a chain, can also be inserted in abscess cavities and infected soft-tissue lesions. Mini-chains are available for jaw and hand surgery. Toxic side effects do not arise since only very low gentamicin concentrations are detected in the serum. The beads are assembled on a wire containing chromium and nickel, and topical hypersensitivity reactions have been reported.

A bone cement containing gentamicin for prosthetic implants is also available (Palacos R). It is used to fix internal prostheses of the hip, knees and other arthroplasties. Gentamicin is released at the site of implantation for prophylaxis of infections.

Gentamicin *overdosage* is treated better by haemodialysis than by peritoneal dialysis, since the former removes gentamicin twice as quickly. A 6–8 h haemodialysis will remove about 50% of the gentamicin from the body.

Preparations: Vials of 10, 20, 40, 80, 120 and 160 mg for injection, vials for intrathecal instillation of 1 mg and 5 mg, skin ointment, cream and powder, ophthalmic solution and ointment, gentamicin-PMMA beads and chains (Septopal), gentamicin-Palacos bone cement and gentamicin-containing sponge (collagen from ox tendon, Sulmycin implant).

Summary: The advantages of gentamicin are its broad spectrum of activity (including Pseudomonas aeruginosa) and its bactericidal action. It is not active against streptococci or anaerobes and has weak activity against haemophilus. Its main uses are in combination with other antibiotics in septicaemia (particularly where gut-related) and endocarditis, gram-negative pneumonia and alone in severe urinary infections with susceptible organisms. The narrow therapeutic range in comparison with penicillins and cephalosporins, and the enhanced risk of side-effects are disadvantages.

References

Chan, K. W., W. L. Ng: Gentamicin nephropathy in a neonate. Pathology *17:* 514 (1985).
Edwards, C., D. C. Low, J. G. Bissenden: Gentamicin dosage for the newborn. Lancet *1:* 508 (1986).
Fee Jr., W. E.: Gentamicin and tobramycin: comparison of ototoxicity. Rev. Infect. Dis. *5 (Suppl. 2):* 304 (1983).
Green, T. P.: Gentamicin elimination during exchange transfusion. J. Pediatr. *98:* 50 (1981).
Koren, G., S. Leeder, E. Harding et al.: Optimization of gentamicin therapy in very low birth weight infants. Pediatr. Pharmacol. *5:* 79 (1985).
Matzke, G. R., C. E. Halstenson, W. F. Keane: Hemodialysis elimination rates and clearance of gentamicin and tobramycin. Antimicrob. Ag. Chemother. *25:* 128 (1984).
Miranda, J. C., M. M. Schimmel, L. S. James: Gentamicin kinetics on the neonate. Pediatr. Pharmacol. *5:* 57 (1985).
Pancorbo, S., C. Comty: Pharmacokinetics of gentamicin in patients undergoing continuous ambulatory peritoneal dialysis. Antimicrob. Ag. Chemother. *19:* 605 (1981).
Richman, J., H. Zolezio, D. Tang-Liu: Comparison of ofloxacin, gentamicin, and tobramycin concentrations in tears and in vitro MICs for 90% of test organisms. Antimicrob. Agents Chemother. *34:* 1602–1604 (1990).
Schentag, J. J., M. E. Plaut, F. B. Cerra: Comparative nephrotoxicity of gentamicin and tobramycin: pharmacokinetic and clinical studies in 201 patients. Antimicrob. Ag. Chemother. *19:* 859 (1981).

TÖRHOLM, C., L. LIDGREN, L. LINDBERG, G. KAHLMETER: Total hip joint arthroplasty with gentamicin-impregnated cement. Clin. Orthop. *181:* 99–106 (1983).
VOGEL, F., M. EXNER, H. V. LILIENFELD-TOAL, N. CATTELAENS, M. EICHELBAUM: Serum gentamicin concentrations during intratracheal administration. Klin. Wschr. *62:* 394–398 (1984).
WAHLIG, H., E. DINGELDEIN, H. W. BUCHHOLZ, M. BUCHHOLZ, F. BACHMANN: Pharmacokinetic study of gentamicin-loaded cement in total hip replacements. J. Bone Joint Surg. *66-B:* 175–179 (1984).

b) Tobramycin

Proprietary name: Nebcin.

Description: An aminoglycoside antibiotic (structural formula see Fig. 36, p. 135), the sulphate of which is water-soluble and heat-stable.

Spectrum of activity: Comparable to gentamicin, but considerably more active against Pseudomonas aeruginosa including some gentamicin-resistant strains. Tobramycin is less active against Serratia marcescens, but similar to gentamicin against other susceptible strains. Combination with penicillins (e. g. piperacillin) or cephalosporins is synergistic and potentiates the activity of both components.

Resistance: Cross-resistance with gentamicin and sisomicin. Tobramycin-resistant strains of pseudomonas are often sensitive to amikacin.

Pharmacokinetics: *Maximal blood concentrations:* 3.7 mg/l after 80 mg i. m. (0.56 mg/l after 6 h) and 2.4 mg/l after 40 mg i. m. (0.26 mg/l after 6 h) (Fig. 38). Continuous i. v. infusion of 6.6 mg/h (160 mg/24 h) produces blood concentrations of 1 mg/l.
Half-life: 1½ h. *Not bound to protein. Excretion* of 93% of the dose in active form through the kidneys within 24 h.

Side-effects: Tobramycin shows no clinically relevant differences from gentamicin in either nephrotoxicity or ototoxicity.

Indications: Proven and suspected infections with Pseudomonas aeruginosa.

Contra-indications: As gentamicin. Do not combine with gentamicin, another aminoglycoside, cisplatin or potent loop diuretics.

Dose and administration: By injection i. m. every 6–12 h or by slow i. v. injection (15 min) or short i. v. infusion of 1–2 mg/kg 2–3 times daily according to the severiy and site of the infection, generally for not longer than 10 days. Do not mix with other drugs, particularly ticarcillin, in the same solution (inactivation). The dose should be reduced, and the dose-interval prolonged in renal failure, as with gentamicin (see p. 139). Premature and full-term neonates should receive 2 mg/kg twice a day.

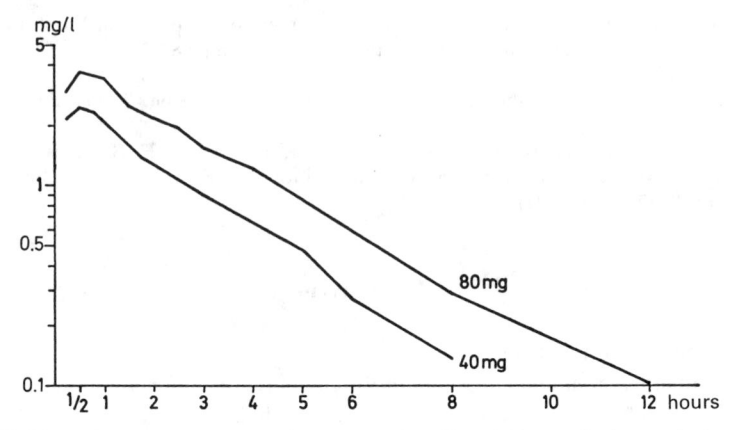

Fig. 38. Mean serum concentration-time curve after 40 and 80 mg of tobramycin i. m. (own data).

Preparations: Injection of 40 and 80 mg; eye drops and eye ointment.

Summary: A similar aminoglycoside to gentamicin with improved activity against pseudomonas. Should be combined with an antipseudomonal penicillin in severe infections with this organism.

References

HORREVORTS, A. M., J. E. DEGENER, G. DZOLJIC-DAMLOVIC et al.: Pharmacokinetics of tobramycin in patients with cystic fibrosis: implications for the dosing interval. Chest *88:* 260 (1985).
MARKS, M. I.: Pharmacokinetics of tobramycin in neonates. J. Pediatr. *104:* 160 (1984).
RYBAK, M. J., S. C. BOIKE, D. P. LEVINE, S. R. ERICKSON: Clinical use and toxicity of high-dose tobramycin in patients with pseudomonal endocarditis. J. Antimicrob. Chemother. *17:* 115 (1986).

c) Sisomicin

Description: A similar aminoglycoside to gentamicin C_{1a}, from which it differs only by the presence of a double bond in one of the glycoside rings (Fig. 39). Colourless or slightly yellow, water-soluble as the sulphate and stable.

Mode of action: Bactericidal in the log phase of bacterial growth but not in the resting phase. Acts by inhibition of protein synthesis.

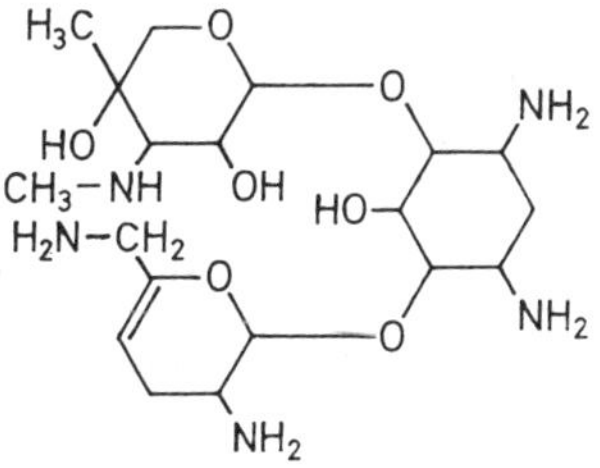

Fig. 39. Structural formula of sisomicin.

Spectrum of action: Almost identical with that of gentamicin. Sisomicin is, however, more active against Proteus species (especially Proteus vulgaris), Pseudomonas aeruginosa and some strains of citrobacter, klebsiella and serratia. Less effective than tobramycin against pseudomonas.

Resistance: Substantial cross-resistance with gentamicin and tobramycin. Like gentamicin, sisomicin is inactivated by 5 of the 9 most important bacterial aminoglycoside-inactivating enzymes. Bacterial strains which elaborate the aminoglycoside acetyltransferase-6' (AAC-6') enzyme are resistant to both sisomicin and amikacin, and amikacin-resistant bacteria are almost all sisomicin-resistant as well. Resistance does not develop rapidly during therapy.

Pharmacokinetics:
Absorption after oral administration is minimal, but is rapid after i. m. injection.
Serum concentrations: Maximum serum concentrations of 3–4 mg/l are found about 45 min after 80 mg i. m. and decline to 0.5 mg/l after 6 h. Continuous infusion of 6.6 mg/h (160 mg/day) gives a serum concentration of 0.64 mg/l in the steady state.
Half-life: 1½–2 h. Not bound to *plasma protein.* Poor *cerebrospinal fluid penetration.* *Tissue penetration* comparable to that of gentamicin.
Excretion: About 80% through the kidneys in 24 h; storage in the renal parenchyma results in measurable urine concentrations for up to 2 weeks after cessation of therapy. Urine concentrations in the first 2 h after 80 mg i. m.: 100–500 mg/l (at 6–9 h: 20–50 mg/l).

Side-effects: As for gentamicin. Potentially nephro- and ototoxic; dosage should therefore be carefully controlled. Reduce dosage in renal failure (see p. 139).

Indications and contra-indications: As for gentamicin (p. 138).

Administration: I. m. injection, very slow i. v. injection or short i. v. infusion over 30 min. Do not mix with other drugs in the solution, particularly with ticarcillin (inactivation). The infusion solution (preferably 5% glucose) should not contain magnesium or calcium. A solution for inhalation containing 4 mg/ml may be given to a total dose of 40–60 mg without significant absorption.

Dosage: As for gentamicin (2–3 mg/kg/day, up to 6 mg/kg for short periods) in 2–3 divided doses. For details see p. 138.

Preparations: Injection of 20, 50, 75 and 100 mg.

Summary: Similar to gentamicin but much less used.

References

SANDERS JR., W. E., C. C. SANDERS: Sisomycin: A review of eight years' experience. Rev. Infect. Dis. *2:* 182 (1980).

d) Netilmicin

Proprietary names: Netillin.

Properties: Netilmicin is the N-ethyl derivative of sisomicin and, as the sulphate, is water-soluble and stable.

Spectrum of action: Largely the same as gentamicin, though some gentamicin-resistant strains of Escherichia coli, Proteus mirabilis, Enterobacter species, Klebsiella pneumoniae, Citrobacter freundii and Serratia marcescens are sensitive to netilmicin. On the other hand, most gentamicin-resistant strains of pseudomonas are resistant to netilmicin, which is only inactivated by four of the nine known bacterial inactivating enzymes, while gentamicin is inactivated by six enzymes. Netilmicin is less active against Pseudomonas aeruginosa but more active against Serratia marcescens than gentamicin.

Resistance: There is incomplete cross-resistance with gentamicin and partial (one-sided) cross-resistance with amikacin (amikacin-resistant strains are always netilmicin-resistant, but not vice versa).

Pharmacokinetics and side-effects: Similar to gentamicin. Oto- and nephrotoxicity in animal tests are less than with gentamicin, but disturbances of hearing, balance and renal function (reversible) have also been observed in man.

Dosage as for gentamicin. The manufacturers recommend that renal function, hearing and balance be monitored in patients during therapy and that peak serum concentrations of more than 16 mg/l and trough concentrations over 4 mg/l be avoided.

Preparations: Injection of 15, 50, 100, 150 and 200 mg.

Conclusion: Netilmicin has few advantages in bacterial sensitivity and general tolerance over gentamicin and is less likely to be effective against gentamicin-resistant bacteria than amikacin.

References

Bhattacharya, B. K., H. Gorringe, M. J. Farr: Netilmicin and nephrotoxicity. Lancet 2: 216 (1983).
Bosso, J. A., P. L. Townsend, J. J. Herbst, J. M. Matsen: Pharmacokinetics and dosage requirements of netilmicin in cystic fibrosis patients. Antimicrob. Ag. Chemother. 28: 829 (1985).
Brauner, L., G. Kahlmeter, T. Lindholm, O. Simonsen: Vancomycin and netilmicin as first line treatment of peritonitis in CAPD patients. J. Antimicrob. Chemother. 15: 751 (1985).
Brückner, O., M. Trautmann, D. Kolodziejczyk et al.: Netilmicin in human CSF after parenteral administration in patients with slightly and severely impaired blood CSF barrier. J. Antimicrob. Chemother. 11: 565 (1983).
Finitzo-Hieber, T., G. H. McCracken Jr., K. C. Brown: Prospective controlled evaluation of auditory function in neonates given netilmicin or amikacin. J. Pediatr. 106: 129 (1985).
Gatell, J. M., J. G. San Miguel, V. Araujo et al.: Prospective randomized double-blind comparison of nephrotoxicity and auditory toxicity of tobramycin and netilmicin. Antimicrob. Ag. Chemother. 26: 766 (1984).
Granati, B., B. M. Assael, M. Chung et al.: Clinical pharmacology of netilmicin in preterm and term newborn infants. J. Pediatr. 106: 664 (1985).
Hjelte, L., A. S. Malmborg, B. Strandvik: Serum and sputum concentrations of netilmicin in combination with acylureidopenicillin and cephalosporins in clinical treatment of pulmonary exacerbations in cystic fibrosis. J. Antimicrob. Chemother. 23: 885–890 (1989).

e) Amikacin

Proprietary names: Amikin, Biklin.

Properties: A semi-synthetic derivative of kanamycin which, as the sulphate, is a colourless or slightly yellow solution which is stable at room temperature for at least 2 years.

Range of action: Since amikacin is not affected by most of the bacterial aminoglycoside-inactivating enzymes, it has a broader spectrum than gentamicin, sisomicin, tobramycin and netilmicin and inhibits most gentamicin-resistant strains of Escherichia coli, klebsiella, enterobacter, serratia, Proteus species (including Proteus rettgeri), providencia, acinetobacter, Citrobacter freundii and Staphylococcus aureus. Mycobacteria and Nocardia asteroides are always sensitive. Amikacin-resistance is extremely rare in gentamicin-sensitive bacteria (gram-negative bacilli and staphylococci). Amikacin is synergistic with azolocillin and ticarcillin against Pseudomonas aeruginosa and other Enterobacteriaceae, but is less active, weight for weight, than gentamicin and so has to be given at a higher dosage. Streptococci (including pneumococci) and Haemophilus influenzae are not sensitive. Amikacin is not active against most anaerobes, Pseudomonas cepacia and Xanthomonas maltophilia.

Resistance: Resistance during treatment is not quite as rare as was thought earlier. Partial cross-resistance in one or both directions with the other aminoglycosides.

Pharmacokinetics:
Absorption after oral administration is minimal, and is somewhat slower than gentamicin after i. m. injection (maximum serum concentration after 1½ h).

Serum concentrations: 21 mg/l (1 h) and 2.1 mg/l (10 h) after 500 mg (0.75 mg/kg) i. m. A short infusion of 500 mg over ½ h gives a mean serum concentration of 38 mg/l at the end of infusion, 18 mg/l 1 h later, and 0.75 mg/l after 10 h. There is no accumulation during a course of treatment when renal function is intact. *Half-life:* 2.3 h (7 h for the newborn in the first week of life). *Plasma protein binding:* 4–10%. Limited *CSF penetration* of 10–20% of the serum concentrations, and up to 50% in meningitis. Amikacin crosses the placenta and is concentrated in amniotic fluid.

Excretion: More than 90% excreted through the kidneys in the first 8 h in active form, primarily by glomerular filtration, and 95–100% in 24 h. Mean urinary concentrations during the first 6 h after 500 mg i. m.: 800 mg/l.

Side-effects: Like other aminoglycosides, amikacin is potentially nephro-, oto- and neurotoxic.
1. *Nephrotoxicity* (urinary loss of protein, cells and casts, azotaemia and oliguria) at normal dosage in the presence of normal renal function and an adequate fluid intake is uncommon and usually reversible.
2. *Ototoxicity* (labyrinthine deafness, dizziness) usually only occurs when the recommended dose is exceeded (see below), with prolonged treatment (longer than 10 days) or with renal failure without a compensatory reduction of dosage. A serum concentration of 35 mg/l should not be exceeded. Permanent auditory damage is rare. When related to the normal therapeutic dosage, the ototoxicity of amikacin (1 g a day) is comparable with that of gentamicin (240–320 mg a day).
3. *Neurotoxicity* (neuromuscular blockade and respiratory paralysis) occurs in combination with anaesthetics and muscle relaxants and also with simultaneous transfusion of large quantities of citrated blood. Neuromuscular blockade can also occur after rapid i. v. administration of amikacin and after local instillation in the abdominal or pleural cavities.
4. *Rare side-effects* are skin rashes, drug fever, tremor, nausea, vomiting, eosinophilia etc.

Main indications: Severe infections where other aminoglycosides have failed and hospital isolates of gentamicin-resistant gram-negative bacilli are common. Specific treatment of severe infections with gentamicin-resistant organisms, particularly Proteus rettgeri or Providencia stuartii, Serratia marcescens and Pseudomonas aeruginosa. Initial treatment of septicaemia and severe organ infections before the causative organism is known in immunologically compromised patients, particularly with malignancies. Also useful in peritonitis, neonatal sepsis and neonatal meningitis, always given in combination with other agents. May be important for infections with resistant mycobacteria.

Inappropriate use: Mild infections, and severe infections where gentamicin or tobramycin would be equally effective. Infections with streptococci, pneumococci or enterococci.

Contra-indications: Pregnancy. Care must be taken in renal failure, when a different aminoglycoside has been given immediately before, and when the patient has inner ear damage. Amikacin should not be combined with other potentially nephro- or ototoxic antibiotics, with other aminoglycosides or with potent loop diuretics such as ethacrynic acid, frusemide or mannitol, because of the increased risk of ototoxicity. Intolerance of other aminoglycosides excludes the use of amikacin also. For further *interactions*, see p. 138.

Administration: Generally by intramuscular injection, i. v. infusion over 1 h, or very slow i. v. injection. Do not mix other drugs with amikacin in the infusion solution (preferably 5% glucose).

Dosage: Daily dose of 15 mg/kg up to a maximum of 1.5 g, given as 2 or 3 i. m. injections or i. v. infusions (7.5 mg/kg every 12 h or 5 mg/kg every 8 h). Length of treatment: up to 7–10 days. If longer courses cannot be avoided, auditory and vestibular function should be checked regularly, performing audiography if possible.

If renal function is impaired, extend the dose interval between single doses of 7.5 mg/kg according to the following rule: Divide the patient's serum creatinine value in µmol/l by 10 to obtain the correct dose interval in hours (e. g. creatinine value of 180 µmol/l divided by 10 = 18, i. e. give 7.5 mg/kg every 18 h). In chronic renal failure, where the maintenance dose to be given every 12 hours is to be determined and the creatinine clearance is known, apply the following formula:

$$\frac{\text{patient's creatinine clearance (ml/min)}}{\text{normal creatinine clearance (ml/min)}} \times 7.5 \text{ mg/kg,}$$

e. g. creatinine clearance of patient (30), divided by normal creatinine clearance (140), × 7.5 mg/kg = maintenance dose of 1.6 mg/kg/12 h. The initial dose should always be 7.5 mg/kg. Rapid assay methods such as enzyme immunoassays greatly facilitate the control of serum concentrations during therapy, particularly in severe renal failure. The peak serum concentration should not exceed 35 mg/l and the trough 3 mg/l. Half the normal single dose of 7.5 mg/kg is given at the end of a session of haemo- or peritoneal dialysis. Give 7.5 mg/kg every 12 h in the newborn during the first week of life to avoid accumulation. In the very premature the dose interval may have to be prolonged to 24 h.

Topical use: Inhalation by aerosol is possible.

In case of **overdose** or toxic reactions, amikacin may be removed by haemodialysis (in neonates by exchange transfusion).

Preparations: Injection of 100 and 500 mg.

Summary: A broad-spectrum, bactericidal antibiotic which is generally reserved for severe systemic infections such as suspected gram-negative septicaemia, when it can be life-saving, particularly when combined with an anti-pseudomonal penicillin or a broad-spectrum cephalosporin, in patients with impaired immunity. Often active against organisms resistant to gentamicin. A valuable agent in severe hospital-acquired infection with gentamicin-resistant bacteria, but the dosage must be carefully controlled because of the risk of toxic side-effects.

References

BLASER, J., S. RÜTTIMANN, H. BHEND, R. LÜTHY: Increase of amikacin half-life during therapy in patients with renal insufficiency. Antimicrob. Ag. Chemother. *23:* 888 (1983).
FADEN, H., G. DESHPANDE, M. GROSSI: Renal and auditory toxic effects of amikacin in children with cancer. Amer. J. Dis. Child. *136:* 223 (1982).
GOMBERT, M. E., T. M. AULICINO: Amikacin synergism with beta-lactam antibiotics against selected nosocomial pathogens. J. Antimicrob. Chemother. *17:* 323 (1986).
KAOJARERN, S., S. MAOLEEKOONPAIROJ, V. ATICHARTAKARN: Pharmacokinetics of amikacin in hematologic malignancies. Antimicrob. Agents Chemother. *33:* 1406–1408 (1989).
LANAO, J. M., A. S. NAVARRO, A. DOMINGUEZ-GIL et al.: Amikacin concentrations in serum and blister fluid in healthy volunteers and in patients with renal impairment. J. Antimicrob. Chemother. *12:* 481 (1983).
PERLIN, M. H., S. A. LERNER: High-level amikacin resistance in Escherichia coli due to phosphorylation and impaired aminoglycoside uptake. Antimicrob. Ag. Chemother. *29:* 216 (1986).
ZINNER, S. H.: Review of amikacin usage in the EORTC trials. Am. J. Med. *79 (Suppl. A):* 17 (1985).

f) Spectinomycin

Proprietary name: Trobicin.

Properties: As an aminocyclitol, closely related to the aminoglycosides. More effective and better tolerated locally as the hydrochloride than as the sulphate, which was formerly used.

Mode of action: Inhibition of bacterial protein synthesis.

Spectrum of activity: A broad-spectrum antibiotic with relatively low activity except against gonococci (minimal inhibitory concentration 7.5–20 mg/l), which is of clinical use. Ureaplasma urealyticum is also sensitive, but not Chlamydia trachomatis (both can cause nongonococcal urethritis).

Resistance development: Can occur in gonococci. Primary resistance now found in gonococcal strains with increasing frequency (up to 10%). There is no cross-resistance with penicillins and cephalosporins.

Pharmacokinetics: Not absorbed by mouth. *Serum concentrations* of 100 mg/l and 15 mg/l occur 1 and 8 h respectively after 2 g i. m., and 160 and 31 mg/l are found 2 and 8 h respectively after 4 g i. m. *Half-life:* 2½ h. *Serum protein binding:* Little or none. High urine concentrations. *Urinary recovery:* over 80%.

Side-effects occur in less than 1% of patients after a single dose, but headache, dizziness, nausea, vomiting and pain at the site of injection have been reported.

Indications: Single-dose therapy of gonorrhoea, especially in patients with allergy to penicillin or where penicillin has failed. Such treatment is ineffective against gonococcal pharyngitis.

Inappropriate use: Other infections. Avoid in pregnant women and neonates.

Dosage: A single deep i. m. injection of 2 g in 3.5 ml diluent is recommended for uncomplicated gonorrhoea in the male and female. Earlier recommendation in the female was a single 4-g dose in 6.5 ml water for injection, possibly divided between 2 injection sites. Syphilis is not affected by spectinomycin and so is not masked either.

Preparations: Injection of 2 g (with diluent).

Summary: An alternative to benzylpenicillin as a single treatment of gonorrhoea, but with a failure rate of about 10%. Increasing resistance and the advent of β-lactamase-stable cephalosporins, which are easier to give, as well as the quinolones have made spectinomycin less important.

References

Ashford, W. A., O. W. Potts, H. J. U. Adams et al.: Spectinomycin-resistant penicillinase producing Neisseria gonorrhoeae. Lancet 2: 1035 (1981).
Centers for Disease Control: Spectinomycin-resistant penicillinase-producing Neisseria gonorrhoeae. Morbid. Mortal. Wkly Rep. 32: 51 (1983).
Gollow, M. M., M. Blums, A. Ismail: Penicillin-sensitive spectinomycin-resistant Neisseria gonorrhoeae. Med. J. Aust. 144: 651 (1986).
Ison, C. A., K. Littleton, K. P. Shannon et al.: Spectinomycin resistant gonococci. Brit. Med. J. 287: 1827 (1983).
Rousseau, D., D. Nadeau, G. Lafontaine: Emergence of spectinomycin-resistant strains of penicillinase-producing Neisseria gonorrhoeae in Quebec. Can. Med. Assoc. J. 141: 423–424 (1989).

7. Macrolides

The macrolides are a group of complex antibiotics with a lactone ring and glycosidic bonds to sugar and/or amino sugar moieties. Individual macrolides are distinguished by the size of the ring, the basic framework and the type of sugar. The lactone ring can have 14, 15 or 16 atoms. Semisynthetic macrolides have recently been developed and a number of new macrolides may be expected in the future. The most active antihelminthic agent at present available, Ivermectin, is a macrolide. The standard substance is erythromycin.

Macrolides are stored in many tissues and give rise to high intracellular concentrations (especially in granulocytes and macrophages). There is, therefore, little correlation between blood levels and clinical efficacy.

a) Erythromycin

Propietary names: Erythrocin, Erythroped.

Properties: The macrocyclic lactone ring in erythromycin is linked by the sugars desosamine and cladinose (Fig. 40). Erythromycin is a weak base which readily forms salts and esters with organic acids. Erythromycin base, the ester erythromycin ethylsuccinate and the salts erythromycin estolate, erythromycin stearate, erythromycin glucoheptonate and erythromycin lactobionate are all used therapeutically.

The erythromycin salts and ester release erythromycin base into the blood. The base is only slightly soluble in water but readily soluble in ethyl alcohol and other organic solvents. Erythromycin base is inactivated by acids so tablets for oral use must be in a form which is resistant to gastric acid. Erythromycin stearate and erythromycin ethylsuccinate are also acid-labile and are given with the addition of buffer or as film tablets. Erythromycin estolate (propionyl erythromycin ester

7. Macrolides

Erythromycin A	Structure showing 14-membered Lactone ring with Desosamine and Cladinose sugars attached.
Clarithromycin	Structure showing 14-membered Lactone ring with Desosamine and Cladinose sugars attached (with OCH$_3$ substitution).
Roxithromycin	Structure showing 14-membered Lactone ring with Desosamine and Cladinose sugars, and H$_3$C–O–CH$_2$–CH$_2$–O–CH$_2$–O–N= side chain.

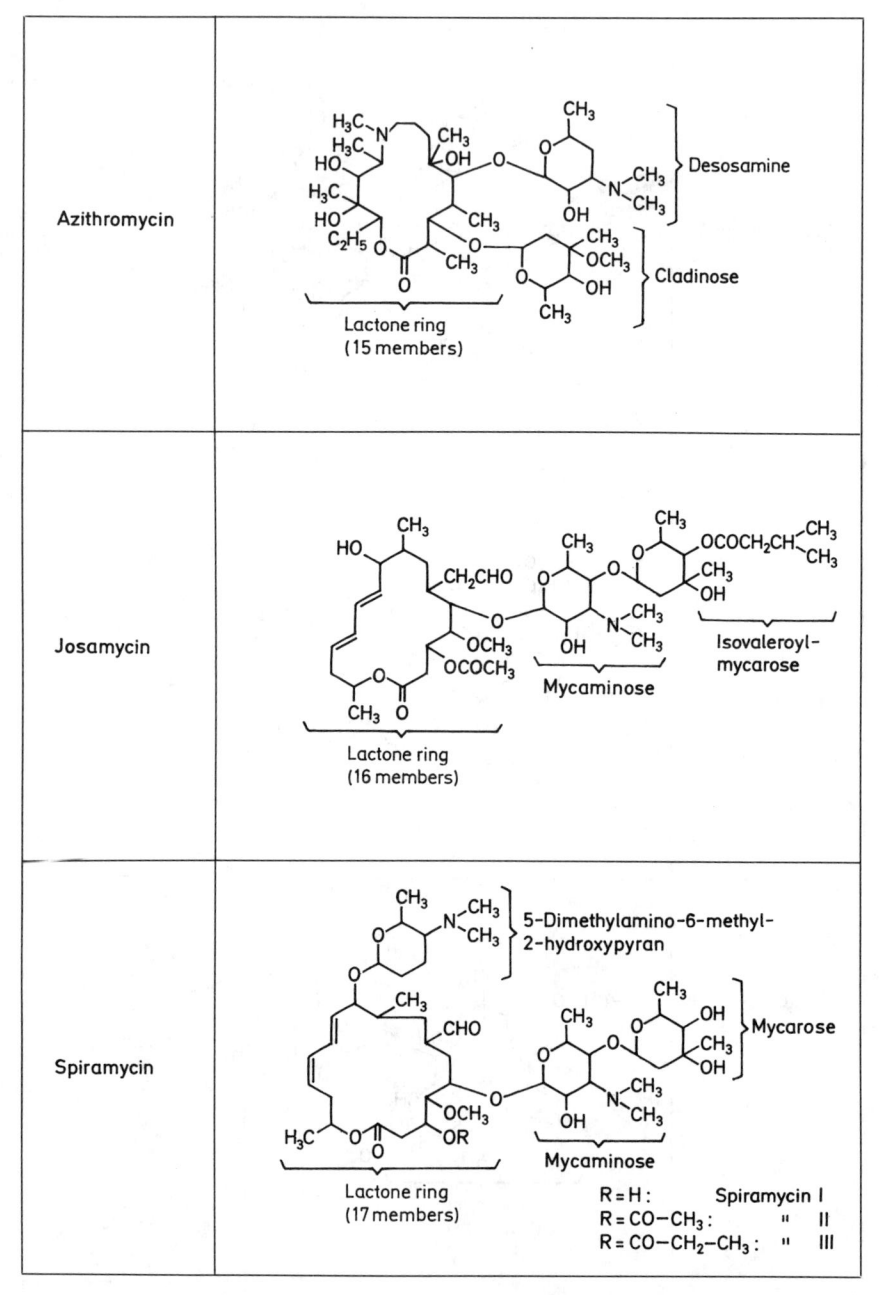

Azithromycin	Lactone ring (15 members); Desosamine; Cladinose
Josamycin	Lactone ring (16 members); Mycaminose; Isovaleroyl-mycarose
Spiramycin	Lactone ring (17 members); 5-Dimethylamino-6-methyl-2-hydroxypyran; Mycaminose; Mycarose R = H : Spiramycin I R = CO–CH$_3$: " II R = CO–CH$_2$–CH$_3$: " III

Fig. 40. Structural formulae of erythromycin and new macrolides.

lauryl sulphate) is, however, resistant to gastric acid. The water-soluble salts, erythromycin glucoheptonate and erythromycin lactobionate, are available for intravenous use, and the very water-soluble ethylsuccinate is suitable for intramuscular use.

Mode of action: Inhibition of ribosomal bacterial protein synthesis. Bacteriostatic at therapeutic concentrations, but some bactericidal activity at higher concentrations on actively dividing bacteria.

Spectrum of activity: Streptococcus pneumoniae (pneumococci), Streptococcus pyogenes (group A streptococci), Bordetella pertussis, Mycoplasma pneumoniae, Ureaplasma urealyticum, Legionella species, Bacillus anthracis, Clostridium perfringens, Clostridium tetani, Actinomyces israeli, Erysipelothrix rhusiopathiae and Listeria monocytogenes are all *very sensitive*.

Campylobacter jejuni, Chlamydia trachomatis, Treponema pallidum, rickettsiae, Coxiella burnetii and many anaerobes including peptostreptococci, most peptococci and Propionibacterium acnes, are *sensitive*.

Streptococcus viridans and Corynebacterium diphtheriae are *moderately sensitive*. The minimal inhibitory concentrations for other bacterial species vary, sometimes low but sometimes over 6 mg/l. These include staphylococci, Enterococcus faecalis (enterococci), Neisseria gonorrheae (gonococci), Neisseria meningitidis (meningococci) and Haemophilus influenzae.

Brucellae, Nocardia asteroides, Chlamydia psittaci, Mycoplasma hominis, Bacteroides fragilis and fusobacteria are almost always *resistant*. The gram-negative enterobacteria and mycobacteria are always resistant.

Resistance: Primary resistance to erythromycin occurs rarely in Streptococcus pneumoniae and Streptococcus pyogenes, but more frequently (5–30%) in staphylococci. 10–20% of Enterococcus faecalis are nowadays resistant. Resistance is rarely seen with Campylobacter jejuni, Mycoplasma pneumoniae and Ureaplasma urealyticum. Penicillin-resistant gonococci are generally resistant to erythromycin. There is partial cross-resistance between erythromycin and the other macrolides and between erythromycin and the lincosamides. Resistance in staphylococci can develop after relatively few *in vitro* passages.

Pharmacokinetics: The degree of absorption of the individual oral forms is somewhat controversial. Oral erythromycin is predominantly absorbed in the duodenum. The oral bioavailability is variable and to some extent dependent on the particular erythromycin compound, its acid stability, the other contents of the gastrointestinal tract and the galenic form. Erythromycin base is very acid-labile, but when formulated as gastric acid-resistant tablets is relatively well absorbed in the small intestine after passage through the stomach. The degree of absorption by this route, however, varies considerably from person to person. Erythromycin stearate is also very acid-labile and is broken down in the intestine to the base.

Erythromycin ethylsuccinate is absorbed as the undissociated ester, which is partially hydrolysed in the blood, giving rise to free active erythromycin base. Erythromycin estolate is acid-stable. It dissociates in the upper small intestine, releasing the inactive propionate ester which, after absorption into the bloodstream, is partially hydrolysed to free erythromycin base. Single oral doses of erythromycin compounds give rise to peak serum concentrations within 2–3 h. Peak concentrations after repeated dosing are higher than after a single dose.

Serum concentrations after a single dose of 0.5 g erythromycin ethylsuccinate by mouth are 1.8 mg/l, and 2.4 mg/l after a dose of 1 g (Fig. 41). A single oral dose of 0.5 g erythromycin estolate gives rise to peak serum concentrations of 2–3 mg/l, which only 20% is present as the antibacterially active base and 80% as the inactive ester. An oral dose of 0.5 g erythromycin base gives rise after 3 h to a maximum concentration of 1.7 mg/l. Erythromycin stearate is very variably absorbed and, in some individuals, not at all. When erythromycin lactobionate is given as an i.v. infusion over 1 h, serum concentrations at the end of infusion of 0.5 g are 10 mg/l, 3 mg/l after 2 h and 1 mg/l after 5 h. Similar values are seen when erythromycin ethylsuccinate is infused i.v. After the i.v. infusion of 500 mg of *lactobionate* over 60 min, serum concentrations of 10 mg/l are found at the end of infusion, 3 mg/l at 2 h and 1 mg/l at 5 h after the end of infusion. Absorption by the rectal route is very unreliable.

Half-life: 2 hours; 8 hours in anuric patients.

Plasma protein binding: 60%.

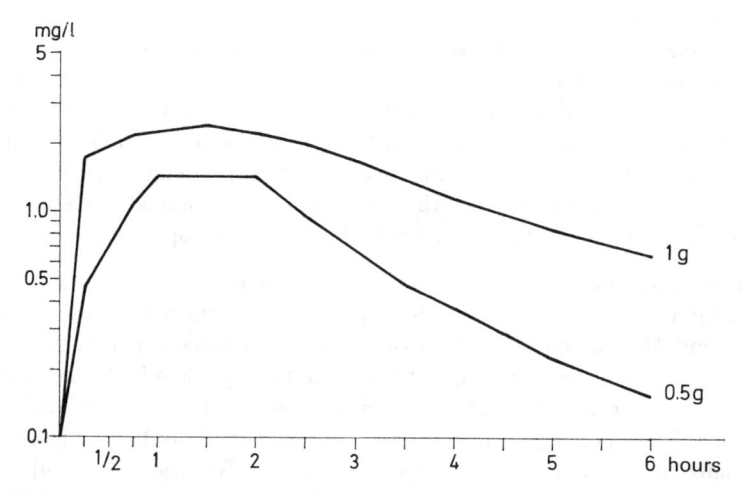

Fig. 41. Mean serum concentrations in 10 healthy adults after 0.5 g and 1 g of erythromycin ethylsuccinate by mouth 1 h after a standard breakfast (bioassay).

CSF penetration: Small (2–5%), but 10–20% of serum concentrations with inflamed meninges.

Tissue concentrations: Good (with relatively high intracellular concentrations). Rapid passage into the saliva (constant relationship to the serum of 1:2). 30% of serum levels are in bronchial secretions.

15–30% of serum concentrations are found in pleural, peritoneal and synovial fluids. Only 10% of the mother's blood concentration is detected in the cord blood. The erythromycin concentrations in breast milk are about 50% of the serum values.

Excretion varies according to the preparation: 20–30% passes out through the bile where concentrations of 6–50 mg/l are found after oral administration and of 50–300 mg/l after an i.v. dose, where hepatic function is normal. Only 2–8% passes into the urine after oral administration, and 12–15% after i.v. administration, giving concentrations of 5–60 mg/l. Concentrations of 300–600 µg/g are found in the faeces. Erythromycin is rapidly metabolised by demethylation into the antibacterially inactive N-methyl erythromycin.

Side-effects: About 5% of patients experience mild gastrointestinal disorders after oral administration (abdominal pain, nausea, loose stools), mainly with high doses. If persistent diarrhoea and colic occur, erythromycin treatment should be stopped and pseudomembranous enterocolitis with Clostridium difficile ruled out. Allergic skin rashes are rare. When given over 2–3 weeks, erythromycin estolate (lauryl sulphate) may give rise to intrahepatic cholestasis with or without jaundice and colicky abdominal pain, particularly with preexisting liver damage, repeated courses and in already sensitised patients. This is a hypersensitivity reaction. The abdominal pain can be severe enough to mimic cholelithiasis, pancreatitis or ulcer perforation. For this reason, the use of erythromycin estolate should be limited to 7–10 days and the estolate not given to patients with liver disease or general allergies. Similar disorders of liver function and elevation of transaminases can occur with the other erythromycin derivatives, but are less common. Reversible hearing disorders are occasionally seen in older patients with renal or hepatic failure and at higher doses (>4 g). The i.v. preparations often cause phlebitis (see below).

Indications: Acute respiratory infections, particularly with streptococci, pneumococci and mycoplasma; Chlamydia pneumoniae and Chlamydia trachomatis pneumonia and conjunctivitis; skin infections with sensitive organisms; erythrasma, rosacea, acne vulgaris. The drug of choice in legionellosis (due to Legionella pneumophila). Used in severe campylobacter enteritis, though quinolones such as ciprofloxacin may be more effective. Erythromycin is an alternative to penicillin in penicillin-allergic patients with scarlet fever, erysipelas, gonorrhoea, syphilis or diphtheria. Effective in trachoma, lymphogranuloma inguinale, non-gonococcal urethritis due to chlamydia, and as a prophylaxis for whooping cough (after exposure).

Inappropriate use: Generalised sepsis and osteomyelitis, against which penicillins, cephalosporins or aminoglycosides act more rapidly and effectively. Ornithosis (psittacosis).

Contra-indications: Erythromycin compounds should be used with care in patients with liver disease, and erythromycin estolate should be avoided altogether.

Interactions: When erythromycin is given concurrently with theophylline, theophylline concentrations are increased, and side-effects of theophylline may appear. When erythromycin is given at the same time as dihydroergotamine or a non-hydrated ergot alkaloid, increased vasoconstriction may occur. Erythromycin may potentiate the nephrotoxic activity of cyclosporin A, particularly in renal failure. The excretion of methyl prednisolone, carbamazepine and coumarin anticoagulants may be retarded by erythromycin. Erythromycin can increase the digoxin level in digitalised patients.

Administration: There are a number of views about the optimal preparation of erythromycin. In our experience, erythromycin ethylsuccinate is preferable for oral use. In severe infections and where the oral route is not possible, erythromycin glucoheptonate or lactobionate may be given parenterally, preferably by short intravenous infusion or slow i.v. injection. Reconstitute the powder in sterile double-distilled water or 5% dextrose solution strictly as instructed, as solutions which are too concentrated can cause thrombophlebitis. Nausea and vomiting, venous pain and circulatory reactions may follow slow i.v. injection of the diluted solution. Intramuscular injection is often painful and therefore not recommended. Rectal administration by suppository is not advisable because of the poor absorption by this route. Erythromycin is also available as a solution and gel for topical use on the skin in acne, and as an eye ointment.

Dosage:
Oral erythromycin: 1–2 g a day for adults, 30 (–50) mg/kg for children, in 2–4 divided doses. The dose should not be reduced in renal failure.
Intravenous administration of erythromycin glucoheptonate or lactobionate as a short infusion (250–500 mg in 30 min) or continuous infusion (1–2 g in 500–1000 ml fluid): 1–2 g a day for adults, 20–30 mg/kg a day for children.
Instillation (intrapleural, intraperitoneal or intra-articular) of erythromycin glucoheptonate or erythromycin lactobionate, dissolved as instructed and then further dissolved to a final concentration of 10 mg/ml (intrapleural), 2.5 mg/ml (intraperitoneal), and 1.25–2.5 mg/ml (intra-articular).

Preparations:
Tablets of 200 mg and 500 mg as ethylsuccinate.
Syrup or drops containing 40 mg/ml and 80 mg/ml of ethylsuccinate.

Tablets of 250 mg and 500 mg of stearate.
Coated tablets of 250 mg as erythromycin base.
Syrup with 25 mg/ml as estolate.
Ampoules with 250 mg as glucoheptonate and 1 g as lactobionate.
Ampoules of 100 mg erythromycin ethylsuccinate for i. m. injection.

Summary:
Advantages: Selective activity against gram-positive bacteria; well tolerated when dose not too high.

Disadvantages: Some resistance amongst staphylococci and Haemophilus influenzae; secondary resistance can arise during prolonged treatment. Incomplete and unreliable absorption, extensive metabolism.

References

BACHMANN, K., J. I. SCHWARTZ, R. FORNEY, A. FROGAMENI, L. E. JAUREGUI: The effect of erythromycin on the disposition kinetics of warfarin. Pharmacology *28:* 171–176 (1984).
BRITTAIN, D. C.: Erythromycin. Med. Clin. North Am. *71:* 1147 (1987).
BRUMMETT, R. E., and K. E. FOX: Vancomycin- and erythromycin-induced hearing loss in humans. Antimicrob. Agents Chemother. *33:* 791 (1989).
CARRANCO, E., J. KAREUS, C. SCHENLEY, V. PEAK, S. AL-RAJEH: Carbamazepine toxicity induced by concurrent erythromycin therapy. Arch. Neurol. *42:* 187–188 (1985).
DETTE, G. A., M. KNOTHE: The binding protein of erythromycin in human serum. Biochemical Pharmacology *35:* 959–966 (1986).
DISSE, B., U. GUNDERT-REMY, E. WEBER, K. ANDRASSY, W. SIETZEN, A. LANG: Pharmacokinetics of erythromycin in patients with different degrees of renal impairment. Internat. J. Clin. Pharmacol. Ther. and Toxicol. *24:* 460–464 (1986).
EICHENWALD, H. F.: Adverse reactions to erythromycin. Pediatric Inf. Dis. *5:* 147–150 (1986).
GRAFFNER, C., K. JOSEFSSON, O. STOCKMAN: Intra- and intersubject variation of erythromycin in healthy volunteers. Eur. J. Clin. Pharmacol. *28:* 231–233 (1986).
HALL, K. W., C. H. NIGHTINGALE, M. GIBALDI, E. NELSON, T. R. BATES, A. R. DI SANTO: Pharmacokinetics of erythromycin in normal and alcoholic liver disease subjects. J. Clin. Pharmacol. *22:* 321–325 (1982).
HAYDON, R. C., J. W. THELIN, W. E. DAVIS: Erythromycin ototoxicity: analysis and conclusions based on 22 case reports. Otolaryngol. Head Neck Surg. *92:* 678 (1984).
HOVI, T., K. JOSEFSSON, O. V. RENKONEN: Erythromycin absorption in healthy volunteers from single and multiple doses of enteric-coated pellets and tablets. Eur. J. Clin. Pharmacol. *25:* 271–273 (1983).
HOVI, T., M. HEIKINHEIMO: Effect of concomitant food intake on absorption kinetics of erythromycin in healthy volunteers. Eur. J. Clin. Pharmacol. *28:* 231–233 (1985).
ILOPOULOU, A., M. E. ALDHOUS, A. JOHNSTON, P. TURNER: Pharmacokinetic interaction between theophylline and erythromycin. Brit. J. Clin. Pharmacol. *14:* 445–499 (1982).
INMAN, W. H. W., N. S. B. RAWSON: Erythromycin estolate and jaundice. Br. Med. J. *28:* 1954 (1983).
JOSEFSSON, K., T. BERGAN, L. MAGNI: Dose-related pharmacokinetics after oral administration of a new formulation of erythromycin base. Brit. J. Clin. Pharmacol. *13:* 685–691 (1983).

Kroboth, P. D., A. Brown, J. A. Lyon, F. J. Kroboth, R. P. Juhl: Pharmacokinetics of single-dose erythromycin in normal and alcoholic liver disease subjects. Antimicrob. Ag. Chemother. *21:* 135–140 (1982).

Laforce, C. F., H. Chai, M. F. Miller: Effect of erythromycin on theophylline clearance of asthmatic children. J. Pediatrics *99:* 153–156 (1981).

Larrey, D., C. Funck-Brentano, P. Breil, J. Vitaux, C. Theodore, G. Babany, D. Pessayre: Effects of erythromycin on hepatic drug-metabolizing enzymes in humans. Biochem. Pharmacol. *32:* 1063–1068 (1983).

Malmborg, A. S.: Bioavailability of erythromycin ethylsuccinate from tablet and mixture forms: A comparison with equivalent doses of erythromycin stearate. Curr. Ther. Res. *27:* 733–740 (1980).

Martell, R., D. Heinrichs, C. R. Stiller et al.: The effects of erythromycin in patients treated with cyclosporine. Ann. Intern. Med. *104:* 660 (1986).

Martin, J. R., P. Johnson, M. F. Miller: Uptake, accumulation, and egress of erythromycin by tissue culture cells of human origin. Antimicrob. Ag. Chemother. *27:* 314–319 (1985).

Miller, M. F., J. R. Martin, P. Johnson, J. T. Ulrich, E. J. Rdzok, P. Billing: Erythromycin uptake and accumulation by human polymorphonuclear leukocytes and efficacy of erythromycin in killing ingested Legionella pneumophila. J. Infect. Dis. *149:* 714–718 (1984).

Otterson, M. F., S. K. Sarna: Gastrointestinal motor effects of erythromycin. Am. J. Physiol. *259:* G355–363 (1990).

Ptachcinski, R. J., B. J. Carpenter, G. J. Burckart, R. Venkataramanan, J. T. Rosenthal: Effect of erythromycin on cyclosporine levels. New Engl. J. Med. *313:* 1416–1417 (1985).

Putzi, R., J. Blaser, R. Lüthy et al.: Side-effects due to the intravenous infusion of erythromycin lactobionate. Infection *11:* 161 (1983).

Richelmio, P., C. Baldi, L. Manzo et al.: Erythromycin estolate impairs the mitochondrial and microsomal calcium homeostasis: correlation with hepatotoxicity. Arch. Toxicol. Suppl. *7:* 298 (1984).

Sacristan, J. A., J. Soto, M. A. de Cos: Erythromycin-induced hearing loss (letter). Lancet *336:* 1080 (1990).

Sato, R. I., D. R. Gray, S. E. Brown: Warfarin interaction with erythromycin. Arch. Intern. Med. *144:* 2413–2414 (1984).

Schreiner, A., A. Digranes: Absorption of erythromycin stearate and enteric coated erythromycin base after a single oral dose immediately before breakfast. Infection *12:* 345–348 (1984).

Schwartz, J. I., K. Bachmann: Erythromycin-warfarin interaction. Arch. Intern. Med. *144:* 2094 (1984).

Tjandramaga, T. B., A. Van Hecken, A. Mullie et al.: Relative bioavailability of enteric coated pellets, stearate and ethylsuccinate formulations of erythromycin. Pharmacology *29:* 305 (1984).

Vereerstraeten, P., J. C. Stolear, E. Schoutens-Serruys, N. Maes, J. P. Thys, C. Liesnard, F. Rost, P. Kinnaert, C. Toussaint: Erythromycin prophylaxis for legionaire's disease in immunosuppressed patients in a contaminated hospital environment. Transplantation *41:* 52–54 (1986).

Weisblum, B.: Inducible resistance to macrolides, lincosamides and streptogramin type B antibiotics: the resistance phenotypes, its biological diversity, and structural elements that regulate expression. A review. J. Antimicrob. Chemother. *16 (Suppl. A):* 63–90 (1985).

Weisblum, B.: Inducible erythromycin resistance in bacteria. Br. Med. Bull. *40:* 47 (1984).

Wroblewski, B. A.: Carbamazepine-erythromycin interaction. JAMA *255:* 1165–7 (1986).

Yakatan, G. J., C. E. Rasmussen, P. J. Feis, S. Wallen: Bioequivalence of erythromycin ethylsuccinate and enteric-coated erythromycin pellets following multiple oral doses. J. Clin. Pharmacol. 25: 36–42 (1985).

b) Josamycin

Proprietary name: Wilprafen.

Properties: Josamycin has a 16-membered lactone ring with an amino and a neutral sugar (Fig. 40). It is available as the propionate (antibacterially inactive) which is hydrolysed in the body to the active base. Poorly soluble in water but readily soluble in ethanol and other organic solvents.

Spectrum of activity: Similar to that of erythromycin (also active against Bordetella pertussis and Mycoplasma pneumoniae) but campylobacter and some strains of clostridia and fusobacteria are resistant. Josamycin is 1–2 times less active *in vitro* than erythromycin against staphylococci, pneumococci, other streptococci and Haemophilus influenzae. A few staphylococcal strains and most haemophilus strains are resistant. There is a partial cross-resistance with other macrolides.

Pharmakokinetics resemble that of erythromycin: incomplete absorption after oral administration, *half-life* 90 min, low *urinary recovery* (<10%), highly metabolised in the liver.

Gastrointestinal **side-effects** (4–5%) are usually mild.

Indication: Acute bacterial infection of the upper respiratory tract.

Contra-indication: Impaired liver function.

Daily dose: 1–2 g for adults, 30–50 mg/kg for children, divided in 3–4 doses.

Preparation: Suspension (30 mg/ml), tablets of 500 mg.

Summary: No advantages in comparison to erythromycin. Unreliable in haemophilus infections.

References

Long, S. S., S. Mueller, R. M. Swenson: In vitro susceptibilities of anaerobic bacteria to josamycin. Antimicrob. Ag. Chemother. 9: 859 (1976).
Reese, E. R.: In vitro susceptibility of common clinical anaerobic and aerobic isolates against josamycin. Antimicrob. Ag. Chemother. 10 (2): 253 (1976).
Simon, C.: Wirksamkeit von Josamycin auf bakterielle Erreger von Atemwegsinfektionen. Pädiat. Praxis 30: 57 (1984).
Strausbaugh, L. J., W. K. Bolton, J. A. Dilworth, R. L. Guerrant, M. A. Sande: Comparative pharmacology of josamycin and erythromycin stearate. Antimicrob. Ag. Chemother. 10: 450 (1976).

c) Roxithromycin

Trade name: Rulid.

Properties: Roxithromycin is a derivative of erythromycin (see Fig. 40). This structural modification improves acid stability in comparison with erythromycin base.

Spectrum of activity: Similar to that of erythromycin. *In vitro* activity generally less than that of erythromycin. Most strains of Haemophilus influenzae are resistant. There is partial cross-resistance with other macrolides.

Pharmacokinetics:
Relatively well absorbed after an oral dose of 150 mg: mean peak serum concentration 6 mg/l (after 12 h 1.8 mg/l). *Half-life* 10 h (doubled in liver failure). *Plasma protein binding* 96%. Rate of metabolism not precisely known; 3 metabolites have been shown in faeces and urine. Relatively good lung penetration. *Elimination* predominantly with the faeces, but a small amount excreted unchanged and as metabolites in urine.

Side-effects: Gastrointestinal upset in about 4% (nausea, colic, diarrhoea) and skin rashes.

Interactions: Simultaneous administration of theophylline can lead to raised blood theophylline concentrations. Roxithromycin and ergotamine together can lead to impaired peripheral circulation (particularly in the fingers and toes).

Indications: As erythromycin.

Dosage: 150 mg by mouth (probably fasting) twice daily (toxicity precludes higher dosage). Despite the prolonged half-life in liver failure, dose reduction is unnecessary because the drug is well tolerated.

Preparation: Tablets of 0.15 g.

Summary: Limited clinical experience at present. As far as can be assessed, roxithromycin is likely to have similar efficacy to that of erythromycin. Its advantage may be a lower dosage and increased dose interval.

References

BARLAM, T., H. C. NEU: In vitro comparison of the activity of RU 28965, a new macrolide, with that of erythromycin against aerobic and anaerobic bacteria. Antimicrob. Ag. Chemother. *Vol. 25:* 4: 529–531 (1984).

BÉGUÉ, P., D. A. KAFETZIS, H. ALBIN, CH. SAFRAN: Pharmacokinetics of roxithromycin in paediatrics. J. Antimicrob. Chemother. *20 (Suppl. B):* 101 (1987).

BERGOGNE-BÉRÉZIN, E.: Tissue distribution of roxithromycin. J. Antimicrob. Chemother. *20 (Suppl. B):* 113 (1987).
BLANC, F., J. D'ENFERT, S. FIESSINGER, A. LENOIR, M. RENAULT, Y. REZVANI: An evaluation of tolerance of roxithromycin in adults. J. Antimicrob. Chemother. *20 (Suppl. B):* 179 (1987).
CEVENINI, R., V. SAMBRI, M. LA PLACA: Comparative in vitro activity of RU 28965 against Chlamydia trachomatis in cell culture. Eur. J. Clin. Microbiol. *5:* 598–600 (1986).
CHAN, J., B. LUFT: Activity of roxithromycin (RU 28965), a macrolide, against Toxoplasma gondii infection in mice. Antimicrob. Ag. Chemother. *30:* 323–324 (1986).
CHANG, H. R., J.-C. F. PECHÈRE: Effect of roxithromycin on acute toxoplasmosis in mice. Antimicrob. Ag. Chemother. *31:* 1147–1149 (1987).
CHANTOT, J. F., A. BRYSKIER, J. C. GASC: Antibacterial activity of roxithromycin: a laboratory evaluation. J. Antibiotics *39:* 660–668 (1986).
GENTRY, LAYNE O.: Roxithromycin, a new macrolide antibiotic, in the treatment of infections in the lower respiratory tract: an overview. J. Antimicrob. Chemother. *20 (Suppl. B):* 145–152 (1987).
HALSTENSON, C. E., J. A. OPSAHL, M. H. SCHWENK, J. M. KOVARIK, S. K. PURI, I. HO, G. R. MATZKE: Disposition of roxithromycin in patients with normal and severely impaired renal function. Antimicrob. Agents Chemother. *34:* 385–389 (1990).
HOFFLIN, J. M., J. S. REMINGTON: In vivo synergism of roxithromycin (RU 965) and interferon against Toxoplasma gondii. Antimicrob. Ag. Chemother. *31:* 346–348 (1987).
JORGENSEN, J. H., J. S. REDDING, W. HOWELL: In vitro activity of the new macrolide antibiotic roxithromycin (RU 28965) against clinical isolates of Haemophilus influenzae. Antimicrob. Ag. Chemother. *29:* 921–922 (1986).
LE NOC, P., J. CROIZE, A. BRYSKIER, D. LE NOC, J. ROBERT: Comparative in vitro bacteriostatic and bactericidal effect of 5 macrolides: roxithromycin, erythromycin, oleandomycin, josamycin and spiramycin against 284 hospital bacterial strains. Pathol. Biol. Paris *37:* 553–559 (1989).
LUFT, B. J.: In vivo and in vitro activity of roxithromycin against Toxoplasma gondii in mice. Eur. J. Clin. Microbiol. 479–481 (1987).
NILSEN, O. G.: Comparative pharmacokinetics of macrolides. J. Antimicrob. Chemother. *20 (Suppl. B):* 81 (1987).
PERITI, P., T. MAZZEI: Pharmacokinetics of roxithromycin in renal and hepatic failure and drug interactions. J. Antimicrob. Chemother. *20 (Suppl. B):* 107 (1987).
PURI, S. K., H. B. LASSMAN: Roxithromycin: a pharmacokinetic review of a macrolide. J. Antimicrob. Chemother. *20 (Suppl. B):* 89 (1987).
SAINT-SALVI, B., D. TREMBLAY, A. SURJUS, M. A. LEFEBVRE: A study of the interaction of roxithromycin with theophylline and carbamazepine. J. Antimicrob. Chemother. *20 (Suppl. B):* 121–129 (1987).
TREMBLAY, D., A. BRYSKIER, M. VUCKOVIC, A. STOCKIS, C. MANUEL: RU 28965, nouveau macrolide semi-synthétique. Biodisponibilité et profil pharmacocinétique après administration par voie orale. Path. Biol. *33:* 502–506 (1985).

d) Clarithromycin

Proprietary name: Klacid.

Properties: Clarithromycin (6-o-methylerythromycin A) is an acid-stable 14-membered macrolide and differs chemically from erythromycin only in the substitution of the hydroxyl group in position 6 by a CH_3O group in the erythromycin lactonic ring (Fig. 40, p. 151). The structural modification explains the improved acid stability in comparison with erythromycin base.

Mode of action: Inhibition of ribosomal bacterial protein synthesis.

Spectrum of activity: Similar to that erythromycin. The activity *in-vitro* against common pathogens (Table 17) is almost equal to that of erythromycin, but clarithromycin is more active against Legionella pneumophila, Chlamydia trachomatis, Chlamydia pneumoniae and Mycobacterium avium-intracellulare. Against Haemophilus influenzae, erythromycin is twice as active as clarithromycin, with MIC_{50} values of 6.2 mg/l, compared with 12.5 mg/l for clarithromycin (MIC_{90} for both is 12.5 mg/l). The 14-hydroxy metabolite of clarithromycin inhibits haemophilus at the same concentrations as erythromycin. Combinations

Tab. 17. *In-vitro* activity of erythromycin and other macrolides against common pathogens (own data). E = erythromycin, D = dirithromycin, R = roxithromycin, A = azithromycin, C = clarithromycin, C (M) = 14-hydroxy clarithromycin, S = spiramycin.

Species	n	$MIC_{50\%}$ (mg/l)						
		E	D	R	A	C	C (M)	S
Staphylococcus aureus	21	0.4	0.8	0.4	0.8	0.2	0.4	6.2
Staphylococcus epidermidis	38	25	50	50	25	12.5	12.5	6.2
Streptococcus pneumoniae	13	0.05	0.1	0.05	0.05	0.025	0.025	0.1
Streptococcus pyogenes	10	0.05	0.1	0.1	0.1	0.025	0.05	0.4
Streptococcus agalactiae	10	0.05	0.2	0.1	0.1	0.05	0.05	0.4
Haemophilus influenzae	27	6.2	12.5	25	1.6	12.5	6.2	>100
Bordetella pertussis	13	0.012	0.025	0.025	0.012	0.006	0.006	0.2
Branhamella catarrhalis	40	0.1	0.1	0.2	0.025	0.05	0.05	1.6
Escherichia coli	56	–	–	–	0.1	–	–	–
Yersinia enterocolitica	16	–	–	–	0.2	–	–	–
Salmonella typhi	1	–	–	–	0.1	–	–	–
Shigella sonnei	1	–	–	–	0.2	–	–	–

of clarithromycin and its metabolite have an additive effect against haemophilus strains.

Resistance: Nowadays, most strains of Staphylococcus epidermidis (>75%) and of Haemophilus influenzae (>50%) are resistant to clarithromycin. There is partial cross-resistance with other macrolides.

Pharmacokinetics: The steady-state peak *serum concentrations* of clarithromycin are 1–1.5 mg/l after a 250-mg dose and 2–3 mg/l after a 500-mg dose. *Half-life:* 5 h (prolonged in impaired renal and impaired hepatic function). At a creatinine clearance of 30–80 ml/min the clarithromycin half-life increases to 12 h and at a creatinine clearance below 30 ml/min to 32 h. *Plasma protein binding:* 1%. Relatively good *lung penetration*. The primary metabolic pathways is n-demethylation with stereospecific hydroxylation at the 14-position of the ring. Half-life of 14-hydroxy clarithromycin: 5 h after a 250-mg dose and 7 h after a 500-mg dose. *Elimination* predominantly with the faeces, but 18% (unchanged) and 12% (as 14-hydroxy clarithromycin) are excreted in the urine.

Side-effects: Gastrointestinal upset in about 4–10% (nausea, colic, diarrhoea) and skin rashes.

Indications: As erythromycin. Infections by Mycobacterium avium-intracellulare (common in terminal stage of AIDS).

Dosage: 250–500 mg by mouth twice daily. In patients with impaired renal function reduced dosage is necessary. In patients with hepatic dysfunction more of the parent drug is cleared through the kidneys; if renal function is normal, the drug can be administered without any adjustment of dose.

Summary: Although there is little clinical experience of clarithromycin at present, the efficacy of clarithromycin is likely to be similar to that of erythromycin. Its advantages are a lower dosage (better absorption) and increased dose interval. Unreliable in haemophilus infections (as is erythromycin).

References

ANDERSON, G., T. S. ESMONDE, S. COLES: A comparative safety and efficacy study of clarithromycin and erythromycin stearate in community-acquired pneumonia. J. Antimicrob. Chemother. 26, Suppl. A, (1990).
CASSELL, G. H., J. DRNEC, K. B. WAITES: Efficacy of clarithromycin against Mycoplasma pneumoniae. J. Antimicrob. Chemother. 27, Suppl. A, 47–59 (1991).
DABERNAT, H., C. DELMAS, M. SEGUY: The activity of clarithromycin and its 14-hydroxy metabolite against Haemophilus influenzae, determined by in-vitro and serum bactericidal tests. J. Antimicrob. Chemother. 27, Suppl. A, 19–30 (1991).
FERNANDES, P. B., D. J. HARDY, D. McDANIEL, C. W. HANSON, R. N. SWANSON: In vitro and in vivo activities of clarithromycin against Mycobacterium avium. Antimicrob. Agents Chemother. 33: 1531–1534 (1989).

FRASCHINI, F., F. SCAGLIONE, G. PIOTUCCI: The diffusion of clarithromycin and roxithromycin into nasal mucosa, tonsil and lung in humans. J. Antimicrob. Chemother. 26, Suppl. C, (1990).
HARDY, D. J., D. M. HENSEY, J. M. BEYER: Comparative in vitro activities of new 14-, 15-, and 16-membered macrolides. Antimicrob. Ag. Chemother. 32: 1710–1719 (1988).
HARDY, D. J., R. N. SWANSON, R. A. RODE, K. MARSH, N. L. SKIPKOWITZ, J. J. CLEMENT: Enhancement of the in vitro and in vivo activities of clarithromycin against Haemophilus influenzae by 14-hydroxy-clarithromycin, its major metabolite in humans. Antimicrob. Agents Chemother. 34: 1407–1413 (1990).
NEU, H. C.: The development of macrolides: clarithromycin in perspective. J. Antimicrob. Chemother. 27, Suppl. A, 1–9 (1991).
OLSSON-LILJEQUIST, B., B.-M. HOFFMANN: In-vitro activity of clarithromycin with its 14-hydroxy metabolite A-62671 against Haemophilus influenzae. J. Antimicrob. Chemother. 27, Suppl. A, 11–17 (1991).
RIDGWAY, G. L., G. MUMTAZ, L. FENELON: The in-vitro activity of clarithromycin and other macrolides against the type strain of Chlamydia pneumoniae (TWAR). J. Antimicrob. Chemother. 27, Suppl. A, 43–45 (1991).
VALLÉE, E., E. AZOULAY-DUPUIS, R. SWANSON: Individual and combined activities of clarithromycin and its 14-hydroxy metabolite in a murine model of Haemophilus influenzae infection. J. Antimicrob. Chemother. 27, Suppl. A, 31–41 (1991).

e) Azithromycin

Proprietary name: Zithromax.

Properties: Azithromycin differs from erythromycin A by the possession of a methyl-substituted nitrogen atom in position 9a of the aglycone ring (see Fig. 40, p. 152), which considerably improves acid stability. It is relatively insoluble in water but freely soluble in ethanol and methanol.

Spectrum of action: Similar to that of erythromycin, but extended to include Esch. coli, salmonellae, shigellae and Yersinia enterocolitica (Table 17). Azithromycin is 4–8 times as active as erythromycin *in vitro* against Haemophilus influenzae, 4 times as active against Branhamella catarrhalis and 8 times as active against gonococci. In contrast, however, azithromycin has only ¼ the activity of erythromycin against Staphylococcus aureus and epidermidis and ⅛th–¹⁄₁₆th the activity against Streptococcus pyogenes and Streptococcus pneumoniae (pneumococci). There is little difference between azithromycin and erythromycin against other bacterial species including Campylobacter jejuni, legionellae and Chlamydia trachomatis. Toxoplasmosis in mice has been cured by azithromycin (200 mg/kg daily).

Pharmacokinetics: Oral administration of 0.25 g and 0.5 g azithromycin gives rise to mean serum concentrations after 2 h of 0.2 and 0.4 mg/l respectively; these are 4 times higher with erythromycin. *Half-life* 12 h. *Plasma protein binding* 20%. High tissue concentrations, several times higher than the simultaneous plasma concentrations. *Urinary recovery* in the first 24 h 3–5% (after oral administration) and 10% (after i. v. administration). As a result of the exceptional extent of tissue storage and slow release, azithromycin is excreted in the urine up to the 4th week after treatment.

Side-effects: Similar to erythromycin, so far as is known.

Possible indications: Haemophilus infections (e. g. suppurative otitis media and suppurative bronchitis). Severe intestinal infections with bloody diarrhoea due to invasive pathogens (campylobacter, yersinia, salmonella, shigella). Possibly useful for toxoplasmosis when pyrimethamine or sulphonamides are poorly tolerated.

Dosage: Initial dose 0.5 g, then 0.25 g orally every 24 h for 5 days.

Summary: Assessment is not yet possible. The long half-life and very good tissue penetration could be an advantage but may also carry some risk.

References

COOPER, M. A.: The pharmacokinetics and inflammatory fluid penetration of orally administered azithromycin, J. Antimicrob. Chemother. *26:* 533–538 (1990).
DEROUIN, F., C. CHASTANG: Activity in vitro against Toxoplasma gondii of azithromycin and clarithromycin alone and with pyrimethamine. J. Antimicrob. Chemother. *25:* 708–710 (1990).
EDELSTEIN, P. H., M. A. C. EDELSTEIN: In vitro activity of azithromycin against clinical isolates of legionella species. Antimicrob. Ag. Chemother. *35:* 407–413 (1991).
FOULDS, G., R. M. SHEPARD, R. B. JOHNSON: The pharmacokinetics of azithromycin in human serum and tissues. J. Antimicrob. Chemother. 25 *(Suppl. A):* 73–82 (1990).
GEVAUDIN, M. J.: Étude de l'activité de l'azithromycine et de la roxithromycine seules et en asociations vis-à-vis de Mycobacterium avium et de Mycobacterium xenopi. Path. et Biologie *38:* 413–419 (1990).
GIRARD, A. E., D. GIRARD, A. R. ENGLISH, T. D. GOOTZ, C. R. CIMOCHOWSKI, J. A. FAIELLA, S. L. HASKELL, J. A. RETSEMA: Pharmacokinetic and in vitro studies with azithromycin (CP-62,993), a new macrolide with an extended half-life and excellent tissue distribution. Antimicrob. Ag. Chemother. *31:* 1948–1954 (1987).
GLADUE, R. P., M. E. SNIDER: Intracellular accumulation of azithromycin by cultured human fibroblasts. Antimicrob. Ag. Chemother. *34:* 1056–1060 (1990).
GOLDSTEIN, F. W., M. F. EMIRIAN, A. COUTROT, J. F. ACAR: Bacteriostatic and bactericidal activity of azithromycin against Haemophilus influenzae. J. Antimicrob. Chemother. *25 (Suppl. A):* 25–28 (1990).
JOHNSON, R. C.: In-vitro and in-vivo susceptibility of Borrelia burgdorferi to azithromycin. J. Antimicrob. Chemother. *25* (Suppl. A): 33–38 (1990).
KITZIS, M. D., F. W. GOLDSTEIN, M. MIEGI, J. F. ACAR: In vitro activity of azithromycin against various Gram-negative bacilli and anaerobic bacteria. J. Antimicrob. Chemother. *25 (Suppl. A):* 15–18 (1990).
LASSUS, A.: Comparative studies of azithromycin in skin and soft-tissue infections and sexually transmitted infections by Neisseria and Chlamydia species. J. Antimicrob. Chemother. *25 (Suppl. A):* 115–121 (1990).
RENAUDIN, H., C. BÉBÉAR: Comparative in vitro activity of azithromycin, clarithromycin, erythromycin and lomefloxacin against Mycoplasma pneumoniae, Mycoplasma hominis and Ureaplasma urealyticum. Europ. J. Clin. Microb. Infect. Dis. *9:* 838–841 (1990).

RETSEMA, J. A., A. E. GIRARD, D. GIRARD, W. B. MILISEN: Relationship of high tissue concentrations of azithromycin to bactericidal activity and efficacy in vivo. J. Antimicrob. Chemother. 25 (Suppl. A): 83–89 (1990).
STEINGRIMSSON, O., J. H. OLAFSSON, H. THORARINSSON, R. W. RYAN, R. B. JOHNSON, R. C. TILTON: Azithromycin in the treatment of sexually transmitted disease. J. Antimicrob. Chemother. 25 (Suppl. A): 109–114 (1990).

f) Spiramycin

Trade names: Rovamycine, Selectomycin.

Properties: Spiramycin is a complex of 3 components, the only active one of which is spiramycin A. Spiramycin A has a 17-membered lactone ring. It is poorly soluble in water but freely soluble in organic solvents.

Spectrum of activity: Spiramycin, like the other macrolides, is bacteriostatic against gram-positive bacteria such as Staphylococcus aureus, Staphylococcus epidermidis, Streptococcus pyogenes (haemolytic streptococci of Lancefield group A), Streptococcus pneumoniae (pneumococci) and Enterococcus faccalis (enterococci) as well as against Branhamella catarrhalis and some strains of Neisseria gonorrheae (gonococci) and Neisseria meningitidis (meningococci). Haemophilus influenzae and all the other gram-negative bacilli, including the Enterobacteriaceae, are resistant. Spiramycin at very high dosage has been shown in animal experiments to have activity against Toxoplasma gondii. Spiramycin is some 16- to 32-fold weaker than erythromycin against Staphylococcus aureus, 8- to 16-fold weaker against Streptococcus pyogenes and 4- to 8-fold weaker against Streptococcus pneumoniae (Table 17, p. 163).

Frequency of resistance: There are few current data on the frequency of resistance. In the past, 10–20% of staphylococci have been resistant to spiramycin. Some staphylococci show complete cross-resistance with erythromycin, although some erythromycin-resistant staphylococci are susceptible to spiramycin. The majority of meningococcal strains are nowadays resistant.

Pharmacokinetics: Spiramycin is incompletely absorbed after oral administration. Maximum serum concentrations are achieved after 2–3 h. Serum concentrations of 2–3 mg/l (after 2 h) and of 1–2 mg/l (after 6 h) are found after repeated oral administration of spiramycin 1 g 6-hourly.

Half-life 2–3 h. Salivary concentrations of spiramycin are 2–3 times higher than in serum and seem to be particularly high in prostatic tissue. 5–10% of the oral dose is excreted in the urine. The biliary concentration is higher than in the blood. Orally absorbed spiramycin is largely inactivated by metabolism in the body.

Possible indications:
1. Staphylococcal infections when erythromycin and bactericidal agents such as penicillins and cephalosporins are inactive. The activity of spiramycin should be tested *in vitro* before use.

2. Ocular toxoplasmosis (chorioretinitis), when the more active pyrimethamine is contraindicated. The efficacy of spiramycin in toxoplasmosis affecting other organs is uncertain.
3. Streptococcal infections of the teeth and gums (dental root infections etc.).
4. Cryptosporidium infections in AIDS patients (efficacy doubtful).

Side-effects: Gastrointestinal disorders occasionally occur, including nausea, vomiting and diarrhoea, particularly at high dosage. Allergic side effects such as rashes are rare.

Interactions: Simultaneous adminstration of dihydroergotamine or other alkaloids can lead to increased vasoconstriction.

Dosage: Staphylococcal infections and bacterial infections of the teeth and gums should be treated with 0.5 g 4 times daily by mouth, and in children up to the age of 6 years 12.5 mg/kg 4 times a day. This dose may be doubled in severe infections: 1 g 4 times a day in adults and 25 mg/kg 4 times a day in children up to the age of 6.

The dose need not be reduced in renal insufficiency. There is no experience of the drug in hepatic impairment.

Toxoplasmosis should be treated in adults with a daily dose of 3 g orally for 4 weeks, and in children in the first year of life with 100 mg/kg/day for 4 weeks. After an interval of 2 weeks, the same treatment can be repeated for a further 4 weeks.

Summary: The interest in the activity of spiramycin on toxoplasmas, as demonstrated in animal experiments, has undoubtedly been stimulated by the increased incidence of toxoplasmosis in AIDS. This activity is only weak, however, and not well established in man.

References

CHAN, E. C., W. AL JOBURI, S. L. CHENG, F. DELORME: In vitro susceptibilities of oral bacterial isolates to spiramycin. Antimicrob. Agents Chemother. *33:* 2016–2018 (1989).

COLLIER, A. C., R. A. MILLER, J. D. MEYERS: Cryptosporidiosis after marrow transplantation: person-to-person transmission and treatment with spiramycin. Ann. Intern. Med. *101:* 205 (1984).

POCIDALO, J. J., F. ALBERT, J. F. DESNOTTES, S. KERNBAUM: Intraphagocytic penetration of macrolides: in-vivo comparison of erythromycin and spiramycin. J. Antimicrob. Chemother. *16 (Suppl. A):* (1985).

PORTNOY, D., M. E. WHITESIDE, E. BUCKLEY III, C. L. MACLEOD: Treatment of intestinal cryptosporidiosis with spiramycin. Ann. Intern. Med. *101:* 202 (1984).

8. Lincosamides

Lincosamides are antibiotics which, although chemically distinct from the macrolides, show many common features in their mechanism of action, spectrum of activity and pharmacological properties. The first representative of this group is lincomycin, from which the semisynthetic drug clindamycin was derived. Lincomycin consists of an amino acid linked by an amide bond to the sugar pyranoside. It bears no resemblance to other antibiotics. Lincomycin and clindamycin hydrochloride are freely soluble in water.

a) Lincomycin

Proprietary names: Lincocin.

Properties: Available as lincomycin hydrochloride in capsules, syrup and a solution for injection.

Mode of action: Lincomycin inhibits intracellular bacterial protein synthesis.

Spectrum of activity: Lincomycin is active against staphylococci, streptococci and non-sporing anaerobes, although its *in vitro* antibacterial activity against staphylococci, Streptococcus pneumoniae (pneumococci) and Bacteroides fragilis is only one-tenth that of clindamycin (chlordesoxy lincomycin). Lincomycin is also active against viridans streptococci, most clostridia, Actinomyces israelii and Corynebacterium diphtheriae. Enterococcus faecalis (enterococci), neisseriae (gonococci, meningococci), Haemophilus influenzae, Mycoplasma pneumoniae and gram-negative intestinal bacteria are completely resistant.

Resistance: Stepwise increase in resistance occurs *in vitro* but is rare during therapy. Primarily resistant strains of staphylococci, Bacteroides and clostridia occur at varying rates. Pneumococci and group A streptococci are very rarely resistant. Partial cross-resistance is found with erythromycin and clindamycin. Lincomycin-resistant strains of Bacteroides fragilis can be sensitive to clindamycin.

Pharmacokinetics:
Absorption after oral administration depends very much on food intake (Fig. 42). The fasting absorption rate is 73% but with food it is less than 25%. *Peak blood levels* occur after 4 hours and are higher with repeated administration. *Serum concentrations* after 600 mg i.m. are 9–12 mg/l (1 h) and 3–4 mg/l (12 h). The mean serum concentrations after a short i.v. infusion over 1 h of 600 mg are 21.5 mg/l at the end of the infusion and 1.7 mg/l at 12 h. *Plasma protein binding:* 20–30%. *Half-life* 5 h (doubled in renal failure). Good *penetration of tissues,* including bone. Poor *CSF penetration* with up to 40% of the plasma concentrations

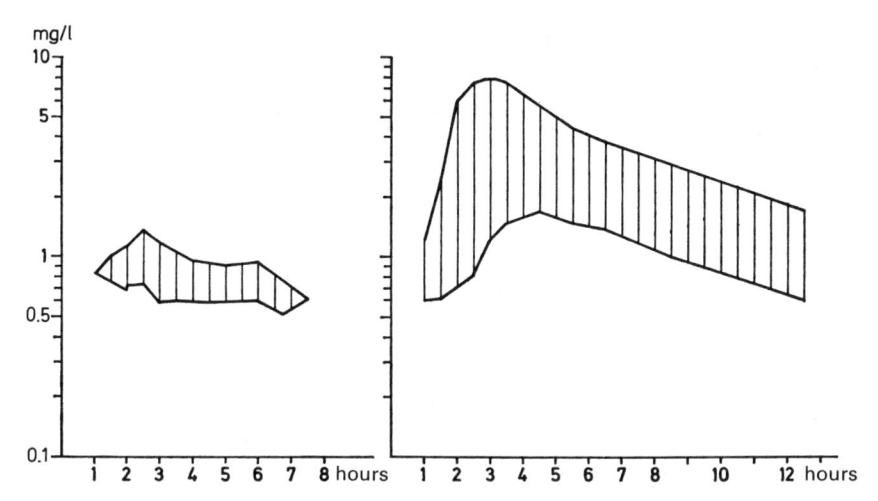

Fig. 42. Serum concentrations of lincomycin in adults after 500 mg of lincomycin by mouth 30 min after a standard breakfast (left) and fasting, i.e. 2 hours before breakfast (right) (own data).

in the CSF in meningitis. 10–60% in cord blood and amniotic fluid and 50–100% of the mother's serum values in breast milk.

Excretion: 38% urine recovery after i.v. administration (9–10% after oral administration on an empty stomach). A small amount is excreted in the bile. Rapidly metabolised (more than 50%). Not dialysable.

Side-effects: Gastrointestinal upset in 5–20% (glossitis, stomatitis, nausea, vomiting, diarrhoea) which can continue after treatment has finished, partly due to the suppression of the anaerobic flora and their replacement by enterococci. Pseudomembranous enterocolitis with persistent mucosanguinous diarrhoea and abdominal pain occurs rarely but can be severe and sometimes fatal. It is related to the proliferation of toxin-producing strains of Clostridium difficile in the large bowel and is resistant to penicillins, cephalosporins, aminoglycosides, tetracyclines, erythromycin, lincomycin and often to clindamycin also. Toxin, which is formed in large quantities, causes mild or severe diarrhoea after 2–25 days which usually stops within 3 weeks but which can recur. Oral vancomycin or metronidazole, to which Clostridium difficile is sensitive, is effective therapy. The frequency of these side-effects varies regionally, being lower in Europe and varying between ≤1 and 10% in the USA. Pseudomembranous enterocolitis is more frequent in the elderly and after intestinal operations. It may also occur during treatment with aminopenicillins and other antibiotics. Allergic reactions also occur. Cardiovascular disturbances (collapse and cardiac arrest) have been reported. Care should be taken in renal and hepatic impairment because of the risk of accumulation.

Interactions: Lincomycin can potentiate the effect of ganglion blockers and should therefore be used with caution in patients receiving these drugs.

Indications: Staphylococcal infections in patients allergic to penicillins, methicillin-resistant staphylococcal infections, and anaerobic infections have all been indications for lincomycin. The more active compound, clindamycin, is now preferred, and metronidazole is suitable for anaerobic infections.

Inappropriate use: Infections due to gram-positive bacteria against which penicillins or erythromycin are equally active.

Contra-indications: Lincomycin should not be used i.v. in the newborn or young infant because the solution contains benzyl alcohol which can give rise to severe respiratory impairment, skin reactions and angioneurotic oedema.

Administration: Oral doses should be given at least 2 hours before or 2 hours after meals. I.m. injection and i.v. infusion are also available.

Dosage: 2 g a day by mouth for adults, and 30–40 mg/kg for children, preferably fasting, in 4 divided doses. I.m. administration (2–4 times a day) or i.v. infusion: 1.2–1.8 g a day for adults, 10–20 mg/kg for children; as a short infusion: 600 mg in 250 ml of 5% dextrose solution (for ½ hour) 2–3 times a day. Reduce dosage by one-half in renal and liver impairment.

Preparations: Capsules of 500 mg, injection of 600 mg and 3 g, and a syrup (50 mg/ml).

Summary: Less active than clindamycin. Absorption after oral intake unreliable. The use of lincomycin is no longer justifiable and should be discontinued in favour of clindamycin.

References

Dornbusch, K., A. Carlström, H. Hugo, A. Lindström: Antibacterial activity of clindamycin and lincomycin in human bone. J. Antimicrob. Chemother. *3:* 153 (1977).
Dyck, W. P., A. L. Viteri, P. H. Howard: Lincomycin, clindamycin, and colitis. Lancet *I:* 272 (1974).
Pittman, F. E., J. C. Pittman, C. D. Humphey: Lincomycin and pseudomembranous colitis. Lancet *I:* 451 (1974).
Scott, A. J., G. I. Nicholson, A. R. Kerr: Lincomycin as a cause of pseudomembranous colitis. Lancet *2:* 1232 (1973).

b) Clindamycin

Proprietary name: Dalacin C.

Properties: Clindamycin is a semisynthetic derivative of lincomycin, from which it differs by substitution of a 7-hydroxy group by a chlorine atom. Its short chemical name is chlordesoxy lincomycin. Clindamycin is available as the hydrochloride (capsules) and the palmitate (syrup) for oral use and as the phosphate for parenteral use and for cutaneous application in acne. Clindamycin hydrochloride, palmitate and phosphate are all white powders which are readily soluble in water and alcohol. 1.7 g of hydrochloride monohydrate, 1.6 g of palmitate and 1.2 g of dihydrogen phosphate correspond to 1 g clindamycin base. The palmitate and phosphate possess no antibacterial activity and are rapidly hydrolysed in the body to active clindamycin. Clindamycin acne solution contains isopropyl alcohol and propylene glycol. The structural formula is shown in Fig. 43.

Mode of action: Clindamycin inhibits protein synthesis in sensitive bacteria and may be bacteriostatic or bactericidal, dependent upon its concentration at the site of infection and on the sensitivity of the causative organisms.

Spectrum of activity: Clindamycin is more active than lincomycin against staphylococci, pneumococci and Bacteroides fragilis. Clindamycin has good activity against group A streptococci (Streptococcus pyogenes), viridans streptococci, Streptococcus durans and Streptococcus bovis, as well as against Corynebacterium diphtheriae, Bacillus anthracis and nocardia. Of the anaerobes, bacteroides, fusobacteria, actinomyces, anaerobic streptococci (peptostreptococci) and anaerobic staphylococci (peptococci) as well as propionibacteria (Propionibacterium acnes), Campylobacter fetus and most strains of Clostridium perfringens are susceptible. Other species of clostridia, enterococci (Enterococcus faecalis and Enterococcus faecium), neisseriae (gonococci, meningococci), aerobic gram-negative bacilli (usually including haemophilus), Mycoplasma

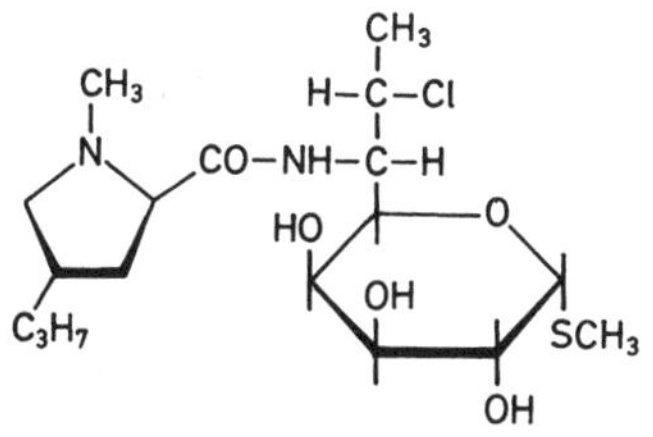

Fig. 43. Structural formula of clindamycin base.

pneumoniae and Ureaplasma urealyticum are resistant. Gentamicin does not antagonise the activity of clindamycin on staphylococci, streptococci (including pneumococci) or clostridia. Clindamycin has activity against toxoplasma and is sometimes used in patients with cerebral toxoplasmosis in AIDS.

Resistance: Some 3% of all staphylococci, including a number of methicillin-resistant strains, are resistant to clindamycin. Resistance is rare in group A streptococci (Streptococcus pyogenes) and pneumococci (Streptococcus pneumoniae). Penicillin-resistant pneumococci are generally also resistant to clindamycin. Viridans streptococci resistant to clindamycin and lincomycin are rarely found. Occasional strains of Bacteroides fragilis, fusobacteria and Clostridium perfringens are resistant. Streptococci and staphylococci may become resistant during treatment, but this is rare. There is partial cross-resistance with the macrolides (e.g. erythromycin) and with lincomycin.

Pharmacokinetics:

Clindamycin is 75% absorbed by the *oral route,* independent of food intake. More rapidly absorbed than lincomycin (*maximal blood concentration* after 45–60 min, though later after meals). Peaks after 150 mg and 300 mg by mouth are 2.8 mg/l, and 4.5 mg/l respectively, falling to 0.2 mg/l and 0.7 mg/l respectively after 8 hours (Fig. 44). No accumulation with repeated administration.

Maximum serum levels of 6 mg/l, 3 h after 300 mg i.m., 3.3 mg/l 1 h after 150 mg i.v. and 0.5 mg/l after 8 h. *Half-life* 2¾ hours. *Plasma protein binding* 84%. Good *tissue penetration* and relatively good penetration into bone. Passes

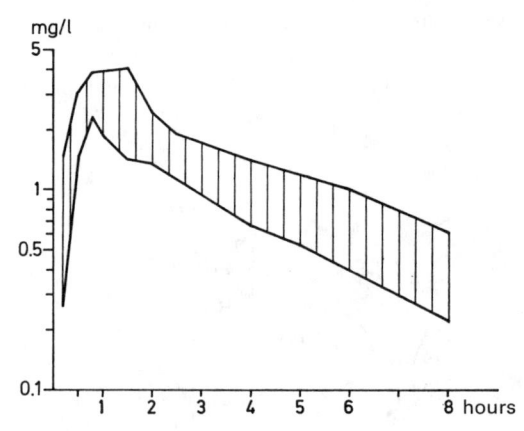

Abb. 44. Serum concentrations of clindamycin in adults after a single oral dose of 150 mg of clindamycin (own data).

into the fetal circulation but not into the *CSF.* Extensively metabolised. Active metabolites are found in the urine in addition to clindamycin (particularly N-dimethyl-clindamycin and clindamycin sulphoxide). *Urinary recovery:* 20–40% compared to 15–35% with oral administration. Not dialysable.

Side-effects: Loose stools occur in 5–20%, often associated with nausea, vomiting and abdominal pain. Severe, ulcerating pseudomembranous enterocolitis is caused by toxin-producing clostridia (Clostridium difficile) which are selected in the intestinal tract by clindamycin treatment. The colitis is characterised by severe, persistent diarrhoea and intense colic with blood and mucus in the stool. Endoscopic examination shows pseudomembranous colitis. The condition is treated with oral vancomycin (250 mg 3 times daily) and clindamycin treatment is immediately stopped.

Allergic reactions with clindamycin are rare. The commonest are itchy maculopapular rashes 1–22 weeks after treatment, but urticaria, erythema multiforme and anaphylactic reactions can also occur.

Abnormal liver function tests and jaundice are sometimes found after i. v. clindamycin. Pain and induration at the injection site may occur after i. m. injection and thrombophlebitis after i. v. injection. Rapid i. v. injection of a large dose can cause circulatory collapse and cardiac arrest.

The propylene glycol in the acne solution may cause reactions in sensitive persons. The isopropyl alcohol which is also present may cause burning and irritation if it accidentally comes into contact with the eyes or other mucous membranes. In such cases the affected part should be thoroughly irrigated with cold water.

Interactions: Clindamycin can potentiate the effect of ganglion blockers and should therefore be used with care in patients receiving these drugs.

Indications: Bacteriologically proven or clinically suspected anaerobic infections (empyema, lung abscess, peritonitis, intra-abdominal abscess, pelvic or tuboovarian abscess or endometritis). Staphylococcal infections with methicillin-resistant strains or in patients with penicillin allergy. Oral medication after i. v. treatment of staphylococcal osteomyelitis. Occasionally used to treat cerebral toxoplasmosis in AIDS.

Inappropriate use: Infections against which penicillins or erythromycin are equally effective.

Contraindications: Clindamycin should not be given i. v. to the newborn or young infants because the solution contains benzyl alcohol as preservative which can give rise to severe breathing disorders and angioneurotic oedema.

Administration and dosage: 600 mg–1.2 g a day by mouth in 3–4 divided doses, and 10–20 mg/kg/day for children. Same dose for parenteral use (i. m. injection, short or continuous i. v. infusion, but not rapid i. v. injection). If liver function is seriously impaired (acute hepatitis), the half-life is sometimes prolonged. Reduce dose to ¼–⅓ of normal in severe renal failure.

Local treatment for several weeks may be given with clindamycin acne solution.

Preparations: Capsules of 75 and 150 mg, syrup (15 mg/ml) and vials for injection of 300, 600 and 900 mg. Solution for external use (in severe acne).

Summary: An important antibiotic for the treatment of severe infections with anaerobes and with staphylococci resistant to other agents. Only use when clearly indicated because of the risk of pseudomembranous enterocolitis.

References

AUCOIN, P. A.: Clindamycin-induced cardiac arrest. South. Med. J. *75:* 768 (1982).
BERGER, S. A., M. KUPFERMINC, J. B. LESSING, A. GOREA, I. GULL, M. R. PEYSER: Penetration of clindamycin, cefoxitin, and metronidazole into pelvic peritoneal fluid of women undergoing diagnostic laparoscopy. Antimicrob. Agents Chemother. *34:* 376–377 (1990).
BRAATHEN, L. R.: Topical clindamycin versus oral tetracycline and placebo in acne vulgaris. Scand. J. Infect. Dis. *16 (S43):* 71 (1984).
ENG, R. H. K., S. GORSKI, A. PERSON, C. MANGURA, H. CHARUEL: Clindamycin elimination in patients with liver disease. J. Antimicrob. Chemother. *8:* 277–281 (1981).
FADEN, H., J. J. HONG, P. L. OGRA: In vivo effects of clindamycin on neutrophil function – a preliminary report. J. Antimicrob. Chemother. *12 (Suppl. C):* 29–34 (1983).
KLEMPNER, M. S., B. STYRT: Clindamycin uptake by neutrophils. J. Inf. Dis. *144:* 472–479 (1981).
LEIGH, D. A.: Antibacterial activity and pharmacokinetics of clindamycin. J. Antimicrob. Chemother. *7 (Suppl. A):* 3–9 (1981).
LENNARD, E. S.: Stratified outcome comparison of clindamycin-gentamicin vs. chloramphenicol-gentamicin for treatment of intra-abdominal sepsis. Arch. Surg. *120:* 889 (1985).
LEVISON, M. E., C. T. MANGURA, B. LORBER et al.: Clindamycin compared with penicillin for the treatment of anaerobic lung abscess. Ann. Intern. Med. *98:* 466 (1983).
REIG, M., M. G. CAMPELLO, F. BAQUERO: Epidemiology of clindamycin resistance in the Bacteroides fragilis group. J. Antimicrob. Chemother. *14:* 595 (1984).
SMITH, C. J., F. L. MACRINA: Large transmissible clindamycin resistance plasmid in Bacteroides ovatus. J. Bacteriol. *158:* 739 (1984).

9. Fusidic Acid

Proprietary name: Fucidin.

Properties: Fusidic acid is a surface-active substance with a steroid structure and lipophilic properties (a cyclopentane perhydrophenanthrene). It bears no relationship to other common antibiotics. The sodium and diethenanolamine salts are stable and readily soluble in water and lipids.

Mode of action: Predominantly bacteriostatic in therapeutically achievable concentrations by inhibition of protein synthesis.

Spectrum of activity: Active against staphylococci, including penicillinase-producing and methicillin-resistant strains (in very low concentrations), as well as against Corynebacterium diphtheriae, gonococci, meningococci, clostridia and Bacteroides fragilis. Most streptococci and pneumococci are only slightly sensitive, and gram-negative bacteria are resistant. Fusidic acid has good in vitro activity against Mycobacterium tuberculosis, although the clinical relevance of this is not yet clear.

Resistance: Develops rapidly *in vitro* but rarely during therapy and can be delayed or prevented by the simultaneous administration of another antibiotic such as penicillin or vancomycin. Primary resistance in staphylococci is occasionally found. No cross-resistance with other antibiotics in general use.

Pharmacokinetics: Absorption after oral administration is somewhat delayed, with *maximal concentrations* after 2–4 hours. *Serum concentrations* of 20 mg/l are found with 500 mg given twice a day over a period of time. *Plasma protein binding:* 90–97%. *Half-life:* 4–6 hours. Good *tissue penetration*. Relatively good *penetration* into inflamed and non-inflamed bone tissue. Synovial fluid concentrations 70–80% of serum levels, and almost 100% when purulent. Virtually no penetration of non-inflamed meninges. Continuous administration of 0.5 g 3 times a day leads to therapeutically useful concentration (up to 1.2 mg/l) in the *aqueous humor*. Repeated doses lead to accumulation through the enterohepatic circulation. *Excretion* is predominantly biliary at high concentrations. Very little (about 1%) is excreted in the urine. The major part is metabolised in the liver to bacteriologically inactive metabolites. Fusidic acid is virtually undialysable.

Side-effects: Oral intake can give rise to epigastric pain, sometimes with nausea and even vomiting. These effects can be largely avoided by giving the drug with meals. Occasional jaundice (reversible).

Indications: Staphylococcal infections (osteomyelitis, septicaemia, staphylococcal pneumonia, skin and wound infections), including follow-up treatment and as an alternative in penicillin allergy or where other anti-staphylococcal agents have failed. In severe cases, clindamycin may be usefully combined with a penicillin or cephalosporin.

Administration: By mouth or as a slow i.v. infusion (up to 50 mg/kg/h) every 4 hours. Do not give i.m. Local treatment with fusidic acid ointment, gel, gauze, powder or solution is available.

Dosage: *Adults:* 1.5 g a day, *children* 20 mg/kg/day in 3 divided doses. Capsules should not be given at the same time as alkalinising substances (sodium bicarbonate, antacids). The dose may be doubled in severe infection and need not be reduced for renal impairment. The bilirubin and liver enzymes should be carefully monitored in patients with impaired liver function.

Preparations: Tablets of 250 mg, suspension of 250 mg/5 ml and intravenous infusion of 580 mg (as diethanolamine fusidate). Preparations for topical use include eye drops (Fucithalmic) and a tulle.

Summary: An antibiotic with good pharmacokinetic features for use in patients with penicillin allergy and against methicillin-resistant strains.

References

BERGERON, M. G., D. DESAULNIERS, C. LESSARD et al.: Concentrations of fusidic acid, cloxacillin, and cefamandole in sera and atrial appendages of patients undergoing cardiac surgery. Antimicrob. Ag. Chemother. 27: 928 (1985).
BRODERSEN, R.: Fusidic acid binding to serum albumin and interaction with binding of bilirubin. Acta Paediatr. Scand. 74: 874 (1985).
CRONBERG, S., B. CASTOR, A. THOREN: Fusidic acid for the treatment of antibiotic-associated colitis induced by Clostridium difficile. Infection 12: 276 (1984).
FOLDES, M., R. MUNRO, T. C. SORRELL et al.: In vitro effects of vancomycin, rifampicin and fusidic acid, alone and in combination, against methicillin-resistant Staphylococcus aureus. J. Antimicrob. Chemother. 11: 21 (1983).
FRIIS-MØLLER, A., C. RECHNITZER, L. NIELSEN, S. MADSEN: Treatment of Legionella lung abscess in a renal transplant recipient with erythromycin and fusidic acid. Eur. J. Clin. Microbiol. 4: 513 (1985).
HANSEN, S.: Intraocular penetration of fusidic acid with topical Fucithalmic. Eur. J. Drug Metab. Pharmacokinet. 10: 329 (1985).
KRAEMER, R., U. B. SCHAAD, G. LEBEK et al.: Sputum penetration of fusidic acid in patients with cystic fibrosis. Eur. J. Pediatr. 138: 172 (1982).

10. Glycopeptide Antibiotics

The glycopeptides are macromolecular antibiotics whose antibiotic effect is exclusively on gram-positive organisms. The substances are readily soluble in water and are stable but, on account of their size, penetrate tissues poorly. The group includes vancomycin and teicoplanin and other derivatives (N-demethyl vancomycin) are under development. The recently developed compound, daptomycin, is a peptolide antibiotic and chemically related to the glycopeptides.

a) Vancomycin

Proprietary names: Vancocin, Vancomycin.

Properties: A glycopeptide of large molecular size which is unrelated to other groups of antibiotics. The hydrochloride is readily soluble in water, and stable.

Mode of action: Vancomycin inhibits bacterial cell wall formation and is bactericidal on growing bacteria.

Spectrum of action: Staphylococci, streptococci (including enterococci and pneumococci), Clostridium difficile, Corynebacterium diphtheriae and a few other gram-positive organisms are sensitive, but gram-negative bacilli are completely resistant.

Resistance: Does not develop during therapy; resistant staphylococcal strains are rare and cross-resistance with other groups of antibiotics is not found.

Pharmacokinetics: Not absorbed by mouth. *Serum concentrations* after 1 g i. v. are 23 mg/l 2 h and 8 mg/l 11 h after the end of the infusion. *Half-life:* 6 hours. Accumulation can occur with repeated dosing. *Plasma protein binding:* 10%.

Poor *CSF penetration,* increasing to 10–20% in meningitis. 50–100% of serum concentrations in pleural, pericardial and synovial fluids.

Excretion after i. v. administration is 80–90% through the kidneys, giving urine concentrations of 100–300 mg/l. A small amount is excreted with the bile, giving concentrations up to 50% of serum values. Not dialysable. When *excretion* is impaired, repeated doses lead rapidly to toxic concentrations in the blood.

Side-effects: Occasional thrombophlebitis. Allergic reactions with fever, urticaria, rashes and even anaphylactic shock occur more frequently. Ototoxicity, particularly when accumulation occurs in renal insufficiency, is a serious risk and renal function should be assessed carefully before treatment. Reversible neutropenia, possibly accompanied by thrombocytopenia, can occur, usually one week or more after starting treatment and after a total dose of 25 g has been exceeded; the blood picture should be monitored. Too rapid administration can evoke a transient release of mediators (red neck or red man syndrome), which is often mistaken for allergy. Hypotension and cardiac arrest are possible with rapid i. v. injection.

Interactions: Care should be taken when combining with other potentially ototoxic or nephrotoxic drugs (e. g. cisplatin).

Indications: Severe staphylococcal infections such as septicaemia, endocarditis or osteomyelitis, where penicillinase-stable penicillins or cephalosporins are contra-indicated because of allergy or methicillin resistance. Staphylococcal infections of foreign body implants (prostheses, CSF shunts etc). Vancomycin is also a useful bactericidal agent in endocarditis with staphylococci, streptococci or enterococci resistant to β-lactam antibiotics, especially when prosthetic heart valves become colonised with multiresistant strains of Staphylococcus epidermidis. In such cases it may be combined with rifampicin in staphylococcal infection and gentamicin in enterococcal endocarditis. Non-specific treatment is justified on suspicion of acute bacterial endocarditis or of endocarditis on an artificial heart

Table 18. Vancomycin dosage in patients with renal failure.

Creatinine clearance (ml/min)	100	90	80	70	60	50	40	30	20	10
Vancomycin daily dose (mg)	1545	1390	1235	1080	925	770	620	465	310	155

valve implant. Vancomycin can also be used to treat resistant corynebacteria (Corynebacterium JK). It may be given by mouth in pseudomembranous enterocolitis due to Clostridium difficile and has been used in combination with other agents for intestinal decontamination.

Contra-indications: Acute renal failure, pre-existing deafness, pregnancy.

Administration: Because vancomycin is not absorbed by mouth, it must be given by continuous i. v. infusion or in 2–4 short infusions a day, either of which may cause phlebitis. Vancomycin should not be injected rapidly i. v. since it gives rise to flushes, nausea and paraesthesiae. Intramuscular administration is very painful and can cause necrosis. Capsules are available for enterocolitis. The mixture of vancomycin with ticarcillin leads to visible precipitation in the infusion solution.

Dosage: 2 g a day *in adults* as a continuous i. v. infusion or 2–4 short i. v. infusions (500 mg in at least 200 ml of 5% glucose solution), 20–40 mg/kg daily in *children,* with a maximum of 20 mg/kg in the first week of life and 30 mg/kg in weeks 2–4 of life, in 2–3 single doses. Treatment should be for no longer than 14 days, except in exceptional circumstances (e. g. endocarditis). Where vancomycin has to be combined with gentamicin, as in enterococcal endocarditis, regular blood levels and audiometric checks should be performed because of the increased risk of ototoxicity. The dose should be reduced from the outset in patients with impaired renal function, and regular assays and hearing tests performed. Peak serum concentrations should be maintained between 10 and 30 mg/l, with an upper limit of 40 mg/l. The recommended daily dose depends on the creatinine clearance (Table 18). When only a serum creatinine value is available, the creatinine clearance in *men* may be estimated by this formula:

$$\frac{\text{Weight (kg)} \times (140 - \text{age in years})}{72 \times \text{serum creatinine (mg/dl)}}.$$

The result is multiplied by 0.85 for *women*. The creatinine clearance should normally be measured afterwards. In anuric patients on haemodialysis, 1 g of vancomycin every 1–2 weeks generally gives adequate levels.

125 mg every 6 h by mouth, and half this dose in children, for 7–10 days is normally sufficient to treat Clostridium difficile infections.

Preparations: Injection of 500 mg; capsules of 125 mg and 250 mg.

Summary: An important bactericidal antistaphylococcal reserve agent with ototoxic side-effects on accumulation. A reliable oral treatment of pseudomembranous enterocolitis.

References

ACKERMAN, B. H., R. W. BRADSHER: Vancomycin and red necks. Ann. Intern. Med. *102:* 724 (1985).
BAILIE, G. R., R. YU, R. MORTON, S. WALDEK: Vancomycin, red neck syndrome, and fits. Lancet *II:* 279 (1985).
BRAUNER, L., G. KAHLMETER, T. LONDHOLM, O. SIMONSEN: Vancomycin and netilmicin as first line treatment of peritonitis in CAPD patients. J. Antimicrob. Chemother. *15:* 751 (1985).
COLE, D. R., M. OLIVER, R. A. COWARD, C. B. BROWN: Allergy, red man syndrome, and vancomycin. Lancet *II:* 280 (1985).
DEAN, R. P., D. J. WAGNER, M. D. TOLPIN: Vancomycin/aminoglycoside nephrotoxicity. J. Pediatr. *106:* 861 (1985).
GARRELTS, J. C., J. D. PETERIE: Vancomycin and the "red man syndrome". New Engl. J. Med. *312:* 245 (1985).
GOLDSTEIN, F. W., A. COUTROT, A. SIEFFER, J. F. ACAR: Percentages and distributions of teicoplanin- and vancomycin-resistant strains among coagulase-negative staphylococci. Antimicrob. Agents Chemother. *34:* 899–900 (1990).
GREEN, M., R. M. WADOWSKY, K. BARBADORA: Recovery of vancomycin-resistant gram-positive cocci from children. J. Clin. Microbiol. 28: 484–488 (1990).
GROSS, J. R., S. L. KAPLAN, W. G. KRAMER, E. O. MASON JR.: Vancomycin pharmacokinetics in premature infants. Pediatr. Pharmacol. *5:* 17 (1985).
GRUER, L. D. et al.: Vancomycin and tobramycin in the treatment of CAPD peritonitis. Nephron. *41:* 279 (1985).
HOLLIMANN, R.: "Red Man Syndrome" associated with rapid vancomycin infusion. Lancet *I:* 1399 (1985).
INGERMAN, M. J., SANTORO, J. VANCOMYCIN: A new old agent. Infect. Dis. Clin. North Am. *3:* 641 (1989).
MACKETT, R. L., D. R. P. GUAY: Vancomycin-induced neutropenia. Can. Med. Assoc. J. *132:* 39 (1985).
MATZKE, G. R., R. W. McGORY, C. E. HALSTENSON, W. F. KEANE: Pharmacokinetics of vancomycin in patients with various degrees of renal function. Antimicrob. Ag. Chemother. *25:* 433 (1984).
MAYHEW, J. F., S. DEUTSCH: Cardiac arrest following administration of vancomycin. Can. Anaesth. Soc. J. *32:* 65 (1985).
MELLOR, J. A., J. KINGDOM, M. GAFFERKEY, C. T. KEANE: Vancomycin toxicity: a prospective study. J. Antimicrob. Chemother. *15:* 773 (1985).
MOELLERING, R. C., D. J. KROGSTAD, D. J. GREENBLATT: Vancomycin therapy in patients with impaired renal function: A nomogram for dosage. Ann. Intern. Med. *94:* 343 (1981).
MOORE, B. J.: Vancomycin dosage recommendations. Lancet *II:* 39 (1985).
MORDENTI, J., C. RIES, G. F. BROOKS et al.: Vancomycin-induced neutropenia complicating bone marrow recovery in a patient with leukemia: case report and reviews of the literature. Am. J. Med. *80:* 333 (1986).
NAQVI, S. H., W. J. KEENAN, R. M. REICHLEY, K. P. FORTUNE: Vancomycin pharmacokinetics in small seriously ill infants. Amer. J. Dis. Child. *140:* 107 (1986).

Odio, C., G. H. McCracken Jr., J. D. Nelson: Nephrotoxicity associated with vancomycin-aminoglycoside therapy in four children. J. Pediatr. *105:* 491 (1984).
Ranson, M. R., B. A. Oppenheim, A. Jackson: Double-blind placebo controlled study of vancomycin prophylaxis for central venous catheter insertion in cancer patients. J. Hosp. Infec. *15:* 95–102 (1990).
Sahai, J. et al.: Influence of anthistamine pretreatment on vancomycin-induced red-man syndrome. J. Infect. Dis. *160:* 876 (1989).
Schaible, D. H., M. L. Rocci Jr., G. A. Alpert et al.: Vancomycin pharmacokinetics in infants: relationships to indices of maturation. Pediatr. Infect. Dis. *5:* 304 (1986).
Schwalbe, R. S., J. T. Stapleton, P. H. Gillingan: Emergence of vancomycin resistance in coagulase-negative staphylococci. New Engl. J. Med. *316:* 927–931 (1987).
Sorrell, T. C., P. J. Collignon: A prospective study of adverse reactions associated with vancomycin therapy. J. Antimicrob. Chemother. *16:* 235 (1985).
Walker, R. W., A. Heaton: Thrombocytopenia due to vancomycin. Lancet *I:* 932 (1985).
Young, G. P. et al.: Antibiotic associated colitis due to Clostridium difficile. Double-blind comparison of vancomycin with bacitracin. Gastroenterology *89:* 1038 (1985).

b) Teicoplanin

Proprietary name: Targocid.

Properties: Teicoplanin is similar to vancomycin. It consists of a mixture of 6 closely related macromolecular glycopeptides. The incorporation of long fatty acid chains makes teicoplanin particularly lipophilic.

Mode of action: Bactericidal, by inhibition of bacterial cell wall synthesis.

Spectrum of activity: Identical with that of vancomycin. Considerably improved *in-vitro* activity. Teicoplanin is active against all the aerobic gram-positive bacteria including methicillin-resistant staphylococci, enterococci, Corynebacterium jeikeium and listeria, but not against gram-negative bacteria. The *in-vitro* activity against Clostridium difficile is ten times as great as that of vancomycin. Teicoplanin is synergistic with imipenem, rifampicin and gentamicin against staphylococci.

Resistance: Resistant staphylococci and enterococci have been found. There is incomplete cross-resistance with vancomycin.

Pharmacokinetics: The mean serum concentrations one hour after i. v. injection of 0.2 g and 0.4 g are 14 mg/l and 32 mg/l respectively; after 24 hours they are 2.1 mg/l and 5.4 mg/l respectively. *Half-life* 3.6 h (in the first 12 hours) with a longer decline phase. On repeated i. v. dosage the serum concentrations are almost twice as high as after single doses, and the half-life is prolonged 2 to 4 times. *Plasma-protein binding* 90%. Good tissue penetration. The concentration in skin blister fluid is 80% of the simultaneous serum concentration. Up to 50% is *excreted* unchanged in the kidneys over 4 days. Teicoplanin is not dialysable.

Side-effects: Teicoplanin is generally well tolerated. In 4–5% of cases mild side-effects such as hypersensitivity (itching, urticaria, rashes), pain at the injection site and occasional tremor occur. One case of high-frequency hearing loss has been reported.

Interactions: The combination with potentially ototoxic drugs (e. g. aminoglycosides) may potentiate the ototoxicity of teicoplanin.

Indications: Severe staphylococcal or enterococcal infection (e. g. foreign body infections or endocarditis where the pathogen has been isolated), particularly when penicillins or cephalosporins are inactive or poorly tolerated.

Contra-indications: Use with caution in acute renal failure and where there is pre-existing hearing loss. Reduce the dose in renal failure. There is no experience to date in pregnancy.

Dosage and administration: Slow intravenous or intramuscular injection of an initial dose of 400 mg and of a maintenance dose of 200 (to 400) mg once daily. In children, an initial dose of 6 mg/kg followed by 3 (to 6) mg/kg per day may be given.

Preparation: Injection vials of 200 mg and 400 mg.

Summary: A development of vancomycin with improved activity and better tolerance. Staphylococci can be resistant.

References

AUBERT, G., S. PASSOT, F. LUCHT, G. DORCHE: Selection of vancomycin- and teicoplanin-resistant Staphylococcus haemolyticus during teicoplanin treatment of S. epidermidis infection (letter). J. Antimicrob. Chemother. 25: 491 (1990).

BIBLER, M. R., P. T. FRAME, D. N. HAGLER et al.: Clinical evaluation of efficacy, pharmacokinetics, and safety of teicoplanin for serious gram-positive infections. Antimicrob. Ag. Chemother. 31: 207–212 (1987).

BRUNET F., G. VEDEL, F. DREYFUS: Failure of teicoplanin therapy in two neutropenic patients with staphylococcal septicemia who recovered after administration of vancomycin. Eur. J. Clin. Microbiol. Infect. Dis. 9: 145–147 (1990).

CALAIN, P., K.-H. KRAUSE, P. VAUDAUX et al.: Early termination of a prospective, randomized trial comparing teicoplanin and flucloxacillin for treating severe staphylococcal infections. J. Infect. Dis. 155 (2): 187–191 (1987).

GOLDSTEIN, F. W., A. COUTROT, A. SIEFFER, J. F. ACAR: Percentages and distributions of teicoplanin- and vancomycin-resistant strains among coagulase-negative staphylococci. Antimicrob. Agents Chemother. 34: 899–900 (1990).

GRANT, A. C., R. W. LACEY, J. H. BROWNJOHN, J. H. TURNEY: Teicoplanin-resistant coagulase-negative staphylococcus. Lancet II: 1166 (1986).

MARTINO, P., M. VENDITTI, A. MICOZZI et al.: Teicoplanin in the treatment of gram-positive bacterial endocarditis. Antimicrob. Agents. Chemother. 33: 1329–1334 (1989).

McElrath, M. J., D. Goldberg, H. C. Neu: Allergic cross-reactivity of teicoplanin and vancomycin. Lancet *I:* 47 (1986).
McNulty, C. A. M., G. M. F. Garden, R. Wise, J. M. Andrews: The pharmacokinetics and tissue penetration of teicoplanin. J. Antimicrob. Chemother. *16:* 743–749 (1985).
Simon, C., M. Simon: Antibacterial Activity of Teicoplanin and Vancomycin in Combination with Rifampicin, Fusidic Acid or Fosfomycin against Staphylococci on Vein Catheters. Scand. J. Infect. Dis. Suppl. *72:* 14–19 (1990).
Stille, W., W. Sietzen, H.-A. Dietrich, J. J. Fell: Clinical efficacy and safety of teicoplanin. J. Antimicrob. Chemother. *21 (Suppl. 17):* 69 (1988).
Tarral, E., F. Jehl, A. Tarral, U. Simeoni: Pharmacokinetics of teicoplanin in children. J. Antimicrob. Chemother. *21:* 47–51 (1988).
Verbist, L., B. Tjandramaga, B. Hendricks, A. van Hecken, P. van Melle, R. Verbesselt, J. Verhaegen, P. J. de Schepper: In vitro activity and human pharmacokinetics of teicoplanin. Antimicrob. Ag. Chemother. *26:* 881–886 (1984).
Wilson, A. P. R., M. D. O'Hare, D. Felmingham, R. N. Grüneberg: Teicoplanin-resistant coagulase-negative staphylococcus. Lancet *II:* 973 (1986).

c) Daptomycin

Properties: A peptolide antibiotic (polypeptide with a fatty acid side-chain), which inhibits bacterial cell wall synthesis at a different site from that attacked by vancomycin and teicoplanin. Daptomycin is a narrow-spectrum antibiotic and, like vancomycin, is active only on gram-positive bacteria (staphylococci, streptococci and enterococci). The *in-vitro* activity is similar to that of vancomycin but with a more rapidly bactericidal action against staphylococci. Daptomycin is synergistic with gentamicin on enterococci. A small proportion of enterococcal strains are only moderately sensitive or resistant.

Pharmacokinetics and tolerability: The mean serum concentration at the end of an i. v. infusion of 1 mg/kg over 30 minutes is 13 mg/l, and 1 mg/l 24 h later. *Half-life* 7 h (prolonged in severe renal insufficiency). *Plasma protein binding* 90–93%. *Urinary recovery* 50% in 24 h. Daptomycin has been shown to be nephrotoxic and neurotoxic at high concentrations in animal experiments. The tolerance in patients has not yet been assessed. A dose of 1 mg/kg daily as a short i. v. infusion has been suggested for clinical trials. The compound may be useful in staphylococcal and enterococcal infections in which other agents are inactive or poorly tolerated.

References

Ehlert, F., H. C. Neu: In vitro activity of LY146032, a new peptolide. Eur. J. Clin. Microbiol. *6:* 84–90 (1987).
Hodinka, R. L., J. Jack-Wait, N. Wannamaker, T. P. Walden, P. H. Gilligan: Comparative in vitro activity of LY146032, a new lipopeptide antimicrobial. Eur. J. Clin. Microbiol. *6:* 100–103 (1987).

JONES, R. N., A. L. BARRY: Antimicrobial activity and spectrum of LY146032, a lipopeptide antibiotic. Antimicrob. Ag. Chemother. *31:* 4 (1987).

JORGENSEN, J. H., L. A. MAHER, J. S. REDDING: In vitro activity of LY146032 against selected aerobic bacteria. Eur. J. Clin. Microbiol. *6:* 91–96 (1987).

KNAPP, C. C., J. A. WASHINGTON: Antistaphylococcal activity of a cyclic peptide, LY146032 and vancomycin. Antimicrob. Ag. Chemother. *30:* 938 (1986).

LOW, D. E., A. MCGEER, R. POON: Activities of daptomycin and teicoplanin against Staphylococcus haemolyticus and Staphylococcus epidermidis, including evaluation of susceptibility testing recommendations. Antimicrob. Agents Chemother. *33:* 585–588 (1989).

MACHKA, K., I. BRAVENY: Comparative in vitro activity of LY146032 against gram-positive cocci. Eur. J. Clin. Microbiol. *6:* 96–99 (1987).

NORD, C. E., A. LINDMARK, I. PERSON: Susceptibility of Clostridium difficile to LY146032. Eur. J. Clin. Microbiol. *6, No. 2:* 189 (1987).

RICE, L. B., G. M. ELIOPOULOS, R. C. MOELLERING JR.: In vitro synergism between daptomycin and fosfomycin against Enterococcus faecalis isolates with high-level gentamicin resistance. Antimicrob. Agents Chemother. *33:* 470–473 (1989).

WATANAKUNAKORN, C.: In vitro activity of LY146032, a novel cyclic lipopeptide alone and in combination with gentamicin or tobramycin against enterococci. J. Antimicrob. Chemother. *19:* 445–448 (1987).

VERBIST, L.: In vitro activity of LY146032, a new lipopeptide antibiotic, against grampositive cocci. Antimicrob. Ag. Chemother. *31:* 340–342 (1987).

11. Fosfomycin

Proprietary name: Fosfocin.

Properties: This broad-spectrum antibiotic was developed in the USA but not marketed there. Its structural formula is shown in Fig. 45.

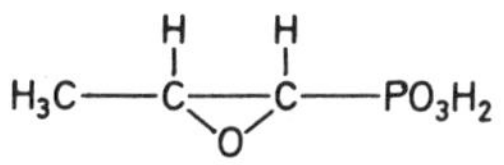

$$H_3C-\underset{\diagdown O \diagup}{\overset{H}{\underset{|}{C}}-\overset{H}{\underset{|}{C}}}-PO_3H_2$$

Fig. 45. Structural formula of fosfomycin.

Fosfomycin is an epoxide and bears no chemical relationship to other antibiotics. It is readily soluble in water but insoluble in ethanol. 1 g fosfomycin contains 14.5 millimol of sodium. An ester formulation for oral use, fosfomycin trometamol, is under development.

Mode of action: Bactericidal in the phase of bactericidal growth. Cell wall synthesis is inhibited by a different mechanism from that of β-lactam antibiotics.

Spectrum of activity: Active *in vitro* against staphylococci, gonococci, Haemophilus influenzae, Escherichia coli, Proteus mirabilis, salmonellae, shigellae, as well as against streptococci, Pseudomonas aeruginosa and Serratia marcescens. A relatively large number of strains of Morganella morganii, Klebsiella pneumoniae and enterobacters are resistant. Fosfomycin is active against peptostreptococci, peptococci, fusobacteria, veillonellas and clostridia but not against any strains of bacteroides. Susceptibility testing is very dependent on the culture medium, bacterial inoculum and test method. The addition of glucose-6-phosphate to the medium improves *in-vitro* activity. Fosfomycin is an antibiotic with poor correlation between *in-vitro* test results and clinical efficacy.

Resistance: Secondary resistance is found *in vitro* and *in vivo* and is due to inhibition of active transport of fosfomycin in the bacterial cell wall. Cross-resistance with other antibiotics is not found.

Pharmacokinetics: Poorly absorbed after oral administration. *Serum concentrations* are 40 mg/l after the i.v. infusion of 3 g and 70 mg/l after 5 g (2 h after the end of the infusion in each case). *Half-life:* 2 h. Not bound to plasma proteins. Good *tissue penetration*. Passes into the CSF and fetal circulation. *Urinary recovery:* 90%. High urine concentrations. Little or no metabolism. Dialysable.

Side-effects: Local pain after i.m. and phlebitis after i.v. injection; nausea and gastric discomfort are reported in 8% of cases, but vomiting, diarrhoea, headache, allergic reactions and transient elevation of alkaline phosphatase and transaminases are less frequent. *Beware* of sodium overload.

Indications: Bacterial infections with sensitive organisms in patients allergic to penicillins and cephalosporins. Do not give as a single agent in severe or life-threatening infection.

Contra-indications: Pregnancy.

Dosage: 3–5 g 2–3 times a day in *adults,* based on susceptibility testing. 50–80 mg/kg 2–3 times a day in *children*.

Dosage should be reduced in renal failure (Table 19). Give as a short i.v. infusion over 30 min. Monitor plasma electrolytes at higher dosage, on account of the danger of hypernatraemia, particularly in cardiac failure, oedema and secondary hyperaldosteronism. Increased potassium excretion may result and potassium substitution may be necessary.

Preparations: Injection vials of 3 and 5 g.

Summary: A broad-spectrum antibiotic which is well tolerated but has been little used to date. Watch for development of resistance during therapy and for hypernatraemia.

Table 19. Fosfomycin dosage in renal failure.

Plasma creatinine (mg/dl)	Dose (g)	Dose interval (h)	% of the normal dose
0.8	3	8	100
2.0	3	12	66
3.5	1.5	8	50
6.0	1.5	12	33
15.0	1.5	24	16

References

GATERMANN, S., E. SCHULZ, R. MARRE: The microbiological efficacy of the combination of fosfomycin and vancomycin against clinically relevant staphylococci. Infection *17:* 35 (1989).

KIRBY, W. M. M.: Pharmacokinetics of fosfomycin. Chemotherapy *23 (Suppl. 1):* 141 (1977).

MEISSNER, A., R. HAAG, R. RAHMANZADEH: Adjuvant fosfomycin medication in chronic osteomyelitis. Infection *17:* 146 (1989).

SICILIA, T., E. ESTÉVEZ, A. RODRÍGUEZ: Fosfomycin penetration into the cerebrospinal fluid of patients with bacterial meningitis. Chemotherapy *27:* 405 (1981).

12. Topical Antibiotics

The **antibacterial activity** of antibiotics used topically depends upon:
1. the active substance (solubility, mode of action, spectrum of activity, intrinsic antibacterial activity, diffusion properties),
2. the galenic properties (release, duration of action, adjuvants, etc.),
3. the danger of rapid development of secondary resistance (e.g. with fusidic acid).

Tolerability is limited with drugs which can be absorbed from wounds and mucous membranes and then exert toxic effects (e.g. bacitracin). A few agents (e.g. β-lactam antibiotics and neomycin) can give rise to allergic reactions in susceptible individuals. When there is a risk of toxicity or the development of secondary bacterial resistance, local antibiotics should be used with great care. Local antibiotics should particularly be avoided in the oropharynx because of poor activity and the possible selection of resistant micro-organisms. Local treatment with certain chemical compounds whose properties and mode of action are well understood is more satisfactory in this situation. Even here, however, the indications need to be clearly defined because, in severe infections, antibiotics should be used systemically if serious complications are to be avoided. There is still a need for the development and testing of precisely defined, serious local therapeutic agents.

a) Bacitracin

Properties: For topical use only; a toxic polypeptide antibiotic which is bactericidal to gram-positive bacteria including staphylococci and enterococci, to neisseria and Haemophilus influenzae but not other gram-negative bacteria or fungi. Resistance develops only slowly, and there is no cross-resistance with other antibiotics. Not absorbed by mouth. No longer used parenterally because of nephrotoxicity.

Topical administration: Alone, or in combination with neomycin, as a skin ointment, powder, solution, eye ointment, styli or tablets for treatment of enteritis. The instillation of bacitracin in combination with neomycin is not recommended because of the risk of side-effects. Systemic antibiotic therapy with other agents is preferable. The administration of bacitracin in lozenges is not recommended.

b) Tyrothricin

Properties: A topical bactericidal antibiotic containing gramicidin and tyrocidin. It is a very stable polypeptide, is only partly soluble in water but dissolves in alcohol and propylene glycol. Predominant activity against gram-positive cocci and bacilli. No cross-resistance with other antibiotics. Because of its high toxicity, it is not used parenterally or instilled into body cavities.

Administration: External only, on superficial infections as an ointment, powder, spray, solution and lozenges. Several commercial preparations. It should never be used alone in streptococcal sore throat since it is inadequate therapy and does not prevent secondary complications.

c) Polymyxins (Colistin and Polymyxin B)

Description: Basic cyclic polypeptides which are unrelated to other antibiotics. Colistin is polymyxin E and so is chemically related to polymyxin B. Colistin is available as colistin sulphate for oral use and as colistin sulphomethate for parenteral administration. Polymyxin B is produced as the sulphate for both oral and parenteral use. On account of their poor tolerability (see below) and unfavourable pharmacokinetics (poor tissue diffusion), they should no longer be used systemically. Many more active and better tolerated systemic agents are now available. The polymyxins may still be used as local agents.

Colistin is dosed by units (1 unit = 0.033 µg of colistin base; 1 mg of colistin base = approx. 30,000 units). Polymyxin B is dosed according to weight (1 mg polymyxin B base = 10,000 U). The sulphates of colistin and polymyxin B are water-soluble and relatively stable.

Mode of action: Bactericidal in both the lag and log phases of bacterial growth, acting on the cytoplasmic membrane as cationic detergents. The polymyxins mainly affect extracellular bacteria and have little or no action on organisms within cells.

Spectrum of activity: Active only against gram-negative bacteria such as Pseudomonas aeruginosa, Escherichia coli, enterobacter, klebsiella and brucella, though some resistant strains are found within these species. Salmonellae, shigellae, pasteurellae and Haemophilus influenzae are always sensitive, while proteus, gonococci, meningococci and gram-positive bacteria are resistant.

Resistance develops slowly *in vitro* and is rare during therapy. There is complete cross-resistance between colistin and polymyxin B.

Pharmacokinetics:

Absorption is minimal after oral administration and high concentrations are found in the intestinal lumen, so that when the mucosa is severely inflamed, a proportion of the administered dose may be absorbed and give rise to toxic effects. Application to skin and mucous membrane infections with ulceration also carries the risk of absorption.

Side-effects after parenteral administration are signs of neuro- and nephrotoxicity, allergic reactions and neuromuscular blockade.

Indications: Given by mouth for intestinal decontamination in leukaemic patients, and topically for superficial infections. Polymyxin B is a component of many topical preparations used in dermatological, ENT and ophthalmological practice.

Contra-indications: Instillation into body cavities (except the bladder) and local treatment of burns and open wounds, which carries the risk of toxic side-effects as a result of absorption.

Administration: By mouth for intestinal decontamination. As an ointment of powder for burns, superficial wound infections etc. and also as eye and ear drops. Instillation into the pleural cavity or joints is not recommended because of the possibility of absorption. Intrathecal administration is contraindicated because of the risk of the cauda equina syndrome.

Dosage: Average daily dose *by mouth* of *colistin sulphate:* 8 million units for adults, 4 million units for children between 1 and 12 years and 0.25 million units/kg in infants; *polymyxin B sulphate:* Adults and children from 6–12 y.: 300–400 mg; children between 2 and 5 y.: 150–225 mg; infants: 20 mg/kg.

Solutions of 1–10 mg of polymyxin B in 2 ml are used for *inhalation therapy,* although polymyxin irritates the mucosa.

Preparations: Colistin is available as tablets of 0.5 million units (= 16.7 mg). Polymyxin B is available as tablets of 25 mg by mouth. Polymyxin B is a component of creams, ointments, gels, powders, sprays, eye ointment, eye drops, ear drops, nasal spray, vaginal pessaries and a solution for bladder irrigation (often in combination with neomycin, bacitracin or a corticosteroid).

Summary: Suitable for topical use in superficial infections with gram-negative bacilli.

References

GODARD, J., C. GUILLAUME, M. E. REVERDY, P. BACHMANN, B. BUI-XUAN, A. NAGEOTTE, J. MOTIN: Intestinal decontamination in a polyvalent ICU. A double-blind study. Intensive Care Med. *16:* 307 (1990).

d) Kanamycin

Locally applied kanamycin is *effective* against staphylococci, Escherichia coli, Enterobacter aerogenes, Klebsiella pneumoniae, and some species of proteus and serratia. Streptococci (including enterococci), pseudomonas, bacteroides, clostridiae and fungi are *resistant.* Primary resistance is common in Escherichia coli and other gram-negative rods. Resistance may develop during therapy. There is complete cross-resistance with neomycin and paromomycin, and partial cross-resistance with streptomycin and gentamicin.

Kanamycin is no longer used systemically because of its *ototoxicity.* It is now available only as skin cream, eye drops and eye ointment.

e) Neomycin

Properties: Neomycin B (framycetin) is a toxic aminoglycoside for topical application only. Its principal activity is against gram-negative bacteria including salmonellae, shigellae, some strains of proteus and Escherichia coli, but very rarely against Pseudomonas aeruginosa. Some staphylococci are sensitive but streptococci and enterococci are resistant. *Resistance* develops slowly in stages.

Cross-resistance is complete with kanamycin and paromomycin and partial with streptomycin and gentamicin.

Little or no *absorption* after oral intake.

Side-effects: Parenteral use is *contraindicated* because of the considerable oto- and nephrotoxicity. Sufficient absorption can also take place from extensive wounds and gastric or duodenal ulcers to create a risk of side-effects. If high doses of neomycin are given for long periods during hepatic coma, small amounts can be absorbed from the bowel and, if there is simultaneous renal failure, accumulate and lead to deafness. Allergic skin rashes (contact dermatitis) are not uncommon with topical administration. Neomycin releases histamine from most cells *in vitro* and *in vivo*. An overgrowth of candida in the bowel sometimes follows oral administration and results in diarrhoea; prophylactic nystatin is therefore recommended. Severe enterocolitis caused by neomycin-resistant staphylococci has been observed after pre-operative preparation (sometimes misnamed "sterilisation") of the large intestine. A malabsorption syndrome with diarrhoea and steatorrhoea can result from mucosal damage after giving high doses by mouth for a long period. It is generally reversible after treatment is discontinued.

Topical administration:

1. As an *ointment, powder, spray, styli, solution, eye and ear drops* and *ophthalmic ointment* for superficial infections of the skin and mucous membranes. Because of the risk of absorption, a maximum total topical dose of 15 mg/kg/day should not be exceeded; length of treatment: 1–3 days; reduce dose over longer periods.

2. *Instillation:* No longer recommended because effective antibiotics are now available which penetrate body cavities well. There is a risk of neuromuscular blockade (apnoea) with intraperitoneal and intrapleural instillation, particularly when muscle relaxants are given at the same time. *Antidote:* prostigmine and calcium gluconate i.v.

3. *Oral administration* for "bacterial diarrhoea" is no longer justifiable because of the lack of clinical effect and risk of side effects. Do not give to patients with ileus or renal failure because small quantities of neomycin absorbed from the bowel can accumulate. Neomycin is still used occasionally as part of the surgical bowel preparation prior to intestinal operations, in leukaemia and hepatic coma. Dosage: 2–4 g orally for adults, 30–60 mg/kg for children, in 4–6 divided doses, possible in combination with nystatin (against candida).

Summary: An old, toxic aminoglycoside which no longer has a place on account of its frequent lack of efficacy, resistance development and risk of allergy.

References

Breen, L. J., R. E. Bryant, J. D. Levinson, S. Schenker: Neomycin absorption in man. Ann. Intern. Med. *76:* 211 (1972).
Weinstein, A. J., M. McHenry, T. L. Gavan: Systemic absorption of neomycin irrigating solution. JAMA *238:* 152 (1977).

f) Paromomycin

Proprietary name: Humatin.

Description: A bactericidal aminoglycoside antibiotic, identical with aminosidin and catenulin, which is soluble in water as paromomycin base and should be used *topically only*.

Activity against Escherichia coli, Enterobacter aerogenes, Klebsiella pneumoniae, salmonellae, shigellae, proteus and staphylococci. Paromomycin has little activity against pseudomonas. Clostridia, fungi and viruses are resistant. Hospital strains of resistant intestinal bacteria have been found. Cross-resistance is found with kanamycin, neomycin and partially with streptomycin also.

Absorption: Very little after oral administration.

Side-effects: Parenteral use is contraindicated because of oto- and nephrotoxicity. Minor gastro-intestinal disorders can occur after oral administration.

Administration: For bacterial enterocolitis, but no longer recommended: *Adults:* 1–2 g daily, *children:* 50 mg/kg daily, in 3–4 divided doses for 7 days.

g) Mupirocin

Proprietary name: Bactroban.

Properties: An antibiotic produced by *Pseudomonas fluorescens* (pseudomonic acid A), active only against staphylococci and streptococci, including methicillin-resistant *Staphylococcus aureus* (MRSA). Predominantly bacteriostatic by inhibition of bacterial protein synthesis. Unrelated to other antibiotics. No danger of rapid development of secondary resistance. Mupirocin is well absorbed by mouth but is rapidly metabolised in the body.

Use: As a skin ointment in staphylococcal and streptococcal skin infections. The ointment should be applied 1–3 times a day on the affected areas of the skin. Occasional side-effects are itching, burning, redness and local dehydration. Do not use in eyes or nose. A special, less irritant nasal preparation is available for the eradication of nasal carriage of staphylococci, including methicillin-resistant strains (MRSA).

Contra-indications: Pregnancy. Application to large areas of skin in patients with impaired renal function.

References

CASEWELL, M. W., R. L. R. HILL: Mupirocin ("Pseudomonic acid") – a promising new topical antimicrobial agent. J. Antimicrob. Chemother. *19:* 1–5 (1987).
EELLS, L. D., P. M. MERTZ, Y. PIOVANETTI, G. M. PEKOE, W. H. EAGLSTEIN: Topical antibiotic treatment of impetigo with mupirocin. Arch. Dermatol. *122:* 1273–1276 (1986).
GILBERT, M.: Topical 2% mupirocin versus 2% fusidic acid ointment in the treatment of primary and secondary skin infections. J. Am. Acad. Dermatol. *20:* 1083–1087 (1989).
Medical Letter. Mupirocin – a new topical antibiotic. Med. Lett. Drugs Ther. *30:* 55 (1988).
RODE, H., D. HANSLO, P. M. DE WET et al.: Efficacy of mupirocin in methicillin-resistant Staphylococcus aureus burn wound infection. Antimicrob. Agents. Chemother. *33:* 1358–1361 (1989).
WHITE, D. G., P. O. COLLINS, R. B. ROWSELL: Topical antibiotics in the treatment of superficial skin infections in general practice – a comparison of mupirocin with sodium fusidate. J. Infect. *18:* 221–229 (1989).
WUITE, J. et al.: Pseudomonic acid, a new antibiotic for topical therapy. J. Amer. Acad. Dermatol. *12:* 1026–1301 (1985).

h) Fusafungin

Proprietary name: Locabiosol.

Properties: A bacteriostatic cyclic depsipeptide antibiotic which is said also to have an anti-inflammatory effect. Active against staphylococci, streptococci (including pneumococci) and candida.

Use: As a dose aerosol into the oropharynx in bacterial tracheitis and bronchitis: *Adults* should inhale 4 aerosol doses every two to three hours, and *children* 2 aerosol doses. The aerosol can be used with a nasal tube in bacterial rhinitis. Side-effects include a feeling of dryness, itching, sneezing or coughing. The clinical importance of fusafungin is controversial.

13. Antifungal Agents

a) Polyenes

α) Amphotericin B

Proprietary names: Fungilin, Fungizone.

Properties: An amphoteric heptaene which, like nystatin and pimaricin, is a member of the polyene group. The amphotericin B-sodium desoxycholate complex with phosphate buffer is more water-soluble and so is preferred for intravenous use. A preparation in liposomes is under development.

Mode of action: Alteration of cytoplasmic membrane permeability (antagonism of sterol synthesis).

Spectrum of action: Active in candidiasis (Candida albicans and other candida species), histoplasmosis, sporotrichosis, cryptococcosis, torulopsosis, blastomycosis, mucormycosis, aspergillosis and coccidioidomycosis. No effect against dermatophytes (Microsporum, Trichophyton and Epidermophyton species) or bacteria, viruses or most protozoa. Synergistic in combination with flucytosine but antagonistic with miconazole and ketoconazole.

Resistance has not developed during therapy. Primary resistance in strains of candida is very rare. Cross-resistance occurs with other polyenes such as nystatin but not always with pimaricin.

Pharmacokinetics: There is virtually no *absorption* after oral administration. *Serum concentrations* of about 2–3 mg/l follow an i.v. infusion of 0.7–1 mg/kg, and these levels fall slowly. *Half-life:* 20 hours. *Plasma protein binding:* >90%. Poor *CSF penetration,* somewhat improved in meningitis (0.1–0.5 mg/l). Slow renal *excretion* (5% in 24 h, 20–40% in 1 week), urine concentrations between 1 and 5 mg/l. Serum levels are not increased even in severe renal failure. Not dialysable.

Side-effects:
1. *Nephrotoxicity:* The increased blood urea is reversible at first, but permanent renal damage can follow higher dosage. Symptoms: haematuria, proteinuria, hyposthenuria, azotaemia, hyperkaliuria and hypokalaemia.
2. *Systemic manifestations:* Fever, rigors, vomiting, circulatory collapse.
3. *Thrombophlebitis* at site of injection.
4. *Rare side effects:* Anaemia, thrombocytopenia, convulsions, hypomagnesaemia, liver damage, reversible paresis, leucocyte stasis with simultaneous leucocyte transfusion. Cardiac arrhythmias occur with rapid infusion.

Indications: Generalised fungal infections such as histoplasmosis, candida septicaemia and meningitis, cryptococcal meningitis, granulomatous candidiasis, coccidioidomycosis. Effective in infections with A. fumigatus (but failure not uncommon); combine with flucytosine if possible.

Inappropriate use: Parenteral administration for superficial fungal skin infections or without good evidence of generalised fungal infection.

Contra-indications: Impending renal failure (nephrotoxicity); concurrent treatment with other potentially nephrotoxic agents.

Administration:

Intravenous infusion in accordance with strict instructions: prepare primary solution by adding 10 ml of distilled water, then dilute with 5% glucose to a concentration of 0.1 mg/ml. Other solutions must not be used as diluents, and the infusion should last at least 6 h. Protect the infusion solution from light during administration.

Topical administration: As ointment, cream, pessaries, vaginal cream, or tablets.

Dosage in parenteral administration:

Give a *test dose* of 1 mg on day 1, then 5 mg on day 2 *(adults)*, 10 mg on day 3, followed by a daily increase of 5–10 mg (1–2 mg in *children*) until the full dose of 1 mg/kg/day is reached. A more rapid regime for acute clinical situations is 0.25 mg/kg body weight initially, increased daily by 0.25 mg/kg up to the daily dose of 1 mg/kg. A smaller dose (0.3–0.6 mg/kg/day) may be adequate when combined with flucytosine if sensitivity to flucytosine *in vitro* has already been established. A total adult dose of 2–4 g, with a maximum daily dose of 1.5 mg/kg, should not be exceeded, and treatment will normally be required for 4–8 weeks. Dosage interval: 24 hours, extended to 48 hours when improvement begins. Toxicity should be monitored 2–3 times weekly by blood urea, creatinine, potassium, magnesium, a full blood count, liver functions tests and urinalysis. Correction of hyponatraemia reduces the nephrotoxicity. Where febrile reactions occur, hydrocortisone (50 mg initially) or prednisone may be added to the infusion. Small quantities of heparin (1000 U) in the infusion may reduce the risk of thrombophlebitis. If signs of nephrotoxicity emerge, stop amphotericin B until they improve. Therapy should be restarted at a low level and slowly built up.

Lumbar intrathecal administration in meningitis: Give 10 mg prednisone initially, followed by a slow injection of 0.5 mg amphotericin B diluted with CSF in the syringe. Repeat after 2 or 3 days. If possible increase the dose progressively (0.1 mg on 1st day, increasing by 0.1 mg every second day to 0.5 mg). Side effects: paraesthesiae, transient paralysis, arachnoiditis, and spinal nerve root inflammation.

Intrapleural and intrapericardial instillation is possible (2 mg) as is intra-articular (5–20 mg every 48 h); in the latter case 25 mg of hydrocortisone at the same time improves tolerance.

Bladder instillation (in candida cystitis): Dissolve 50 mg in 1 litre of sterile water, or take 3 ml of stock solution (50 mg amphotericin B dissolved in 10 ml distilled water) diluted in 100 ml of distilled water, and infuse for a day through a 3-way catheter.

Peritoneal lavage with amphotericin B (1 mg/l) may be performed in candida peritonitis.

Aerosol treatment of fungal respiratory infections including pneumonia: 2 ml stock solution (50 mg amphotericin B dissolved in 10 ml distilled water), 2–4 inhalation sessions a day. Absorption through the mucosa does not occur.

Topical administration for gastro-intestinal fungal infection: one 100-mg tablet 4 times a day (1 ml suspension 4 times a day in infants); for oral thrush: 1-mg lozenge 4 times a day; for vaginal thrush: 10-mg pessary 1–2 times a day, or the introduction of a proprietary applicator filling of vaginal cream.

Preparations: Vials for injection containing 50 mg, tablets of 100 mg, lozenges of 10 mg, suspension of 100 mg/ml as well as a lotion, cream, ointment, dry substance (with diluting solution), pessary and vaginal cream. An ointment and cream in combination with triamcinolone, neomycin and gramicidin, and a combination with tetracycline as mystecline (capsules of 250 mg with the addition of 50 mg of amphotericin B).

Summary: A highly effective parenteral anti-fungal antibiotic which carries a risk of serious side effects. Systemic administration is only justifiable in systemic mycoses and severe organ infections where the diagnosis can be made with reasonable certainty. Administration as liposomes may improve tolerance and efficacy.

References

BALEY, J. E., C. MEYERS, R. M. KLIEGMAN, M. R. JACOBS, J. L. BLUMER: Pharmacokinetics, outcome of treatment, and toxic effects of amphotericin B and 5-fluorocytosine in neonates. J. Pediatr. *116:* 791–797 (1990).

BERLINER, S., M. WEINBERGER, M. BEN-BASSAT et al.: Amphotericin B causes aggregation of neutrophils and enhances pulmonary leukostasis. Am. Rev. Resp. Dis. *132:* 602 (1985).

BOW, E. J., M.-L. SCHROEDER, T. J. LOUIE: Pulmonary complications in patients receiving granulocyte transfusions and amphotericin B. Can Med. Assoc. J. *130:* 593 (1984).

CRAVEN, P. C., D. H. GREMILLION: Risk factors of ventricular fibrillation during rapid amphotericin B infusion. Antimicrob. Ag. Chemother. *28:* 868 (1985).

DE GREGORIO, M. W., W. M. F. LEE, C. A. RIES: Pulmonary reactions associated with amphotericin B and leukocyte transfusions. New Engl. J. Med. *305:* 585 (1981).

FISHER, J. F., A. T. TAYLOR, J. CLARK et al.: Penetration of amphotericin B into the human eye. J. Infect. Dis. *147:* 164 (1983).

FEELY, J., H. HEIDEMANN, J. GERKENS et al.: Sodium depletion enhances nephrotoxicity of amphotericin B. Lancet *I:* 1422 (1981).

HEIDEMANN, H. TH., J. F. GERKENS, W. A. SPICKARD et al.: Amphotericin B nephrotoxicity in humans decreased by salt repletion. Amer. J. Med. *75:* 476 (1983).

HUGHES, C. E., C. HARRIS, J. A. MOODY et al.: In vitro activities of amphotericin B in combination with four antifungal agents and rifampin against Aspergillus species. Antimicrob. Ag. Chemother. *25:* 560 (1984).

KOREN, G., et al.: Pharmacokinetics and adverse effects of amphotericin B in infants and children. J. Pediatr. *118:* 559 (1988).

LOPEZ-BERESTEIN, G., V. FAINSTEIN, R. HOPFER et al.: Liposomal amphotericin B for the treatment of systemic fungal infections in patients with cancer: a preliminary study. J. Infect. Dis. *151:* 704 (1985).

MEHTA, R., G. LOPEZ-BERESTEIN, R. HOPFER et al.: Liposomal amphotericin B is toxic to fungal cells but not to mammalian cells. Biochim. Biophys. Acta *770:* 230 (1984).

MILLER, M. A.: Reversible hepatotoxicity related to amphotericin B. Can. Med. Assoc. J. *131:* 1245 (1984).

Rahko, P. S., W. P. Davey, J. Wheat, M. Bartlett: Treatment of Torulopsis glabrata peritonitis with intraperitoneal amphotericin B. JAMA *249:* 1187 (1983).

Rodenhuis, S., F. Beaumont, H. F. Kauffman, H. J. Sluiter: Invasive pulmonary aspergillosis in a non-immunosuppressed patient: successful management with systemic amphotericin and flucytosine and inhaled amphotericin. Thorax. *39:* 78 (1984).

Sorensen, L. J., E. G. McNally, T. H. Sternberg: The development of strains of Candida albicans and Coccidioides immitis, which are resistant to amphotericin B. Antibiot. Annual *1958–1959:* 920 (1959).

Wright, D. G.: Lethal pulmonary reactions associated with the combined use of amphotericin B and leukocyte transfusions. N. Engl. J. Med. *304:* 1185 (1981).

β) Nystatin

Proprietary name: Nystan.

Properties: An amphoteric tetraene of the polyene group. Insoluble in water but soluble in propylene glycol.

Mode of action: Nystatin increases the permeability of the cytoplasmic membrane of fungi.

Spectrum of action: Active against Candida albicans and other candida species, Blastomyces dermatitidis and B. brasiliensis, Coccidioides immitis, Cryptococcus neoformans, Histoplasma capsulatum, geotrichum, aspergillus. No effect on bacteria, viruses, actinomycetes or dermatophytes.

Resistance: Development of resistance during therapy has not been observed. Primary resistant strains are very rare. Cross-resistance with amphotericin B occurs.

Pharmacokinetics: No significant *absorption* after oral or topical administration. A parenteral form is not available.

Side-effects: Uncommon (nausea, vomiting and loose stools may all follow a large oral dose).

Indications: Candidiasis of the skin, mouth, genital or intestinal mucosa, candida balanitis, other topical fungal diseases (see spectrum of action), topical treatment in generalised fungal infection. Long-term therapy for susceptible patients such as neonates, infants treated with antibiotics, diabetics and patients with malignancies, particularly leukaemia to prevent systemic infection.

Administration: As an oral suspension containing 100,000 units/ml, or sugar-coated tablets, as a powder or ointment for topical use and as a pessary in vaginitis. A suspension for irrigation and aerosol treatment can be made from an ampoule of sterile pure substance by shaking with 5 ml of physiological saline. The patient inhales 1 ml (= 100,000 U) twice a day as an aerosol. Since nystatin is inactivated by heat, a pressurised inhaler should be used.

Dosage: Adults and children with intestinal candidiasis should be given 1.5–3 million units a day, in three divided doses (0.5–1 million units in infants). 1–2 pessaries a day for at least 2 weeks are recommended for candida vaginitis, and in pregnancy this should be started 3–6 weeks before the estimated date of delivery. Used in this way, prophylaxis of neonatal candidiasis can be achieved.

Preparations: Coated tablets, oral suspension, ointment, paste, powder, pessaries, vaginal cream, pure substance, vaginal tablets, eye drops, ear drops, compound gel and ointment (with neomycin, gramicidin and triamcinolone acetonide), paste with zinc oxide etc.

Summary: An antifungal agent for *local use only* in candidiasis of the skin and mucous membranes, with a low risk of side-effects.

γ) Natamycin (Pimaricin)

Properties: Natamycin is a tetraene of the polyene group and is mainly fungistatic; it is sensitive to light and insoluble in water. It may be used in skin infections with Candida, Trichophyton and Microsporum species, and is active against trichomonads also.

Topical administration: As a cream, powder, lotion, lozenge, coated tablet, suspension, vaginal tablets: as an eye ointment in combination with neomycin and hydrocortisone; as a cream in combination with benzalkonium chloride and hydrocortisone for anal mycosis and anal fissures.

b) Azoles

An important group of antifungal agents, somewhat variable chemically, with either an imidazole or a triazole structure but identical mode of action (inhibition of ergosterol synthesis). The first representative to be developed was clotrimazole. Some of the derivatives may be used systemically. A distinction between systemic and topical azoles (Table 20) is of practical value. Systemic azoles can also be used locally.

Table 20. Systemic and topical azoles.

Systemic treatment	Local treatment
Miconazole	Clotrimazole
Ketoconazole	Econazole
Fluconazole	Isoconazole
Itraconazole	Oxiconazole etc.

Azoles for systemic use

α) Miconazole

Proprietary names: Daktarin, Gyno-Daktarin, Gyno-Monistat, Monistat.

Properties: Miconazole is a poorly water-soluble imidazole derivative. It has a wide range of action including epidermophyton, trichophyton, candida and aspergillus as well as Malassezia furfur (the cause of tinea versicolor). Histoplasma capsulatum, Coccidioides immitis, Pseudallescheria boydii and several rare fungi are also sensitive. There is also activity against some gram-positive bacteria (nocardia, streptococci). No activity against gram-negative bacteria. The structural formula is shown in Fig. 46.

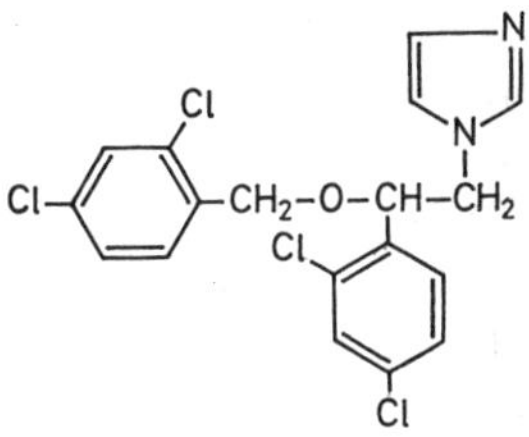

Fig. 46. Structural formula of miconazole.

Pharmacokinetics: Miconazole is not absorbed when applied to skin or mucous membranes and only slightly absorbed when given orally. Intravenous dosage achieves *maximal serum concentrations* which are tenfold greater than after oral administration (5–7 mg/l after 0.8 g i. v.). *Half-life:* 2–4 h (in the first 12 h) and 24 h (in the second 12 h). *Plasma protein binding:* 90%. *Urinary recovery:* 10% (only 1% unchanged). Highly metabolised in the body. Low concentrations in CSF and aqueous humor. Half-life is not prolonged in renal failure. Only dialysable to a small extent.

Side-effects: Thrombophlebitis not uncommonly complicates i. v. administration. Vomiting, diarrhoea, allergic reactions, fever and hot flushes are also reported. Tachycardia and arrhythmias can follow rapid injection. The proprietary solvent Cremophor in the intravenous preparation can cause hyperlipaemia and changes in the blood picture (erythrocyte rouleaux, anaemia and thrombocytosis), also pruritus and allergic shock (rarely). Local treatment in the vagina can give rise to burning or itching (in part due to infection).

Interactions: Miconazole has a marked inhibitory effect on liver enzymes, potentiating the activity of some drugs given concurrently, e. g. antidiabetic agents, antiepileptic drugs and anticoagulants, the dose of which should be reduced accordingly.

Indications: Topical treatment of infections with dermatomycetes and candida. Systemic treatment of localised organ involvement, disseminated fungal infection and severe cutaneous mycoses, especially candidiasis, aspergillosis, cryptococcosis, as well as blastomycosis and coccidioidomycosis. Should not be combined with amphotericin B in systemic use because of the possibility of antagonism.

Administration and dosage: Powders and ointment may be used for the *topical treatment of skin infections*. Prolonged treatment with occlusive dressings is necessary for *nail infections*. *Candidal vaginitis* should be treated for at least 2 weeks, despite rapid improvement, to prevent recurrence. Miconazole gel may be given for *oral thrush* for 1–2 weeks (1.25 ml four times a day in infants, and 2.5 ml four times daily for older children). Adults with oral thrush should dissolve a tablet in the mouth several times a day.

Systemic and organic mycoses in adults are treated with a daily dose of 0.6 g by i. v. infusion in 60 min; children should receive 15 mg/kg. The dosage can be increased without risk up to 1.8 g a day (in children 20–30 mg/kg) in 2 or 3 doses. Phlebitis may be avoided by adequate dilution or by infusion through a central venous line. Treatment should last at least 12 days. Miconazole should not be given orally in systemic mycoses.

Bladder instillations: 200 mg in 20 ml of undiluted solution 2–4 times a day.
Sinus instillations: 20 ml of solution twice a day.

Preparations: Powder, ointment (2%), gel, lotion, solution, vaginal cream, pessaries, tampons, solution for i. v. infusion in 0.2 g vials, tablets.

Summary: Broad-spectrum antimycotic for topical and systemic use. Treatment should last long enough to prevent recurrence. Failures of treatment of systemic fungal infections occur. Miconazole was an alternative to amphotericin B because of its better i. v. tolerance, but unreliable efficacy in aspergillosis. Now often replaced by flu- or itraconazole. Drug of choice in infections with Pseudallescheria boydii.

References

FEINSTEIN, V., G. P. BODEY: Cardiorespiratory toxicity due to miconazole. Ann. Intern. Med. *93:* 432 (1980).
HOLT, R. J. A. AZMI: Miconazole-resistant Candida. Lancet *1:* 50 (1978).
ROLAN, P.E., A. A. SOMOGYI, M. J. R. DREW et al.: Phenytoin intoxication during treatment with parenteral miconazole. Brit. Med. J. *287:* 1760 (1983).

β) Ketoconazole

Proprietary name: Nizoral.

Properties: An imidazole dioxolane derivative with a similar range of activity to miconazole, namely dermatophytes, candida and other fungal pathogens. Poorly water-soluble except at a pH of 3.0 or less, highly lipophilic (structural formula in Fig. 47).

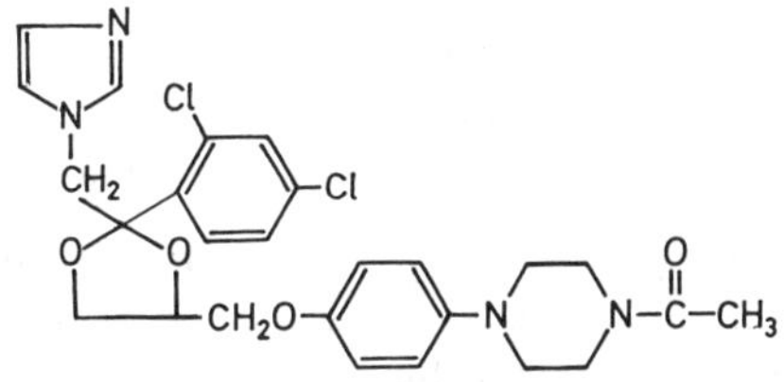

Fig. 47. Structural formula of ketoconazole.

Pharmacokinetics: *Absorption* is best in the fasting state and is reduced in achlorhydria because ketoconazole is only soluble in an acid medium. Maximal *serum concentrations* of 3.4 mg/l occur 1 to 2 h after 0.2 g orally. *Half-life:* 2 h in the first 10 h, 8 h thereafter. *Plasma-protein binding:* 99%. *Urinary recovery:* 2–4% (*unchanged*). 20–65% excreted in bile into the intestine. Extensively metabolised, little CSF penetration and not generally absorbed after topical application.

Side-effects: Itching, nausea, vomiting, abdominal pain and urticaria occur frequently; headache, giddiness, drowsiness, photophobia, fever with rigors and diarrhoea are less common. Transient increase in hepatic enzymes and cholestatic jaundice are possible, as is rare but fatal hepatotoxicity (estimated frequency 1 in 10,000). Liver function should therefore be tested before starting the course and monitored frequently during treatment. Ketoconazole should be stopped immediately if the liver enzymes rise markedly. Higher doses of ketoconazole can inhibit cortisol and testosterone formation and can also lead to oligospermia and gynaecomastia. Anaemia, leukocytopenia and thrombocytopenia are rare. Topical use of the cream gives rise to local irritation (burning, itching etc.).

Interactions: Antacids, anticholinergic agents and H_2-blockers impair the absorption of ketoconazole. Ketoconazole interferes with cytochrome P 450 – dependent metabolism in the liver. Potentiation of anticoagulants, phenytoin and oral antidiabetic agents should be taken into account. Ketoconazole can increase the blood concentration of cyclosporin A. The simultaneous administration of rifampicin or INH can reduce the blood concentration of ketoconazole.

Indications: Chronic mucocutaneous candidiasis and systemic and local mycoses (Candida septicaemia, coccidioidomycosis, histoplasmosis) and also severe recurrent vaginal mycoses. In severe trichophytosis, ketoconazole should only be used when topical treatment has failed. Unreliable activity in aspergillosis. The cream can be used for local treatment of severe tinea, microsporum infection and pityriasis versicolor. Ketoconazole is important in the treatment of candida infections in AIDS, for which a higher dosage (0.4 g – 0.6 g daily) and often prolonged treatment are necessary because of the risk of relapse. In oral candidiasis the tablets are combined with local ketoconazole suspension. Ketoconazole is suitable for the prophylaxis of fungal infections in leukaemia.

Contra-indications: Pregnancy, as ketoconazole has been shown to be teratogenic and embryotoxic in animal experiments. Contraceptive measures are therefore necessary during treatment. Since ketoconazole passes into the breast milk, breast feeding is not permitted. Do not use in the first two years of life. Use with caution in patients who have received griseofulvin in the previous four weeks. Do not use for uncomplicated superficial infections which would respond readily to topical treatment.

Dosage: The standard dosage in epidermophytosis is 200 mg once daily by mouth (always with meals), and in children 3 mg/kg. Increase the dose to 400 mg (6 mg/kg) once daily for severe infections. *Duration of therapy:* 10 days for oral trush, one to two months for deep-seated cutaneous mycoses and generalised candidiasis, and two to six months in coccidioidomycosis and histoplasmosis. The cream (which contains additional propylene glycol and polysorbates) should be applied once a day to the infected skin area. The duration of tinea is 2–4 weeks according to the site, and up to six weeks for tinea pedis.

Preparations: Tablets (200 mg); cream.

Summary: Ketoconazole is better avoided on account of its serious side-effects and drug interactions; safer alternatives (e.g. fluconazole, itraconazole) are now available.

References

AYUB, M., M. J. LEVELL: The effect of ketoconazole related imidazole drugs and antiandrogens on [3H] R 1881 binding to the prostatic androgen receptor and [3H] 5 alpha-dihydrotestosterone and [3H] cortisol binding to plasma proteins. J. Steroid Biochem. *33:* 251–255 (1989).
BLATCHFORD, N. R., M. B. EMANUEL, G. CAUWENBERGH: Ketoconazole resistance. Lancet *II:* 770 (1982).

Daneshmend, T. K.: Ketoconazole-cyclosporin interaction. Lancet *II:* 1342 (1982).
De Felice, R., D. G. Johnson, J. N. Galgiani: Gynecomastia with ketoconazole. Antimicrob. Ag. Chemother. *19:* 1073 (1981).
Dieperink, H., J. Møller: Ketoconazole and cyclosporin. Lancet *II:* 1217 (1982).
Engelhard, D., H. R. Stutman, M. I. Marks: Interaction of ketoconazole with rifampin and isoniazid. New Engl. J. Med. *311:* 1681 (1984).
Firebrace, D. A. J.: Hepatitis and ketoconazole therapy. Brit. Med. J. *283:* 1058 (1981).
Grosso, D. S., T. W. Boyden, R. W. Pamenter et al.: Ketoconazole inhibition of testicular secretion of testosterone and displacement of steroid hormones from serum transport proteins. Antimicrob. Ag. Chemother. *23:* 207 (1983).
Heiberg, J. K., E. Svejgaard: Toxic hepatitis during ketoconazole treatment. Brit. Med. J. *283:* 825 (1981).
Horsburgh Jr., C. R., C. H. Kirkpatrick, C. B. Teutsch: Ketoconazole and the liver. Lancet *1:* 860 (1982).
Janssen, P. A. J., J. E. Symoens: Hepatic reactions during ketoconazole treatment. Amer. J. Med. *74:* 80 (1983).
MacNair, A. L., E. Gascoigne, J. Hear et al.: Hepatitis and ketoconazole therapy. Brit. Med. J. *283:* 1058 (1981).
Maksymiuk, A. W., H. B. Levine, G. P. Bodey: Pharmacokinetics of ketoconazole in patients with neoplastic diseases. Antimicrob. Ag. Chemother. *22:* 43 (1982).
Morgenstern, G. R., R. Powles, B. Robinson, T. J. McElwain: Cyclosporin interaction with ketoconazole and melphalan. Lancet *II:* 1342 (1982).
National Institute of Allergy and Infectious Diseases Mycoses Study Group: Treatment of blastomycosis and histoplasmosis with ketoconazole. Results of a prospective randomized clinical trial. Ann. Intern. Med. *103:* 861–872 (1985).
Pillans, P. I., P. Cowan, D. Whitelaw: Hyponatraemia and confusion in a patient taking ketoconazole. Lancet *I:* 821 (1985).
Pont, A., J. R. Graybill, P. C. Graven et al.: High-dose ketoconazole therapy and adrenal and testicular function in humans. Arch. Intern. Med. *144:* 2150 (1984).
Pont, A., P. L. Williams, S. Azhar et al.: Ketoconazole blocks testosterone synthesis. Arch. Intern. Med. *142:* 2137 (1983).
Pont, A., E. S. Goldman, A. M. Sugar et al.: Ketoconazole-induced increase in estradiol-testosterone ratio. Probable explanation for gynecomastia. Arch. Intern. Med *145:* 1429 (1985).
Schurmeyer, Th., E. Nieschlag: Ketoconazole-induced drop in serum and saliva testosterone. Lancet *II:* 1998 (1982).
Smith, A. G.: Potentiation of oral anticoagulants by ketoconazole. Brit. Med. J. *288:* 188 (1985).
Tavihan, A., J.-P. Raufman, L. E. Rosenthal et al.: Ketoconazole-resistant Candida esophagitis in patients with acquired immunodeficiency sydrome. Gastroenterology *90:* 443 (1986)
Tucker, W. S., B. B. Snell, D. P. Island, C. R. Gregg: Reversible adrenal insufficiency induced by ketoconazole. J. Am. Med. Assoc. *253:* 2413 (1985).
Van den Bossche, H., G. Willemsens, W. Cools et al.: In vitro and in vivo effects of the antimycotic drug ketoconazole on sterol synthesis. Antimicrob. Ag. Chemother. *17:* 922 (1980).
Van Duke, C. P. H., F. R. Veerman, H. Ch. Haverkamp: Anaphylactic reactions to ketoconazole. Brit. Med. J. *287:* 1673 (1983).

WATANABE, H., J. A. MENZIES: Depression of ovarian estradiol-17beta following single oral dose of ketoconazole. Res. Commun. Chem. Pathol. Pharmacol. *48:* 141 (1985).
WHITE, M. C., P. KENDALL-TAYLOR: Adrenal hypofunction in patients taking ketoconazole. Lancet *I:* 44 (1985).

γ) Itraconazole

Proprietary names: Sempera, Sporanox.

Properties: A newly developed systemic azole derivative (triazole) which is considerably more active than the other azoles (including ketoconazole) against aspergilli, including Aspergillus fumigatus. It is a broad-spectrum antifungal agent and is active also against dermatophytes, Candida species, cryptococcus, sporothrix, cladosporium and phialophora. It may be used orally in systemic and severe local fungal infections.

Pharmacokinetics: Absorption during or after a meal is better than in the fasting state. Continuous oral treatment of 0.1 or 0.2 g once daily results after one week in constant mean serum concentration of 0.6 mg/l. Half-life: 24 h, plasma protein binding: 99%. High tissue levels (also in the brain). Does not penetrate CSF or aqueous humor. Unchanged itraconazole cannot be detected in the urine. Hepatic metabolism predominates. Renal dysfunction, haemodialysis and continuous peritoneal dialysis do not alter metabolism. Concurrent administration of rifampicin or phenytoin reduces the serum concentration of itraconazole.

Side-effects: Occasional nausea, vomiting, abdominal pain, rash, headache, giddiness and heartburn.

Indications: Pityriasis versicolor, dermatomycoses, fungal keratitis (caused by aspergillus, candida, fusarium). Severe fungal infections in patients with AIDS (caused by cryptococcus, histoplasma and other fungi).

Contra-indications: Pregnancy (because of teratogenicity shown in animal experiments), lactation, severe hepatic dysfunction. When given together with cyclosporin A, serum levels of cyclosporin should be monitored.

Dosage: 0.2 g once daily for one week (pityriasis) or 3 weeks (fungal keratitis), and 0.1 g once daily for 2–4 weeks (dermatomycoses). No dose reduction is necessary in impaired renal function.

Summary: Newly developed antifungal agent for systemic use with good tolerance.

References

BORELLI, D.: A clinical trial of itraconazole in the treatment of deep mycoses and leishmaniasis. Rev. Infect. Dis. *9:* 57–63 (1987).

BORGERS, M., M. A. VAN DE VEN: Degenerative changes in fungi after itraconazole treatment. Rev. Infect. Dis. *9:* 33 (1987).
CAUWENBERGH, G., P. DE DONCKER: Itraconazole (R 51.211): a clinical review of its antimycotic activity in dermatology, gynecology, and internal medicine. Drug. Dev. Res. *8:* 317–323 (1986).
DEL PALACIO HERNANZ, A., S. V. DELGADO, F. R. MENENDEZ, A. B. RODRIGUEZ-NORIEGA: Randomized comparative clinical trial of Itraconazole and selenium sulfide shampoo for the treatment of pityriasis versicolor. Rev. Infect. Dis. *9* (Suppl. 1): 121–127 (1987).
DENNING, D. W. et al.: Itraconazole therapy for cryptococcal meningitis and cryptococcosis. Arch. Intern. Med. *149:* 2301, 1989.
DUPONT, B., E. DROUHET: Early experience with itraconazole in vitro and in patients – pharmacokinetic studies and clinical results. Rev. Infect. Dis. *9:* 71–76 (1987).
ESPINEL-INGROFF, A., S. SHADOMY, R. J. GEBHARDT: In vitro studies with R 51.211 (itraconazole). Antimicrob. Ag. Chemother. *26:* 5–9 (1984).
GANER, A., E. ARATHOON, D. A. STEVENS: Initial experience in therapy for progressive mycoses with itraconazole, the first clinically studied triazole. Rev. Infect. Dis. *9:* 77–88 (1987).
HEYKANTS, J., M. MICHIELS, W. MEULDERMANS, J. MONBALIU, K. LAVRIJSEN, A. VAN PEER, J. C. LEVRON, R. WOESTENBORGHS, G. CAUWENBERGH: The pharmacokinetics of itraconazole in animals and man: an overview, S. 1–29. In: FROMTLING, R. A. (Hrsg.) Recent Trends in the Discovery, Development and Evaluation of Antifungal Agents. Telesymposia Proceedings, Barcelona, Spain 1987.
MCEWEN, J. G., G. R. PETERS, T. F. BLASCHKE, E. BRUMMER, A. M. PERLMAN, A. RESTREPO, D. A. STEVENS: Treatment of paracoccidioidomycosis with itraconazole in a murine model. J. Trop. Med. Hyg. *88:* 295–299 (1985).
NEGRONI, R., O. PALMIERI, F. KOREN, I. N. TIRABOSCHI, R. L. GALIMBERTI: Oral treatment of paracoccidioidomycosis and histoplasmosis with itraconazole in humans. Rev. Infect. Dis. *9:* 47–50 (1987).
ODDS, F. C., C. E. WEBSTER, A. B. ABBOTT: Antifungal relative inhibition factors: BAY 19139, bifonazole, butoconazole, isoconazole, itraconazole (R 51211), oxiconazole. Ro 14-4767/002, sulconazole, terconazole and vibunazole (BAY n-7133) compared in vitro with nine established antifungal agents. J. Antimicrob. Chemother. *14:* 105–114 (1984).
PERFECT, J. R., D. V. SAVANI, D. T. DURACK: Comparison of itraconazole and fluconazole in treatment of cryptococcal meningitis and candida pyelonephritis in rabbits. Antimicrob. Agents. Chemother. *29:* 579–583 (1986).
RESTREPO, A., I. GOMEZ, J. ROBLEDO, M. M. PATINO, L. E. CANO: itraconazole in the treatment of paracoccidioidomycosis: a preliminary report. Rev. Infect. Dis. *9:* 51–56 (1987).
SACHS, M. K., R. G. PALUZZI, J. H. MOORE: Amphotericin-resistant aspergillus osteomyelitis controlled by itraconazole (letter). Lancet. *335:* 1475 (1990).
VAN CAUTEREN, H., J. HEYKANTS, R. DE COSTER, G. CAUWENBERGH: Itraconazole: pharmacologic studies in animals and humans. Rev. Infect. Dis. *9:* 43–46 (1987).
VAN CUTSEM, J., F. VAN GERVEN, M.-A. VAN DE VEN, M. BORGERS, P. A. J. JANNSEN: Itraconazole, a new triazole that is orally active in aspergillosis. Antimicrob. Ag. Chemother. *26:* 527–534 (1984).
VAN'T WOUT, J. W., E. J. RAVEN, J. W. VAN DER MEER: Treatment of invasive aspergillosis with itraconazole in a patient with chronic granulomatous disease. J. Infect. *20:* 147–150 (1990).
WARNOCK, D. W.: Itraconazole and fluconazole: new drugs for deep fungal infection. J. Antimicrob. Chemother. *24:* 275–277 (1989).

δ) Fluconazole

Proprietary name: Diflucan.

Properties: A new systemic azole derivative (triazole) for systemic use with good activity against Candida spp. and Cryptococcus neoformans. Fluconazole is readily soluble in water but only slightly lipophilic.

Spectrum of activity: Active in vitro mainly against Candida species (except C. krusei) and Cryptococcus neoformans. Aspergillus spp. are resistant in vitro.

Pharmacokinetics: Fluconazole is well absorbed after oral administration. After a single oral dose of 2.5–3.0 mg/kg, the mean serum concentration is 1.3 mg/l. After a single 30-minute i. v. infusion of 0.05 g or 0.1 g, serum concentrations are 0.9 mg/l and 2.1 mg/l respectively (15 minutes after the end of the infusion).

Half-life: 25 h. Plasma protein binding: 12%. Good *tissue penetration* (also into skin). Relatively high concentrations in urine, saliva, sputum, ocular fluids and CSF (CSF concentrations are almost as high as in serum). *Urinary recovery:* 60–75% of an oral dose (unchanged) and 80% of an i. v. administered dose.

Side-effects: Fluconazole is generally well tolerated. Gastrointestinal effects (nausea, abdominal pain, diarrhoea) are more frequent than rashes and CNS effects (headache, vertigo, convulsions, insomnia). Hepatic dysfunction occurs very rarely.

Indications: Systemic infections with Candida albicans, meningitis caused by Cryptococcus neoformans and severe mucocutaneous candida infections (stomatitis, oesophagitis) particularly in AIDS patients and in the compromised host. Also used for prophylaxis of candida infections in immunosuppressed patients.

Contra-indications: Pregnancy and lactation.

Administration and dosage: For systemic infections and cryptococcal meningitis, 0.4 g initially then 0.2 g once daily by i.v. infusion over 30 minutes, later orally. For mucosal infections and for prophylaxis, 0.05–0.1 g once daily are recommended. Reduced dosage in renal insufficiency: the single dose is given every 48 h (creatinine clearance 21–40 ml/min.) or every 72 h (creatinine clearance 10–20 ml/min.). Duration of treatment: in patients with systemic infection and meningitis up to 3 months, in patients with severe mucosal infections up to 2 weeks.

Preparations: Capsules of 50 mg, 100 mg and 200 mg, suspension for oral use (0.5%), infusion bottles of 100 mg and 200 mg.

Summary: Effective drug in systemic candida and cryptococcal infections. Can by given i. v. and orally. Well tolerated.

References

BRAMMER, K. W., P. R. FARROW, J. K. FAULKNER: Pharmacokinetics and tissue penetration of fluconazole in humans. Rev. Infect. Dis. *12 Suppl. 3:* S 318–326 (1990).
COLLIGNON, P.: Interaction of fluconazole with cyclosporin. Lancet *1:* 1262 (1989).
DAVE, J., M. M. HICKEY, E. G. L. WILKINS: Fluconazole in renal candidosis. Lancet *1:* 163–164 (1989).
EBDEN, P., P. NEILL, P. R. FARROW: Sputum levels of fluconazole in humans. Antimicrob. Agents. Chemother. *33:* 963–964 (1989).
ESPOSITO, R., C. U. FOPPA, S. ANTINORI: Fluconazole for cryptococcal meningitis. Ann. Intern. Med. *110:* 170 (1989).
LARSEN, R. A., M. A. LEAL, L. S. CHAN: Fluconazole compared with amphotericin B plus flucytosine for cryptococcal meningitis in AIDS. A randomized trial. Ann. Intern. Med. *113:* 183–187 (1990).
LAZAR, J. D., K. D. WILNER: Drug interactions with Fluconazole. Rev. Inf. Dis. *12* (Suppl. 3): 327–333 (1990).
MEUNIER, F., M. AOUN, M. GERARD: Therapy for oropharyngeal candidiasis in the immunocompromised host: a randomized double-blind study of fluconazole vs. ketoconazole. Res. Infect. Dis. *12 Suppl. 3:* S 364–368 (1990).
STERN, J. J. et al.: Fluconazole therapy for patients with acquired immunodeficiency syndrome and cryptococcosis: Experience with 22 patients. Am. J. Med. *85:* 477 (1988).
TUCKER, R. M., J. N. GALGIANI, D. W. DENNING et al.: Treatment of coccidioidal meningitis with fluconazole. Rev. Infect. Dis. *12 Suppl. 3:* S 380–389 (1990).

c) Azoles for Topical Use

α) Clotrimazole

Proprietary names: Canesten etc.

Properties: A tritylimidazole derivative, slightly alkaline, insoluble in water but soluble in lipoid solvents. The structural formulae of clotrimazole and other azoles for topical use are shown in Fig. 48 (p. 207).

Spectrum of action: Fungistatic against dermatomycetes (Trichophyton and Microsporum species, Epidermophyton floccosum), blastomycetes (Candida), chromomycetes (Hormodendrum and Phialophora species) and some causes of systemic mycoses. Inactive against most bacteria and all viruses.

Resistance: Apparently no primary resistance in Candida albicans and trichophyton. Secondary resistance has not been observed so far.

Side-effects: Skin irritation (redness, swelling, burning, itching) occur occasionally as do skin reactions to additives (e. g. propylene or polyethylene glycol, isopropanol or cetyl stearyl alcohol). Irritation can occur with vaginal pessaries.

Indications: Suitable for topical treatment (with a 1% solution, ointment or spray) of dermatomycoses due to candida, trichophyton, microsporum, Epidermophyton floccosum and Malassezia furfur, as well as erythrasma and pityriasis versicolor. Pessaries and vaginal cream are available for the local treatment of candida vaginitis. May be used in pregnancy.

Dosage and duration of treatment: Skin cream or ointment should be thinly applied and rubbed in two to three times a day to the affected area. Use spray twice daily. Pessaries (100 mg) should be inserted once or twice every evening for 7 days or 200 mg tablets given once each evening for 3 days or 500 mg tablets in a single dose. During pregnancy, treatment for 3 or 7 days is more effective. For candida and trichophyton infections of the skin treat for 4–6 weeks, for erythrasma and pityriasis versicolor about 3 weeks and for onychomycosis for not less than four months.

Summary: A highly effective topical antimycotic with a broad spectrum and good local tolerance.

References

COHEN, L.: Single dose treatment of vaginal candidosis: comparison of clotrimazole and isoconazole. Brit. J. Vener. Dis. *60:* 42 (1984).
MILSOM, I., L. FORSSMAN: Treatment of vaginal candidosis with a single 500-mg clotrimazole pessary. Brit. J. Vener. Dis. *58:* 124 (1982).
OWENS, N. J., C. H. NIGHTINGALE, R. T. SCHWEIZER et al.: Prophylaxis of oral candidiasis with clotrimazole troches. Arch. Intern. Med. *144:* 290 (1984).
RITTER, W. K. PATZSCHKE, U. KRAUSE, S. STETTENDORF: Pharmacokinetic fundamentals of vaginal treatment with clotrimazole. Chemotherapy *28 (Suppl. 1):* 37–42 (1982).
ROLLER, J. A.: Contact allergy to clotrimazole. Brit. Med. J. *II:* 737 (1978).
SCHECHTMAN, L. B., L. FUNARO, T. ROBIN et al.: Clotrimazole treatment of oral candidiasis in patients with neoplastic disease. Amer. J. Med. *76:* 91 (1984).

β) Econazole

Proprietary name: Ecostatin.

Properties: Imidazole derivative, closely related chemically to miconazole (1 chlorine atom less). The structural formula is shown in Fig. 48. Econazole is somewhat more active *in vitro* against fungi than miconazole. Effective in topical treatment of cutaneous mycoses and vaginal thrush.

Administration: Topical as a powder, cream, ointment, lotion, solution, pessaries and spray. Redness, burning and itching can occur as side-effects.

References

BENIJTS, G., M. VIGNALLI, W. KREYSING, S. STETTENDORF: Three-day therapy of vaginal candidiasis with clotrimazole vaginal tablets and econazole ovules: a multicentre comparative study. Curr. Med. Res. Opin. *7:* 55 (1980).
BINGHAM, J. S., C. E. STEELE: Treatment of vaginal candidosis with econazole nitrate and nystatin. A comparative study. Brit. J. Vener. Dis. *57:* 204 (1981).

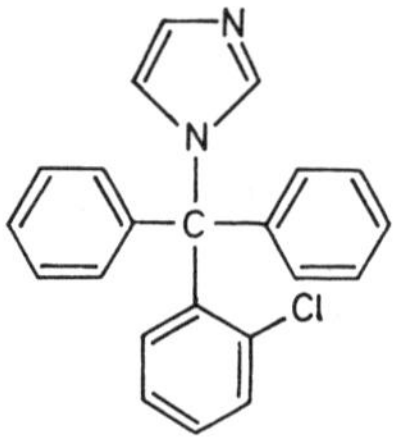

13. Antifungal Agents

Clotrimazole

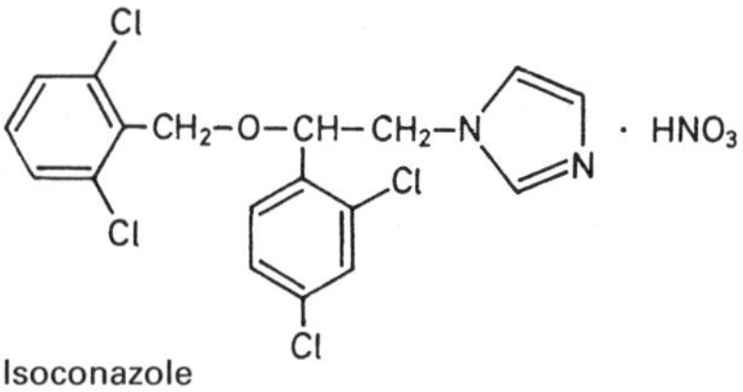

Isoconazole

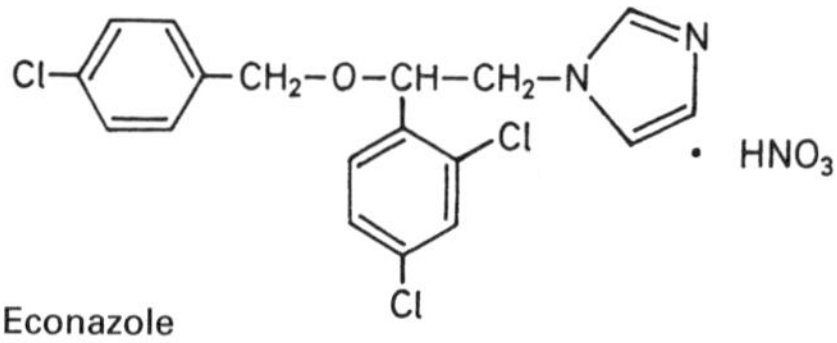

Econazole

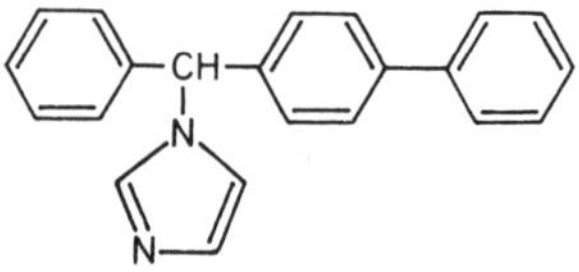

Bifonazole

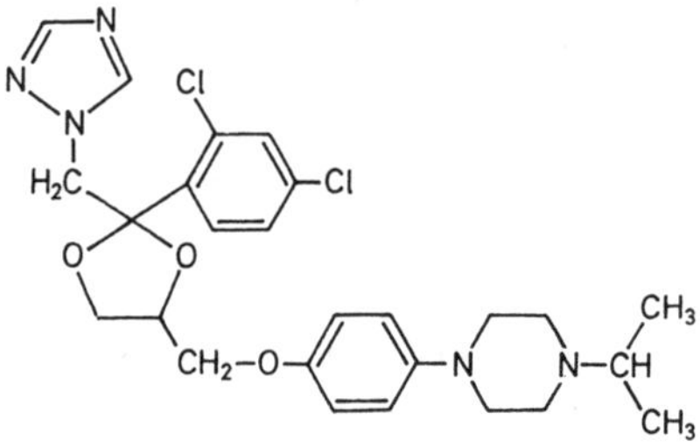

Terconazole

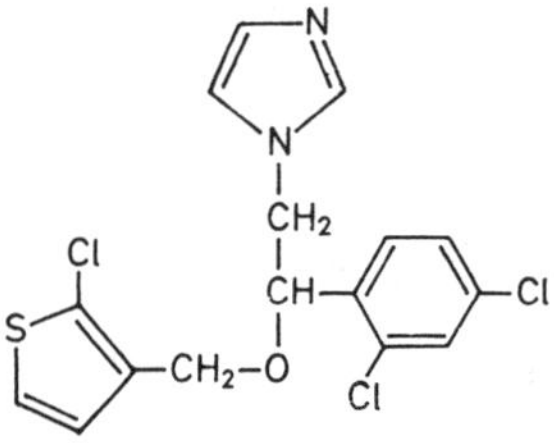

Tioconazole

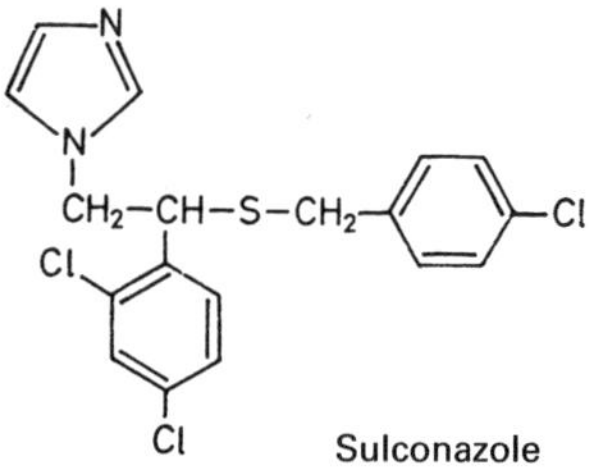

Sulconazole

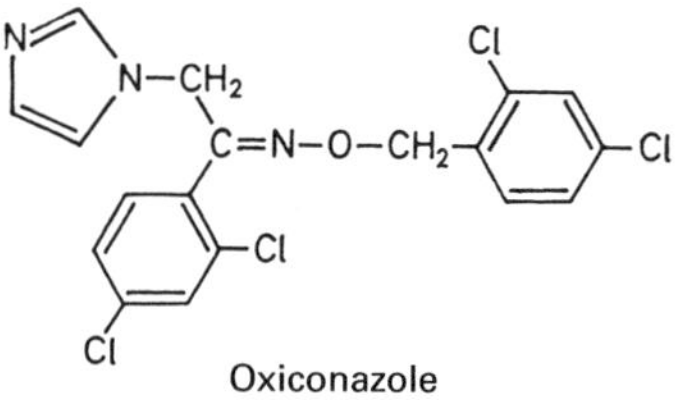

Oxiconazole

Fig. 48. Structural formulae of azoles for topical use.

γ) Isoconazole

Proprietary names: Travogen, Gyno-Travogen.

Properties: An azole for *local use* with activity against candida, dermatophytes and sporing fungi. Used in superficial mycoses of the skin (also in erythrasma and pityriasis versicolor) as a 1% cream (Travogen) or 1% solution. The corticosteroid-supplemented cream (Travocort cream) should not be given for more than 2 weeks. Hypersensitivity may arise against cetyl stearyl alcohol in the cream or propylene glycol in the spray. Avoid contact with eyes. Gyno-Travogen is used as pessaries (300 mg) and cream for local treatment of vulvovaginal mycoses. Do not use in the eye.

Contra-indications: The first trimester of pregnancy. Do not use over extensive areas for long periods.

Side-effects: Skin and mucosal irritation.

References

Cohen, L.: Single dose treatment of vaginal candidosis: Comparison of clotrimazole and isoconazole. Brit. J. Vener. Dis. *60:* 42–44 (1984).

Taeuber, U.: Availability of isoconazole in human skin after dermal application as free base and as nitrate in vitro. Arzneim.-Forsch. *37/1, 4:* 461–463 (1987).

δ) Oxiconazole

Proprietary name: Oceral.

Properties: An azole for local use with a broad spectrum of activity against Trichophyton, Epidermophyton and Microsporum species, Candida species, Malassezia furfur (the causative agent of pityriasis versicolor) and sporing fungi. Oxiconazole is also active against gram-positive bacteria (staphylococci and streptococci). Oxiconazole is virtually not absorbed from the skin. Burning and irritation may occasionally arise in the area of skin treated, as can dehydration with use over longer periods.

Application: The cream, the powder or the solution (to apply directly or spray on) should be applied to the affected area of skin for at least 3 weeks. To prevent relapse, local treatment should continue for 1–2 weeks after the skin manifestations have fully healed.

ε) Bifonazole

Proprietary name: Mycospor.

Properties: An azole with a broad spectrum against different fungi: dermatophytes, Candida and Aspergillus species, Malassezia furfur (Pityriasis versicolor) and also against Corynebacterium minutissimum (Erythrasma).

Application: As cream or lotion (contains cetylstearyl alcohol), powder, solution or spray. For topical use in fungal infections of the skin. Duration of treatment: 2–4 weeks. Redness, burning and itching can occur as side-effects.

d) Flucytosine

Proprietary name: Alcobon.

Properties: Flucytosine (5-fluorocytosine) is a fluorinated pyrimidine (for structural formula, see Fig. 49) and acts as an antimetabolite of cytosine by being transformed into the cytotoxic agent 5-fluorouracil within the cells of sensitive fungi. Flucytosine is little metabolised in man. Very little metabolite is excreted in the urine.

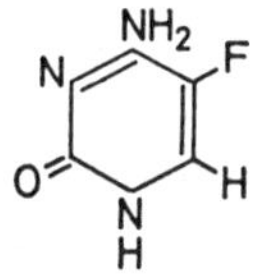

Fig. 49. Structural formula of flucytosine.

Spectrum of action: Good or excellent activity against Candida albicans, most other species of candida, Cryptococcus neoformans, Geotrichum candidum, some of the aspergilli (particularly Aspergillus fumigatus) and the pathogens of chromoblastomycosis (phialophora, cladosporium). There is synergy with amphotericin B against candida, cryptococcus and aspergillus. There is no activity against Histoplasma capsulatum, Blastomyces dermatitidis, Coccidioides immitis, sporotrichon, epidermophyton, mucor and other filamentous fungi, nor against any bacteria.

Resistance: Primary resistance is found in candida (from 20–50%), cryptococcus and aspergillus strains. Disc-sensitivity testing is therefore advisable prior to therapy using antagonist-free culture media in order to avoid false negative results. Secondary resistance often arises during treatment (risk of relapse), especially with infections due to Candida species and Cryptococcus neoformans. No cross-resistance with other antifungal agents.

Pharmacokinetics: Well absorbed after oral administration (80–90%). *Serum levels* of 10–30 mg/l (for 6–10 h) follow the oral administration of 100 mg/kg daily (single dose of 2 g), and CSF levels of 8–20 mg/l. Flucytosine is well distributed and penetrates the aqueous humor, peritoneal exudate and synovial fluid. Maximum serum concentrations of 30–50 mg/l follow the i.v. administration of 1.5–2 g. *Half-life:* 3–4 hours. Little *plasma protein binding*. *Urinary recovery:* 90% (as the unchanged substance). 1–10% eliminated with the faeces. Considerable accumulation in renal failure.

Side-effects: Fairly well tolerated even at high dosage. Reversible blood dyscrasias (leukocytopenia, thrombocytopenia and/or anaemia) in about 10% and temporary rise in blood liver enzymes. Gastrointestinal upset, hallucinations, dizziness, headache and fatigue are rare, and fatal cases of agranulocytosis and hepatic necrosis have been described.

Interactions: Concurrent administration of the cytotoxic agent, cytosine arabinoside, abolishes the antimycotic effect of flucytosine.

Indications: Disseminated infection and severe organ involvement with Cryptococcus neoformans, Candida albicans, Aspergillus fumigatus, Candida (Torulopsis) glabrata and chromoblastomycosis. Fungal infections in bone-marrow insufficiency (leukaemia etc.) sometimes require urgent treatment without prior testing. Combined treatment with amphotericin B prevents the emergence of secondary resistance in cryptococcosis, aspergillosis and candidiasis, allows a lower dosage of amphotericin B and gives the best clinical results.

Contra-indication: Pregnancy. Use with caution in renal failure (increased risk of blood toxicity), in liver damage and in pre-existing bone-marrow suppression (due to malignancy).

Administration and dosage: Oral administration of 100–150 (and exceptionally 200) mg/kg body weight daily (6–10 g in adults) in 4 divided doses. Taking the tablets over 15 min reduces nausea and vomiting. Length of treatment: 4–6 weeks, up to 12 weeks for cryptococcosis (risk of relapse). Blood count and liver function need regular monitoring. The tablets dissolve readily in water and can then be taken as a tasteless suspension.

Dosage for short i.v. infusion (30 min) as for oral administration. The low concentration (1%) necessitates a high volume of infusion. No other drugs should be mixed with the infusion solution. Reduce dosage in impaired renal function to a single dose of 50 mg/kg 12-hourly (creatinine clearance 20–40 ml/min) and 24-hourly (creatinine clearance 10–20 ml/min). Where there is severe renal impairment, the dose interval must be established by measuring serum concentrations which should lie between 25–40 mg/l and not exceed 100 mg/l. Flucytosine is readily dialysable. A peritoneal lavage with flucytosine (50 mg/l) is useful in candida peritonitis, which sometimes complicates peritoneal dialysis.

For combined therapy with amphotericin B, give 150 mg/kg/day of flucytosine on day 1 with 0.05 mg/kg/day of amphotericin B, 0.10 mg/kg/day on day 2 and 0.25 mg/kg/day on day 3. The 10% ointment is only recommended to supplement the oral or i. v. treatment of chromoblastomycosis preferably with an occlusive dressing.

Preparations: Tablets of 0.5 g, infusion of 2.5 g in 250 ml.

Summary: A reliable antimycotic agent against susceptible strains which is quite well tolerated when used systemically in fungal infections. Should not be used prophylactically because of the risk of secondary resistance. Penetrates well into the cerebrospinal fluid. Only effective in combination with amphotericin B (except in chromoblastomycosis).

References

DeFever, K. S., W. L. Whelan, A. L. Rogers et al.: Candida albicans resistance to 5-fluorocytosine: frequency of partially resistant strains among clinical isolates. Antimicrob. Ag. Chemother. *22:* 810 (1982).
Smego, R. A., J. R. Perfect, D. T. Durack: Combined therapy with amphotericin B and flucytosine for Candida meningitis. Rev. Infect. Dis. *6:* 791 (1984).
Speller, D. C. E., R. Y. Cartwright, E. G. V. Evans et al.: Laboratory methods for flucytosine (5-fluorocytosine): report of a working group of the British Society for Mycopathology. J. Antimicrob. Chemother. *14:* 1 (1984).
Washburn, R. G., D. M. Klym, M. H. Kroll, J. E. Bennett: Rapid enzymatic method for measurement of serum flucytosine levels. J. Antimicrob. Chemother. *17:* 673 (1986).
White, C. A., J. Traube: Ulcerating enteritis associated with flucytosine therapy. Gastroenterology *83:* 1127 (1982).

e) Griseofulvin

Proprietary names: Fulcin, Grisovin.

Properties: A benzofuran derivative which is soluble in water but stable at acid pH.

Mode of action: Fungistatic (affects fungal guanine metabolism). No antibacterial activity.

Spectrum of action: Active against all Trichophyton species, Microsporum audouinii, M. canis, M. gypseum, M. distortum, Epidermophyton floccosum and Tinea species except Tinea (Pityriasis) versicolor. Ineffective against blastomyces, candida, aspergillus, coccidioides, cryptococcus, histoplasma and mucor. No activity in actinomycosis or erythrasma.

Resistance: Rarely arises during therapy. Cross-resistance with other antibiotics has not been observed.

Pharmacokinetics:
Absorption after oral administration depends on particle size (optimal diameter 0.8–2.7 µm) and is better after a high-fat meal than fasting. *Maximum blood level* occurs 4–5 hours after oral administration.

Serum concentrations: Maximum serum concentrations after griseofulvin (microfine) 0.5 g are 0.5–2.0 mg/l after 4 h, but after the same dose of ultramicronised griseofulvin they are some 50% higher. *Half-life:* about 20 h. Partly metabolised to the inactive demethyl griseofulvin.

There is selective deposition in the newly formed keratin of the hair root, nail matrix and epidermis, but only gradual progression from these deep layers to the skin surface. Prolonged therapy is therefore required to eradicate the fungal infection. *Excretion* is largely faecal, with about 1% in the urine.

Side-effects (relatively rare despite prolonged administration):
1. Central nervous disorders such as headaches, dizziness, fatigue, psychological disturbances, impaired vision, alcohol intolerance.
2. Gastrointestinal upset.
3. Allergic rash or photosensitivity.
4. Reversible leukocytopenia, monocytosis,
5. Transient albuminuria.
6. Impairment of spermatogenesis.

Interactions: Simultaneous administration of barbiturates can, as a result of hepatic enzyme induction, impair the action of griseofulvin, and the concurrent use of coumarin derivatives can adversely affect anticoagulant activity. Griseofulvin may make oral contraception unreliable on account of increased metabolism.

Indications: Infections with filamentous fungi, i.e. trichophytosis, microsporosis, onychomycosis, favus and epidermophytosis, where the fungi concerned are sensitive.

Incorrect usage: Candida infections, Tinea versicolor and mild dermatophytoses which should respond to tolnaftate or topical miconazole.

Contra-indications: Pregnancy, severe liver disease, porphyria.

Dosage: 0.5 g daily for *adults,* 10(–15) mg/kg for *children,* in (1–)2 and preferably 4 single doses. Higher initial dose for extensive lesions (0.75–1 g daily). Halve dose upon first signs of improvement, or continue full dose on alternate days. With ultramicronised griseofulvin, a daily dose of 0.33 g is sufficient (or 0.66 g in foot and nail mycoses). Length of therapy: 1–6 months according to localisation and severity of fungal infection; about 4–6 weeks for tinea capitis, 2–4 weeks for tinea corporis, 4–8 weeks for tinea pedis, 4 months for fingernails, and 6 months for toenails. Monitor therapy by regular fungal culture. Simultaneous topical therapy with other antifungal agents and keratolytic agents is always recommended, and the removal of the infected hair or nails may be necessary. Avoid extensive exposure to light during therapy because of possible skin photosensitivity. Reactions may be slowed.

Preparations: Tablets of 125 and 500 mg; oral suspension.

Summary: A suitable agent for the systemic treatment of severe fungal infections such as trichophytosis, epidermophytosis, microsporosis and onychomycosis, but not for yeast or mould infections. Good results can only be achieved with prolonged treatment. The presence of infection with one of the filamentous fungi should always be confirmed by prior mycological examination. Now largely superceded by more active azoles.

References

ARTIS, W. M., B. M. ODLE, H. E. JONES: Griseofulvin-resistant dermatophytosis correlates with in vitro resistance. Arch Dermatol. *117:* 16 (1981).
COTE, J.: Interaction of griseofulvin and oral contraceptives. J. Am. Acad. Dermatol. *22:* 124–125 (1990).

f) Ciclopiroxolamine

Proprietary name: Batrafen.

Properties: A topical antifungal agent. It is not an azole but a *pyridone derivative,* and so is unrelated to other antifungal agents. When given as the amino-ethyl salt, it is active against dermatophytes and pathogenic yeasts and moulds. Penetrates the deeper layers of the skin and nails well.

Percutaneous absorption: about 1%. Absorbed better from the vaginal mucosa, so should be avoided in pregnancy. Generally well tolerated; itching and skin burning are rare. Avoid contact with eyes. The ointment and vaginal cream contain cetyl and stearyl alcohols which may cause hypersensitivity.

Effective against superficial cutaneous fungal infections, mycosis of the nail, and vaginal thrush. Available as a lotion, ointment, powder and vaginal cream (apply sparingly 2–3 times a day). Treat dermatomycoses for 2 weeks and vaginal thrush for 6 days. Prolonged therapy is only justified for infections of the nails.

Summary: A non-imidazole broad-spectrum antimycotic for the treatment of dermatomycoses and fungal infections of the nails.

References

ALPERMANN, H. G., E. SCHÜTZ: Zur Pharmakologie und Toxikologie von Ciclopiroxolamin. Arzneimittel-Forsch. *31:* 1328 (1981).
GOUDARD, M., P. REGLI, N. LUBRANO: In vitro antifungal spectrum of ciclopiroxolamine. Pathol. Biol. Paris *37:* 621–623 (1989).
JUE, S. G., G. W. DAWSON, R. N. BROGDEN: Ciclopirox Olamine 1% cream; a preliminary review of its antimicrobial activity and therapeutic use. Drugs *29:* 330–341 (1985).
ROLLMAN, O., S. JOHANSSON: Hendersonula toruloidea infection: Successful response of onychomycosis to nail avulsion and topical Ciclopiroxolamine. Acta derm.-venereol. *67:* 506–510 (1987).
SZEPES, E., I. SCHNEIDER: Ciclopiroxolamine in the treatment of dermatomycoses. Mykosen *29:* 382–386 (1986).

g) Naftifin

Proprietary name: Exoderil.

A topical antifungal agent, unrelated to other antifungals. Active in dermatomycoses due to dermatophytes, yeasts and moulds and also against some bacteria. The cream, gel and solution contain naftifin in a concentration of 1%. Naftifin is well tolerated. Local inflammation may occasionally occur, including burning and dryness of the skin. These effects may also be due to hypersensitivity to cetyl and stearyl alcohol in the cream and propylene glycol in the solution. Do not use in the eyes. Naftifin should be sparingly applied once or twice a day. Use the solution for onychomycoses.

References

GEORGOPOULOS, A., G. PETRANYI, H. MIETH, J. DREWS: In vitro activity of naftifine, a new antifungal agent. Antimicrob. Ag. Chemother. *39:* 386 (1981).
HAAS, P. J., H. TRONNIER, G. WEIDINGER: Naftifin bei Fußmykosen – Doppelblinder Therapievergleich mit Clotrimazol. Mykosen *28:* 33 (1985).

h) Tolnaftate

Proprietary name: Timoped.

Properties: A colourless, flavourless, synthetic antifungal agent. Fungicidal against trichophyton, microsporum, epidermophyton, Aspergillus niger, but not against Candida species.

Indications: Skin infections with filamentous fungi, pityriasis versicolor, erythrasma and onychomycosis. Alternate treatment with 10% salicylic acid ointment in hyperkeratosis. Available as an ointment, solution, spray and powder.

Combined preparations containing nystatin, against candida, are also available. Avoid contact with the eyes.

References

BARRETT-BEE, K. J.: The mode of antifungal action of tolnaftate. J. med. vet. mycol. *24:* 155–60 (1986).
LANG, E.: Combined allergy to tolnaftate and nystatin. Contact dermatitis *12:* 182 (1985).
LOWY, M.: A new combination of Tolnaphtate and Methylpartricine (SPA-S-345, tritol) for mycotic skin infections. Mykosen *28:* 452–56 (1985).
RYDER, N. S.: Ergosterol biosynthesis inhibition by the thiocarbamate antifungal agents tolnaftate and tolciclate. Antimicrob. Ag. Chemother. *29:* 858–60 (1986).

14. Chemotherapeutic Agents

a) Sulphonamides

The sulphonamides were in many ways important prototypes on which many of the principles of antibacterial chemotherapy were worked out. Their low activity and the rapid development of resistance were the reasons for generally abandoning sulphonamides as single-agent therapy. Sulphonamides are, however, still important as partners in combination with bacterial folic acid antagonists such as trimethoprim or pyrimethamine. Of the large number of the earlier sulphonamides, only a few derivatives are now worthy of mention.

Classification: They are grouped according to their *half-lives* as follows:
Short-acting sulphonamides: Sulphaurea (Euvernil, Uramide).
Medium-acting sulphonamides: Sulphadiazine, sulphamethoxazole, sulphamoxole.
Long-acting sulphonamides: Sulphamethoxydiazine (Durenate).
Ultra-long-acting sulphonamides: Sulphametopyrazine = sulphalen (Kelfizine W), sulphadoxine (contained in Fansidar).
Poorly absorbed sulphonamides: Formophthalylsulphacarbamide, sulphaguanidine.

Properties: All sulphonamides are derivatives of para-aminobenzene-sulphonamide with a benzene nucleus consisting of an amino (NH_2) and an amido (SO_2NH_2) group (Fig. 50).

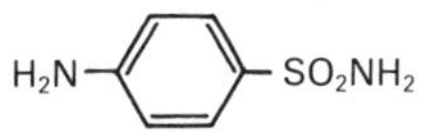

$$H_2N-\langle\rangle-SO_2NH_2$$

Fig. 50. Structural formula of sulphanilamide.

Mode of action: Bacteriostatic for proliferating bacteria by inhibition of folic acid synthesis (blocking the enzyme which forms folic acid from para-aminobenzoic acid), and partly also by inactivation of other enzymes, e. g. dehydrogenase or carboxylase (inhibition of bacterial respiration). Since all bacteria have a certain supply of folic acid, the onset of action of the sulphonamide is always delayed.

Spectrum of action: Good activity against streptococci (except enterococci), pneumococci, meningococci, actinomycetes, nocardia and chlamydiae.

Moderate, slight or variable activity against Escherichia coli, proteus, Klebsiella pneumoniae, Enterobacter aerogenes, Haemophilus influenzae, Pseudomonas aeruginosa, brucella, enterococci, gonococci, staphylococci and shigellae. Sulphonamides are also active against certain protozoa (pneumocystis, toxoplasma, malarial plasmodia). Rickettsiae, spirochaetes, mycobacteria and common fungi are *resistant*.

Resistance: Streptococci, pneumococci and gonococci can become resistant during prolonged therapy (more than 3 weeks). Meningococci are nowadays often resistant to sulphonamides (up to 75%) as are shigella, proteus and Escherichia coli. There is almost total cross-resistance between individual sulphonamides but no cross-resistance with antibiotics. *In vitro* tests, particularly disc-sensitivity determinations, are unreliable with sulphonamides; the marked inoculum effect and influence of antagonists in the culture medium can give a false picture of resistance.

Pharmacokinetics: Sulphonamides are *well absorbed* in the stomach and small intestine (80–100%) after oral administration, with a maximal blood concentration after 4–6 hours.

Blood concentrations of individual sulphonamides after oral administration vary between 50 and 150 mg/l; the decisive factor is the content of free, non-acetylated and non-protein-bound sulphonamide.

The *half-life* in the blood is less than 8 hours for short-acting sulphonamides, 24 to 48 hours for the long-acting sulphonamides, 5 days for sulfadoxine and about 65 hours for sulphametopyrazine.

Plasma protein binding: Some sulphonamides are reversibly bound to protein in the blood and have no antibacterial activity; the irreversibly acetylated sulphonamides behave similarly. The level of protein binding depends on the blood level and is generally lower in short-acting sulphonamides than in most of the medium-acting and long-acting sulphonamides (70–90% and above). However, sulphametopyrazine, which is an ultra-long-acting sulphonamide, has a protein binding of only 34%. The degree of acetylation of sulphonamides in the blood varies between 5 and 20%.

Cerebrospinal fluid penetration is quite good with sulfasomidine, sulphamethoxydiazine and sulfamoxole, but is best with sulphadiazine (CSF serum distribution coefficient: 0.3–0.8). The sulphonamides pass more readily into the CSF when the meninges are inflamed and the protein content of the CSF is increased.

Tissue concentrations: Sulphonamides are concentrated well in the stomach, kidneys, and skin, moderately in the liver, lungs, uterus and muscle and poorly in the brain, bones, adrenals and intestines. They diffuse well into the aqueous humor of the eye, readily into the fetal circulation, but pass poorly into the breast milk. 50–70% of the serum values are found in pleural and pericardial effusions and ascites. Biliary concentrations are low.

Excretion: Predominantly urinary (60–90% with most preparations) and the remainder in the faeces. Present in urine as free sulphonamide and also as an antibacterially inert acetyl derivative and glucuronide. Excretion is mostly by glomerular filtration but partly by tubular secretion, and free sulphonamide is reabsorbed through the tubules. There is rapid excretion of the short-acting sulphonamides and almost no reabsorption through the kidneys, while the excretion of long-acting sulphonamides is retarded and reabsorption is greater (e. g. 60–85% with sulphamethoxydiazine). Urine concentrations of short-acting sulphonamides (daily dose of 3 g): about 1–2 g/l; long-acting sulphonamides (daily dose of 0.5 g): about 0.1–0.5 g/l.

Side-effects:
1. *Allergic reactions:* Occur in 1–3% of cases as fever, conjunctivitis and rashes (macular, nodular or urticarial), mostly between the 5th and 9th day of treatment. They may be more severe with medium and long-acting sulphonamides than with the rapidly excreted short-acting compounds and are more frequent when sulphonamides are used for the topical treatment of the skin. Sulphonamide allergy can be demonstrated by patch tests with sulphonamide ointment performed after scarification of the skin. Sulphonamide medication can also cause photosensitivity of the skin, bullous dermatitis, the Stevens-Johnson syndrome, erythema multiforme, erythema nodosum, exfoliative dermatitis and toxic epidermolysis (Lyell's syndrome), which may be fatal. AIDS patients frequently develop skin reactions during sulphonamide therapy.
2. *Renal damage:* Deposition of crystals of poorly soluble sulphonamides and particularly of acetyl derivatives in the kidneys can cause renal colic, haematuria, the passage of casts, albuminuria, oliguria and anuria. The occurrence of these side-effects depends on the solubility of the related sulphonamide in the urine, which is normally acid (pH 5.5–6.5), the rate of acetylation in the urine (preferably not more than 50%), the dosage and the fluid intake. Modern sulphonamides carry almost no risk of renal damage by crystallisation because of the low degree of acetylation and improved solubility, even in slightly acid urine. Crystalluria can still occur with the poorly soluble sulphadiazine, however. Great care must be taken in patients with dehydration and renal insufficiency. Because of their immature hepatic and renal function,

premature and newborn infants should not be given sulphonamides except for the treatment of toxoplasmosis.
3. *Gastrointestinal upset* with nausea and vomiting are less frequent with the new sulphonamides because of their reduced dosage.
4. There is a risk of *hyperbilirubinaemia* in premature and full-term neonates because the bilirubin is insufficiently bound to glucuronic acid. Bilirubin is also displaced by sulphonamides from its albumin-binding site and can therefore diffuse more easily through the vascular walls.
5. *Abnormal blood counts* resulting from toxic or allergic bone marrow lesions (agranulocytosis, aplastic anaemia) are rare; they generally develop after longer courses of treatment, from the third week onwards, and are also occasionally associated with long-acting sulphonamides.
6. *Cyanosis* due to sulph- or methaemoglobinaemia is very uncommon nowadays except in cases of congenital erythrocyte glucose-6-phosphate dehydrogenase deficiency and haemoglobinopathies, e. g. Hb Köln and Hb Zürich.
7. Cholestatic *jaundice* is rare.

Interactions: Sulphonamides can prolong the prothrombin time when given at the same time as coumarin derivatives, intensify the hypoglycaemic effect when given at the same time as sulphonylurea and increase the concentration of free amethopterin by displacement from the serum protein-binding sites when given at the same time as amethopterin (methotrexate).

Indications: Toxoplasmosis (in combination with pyrimethamine), pneumocystis pneumonia (in combination with trimethoprim), local and systemic treatment of trachoma, nocardiosis (in combination with other agents), chloroquine-resistant malaria (in combination with pyrimethamine etc.) and bacterial infections (in combination with trimethoprim). Other indications have been superceded. The topical use of sulphonamides other than ocular preparations is now no longer justifiable. This also applies to bladder washouts with sulphonamides. Silver sulphadiazine (Flamazine cream 1%) is sometimes used for the local treatment of burns, although it has considerable side-effects. The antibacterial effect depends upon the release of silver ions.

Contra-indications: Hypersensitivity to sulphonamides, renal failure, liver damage, pregnancy (sulphonamides are teratogenic in animal experiments), the puerperium until the end of the first month, the premature and full-term newborn (except for toxoplasmosis), glucose-6-phosphate dehydrogenase deficiency, certain haemoglobinopathies.

Dosage *for oral administration* varies for short-, medium- and long-acting sulphonamides (Table 21). The upper dosage limit should not be exceeded because of the risk of accumulation, particularly with the long-acting sulphonamides. The intervals depend on the rates of excretion: 4–6 hours with short-

Table 21. Dosage of sulphonamides.

	Age	Average daily dose	Maximum daily dose
Short-acting sulphonamides (e. g. sulphaurea)	Adults	4.0–6.0 g	6.0–8.0 g
Medium-acting sulphonamides (e. g. sulphadiazine)	Adults	1.0 g[1]	2.0
	Children of 6–12 y.	1.0 g[1]	1.5 g
	1– 6 y.	0.5 g[1]	1.0 g
	0– 1 y.	0.25 g[1]	0.5 g
Long-acting sulphonamides (e. g. sulphamethoxydiazine)	Adults	0.5 g[1]	1.0 g
	Children of 6–12 y.	0.37 g[1]	0.5 g
	1– 6 y.	0.25 g[1]	0.25 g
	0– 1 y.	0.06–0.12 g[1]	0.12 g
Ultra-long-acting sulphonamides (sulfametopyrazine)	Adults	2.0 g 1 dose per week	

[1] Double dose initially.

acting sulphonamides, 12 hours with medium-acting sulphonamides, 24 hours with long-acting sulphonamides and 6–8 hours with poorly absorbable sulphonamides. A single dose of 2 g of sulphametopyrazine generates an adequate level for two weeks.

Preparations: Tablets of 0.5 g
Coated tablets of 0.5 g
10% Syrup
Eye drops and eye ointment

Summary: Because of their relatively poor activity and the widespread bacterial resistance to them, the sulphonamides have greatly declined in importance and are now only rarely considered for single agent therapy.

References

BELL, E. T., M. L. TAPPER, A. A. POLLOCK: Sulphadiazine desensitisation in AIDS patients. Lancet *I:* 163 (1985).
BUCHANAN, N.: Sulphamethoxazole, hypoalbuminaemia, crystalluria, and renal failure. Brit. Med. J. *2:* 172 (1978).
BUCKWOLD, F. J., P. LUDWIG, G. K. M. HARDING, L. THOMPSON, M. SLUTCHUK, J. SHAW, A. R. RONALD: Therapy for actue cystitis in adult women – randomized comparison of single-dose sulfisoxazole vs trimethoprim-sulfamethoxazole. JAMA *247:* 1839–1842 (1982).

HORNSTEIN, O. P., K. W. RUPRECHT: Fansidar-induced Stevens-Johnson syndrome. New Engl. J. Med. *307:* 1529 (1982).
LYELL, A.: Sulphonamides and Stevens-Johnson syndrome. Lancet *II:* 1460 (1982).
MÄNNISTÖ, P. T., R. MÄNTYLÄ, J. MATTILA et al.: Comparison of pharmacokinetics of sulphadiazine and sulphamethoxazole after intravenous infusion. J. Antimicrob. Chemother. *9:* 461 (1982).
MANDELL, G. L., M. A. SANDE: Antimicrobial agents – sulfonamides, trimethoprim-sulfamethoxazole, and agents for urinary tract infections. In: GOODMAN GILMAN, A., L. S.: Goodman and Gilman's The Pharmacological Basis of Therapeutics. 8. Aufl., S. 1047–1064. Macmillan, New York 1990.
SELBY, C. D., E. J. LADUSANS, P. G. SMITH: Fatal multisystemic toxicity associated with prophylaxis with pyrimethamine and sulfadoxine (Fansidar). Brit. Med. J. *290:* 113 (1985).

b) Co-trimoxazole

Proprietary names: Bactrim, Septrin.

Properties: A combination of the chemotherapeutic agent trimethoprim with the sulphonamide sulphamethoxazole. Trimethoprim is a weak base, is poorly water-soluble, and is, like the antimalarial drug pyrimethamine, a diaminopyrimidine (Fig. 51).

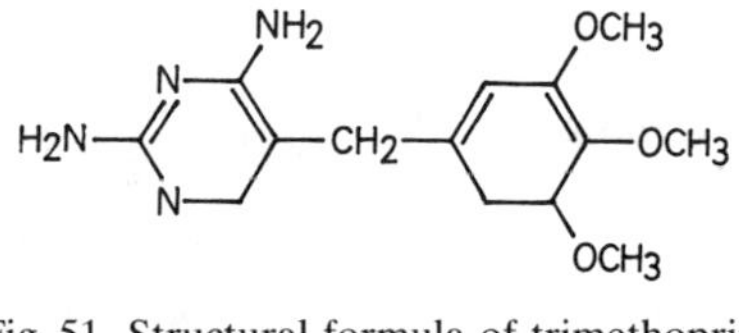

Fig. 51. Structural formula of trimethoprim.

Sulphamethoxazole is a medium-acting sulphonamide. Other sulphonamides, such as sulphadiazine or sulphametrole may be used in place of sulphamethoxazole.

Mode of action: Inhibition of bacterial folic acid synthesis. Sulphamethoxazole inhibits the use of the p-aminobenzoic acid and trimethoprim blocks the reduction of dihydrofolic acid to tetrahydrofolic acid. Sulphamethoxazole and trimethoprim alone act bacteriostatically and the combination of both has been claimed by some to produce a bactericidal effect although this claim has been disputed. The activity against most pathogens is increased with a concentration of 1 part trimethoprim and 20 parts of sulphamethoxazole which, after oral administration, the body absorbs in a ratio of 1:5. The synergistic (potentiated) activity is explained by the sequential sites of action of each component in the bacterial metabolic pathway. This synergy is greatest when the pathogen is sensitive to both drugs. The potentiation of trimethoprim activity by the sulphonamide (and vice versa) varies in intensity with the bacterial species and also within the same species, i.e. it can differ from strain to strain. Synergy is sometimes absent, even when the bacteria are sensitive to both agents. Folic acid deficiency does not generally rise in man because the body's folic acid requirement is supplied in the food and human folic acid reductase is not inhibited until trimethoprim concentrations are 50,000 times in excess.

Spectrum of action: Trimethoprim is active against a broad range of pathogenic bacteria except clostridia, Treponema pallidum, leptospiras, rickettsiae, Chlamydia psittaci, tubercle bacilli and Pseudomonas aeruginosa; it has no effect against mycoplasmas and fungi. The combination extends the range of activity of the sulphonamide component.

An increasing percentage of local and urinary infections may be resistant to co-trimoxazole, however, and sensitivities should be tested before beginning treatment. Species in which resistance is found include Staphylococcus aureus, enterococci, pneumococci, klebsiella and enterobacter. Resistant strains of Haemophilus influenzae are rare. Co-trimoxazole is also active against malarial parasites, but not as effective as chloroquine. It is active, in combination, against chloroquine-resistant falciparum malaria, and also against Pneumocystis carinii.

Resistance: Secondary resistance *in vitro* can be selected for by serial passage through trimethoprim-containing media. Resistance has developed during treatment of infections caused by Escherichia coli and haemophilus. The proportion of resistant strains of Enterobacteriaceae has increased in recent years on account of the increasing use of co-trimoxazole. Culture media free of antagonists (e.g. Oxoid DST medium) must be used when testing bacterial sensitivity *in vitro*. They should have as low a thymidine content as possible.

Pharmacokinetics: Trimethoprim is almost completely absorbed after oral administration. *Maximal blood levels* occur after 1½–3½ hours (0.9–1.2 mg/l after 100 mg orally, and about 2 mg/l after 160 mg). During therapy with i.v. infusion of 0.16 g trimethoprim + 0.8 g sulphamethoxazole (over 1 h) repeated every 8 hours serum concentrations are 2 mg/l (trimethoprim) and 30 mg/l (free sulphamethoxazole). *Protein binding* 45%, *half-life* 12 hours. High tissue levels, especially in the lungs and kidneys. Diffuses relatively well in the saliva, bronchial secretions, aqueous humor, bile and prostatic secretions. Relatively high concentrations are found in the lungs, kidneys, prostate and bones. Low *CSF concentrations*, but antibacterial activity present. Up to 60% glomerular and tubular *excretion* by the kidneys (in 24 h), 8% as conjugated, inactive forms. Urine concentrations are about 100 times higher than serum levels. A small quantity is excreted through the bile, and part is metabolised in the body. Trimethoprim is removed to some extent by haemodialysis, but not at all by peritoneal dialysis.

The pharmacokinetic characteristics of **sulphamethoxazole** resemble those of trimethoprim, and this maintains the good activity of both components in the body. *Half-life:* 10 hours, *plasma protein binding:* 70%, without displacement by trimethoprim or vice versa. 80–90% excreted in the urine in 24 h, ⅓ as the unconjugated form. Dialyses well.

Side-effects: Trimethoprim has very little toxicity in man. There is no haemotoxicity in the short term, though reversible bone-marrow depression (granulo- or thrombocytopenia) can occur with prolonged administration. Fatal agranulocytosis and anaemia (aplastic, haemolytic or megaloblastic) are extremely rare. Thrombocytopenia with purpura has been observed in older patients who received diuretics simultaneously, especially thiazides. As with other sulphonamides, allergic reactions may occur with sulphamethoxazole, including the very serious Stevens-Johnson syndrome. Where renal function is already impaired or the patient is dehydrated, co-trimoxazole can worsen these conditions reversibly, but recovery usually occurs after discontinuation. There have been individual cases of gastrointestinal upset (nausea, vomiting). Infusions may cause local pain or phlebitis. Pain and infiltration at the injection site occurs not infrequently after i.m. injection. At the high dosage used to treat pneumocystis pneumonia in AIDS patients, rashes, fever, neutropenia, thrombocytopenia and raised liver enzyme concentrations are often seen and may prevent further treatment.

Interactions: The simultaneous administration of anticoagulants of the dicoumarol type can intensify hypoprothrombinaemia. Concurrent phenytoin can cause a rise in blood phenytoin concentrations and the concurrent administration of cyclosporin A may impair renal function. Hypoglycaemia can occur in patients taking oral antidiabetic agents of the sulphonylurea group. Concurrent pyrimethamine may lead to changes in the blood count. The toxicity of trimethroprim can be intensified by the simultaneous administration of para-aminosalicylic acid, barbiturates or primidone. Thrombocytopenia with purpura can occur in the elderly during the concurrent administration of diuretics, especially the thiazides. Sulphamethoxazole (in combination) can intensify the toxicity of amethopterin (methotrexate) by displacing it from its serum protein binding site.

Indications: Acute and chronic urinary infections, including pyelonephritis, acute and chronic bronchitis, sinusitis, wound and biliary infections, prostatitis and prostatic abscess. Co-trimoxazole is as active as chloramphenicol in typhoid and paratyphoid fever and may be preferable because of the reduced risk of side-effects. The combination is also effective in enteric infections (dysentery, cholera and salmonellosis), as well as in brucellosis, nocardiosis and skin granulomas due to Mycobacterium marinum. Treatment and prophylaxis of proven or clinically typical pneumocystis pneumonia, for which 3 times the dose is required. Also used for selective gastrointestinal decontamination (see p. 609).

Incorrect use: Viral pneumonia, pseudomonas infections, ornithosis, syphilis, tuberculosis, streptococcal sore throat (penicillin is more effective).

Contra-indications: Megaloblastic anaemia due to folic acid deficiency, allergy to sulphonamides, acute hepatitis and severe hepatic diseases, blood dyscrasias, pregnancy (co-trimoxazole is teratogenic in animals), 1st month of life, lactation (during child's first four weeks). Caution should be exercised in cases of granulocytopenia and severe renal failure as well as in long-term treatment, which should be monitored with regular blood and platelet counts.

Administration and dosage: Tablets, syrup and suspension for oral use. Four tablets of 480 mg twice a day for *adults* (maximum of 3 tablets twice a day, and 1 tablet twice a day for long-term treatment). A syrup is available for adults (5 ml = 1 adult tablet) as well as forte tablets (= 2 normal adult tablets). Four paediatric tablets twice a day for *children* aged 6–12 months, and 2.5 ml of paediatric syrup twice a day for children aged 2–5 months (5 ml = 2 paediatric tablets).

Uncomplicated cystitis in women may be treated by a *single dose* of 4 adult tablets or 2 forte tablets, i. e. the usual daily dose of 1.92 g, on a single occasion.

May also be administered as a one-hour *i. v. infusion* (2 vials twice a day in adequate dilution for up to 3 days). Avoid rapid i. v. injection. The vials contain solvents including ethanol and benzyl alcohol. The vial solution must be mixed with the infusion solution immediately before use. Regular full blood counts should be checked when administered for more than 10 days.

Use half the daily dose (2 tablets once a day) in *renal failure* (creatinine clearance 15–30 ml/min). Co-trimoxazole should not be given in severe renal failure.

For *Pneumocystis carinii pneumonia,* give 3–4 times the usual dose, i. e. 20 mg/kg of trimethoprim and 100 mg/kg sulphamethoxazole daily by mouth in 4 divided doses; for prophylaxis, give a daily dose of 8 mg/kg of trimethoprim and 40 mg/kg sulphamethoxazole in 2 divided doses.

Preparations: Tablets and vials containing 80 mg trimethoprim and 400 mg sulphamethoxazole;

syrup or suspension for adults (5 ml contain 80 mg trimethoprim and 400 mg sulphamethoxazole;

forte tablets of 160 mg trimethoprim and 800 mg sulphamethoxazole; paediatric tablets with 20 mg trimethoprim and 100 mg sulphamethoxazole;

paediatric syrup and suspension (5 ml contain 40 mg trimethoprim and 200 mg sulphamethoxazole).

Summary: A combination of chemotherapeutic agents with a broad spectrum of activity and good clinical results. The treatment of choice in urinary tract infections and pneumocystis pneumonia. A therapeutic alternative in acute and chronic bronchitis, sinusitis and enteritis.

References

ASMAR, B. I., S. MAQBOOK, A. S. DAJANI: Hematologic abnormalities after oral trimethoprim-sulfamethoxazole therapy in children. Amer. J. Dis. Child. *135:* 1100 (1981).
BOWDEN, F. J., P. J. HARMAN, C. R. LUCAS: Serum trimethoprim and sulphamethoxazole levels in AIDS. Lancet *I:* 853 (1986).
CARMICHAEL, A. J., C. Y. TAN: Fatal toxic epidermal necrolysis associated with co-trimoxazole (letter). Lancet *2:* 808–809 (1989).
CRUCIANI, M., E. CONCIA, A. NAVARRA, L. PERVERSI, F. BONETTI, M. ARICO, L. NESPOLI: Prophylactic co-trimoxazole versus norfloxacin in neutropenic children-perspective randomized study. Infection *17:* 65–69 (1989).
DUDLEY, M. N., R. E. LEVITZ, R. QUINTILIANI et al.: Pharmacokinetics of trimethoprim and sulfamethoxazole in serum and cerebrospinal fluid of adult patients with normal meninges. Antimicrob. Ag. Chemother. *26:* 811 (1984).
Editorial: Co-trimoxazole resistance. Lancet *I:* 364 (1986).
GORDIN, F. M. et al.: Adverse reactions to trimethoprim-sulfamethoxazole in patients with the acquired immunodeficiency syndrome. Ann. Intern. Med. *100:* 495 (1984).
GOORIN, A. M., B. J. HERSHEY, M. J. LEVIN et al.: Use of trimethoprim-sulfamethoxazole to prevent bacterial infections in children with acute lymphoblastic leukemia. Pediatr. Infect. Dis. *4:* 265 (1985).
GUTMAN, L. T.: The use of trimethoprim-sulfamethoxazole in children: A review of adverse reactions and indications. Pediatr. Infect. Dis. *3:* 349 (1984).
HEER, M., J. ALTORFER, H. R. BURGER, M. WALTI: Bullous esophageal lesions due to cotrimoxazole: an immune-mediated process? Gastroenterology *88:* 1954 (1985).
JICK, S. S., H. JICK, J. S. HABAKANGAS, B. J. DINAN: Co-trimoxazole toxicity in children. Lancet *II:* 631 (1984).
LIMSON, B., R. LITTAUA: Comparative study of ciprofloxacin versus co-trimoxazole in the treatment of Salmonella enteric fever. Infection *17:* 105–6 (1989).
MURRAY, B. E., T. ALVARADO, K.-H. KIM, M. VORACHIT, P. JAYANETRA, M. LEVINE, I. PRENZEL, M. FLING, L. ELWELL, G. H. MCCRACKEN, G. MADRIGAL, C. ODIO, L. R. TRABULSI: Increasing resistance to trimethoprim-sulfamethoxazole among isolates of Escherichia coli in developing countries. J. Infect. Dis. *152:* 1107–1113 (1985).
RINGDÉN, O., P. MYRENFORS, G. KLINTMALM et al.: Nephrotoxicity by co-trimoxazole and cyclosporin in transplanted patients. Lancet *I:* 1016 (1984).
SIBER, G. R., C. C. GORHAM, J. F. ERICSON, A. L. SMITH: Pharmacokinetics of intravenous trimethoprim-sulfamethoxazole in children and adults with normal and impaired renal function. Rev. Infect. Dis. *4:* 566 (1982).
VERNE-PIGNATELLI, J., G. SPICKETT, A. DALGLEISH, A. DENMAN: Thrombophlebitis migrans following co-trimoxazole therapy. Postgrad. Med. J. *65:* 51–52 (1989).
WELLS, C. L., R. P. PODZORSKI, P. K. PETERSON et al.: Incidence of trimethoprim-sulfamethoxazole-resistant Enterobacteriaceae among transplant recipients. J. Infect. Dis. *150:* 699 (1984).
WHITTINGTON, R. M.: Toxic epidermal necrolysis and co-trimoxazole (letter). Lancet *2:* 574 (1989).

Woods, W. G., A. E. Daigle, R. J. Hutchinson: Myelosuppression associated with co-trimoxazole as a prophylactic antibiotic in the maintenance phase of childhood acute lymphocytic leukemia. J. Pediatr. *105:* 639 (1984).

c) Other Diaminopyrimidine-Sulphonamide Combinations

Trimethoprim has also been **combined with sulphonamides other than sulphamethoxazole** (Table 22). Their characteristics are similar to sulphamethoxazole: *Sulphametrole* has a half-life of 8 h, is 80% bound to serum protein and 90% is excreted in the urine (18% in an unchanged form). *Sulphadiazine* has the same half-life but is less protein-bound (50%) and 65% is excreted unchanged in the urine. The water-solubility *in vitro* of sulphamethoxazole, sulphametrole and sulphamoxole is better than that of sulphadiazine; it is of course dependent on pH and temperature. The primary metabolite of sulphadiazine is more water-soluble at acid pH than that of sulphamethoxazole.

Table 22. Diaminopyrimidine-sulphonamide combinations. Initial dose of 2 tablets for trimethoprim plus sulphadiazine and tetroxoprim plus sulphadiazine.

Generic name	Combination	Recommended daily dose (g)			No. of tablets per day of common proprietary preparation
		Diamino-pyrimidine	Sulphon-amide	Total	
Co-trimoxazole	Trimethoprim + sulphamethoxazole	0.32	1.6	1.92	2 × 2
Co-trimetrole	Trimethoprim + sulphametrole	0.32	1.6	1.92	2 × 2
Co-trimazine	Trimethoprim + sulphadiazine	0.18	0.82	1.0	1 × 1
Co-tetroxazine	Tetroxoprim + sulphadiazine	0.2	0.5	0.7	2 × 1

Tetroxoprim has a shorter half-life (6 h) than trimethoprim, is less bound to serum protein (15%) and has a higher rate of excretion (50% in an active form); 30% of the dose passes out with the faeces. Tetroxoprim is less active *in vitro* on gram-negative rods than trimethoprim and in combination with sulphadiazine (co-tetroxazine) is 2–3 times less effective than co-trimoxazole. Tetroxoprim is only approved for urinary and respiratory tract infections.

Dosage recommendations for various diaminopyrimidine-sulphonamide combinations are given in Table 22. An additional lower dose recommendation of 1 tablet twice daily (0.96 g daily) is made for long-term treatment with co-trimoxazole.

d) Trimethoprim

Properties: Trimethoprim alone (trade names: Monotrim, Ipral, Syraprim, Trimogal, Trimepan) is less active *in vitro* than in combination with a sulphonamide. Trimethoprim is increasingly replacing co-trimoxazole in the treatment of urinary and respiratory infections. Side-effects are less than with co-trimoxazole, especially in older patients, and trimethoprim should be used instead of co-trimoxazole where there is allergy to sulphonamides. Trimethoprim has been used successfully to treat patients with enteric fever (Salmonella typhi, Salmonella paratyphi A and B). It can also be used to treat pneumocystis pneumonia in patients allergic to sulphonamides.

There is little evidence that the use of trimethoprim alone has resulted in an increase in the incidence of trimethoprim-resistant organisms. Moreover, although the combination of trimethoprim and sulphamethoxazole suppresses the appearance of resistant mutants *in vitro,* such studies may not reflect events *in vivo.* Long-term, low-dose trimethoprim prophylaxis has been effective in adult patients with recurrent urinary infections.

Side-effects are comparable to those of co-trimoxazole (see p. 222), except for those typically due to the sulphonamide component alone (skin reactions).

Interactions: Trimethoprim can prolong the half-life of phenytoin and potentiate its activity. The simultaneous administration of p-aminosalicylic acid, barbiturates or primidone can exacerbate the toxicity of trimethoprim.

Contra-indications: As for co-trimoxazole (see p. 223).

Dosage: 100 mg twice daily for one week in *adults* and 50 mg twice daily for *children* of 6 to 12 years. In enteric fever 300 mg every 12 h initially, reducing to 200 mg every 12 h after 2 to 3 days has proved effective in adults. For *long-term therapy* adults are given 100 mg each evening and children of 6–12 years 50 mg. In *impaired renal function* (creatinine clearance 15–30 ml/min), adults receive 50 mg twice daily.

References

AHLMÉN, J., J.-E. BRORSON: Pharmacokinetics of trimethoprim given in single daily doses for three days. Scand. J. Infect. Dis. *14:* 143 (1982).

ASHFORD, J. J., L. J. DOWNEY: A multi-centre study comparing trimethoprim with co-trimoxazole in the treatment of respiratory tract infection in general practice. Brit. J. Clin. Prac. *36:* 551 (1982).

Gibson, J. R.: Recurrent trimethoprim-associated fixed skin eruption. Brit. Med. J. *284:* 1529 (1982).
Goldstein, F. W. et al.: The changing pattern of trimethoprim resistance in Paris, with a review of worldwide experience. Rev. Infect. Dis. *8:* 725 (1986).
Huovinen, P., O.-V. Renkonen, L. Pulkkinen et al.: Trimethoprim resistance of Escherichia coli in outpatients in Finland after ten years' use of plain trimethoprim. J. Antimicrob. Chemother. *16:* 435 (1985).
Huovinen, P., T. Mattila, O. Kiminki et al.: Emergence of trimethoprim resistance in fecal flora. Antimicrob. Ag. Chemother. *28:* 354 (1985).
Huovinen, P., L. Pulkkinen, H.-L. Helin et al.: Emergence of trimethoprim resistance in relation to drug consumption in a Finnish hospital from 1971 through 1984. Antimicrob. Ag. Chemother. *29:* 73 (1986).
Kraft, C. A., D. J. Platt, M. C. Timburry: Trimethoprim resistance in urinary coliforms from patients in the community: plasmids and R transfer. J. Antimicrob. Chemother. *15:* 311 (1985).
Murray, B. E., E. R. Rensimer, H. L. DuPont: Emergence of high-level trimethoprim resistance in fecal Escherichia coli during oral administration of trimethoprim or trimethoprim-sulfamethoxazole. New Engl. J. Med. *306:* 130 (1982).
Nolan, T., L. Lubitz, F. Oberklaid: Single dose trimethoprim for urinary tract infection. Arch. Dis. Child. *64:* 581–586 (1989).
Nyberg, G., H. Gäbel, P. Althoff et al.: Adverse effect of trimethoprim on kidney function in renal transplant patients. Lancet *I:* 394 (1984).

e) Nitrofurans

α) Nitrofurantoin

Proprietary names: Furadantin, Furadantin retard.

Properties: A synthetic nitrofuran derivative, N-(5-nitro-2-furfuryliden)-1-aminohydantoin, which is only slightly water-soluble, is stable and has a bitter taste.

Mode and spectrum of action: Nitrofurantoin is predominantly bacteriostatic but may be bactericidal at higher concentrations, presumably through the inhibition of enzymes involved in bacterial carbohydrate metabolism. Nitrofurantoin is active against most of the common causes of urinary infection. Esch. coli, citrobacter and most strains of klebsiella and enterobacter are susceptible. Proteus, providencia and serratia vary in sensitivity (some 25% of strains are resistant). Pseudomonas aeruginosa and acinetobacter are almost always resistant. Nitrofurantoin also has good activity against gram-positive cocci such as Enterococcus faecalis, Staphylococcus aureus and Staphylococcus epidermidis, as well as against less common causes of urinary infection (salmonella and other Streptococcus species). Secondary resistance does not arise during nitrofurantoin therapy. There is no cross-resistance between nitrofurantoin and other chemotherapeutic agents.

Pharmacokinetics: Nitrofurantoin is rapidly and almost completely absorbed in the intestine and distributed to all tissues and body fluids, including breast milk and the placenta. It fails to achieve therapeutically effective concentrations in either serum or tissues, however. The use of a macrocrystalline form retards the absorption of nitrofurantoin and hence reduces the central-nervous side effects (nausea and giddiness). Dosing with meals achieves the same end.

Excretion is predominantly renal (up to 40%) with a smaller amount excreted in the bile and the remainder broken down to inactive metabolites. Urinary concentrations between 50 mg/l and 250 mg/l are found with normal renal function. The urinary concentrations are reduced with impaired renal function, and the serum concentrations may increase to toxic levels. Only 2% of the active nitrofurantoin is recovered in the faeces and no significant changes in intestinal flora occur during long-term therapy.

Indications: The most important indication is the *suppressive therapy* of chronic obstructive urinary tract infection in patients with congenital or acquired outflow obstruction in whom more effective and lower risk antibacterial agents cannot be used (principally in children with congenital malformations of the urinary tract who seem to suffer fewer side-effects).

Nitrofurantoin may be used as a *bladder instillation* during urological procedures.

Inappropriate indications: Nitrofurantoin is not indicated in urinary infections which involve the renal parenchyma or which have given rise to bacteraemia (pyelonephritis, acute cystitis in the male) or in urethritis (which is mostly due to gonococci, chlamydiae and mycoplasmas) or in prostatitis (nitrofurantoin does not penetrate prostatic secretions). Uncomplicated urinary infections in women should no longer be treated primarily with nitrofurantoin.

Contra-indications:
1. Premature and newborn infants up to the end of the first month of life (because of the danger of haemolytic anaemia).
2. Nitrofurantoin is poorly tolerated in pregnant and lactating mothers, in whom any potentially mutagenic substance should be avoided where possible.
3. Renal insufficiency (even mild), because the accumulation of nitrofurantoin in the serum increases the risk of polyneuropathy.
4. A history of hypersensitivity to nitrofurantoin or other nitrofurans.
5. Caution is advised in diseases which may also give rise to the side-effects of nitrofurantoin, e.g. chronic pulmonary fibrosis, cholestasis or chronic hepatitis, haemolytic anaemia, G-6-PDH-deficiency, polyneuropathy.

Side-effects: Nitrofurantoin quite frequently gives rise to a range of undesirable reactions which can be severe. The commonest side-effects are gastrointestinal upset and allergic skin reactions, but polyneuropathies and pulmonary reactions can also occur. Nausea, loss of appetite and vomiting are frequently seen during nitrofurantoin treatment. These side-effects are due to a direct toxic effect on the CNS and are dose-dependent. Gastro-intestinal tolerance is better at lower dosage, when the drug is taken with meals or when given in macrocrystalline form.

Nitrofurantoin polyneuropathy is a serious complication of nitrofurantoin therapy which particularly occurs with long-term use. Predisposing factors are chronic renal insufficiency and diabetes mellitus. The symptoms regress to some extent after cessation of therapy but occasional fatal cases have been described.

Occasionally serious *pulmonary reactions* occur during nitrofurantoin therapy. The commoner acute form occurs a few hours after the last dose of nitrofurantoin, and involves allergic pulmonary oedema and sudden breathlessness, cough and fever, and pulmonary infiltrations (nitrofurantoin pneumonia). These symptoms are reversible once nitrofurantoin is stopped. *Chronic* pulmonary reactions (interstitial pneumonia, pulmonary fibrosis) can arise after long-term therapy (longer than 6 months) and are only partially reversible. The efficacy of steroid treatment is debatable.

Allergic reactions, particularly skin reactions (pruritus, urticaria), drug fever and angioneurotic oedema are relatively common but usually harmless. Sporadic cases of Stevens-Johnson or Lyell's syndrome and of anaphylactic shock have been described after nitrofurantoin.

Nitrofurantoin can occasionally cause *liver reactions* of varying severity. These reactions range from reversible cholestasis during short-term therapy to chronic active or granulomatous hepatitis, sometimes with fatal outcome, in long-term therapy. Patients with glucose-6-phosphate dehydrogenase deficiency may develop haemolytic crises. A few cases of reversible *agranulocytosis* and *megaloblastic anaemia* have been reported with nitrofurantoin.

Occasional *auto-immune reactions* after nitrofurantoin (generally in association with chronic liver or lung reactions) have been reported as a "lupus like" syndrome with fever, rash, arthralgias and eosinophilia. At least three of the following serum indices were positive: antinuclear antibodies, antibodies to smooth muscle or glomeruli, Coombs test. Transient alopecia, crystalluria, parotitis, pancreatitis, asthma attacks and erythema nodosum are all possible.

At high doses (10 mg/kg) nitrofurantoin can cause reversible *inhibition of spermatogenesis.*

Nitrofurantoin is mutagenic in bacterial and human fibroblast culture by the inhibition of DNA synthetase and is strongly positive in the Ames test (Salmonella/microsome test). Nitrofurantoin itself has not been shown to be carcinogenic, but it gives rise in the body to a metabolite with potentially carcinogenic properties (aminofurantoin). In animal experiments an increased rate of congenital malformation has been observed.

Special precautions: Nitrofurantoin should only be given with or after meals in order to reduce the nausea associated with its intake. Nitrofurantoin solutions must be protected from light. During nitrofurantoin treatment the blood count and hepatic and renal function should be monitored. If life-threatening side-effects occur (e.g. acute dyspnoea, fever, rashes, cholestasis or signs of polyneuropathy) nitrofurantoin treatment should immediately be discontinued.

Interactions: Nitrofurantoin antagonises the effect of nalidixic acid and other quinolones *in vitro*. It can induce liver enzymes which reduce the activity of certain drugs e.g., diphenylhydantoin. Concurrent administration of propantheline bromide increases the absorption of nitrofurantoin. Certain biochemical data (glucose, urea, alkaline phosphatase, bilirubin, creatinine) can be falsely elevated during nitrofurantoin therapy.

Administration and dosage: Nitrofurantoin is given orally as tablets, capsules or coated tablets, preferable in macrocrystalline form (for children also as syrup or drops).
Dosage is usually as follows:
For the treatment of *acute urinary infection:* 300 mg daily (in children, 5 mg/kg) in three divided doses for 1–2 weeks.
For *suppressive therapy* of chronic obstructive urinary infection: 100–150 mg per day (children from 2–3 mg/kg) in 2–3 divided doses for several months.
In conjunction with urological procedures nitrofurantoin may be instilled into the bladder. One ampoule for instillation contains 100 mg of nitrofurantoin in 20 ml polyethylene glycol and should be diluted in 200 ml of distilled water.

Summary: A dangerous urinary chemotherapeutic agent with numerous side-effects, some potentially severe. Safer alternatives are now preferable.

References

BACK, O., R. LUNDGREN, L.-G. WIMAN: Nitrofurantoin induced pulmonary fibrosis and lupus syndrome. Lancet *I:* 930 (1974).
BLACK, M., L. RABIN, N. SCHATZ: Nitrofurantoin-induced chronic active hepatitis. Ann. Intern. Med. *92:* 62 (1980).
CORAGGIO, M. J., T. P. GROSS, J. D. ROSCELLI: Nitrofurantoin toxicity in children. Pediatr. Infect. Dis. J. *8:* 163 (1989).
HOLMBERG, L., G. BOMAN, L. E. BOTTIGER et al.: Adverse reactions to nitrofurantoin: analysis of 921 reports. Am. J. Med. *69:* 733 (1980).
ISRAEL, K. S., R. E. BRASHEAR, H. M. SHARMA, M. N. YUM, J. L. GLOVER: Pulmonary fibrosis and nitrofurantoin. Amer. Rev. resp. Dis. *108:* 353 (1973).
JICK, S. S., H. JICK, A. M. WALKER, J. R. HUNTER: Hospitalizations for pulmonary reactions following nitrofurantoin use. Chest *96:* 512–515 (1989).
MARTIN, W. J.: Nitrofurantoin: evidence for the oxidant injury of lung parenchymal cells. Ann. Rev. Resp. Dis. *127:* 482 (1983).
MEYBOOM, R. H. B., A. VAN GENT, D. J. ZINKSTOK: Nitrofurantoin-induced parotitis. Brit. Med. J. *285:* 1049 (1982).
NELIS, G. F.: Nitrofurantoin-induced pancreatitis: report of a case. Gastroenterology *84:* 1032 (1983).

Pellinen, T. J., J. Klaske: Nitrofurantoin-induced parotitis. Brit. Med. J. *285:* 344 (1982).
Penn, R. G., J. P. Griffin: Adverse reactions to nitrofurantoin in the United Kingdom, Sweden, and Holland. Brit. Med. J. *284:* 1440 (1982).
Robinson, B. W. S.: Nitrofurantoin-induced interstitial pulmonary fibrosis. Presentation and outcome. Med. J. Aust. *1:* 72 (1983).
Sharp, J. R., K. G. Ishak, H. J. Zimmerman: Chronic active hepatitis and severe hepatic necrosis associated with nitrofurantoin. Ann. Intern. Med. *92:* 14 (1980).
Stefanini, M.: Chronic hemolytic anemia association with erythrocyte enolase deficiency exacerbated by ingestion of nitrofurantoin. Amer. J. clin. Path. *58:* 408 (1972).
Toole, J. F., M. L. Parrish: Nitrofurantoin polyneuropathy. Neurology *23:* 554 (1973).
Yiannikas, C., J. D. Pollard, J. G. McLeod: Nitrofurantoin neuropathy. Aust. N. Z. J. Med. *11:* 400 (1981).

β) Nitrofurazone

Proprietary name: Furacin.

Properties: A topical drug which may be absorbed in small quantities for wounds, but not through intact skin. When used topically, bactericidal activity against staphylococci, streptococci, Escherichia coli, enterobacter, klebsiella and proteus may be expected, but not against Pseudomonas aeruginosa or Candida albicans. Sensitisation (allergic contact dermatitis) sometimes occurs. Avoid long-term treatment because of possible oncogenicity and other side-effects, as for nitrofurantoin. Contraindicated in pregnancy.

Administration and indications: Used as ointment or powder for skin and wound infections and as ear drops in otitis.

f) Quinolones

Nalidixic acid, which was introduced in 1962 for the treatment of urinary infections, is no longer clinically important because of its unfavourable pharmacokinetic properties, low activity and tendency to rapid development of resistance. The other *older quinolones* of the nalidixic acid group (pipemidic acid, cinoxacin and rosoxacin) are markedly inferior in their activity and spectrum of action to the *newer fluoquinolones,* currently represented by norfloxacin, ofloxacin and ciprofloxacin. Other new quinolones are undergoing development (fleroxacin, lomefloxacin, pefloxacin, temafloxacin etc.).

All quinolones are carboxylic acid derivatives with an associated carboxylic acid group which is important for their antibacterial activity.

Compounds in this group inhibit bacterial DNA-topoisomerases (or gyrases), which are required for nucleic acid synthesis; they are sometimes referred to as 4-quinolones or gyrase inhibitors. The quinolones can be subdivided on the basis of their chemical structure (Figs. 52 and 53) into:

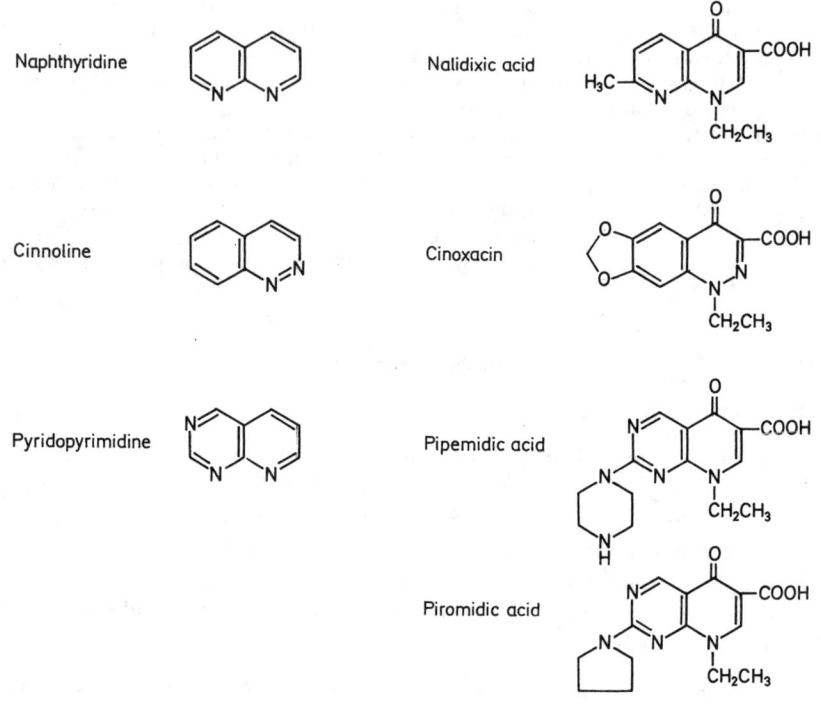

Fig. 52. Structural formulae of older quinolones.

1. Napthyridine carboxylic acids (nalidixic acid, enoxacin)
2. Cinnoline carboxylic acid (Cinoxacin)
3. Pyridopyrimidine carboxylic acids (pipemidic acid)
4. Quinoline carboxylic acids (ciprofloxacin, norfloxacin, ofloxacin, lomefloxacin, temafloxacin, pefloxacin, rosoxacin).

The new quinolone compounds are quinolone carboxylic acids with an attached carboxylic group and a fluorine atom in the 6 position, which considerably improves antibacterial activity and broadens the spectrum to include gram-positive bacteria. The newer quinolones are therefore designated fluoquinolones (with the exception of enoxacin, which is a napthyridine carboxylic acid). Like pipemidic acid, all new quinolones possess a piperazinyl group (an N-methylpiperazine ring in pefloxacin and ofloxacin) which is responsible for their antipseudomonal activity. A particular feature of ofloxacin is an oxacin ring which improves its pharmacokinetic properties, in particular its lack of metabolism in the human body. Ciprofloxacin has no ethyl group in position 1 but has instead a three-carbon ring (cyclopropyl residue) at this position which enhances its *in-vitro*

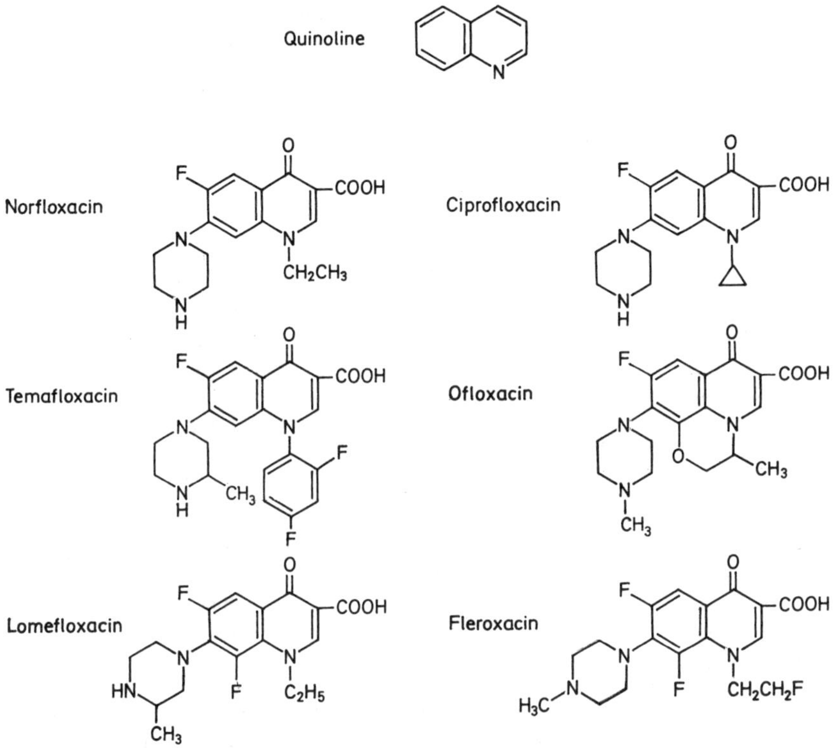

Fig. 53. Structural formulae of newer quinolones.

antibacterial activity. In contrast to the older quinolones of the nalidixic acid group, these newer substances are bactericidal, can be used at lower dosage and are suitable not only for urinary infections but also for infections of other organs. The quinolones are more or less completely absorbed after oral administration and are metabolised to varying degrees in the liver. Ciprofloxacin and ofloxacin can also be given parenterally. The side-effects of the newer quinolones are much less marked than those of the old.

α) Older Quinolones (Nalidixic Acid Group)

Proprietary names:
Nalidixic acid: Negram, Mictral
Pipemidic acid: Deblaston
Cinoxacin: Cinobac
Acrosoxacin (rosoxacin): Eradacin

Properties: Nalidixic acid is a synthetic napthyridine derivative which is unrelated to other antibiotics. Pipemidic acid and rosoxacin possess a piperazinyl ring; cinoxacin has a methylene dioxy group (in the 6,7 position as a five-membered ring). Nalidixic acid is stable and poorly soluble in water and alcohol; it is soluble in acid and alkaline solvents. The sodium salt of cinoxacin is freely soluble.

Mode of action: The inhibition of bacterial gyrases (or DNA topoisomerases) markedly impairs bacterial DNA metabolism. They prevent incorporation of nucleotides into the chromosomes, and DNA replication continues in an unphysiological way. When RNA synthesis is inhibited by high concentrations of a gyrase inhibitor, bacterial replication can no longer occur. There may well be other mechanisms of action of the DNA gyrase inhibitors which could explain certain differences between the individual compounds.

Spectrum of action: Most gram-negative organisms are susceptible (Escherichia coli, enterobacter, klebsiella, proteus, etc). In comparison with nalidixic acid, the activity of the other representatives of this group is often better. A variable percentage of bacterial isolates are resistant. Pipemidic acid has some activity against Pseudomonas aeruginosa but the other substances do not. No derivatives of this group have activity against gram-positive bacteria such as staphylococci and streptococci (including E. faecalis) except for pipemidic acid, which has weak activity against staphylococci.

Resistance: Bacterial resistance develops rapidly during the use of nalidixic acid, whereas pipemidic acid and cinoxacin rarely give rise to resistance. There is complete cross-resistance within the nalidixic acid group, with the exception of pipemidic acid against Pseudomonas aeruginosa, and partial, though uncommon, cross resistance with the new quinolones.

Pharmacokinetics: Rapid, though incomplete, *absorption* after oral administration. Relatively low *serum concentrations*. *Plasma protein binding* is most marked (up to 97%) with nalidixic acid and lowest with pipemidic acid (20–30%). *Half-life* 1.5 h. Nalidixic acid is extensively metabolised in the body; in the urine, 60–80% is excreted as an inactive conjugate, the remainder as active nalidixic and hydroxynalidixic acid. Urinary concentrations of nalidixic acid (1 g four times a day) are between 50 and 500 mg/l. Urinary recovery of pipemidic acid and cinoxacin is 50–60%.

Side-effects: The substances of the nalidixic acid group can give rise to a wide range of side-effects. The commonest symptoms are gastro-intestinal disorders such as nausea, vomiting, diarrhoea and gastric pain. Allergies (rashes, eosinophilia) or phototoxic reactions are less common, as are central nervous disorders such as convulsions, depression of respiration, drowsiness, psychosis, visual disturbances (blurred vision, disorders of colour vision, diplopia) as well as metabolic acidosis, neutropenia and haemolytic anaemia. In children intracranial hypertension has been observed. Symptoms such as tinnitus and photophobia sometimes occur during cinoxacin treatment. In young beagle dogs, high doses of quinolones (100 mg/kg per day) have given rise to cartilage damage (overgrowth and erosions) in weight-bearing joints. Similar changes have been found in rats but not in mice. No evidence of joint damage has been found in children who have received nalidixic acid in the past.

Interactions: The absorption of quinolones is reduced by mineral antacids. Nalidixic acid can increase the activity of oral anticoagulants. Pipemidic acid retards the excretion of theophylline and caffeine and thereby raises the blood concentrations of these substances. Theophylline doses should therefore be reduced and analgesics and drinks containing caffeine should be avoided.

Indications: Before the introduction of the new quinolones, the only indication for this group was in uncomplicated urinary infections with sensitive organisms (Escherichia coli, klebsiella, enterobacter and proteus).

Contra-indications: Oliguria, anuria, epilepsy and cerebral arteriosclerosis. Generally contraindicated in children and adolescents because of the possibility of arthropathies (so far only shown in animal experiments) and in pregnancy. Do not give to nursing mothers. Nalidixic acid should not be used in patients with glucose 6-phosphate dehydrogenase deficiency (favism) because of the danger of haemolysis.

Caution is advised in severe liver damage (as nalidixic acid is metabolised in the liver) and in renal failure (critical level: 80 mg/dl urea in serum). Direct sunlight should be avoided. Nalidixic acid can displace anticoagulants of the coumarin type from their plasma protein binding and thereby potentiate their effect.

Administration, dosage, presentation:

Nalidixic acid:	orally	1 g 4 times a day for 7–10 days (not longer, because of the danger of resistance development)	Tablets of 0.5 g
Pipemidic acid:	orally	0.4 g twice daily	Capsules of 0.2 g
Cinoxacin:	orally	0.5 g twice daily	Capsules of 0.25 g
Acrosoxacin:	orally	0.15 g twice daily	Capsules of 0.15 g

Summary: The older quinolones of the nalidixic acid group should now be replaced by the newer fluoquinolones on account of their poorer antibacterial activity, less favourable pharmacokinetic properties and rapid development of bacterial resistance.

References

Brumfitt, W., G. W. Smith, J. M. T. Hamilton-Miller, R. Bax: Successful use of reduced dosage of cinoxacin in the treatment of recurrent urinary infection. J. Antimicrob. Chemother. *16:* 781 (1985).
Harrison, W. O., F. S. Wignall, S. B. J. Kerbs, S. W. Berg: Oral rosoxacin for treatment of penicillin-resistant gonorrhoea. Lancet *I:* 566 (1984).
Jones, C., L. Cohen: Acrosoxacin-resistant gonococci. Lancet *I:* 855 (1982).
Kilpatrick, C., P. Ebeling: Intracranial hypertension in nalidixic acid therapy. Med. J. Aust. *1:* 252 (1982).
Klinge, E., P. T. Männistö, R. Mäntylä et al.: Single- and multiple-dose pharmacokinetics of pipemidic acid in normal human volunteers. Antimicrob. Ag. Chemother. *26:* 69 (1984).
Meyboom, R. H. B.: Thrombocytopenia induced by nalidixic acid. Brit. Med. J. *289:* 962 (1984).
Murray, E. D. S.: Nalidixic acid in pregnancy. Brit. Med. J. *282:* 224 (1981).
Tafani, O., M. Mazzoli, G. Landini, B. Alterini: Fatal acute immune haemolytic anaemia caused by nalidixic acid. Brit. Med. J. *285:* 936 (1982).

β) Newer Quinolones (Fluoquinolones)

(1) Norfloxacin

Proprietary names: Barazan, Utinor.

Properties: A fluorated quinoline-carboxylic acid derivative (with a piperazinyl group). Parent compound of the new quinolones. Poorly soluble in water.

Spectrum of activity: Norfloxacin is active against most organisms that cause urinary infection, particularly gram-negative bacilli including Pseudomonas aeruginosa. It has weaker activity against staphylococci and enterococci (Table 23). Streptococci of Lancefield groups A and B (Streptococcus pyogenes and S. agalactiae) are not susceptible. Anaerobes (e.g. Bacteroides fragilis), mycoplasmas and chlamydiae are also resistant.

Resistance: Some strains of Pseudomonas, Acinetobacter, Serratia, Providencia and Klebsiella species as well as of Proteus rettgeri and enterococci are resistant. There is partial cross-resistance with the new fluoquinolones. Bacterial strains resistant to nalidixic acid can be susceptible to norfloxacin. Secondary resistance may develop.

Pharmacokinetics: About 35–40% of norfloxacin is absorbed after oral administration. The mean serum concentration one hour after 0.4 g by mouth is 1.5 mg/l. *Half-life:* 4 h (Table 24, p. 244). *Plasma-protein binding:* 14%. *Excretion:* 30–40% unchanged through the kidneys and about 20% as metabolites. Maximum urinary concentration after 0.4 g by mouth is approximately 600 mg/l (more than 60 mg/l after 6 to 12 h).

Table 23. Minimum inhibitory concentrations of older and newer quinolones in ≤90% of bacterial strains studied ($MIC_{90\%}$) (own data).

Bacterial species	$MIC_{90\%}$ (mg/l) of					
	Nalidixic acid	Norfloxacin	Enoxacin	Ofloxacin	Ciprofloxacin	Temafloxacin
E. coli	8	0.06	0.5	0.06	0.016	0.06
Klebsiella pneumoniae	64	0.5	1.0	0.5	0.06	1.0
Enterobacter aerogenes	16	0.25	0.8	0.12	0.03	0.5
Proteus mirabilis	16	0.12	1.0	0.12	0.03	1.0
Proteus vulgaris	4	0.12	0.5	0.12	0.03	0.5
Pseudomonas aeruginosa	>100	2.0	2.0	2.0	0.5	4.0
Serratia marcescens	4	0.5	2.0	0.5	0.12	2.0
Streptococcus pyogenes	>100	16.0	32.0	0.6	0.6	0.6
Streptococcus pneumoniae	>100	8.0	16.0	1.0	1.0	0.5
Enterococcus faecalis	>100	8.0	16.0	2.0	2.0	2.0
Staphylococcus aureus	>100	2.0	2.0	0.5	0.5	0.25
Staphylococcus epidermidis	>100	2.0	2.0	0.5	0.5	0.25
Mycoplasma pneumoniae	>100	12.5	12.5	1.5	1.5	1.5
Legionella pneumophila	–	–	–	0.25	0.25	0.25
Ureaplasma urealyticum	>100	12.5	12.5	3.0	3.0	4.0
Chlamydia trachomatis	1600	16.0	16.0	1.0	1.0	0.25
Bacteroides fragilis	512	32.0	64.0	8.0	8.0	2.0
Other species of Bacteroides	512	8.0	64.0	4.0	8.0	8.0

Side-effects: Overall rate about 5%. The commonest are gastro-intestinal disorders (about 3%). Central-nervous disorders (headache, giddiness, dulled senses, altered mood, confusional states, hallucinations, paraesthesiae, disorders of vision) occur in fewer than 1%. Reaction times in motoring or machine operation can be impaired. Allergic reactions (urticaria, rashes), joint pain and tenovaginitis are rare, as are increases in liver enzymes and serum bilirubin and changes in the blood count (leukocytopenia, eosinophilia).

Indications: Infections of the upper and lower urinary tract (pyelonephritis, cystitis, urethritis).

Contra-indications: Epilepsy, pregnancy, lactation, children and adolescents during the phase of growth (because of arthropathies in young experimental animals).

Dosage: 0.4 g by mouth every 12 h for 7 to 10 days. In women with uncomplicated cystitis, a single dose of 0.4 g is sufficient. In impaired renal function (creatinine clearance below 30 ml/min) 0.4 g should be given every 24 h.

Preparations: Tablets of 0.4 g.

Summary: A reliable and effective agent for urinary tract infection.

References

ADHAMI, Z. N., R. WISE, D. WESTON, B. CRUMP: The pharmacokinetics and tissue penetration of norfloxacin. J. Antimicrob. Chemother. *13:* 87 (1984).
BERGAN, T.: Norfloxacin: a review of clinical experiences. J. Am. Med. Assoc. *(SE Asia Spec. Suppl. April:* 57 (1986).
BERGERON, M. G., M. THABET, R. ROY et al.: Norfloxacin penetration into human renal and prostatic tissues. Antimicrob. Ag. Chemother. *28:* 349 (1985).
CHRISTIANO, P., M. R. IOVENE, R. LOBELLO et al.: Biliary pharmacokinetics of norfloxacin. Chemioterapia *4 (2) (Suppl.):* 494 (1985).
DAVIS, R. L., H. W. KELLY, R. W. QUENZER, J. STANDEFER, B. STEINBERG, J. GALLEGOS: Effect of norfloxacin on theophylline metabolism. Antimicrob. Agents Chemother. *33:* 212–214 (1989).
FILLASTRE, J. P., TH. HANNEDOUCHE, A. LEROY, G. HUMBERT: Pharmacokinetics of norfloxacin in renal failure. J. Antimicrob. Chemother. *14:* 439 (1984).
GIULIANO, M., A. PANTOSTI, G. GENTILE, M. VENDITTI, W. ARCESE, P. MARTINO: Effects on oral and intestinal microfloras of norfloxacin and pefloxacin for selective decontamination in bone marrow transplant patients. Antimicrob. Agents Chemother. *33:* 1709–1713 (1989).
GOLDSTEIN, E. J. C., M. L. ALPERT, B. P. GINSBERG: Norfloxacin versus trimethoprim-sulfamethoxazole in the therapy of uncomplicated, community-acquired urinary tract infections. Antimicrob. Ag. Chemother. *27:* 422 (1985).
PONTICAS, S., D. L. SHUNGU, C. J. GILL: Comparative in vitro activity of norfloxacin against resistant Neisseria gonorrhoeae. Eur. J. Clin. Microbiol. Infect. Dis. *8:* 626–628 (1989).
ROMANOWSKI, B.: Norfloxacin in the therapy of gonococcal infections. Scand. J. Infect. Dis. *48:* 40–45 (1986).

SABBAJ, J., V. L. HOAGLAND, W. J. SHIH: Multiclinic comparative study of norfloxacin and trimethoprim-sulfamethoxazole for the treatment of urinary tract infections. Antimicrob. Ag. Chemother. 27: 297 (1985).
SIMON, C., U. LINDNER: In vitro activity of norfloxacin against Mycoplasma hominis and Ureaplasma urealyticum. Eur. J. clin. Microbiol. 2: 479 (1983).

(2) Ofloxacin

Proprietary name: Tarivid.

Properties: A quinoline carboxylic-acid derivative with a closed ring (responsible for the improved pharmacokinetics). Yellow opalescent crystals or crystalline powder with a bitter taste; readily soluble in acetic acid but soluble with difficulty in water, ethyl alcohol and acetone.

Spectrum of activity: Very broad spectrum including almost all the gram-positive and gram-negative bacteria, identical with that of ciprofloxacin. In vitro only one-quarter as active as ciprofloxacin against *gram-negative bacilli,* and somewhat weaker against *gram-positive bacilli*. Little difference from ciprofloxacin in activity against certain anaerobes (e.g. Bacteroides fragilis), mycoplasmas and chlamydiae (Table 23). Ofloxacin is sometimes ineffective against Proteus rettgeri, providencia and pseudomonas cepacia. Of the anaerobes, some species are resistant, such as certain clostridia (e.g. Clostridium difficile), certain bacteroides (e.g. B. thetaiotaomicron and B. vulgatus) and Peptococcus species (e.g. P. asaccharolyticus).

Resistance: Primary resistance is found in pneumococci and enterococci. The frequency of resistance in Pseudomonas aeruginosa has now risen to 15–20%. Secondary resistance in Pseudomonas aeruginosa and staphylococci may occur in vitro and during treatment. There is some cross-resistance among the new quinolones. Nalidixic acid-resistant bacteria, on the other hand, are generally susceptible to ofloxacin.

Pharmacokinetics: Well absorbed after oral dosage. Mean peak serum levels after 0.2 g and 0.4 g by mouth are 2.2 and 3.5 mg/l (after 1.1 and 1.9 h respectively), which fall after 12 h to 0.4 and 1.0 mg/l respectively. After i.v. infusion of 0.1 g and 0.2 g (in 30 min) the mean serum concentrations are 2.9 and 5.2 mg/l respectively (at the end of infusion) and 0.15 and 0.3 mg/l respectively (after 12 h). *Half-life:* 7 h (Table 24, p. 244).
Plasma-protein binding 25%. *CSF penetration* relatively good: in bacterial meningitis a CSF concentration of 50–60% of the serum concentration (1–2 mg/l) is achieved with 0.2 g orally twice daily. Good *tissue penetration* (e.g. in lung, bone, cartilage and prostatic tissue). High concentrations are also found in saliva and seminal fluid. *Excretion:* 74% excreted unchanged through the kidneys after

oral administration, and 77% after i.v. administration (in 24 h), increasing to 86% (in 72 h). Two metabolites can be shown in the urine, namely desmethyl ofloxacin (1.6% of the administered dose) and ofloxacin N-oxide (0.9%). In the bile and faeces the glucuronide derivative (4%) is a further metabolite.

Side-effects: Frequency 3% to 4%. The commonest are gastro-intestinal disorders (nausea, vomiting, abdominal pain, diarrhoea). Central nervous disorders are not uncommon (headache, dizziness, sleep disorders, disorders of gait, tremor, paraesthesiae, diplopia, hallucinations) as are psychotic reactions (agitation, hyperactivity, confusion). Reaction can therefore be impaired in driving or machine operation. Severe allergic reactions occasionally arise (rashes, photosensitivity, petechial haemorrhages and occasionally shock). These are reasons for immediately discontinuing the drug. Joint pain has occasionally been reported, particularly at high dosage. In individual cases, changes in the blood count (leukocytopenia, thrombocytopenia, anaemia) and transient increases in the liver enzymes and bilirubin have been reported.

Interactions: Simultaneous intake of mineral antacids reduces the absorption of ofloxacin. Slight interaction with theophylline.

Indications: Systemic infections with micro-organisms of proven or suspected susceptibility. An important indication is infection of the urinary tract in the urological patient. Ofloxacin may be used particularly when other agents are ineffective or poorly tolerated. Special indications are gonorrhoea, chlamydia and mycoplasma infections, as well as legionellosis or salmonellosis. In severe pseudomonas infections ofloxacin should be combined with an aminoglycoside because of the improved activity and the risk of emergence of resistance.

Inappropriate use: Meningitis, endocarditis, septicaemia (as a single agent), streptococcal sore throat, erysipelas, scarlet fever and pneumococcal infections of the respiratory tract, the middle ear and the sinuses. In general, ofloxacin should not be given for long periods for reasons of tolerance and the possible development of resistance. Not for uncritical or indiscriminate use in hospitals.

Contra-indications: Epilepsy, pregnancy, lactation, children and adolescents during the phase of growth (because of arthropathies in young experimental animals).

Use and dosage: 0.2 g (maximally 0.4 g) by mouth every 12 h for 7 to 10 days (where necessary, up to four weeks). In *impaired renal function* the normal single dose is given every 24 h (creatinine clearance 10–30 ml/min); patients with a creatinine clearance of less than 10 ml/min receive half the normal individual dose every 24 h. Parenterally 0.1 g every 12 h as i.v. infusion over 30–60 min.

Presentation: Tablets of 0.2 g; injection of 0.1 g.

Summary: An important chemotherapeutic agent with a broad spectrum of action and favourable pharmacokinetics. Watch for side effects, as with the other quinolones.

References

Ariyarit, C., K. Panikabutra, A. Chitwarakorn, C. Wongba, A. Buatiang: Efficacy of ofloxacin in uncomplicated gonorrhoea. Infection *14S:* 311–313 (1986).
Chan, A. S. C., K. G. Tang, K. K. Fung, T. K. Ng: Single dose ofloxacin in treatment of uncomplicated gonorrhoea. Infection *14S:* 314–315 (1986).
Goldstein, E. J. C., D. M. Citron: Comparative activity of the quinolones against anaerobic bacteria isolated in community hospitals. Antimicrob. Ag. Chemother. *27:* 657–659 (1985).
Grosset, J. H., B. H. Ji, C. C. Guelpa-Lauras, E. G. Perani, L. N. N'Deli: Clinical trial of pefloxacin and ofloxacin in the treatment of lepromatous leprosy. Int. J. Lepr. Other Mycobact. Dis. *58:* 281–295 (1990).
Judson, F. N., B. S. Beals, K. J. Tack: Clinical experience with ofloxacin in sexually transmitted disease. Infection. *14 (Suppl.):* 309–310 (1986).
Kalager, T., A. Digranes, T. Bergan, T. Rolstad: Ofloxacin: serum and skin blister fluid pharmacokinetics in the fasting and non-fasting state. J. Antimicrob. Chemother. *17:* 795 (1986).
Lode, L., et al.: Pharmacokinetics of ofloxacin after parenteral and oral administration. Antimicrob. Ag. Chemother. *31:* 1338 (1987).
Moellering, R. C., Jr., H. C. Neu. Ofloxacin: A pharmacodynamic advance in quinolone antimicrobial therapy. Am. J. Med. *87* (Suppl. 6C): 1S–81S (1989).
Osato, M. S., H. G. Jensen, M. D. Trousdale, J. A. Bosso, L. R. Borrmann, J. Frank, P. Akers: The comparative in vitro activity of ofloxacin and selected ophthalmic antimicrobial agents against ocular bacterial isolates. Am. J. Ophthalmol. *108:* 380–386 (1989).
Saito, A., K. Sawatari, Y. Fukuda et al.: Susceptibility of Legionella pneumophila to ofloxacin in vitro and in experimental Legionella pneumonia in guinea pigs. Antimicrob. Ag. Chemother. *28 (1):* 15–20 (1985).
Stahl, J. P., J. Croize, J. P. Akbaral, J. P. Bru, A. Guydi, D. Leduc, J. B. Fourtillan, M. Micoud: Diffusion of ofloxacin into cerebrospinal fluid of patients with bacterial meningitis. Infection *14 (Suppl. 4):* 256–258 (1986).
Stubner, G., W. Weinrich, U. Brandis: Study of the cerebrospinal fluid penetrability of ofloxacin. Infection *14 (Suppl. 4):* 250 (1986).
Wang, F., X. J. Gu, M. F. Zhang, T. Y. Tai: Treatment of typhoid fever with ofloxacin. J. Antimicrob. Chemother. *23:* 785–788 (1989).
Yew, W. W., S. Y. Kwan, W. K. Ma, M. A. Khin, P. Y. Chau: In vitro activity of ofloxacin against Mycobacterium tuberculosis and its clinical efficacy in multiply resistant pulmonary tuberculosis. J. Antimicrob. Chemother. *26:* 227–236 (1990).

(3) Ciprofloxacin

Proprietary names: Ciproxin, Cipro.

Properties: A fluorinated quinoline carboxylic-acid derivative with a piperacinyl and cyclopropyl group. The tablets contain ciprofloxacin hydrochloride and the ampoules ciprofloxacin lactate; both are water-soluble.

Spectrum of action: Active against almost all gram-positive and gram-negative bacteria (as ofloxacin). The *in-vitro* activity against *gram-negative* bacilli is some four times greater than that of ofloxacin, but approximately the same against *gram-positive* bacteria. Ciprofloxacin is not active against certain strains of Xanthomonas maltophilia, Proteus rettgeri, Serratia species and providencia. A number of strains of clostridia (e. g. Clostridium difficile) and bacteroides (e. g. Bacteroides fragilis) as well as Nocardia asteroides and Ureaplasma urealyticum are resistant.

Resistance: Some strains of pseudomonas and enterococci are resistant. Secondary resistance can develop during prolonged treatment with ciprofloxacin of infections caused by staphylococci, pseudomonas, Enterobacter cloacae and Klebsiella pneumoniae. It can also be demonstrated with certain species *in vitro* by daily subculturing. There is some cross-resistance between all members of the fluoquinolone group, while bacteria resistant to nalidixic acid are still generally sensitive to ciprofloxacin.

Pharmacokinetics: Ciprofloxacin is incompletely absorbed after oral administration. Mean serum levels of 1.4, 2.8 and 3.6 mg/l are found 60 to 90 min after 0.25 g, 0.5 g and 0.75 g by mouth respectively (Table 24, p. 244). The serum concentrations at the end of a short i. v. infusion of 0.1 g are 3–4 mg/l. *Half-life* (after i. v. administration): 3–4 h. *Plasma-protein binding:* 30%. *CSF penetration* relatively good (CSF concentrations approximately 20% of the serum concentrations). Good *tissue penetration* (higher concentrations particularly in genital tissue, muscle, skin, lung, liver, intestinal wall, gall bladder wall, prostate, bronchial and seminal fluids and the aqueous humor). An as yet unknown proportion of ciprofloxacin is metabolised in the body.

Excretion is predominantly via the kidneys, up to 30–40% unchanged after oral administration and up to 55% unchanged after i. v. dosage. Several metabolites (at least four) can be demonstrated in the urine. A part of the intake of ciprofloxacin is excreted in the bile; another fraction is secreted by the intestinal wall and eliminated with the faeces. There is a significant enterohepatic cycle.

Side-effects: Total incidence about 6%. The most common are gastro-intestinal reactions (nausea, vomiting, diarrhoea, abdominal pain), whereas central nervous reactions are less common (dizziness, headache, fatigue, irritability, anxiety, disorders of peripheral sensitivity, visual disturbances, fits), hypersensitivity reactions (rashes, itching, facial oedema) and circulatory reactions (rises in blood pressure, tachycardia, flushes). Reaction time when driving or operating machinery may be impaired during ciprofloxacin therapy. Arthropathy is rare; so are pain and redness at the injection site and thrombophlebitis. Transient increases in serum transaminases, alkaline phosphatase and bilirubin may occur, as well as hypercholesterolaemia and hypertriglyceridaemia, and changes in the blood count (e.g. eosinophilia). Of the possible side-effects, only the gastro-intestinal disturbances are dose-dependent (more frequent with daily doses exceeding 1.5 g).

Interactions: Mineral antacids reduce the absorption of ciprofloxacin from the gastro-intestinal tract. The theophylline levels in blood may be slightly raised when ciprofloxacin is given concurrently. Cardiac and circulatory function should be monitored when ciprofloxacin is given simultaneously with barbiturate-containing drugs.

Indications: Systemic infections with micro-organisms of proven or suspected susceptibility, particularly when a quinolone is the only orally effective agent. Oral or parenteral use is also indicated when other antibiotics fail or are poorly tolerated. Ciprofloxacin is also an alternative to other agents that are potentially nephro- or hepatotoxic. Special indications include gonorrhoea, chlamydia and mycoplasma infections as well as legionellosis. In pseudomonas infections, ciprofloxacin may be combined with an aminoglycoside because of the enhanced effect and to avoid development of resistance. Ciprofloxacin is suitable for treatment of typhoid and enteric fever, in the eradication of chronic salmonella excretion and in selective intestinal decontamination in immunosuppressed patients. The use of a single dose of ciprofloxacin in eliminating asymptomatic nasopharyngeal carriage of meningococci appears promising.

Inappropriate use: Meningitis, endocarditis, septicaemia (as single agent therapy), also pneumococcal infection of the respiratory tract, the middle ear and the sinuses. In general, long-term treatment with ciprofloxacin should be avoided on the grounds of tolerability and the possible emergence of resistance. The drug should not be used uncritically nor indiscriminately in hospitals because of the danger of resistance. Experience in prophylactic use is not yet sufficient.

Contra-indications: Epilepsy, pregnancy, lactation, children and adolescents during the period of growth (because of arthropathies in young experimental animals).

Dosage and administration: Oral (250–) 500 (–750) mg every 12 h (in gonorrhoea a single dose of 250 mg), 100–200 mg every 12 h as a *short i. v. infusion* over 30–60 min (in gonorrhoea, a single dose of 100 mg i. v.). Do not mix with other drugs in the infusion solution. Ensure adequate hydration to prevent crystalluria. Duration of treatment: usually one to two weeks (occasionally longer). In *renal*

Table 24. Pharmacokinetic data on newer quinolones (compilation of data from the literature).

Drug	Maximum serum levels (mg/l)	Time (h)	Half-life (h)	Urinary recovery (%)	Serum protein binding (%)
Ofloxacin					
0.2 g orally	2.2	1.1		74	
0.4 g orally	3.5	1.9	7	74	25
0.2 g i. v.	5.2	End of infusion (30 min)		77	
Ciprofloxacin					
0.25 g orally	1.4	1.0		40	
0.5 g orally	2.8	1.2		30	
0.75 g orally	3.6	1.3	3–4	28	30
0.1 g i. v.	~3.0	End of infusion		54	
0.2 g i. v.	~4.0			56	
Norfloxacin					
0.4 g orally	1.5	1	4	40	14
Enoxacin					
0.2 g orally	1.2	1.0	4–6	60	40
0.4 g orally	3.1	1.5			
Temafloxacin					
0.4 g orally	4.0	2.5	7–8	65	26
0.6 g orally	6.0	3.0			

impairment (creatinine clearance <20 ml/min) give the normal single dose every 24 h (or half the normal dose every 12 h).

Preparations: Tablets of 250 mg, 500 mg, 750 mg. Infusion bottles of 100 mg and 200 mg.

Summary: *In-vitro* activity against gram-negative rods is considerably better than that of ofloxacin, but pharmacokinetics are less favourable. The broad spectrum provides many possible uses for this agent, including infections which are difficult to treat by other means.

References

BOELAERT, J., Y. VALCKE, M. SCHURGERS, R. DANEELS, M. ROSSENEU, M. T. ROSSEEL, M. G. BOGAERT: The pharmacokinetics of ciprofloxacin in patients with impaired renal function. J. Antimicrob. Chemother. 16: 87–93 (1985).
CHAPMAN, S. T., D. C. E. SPELLER, D. S. REEVES: Resistance to ciprofloxacin. Lancet *II:* 39 (1985).

CHOW, A. W., J. WONG, K. H. BARTLETT, S. D. SHAFRAN, H. G. STIVER: Cross-resistance of Pseudomonas aeruginosa to ciprofloxacin, extended-spectrum beta-lactams, and aminoglycosides and susceptibility to antibiotic combinations. Antimicrob. Ag. Chemother. *33:* 1368–1372 (1989).
COKER, D. M., I. AHMED-JUSHUF, O. P. ARYA, J. S. CHESSBROUGH, B. C. PRATT: Evaluation of single dose ciprofloxacin in the treatment of rectal and pharyngeal gonorrhoea. J. Antimicrob. Chemother. *24:* 271–272 (1989).
COOPER, B., M. LAWLOR: Pneumococcal bacteremia during ciprofloxacin therapy for pneumococcal pneumonia. Am. J. Med. *87:* 475 (1989).
CROOK, S. M., B. SELKON, P. D. MCLARDY SMITH: Clinical resistance to long term ciprofloxacin. Lancet *I:* 1275 (1985).
CULLMANN, W., M. STIEGLITZ, B. BAARS, W. OPFERKUCH: Comparative evaluation of recently developed quinolone compounds, with a note on the frequency of resistant mutants. Chemotherapy *31:* 19 (1985).
FALLON, R. J., W. M. BROWN: In vitro sensitivity of legionellas, meningococci and mycoplasmas to ciprofloxacin and enoxacin. J. Antimicrob. Chemother. *15:* 787–789 (1985).
FENLON, C. H., M. H. CYNAMON: Comparative in vitro activities of ciprofloxacin and other 4-quinolones against Mycobacterium tuberculosis and Mycobacterium intracellulare. Antimicrob. Ag. Chemother. *29:* 386 (1986).
FITZGEORGE, R. B., D. H. GIBSON, R. JEPRAS, A. BASKERVILLE: Studies on ciprofloxacin therapy of experimental Legionnaires' disease. J. Infection *10:* 194–203 (1985).
GARLANDO, F., M. G. TÄUBER, B. JOOS et al.: Ciprofloxacin-induced hematuria. Infection *13:* 177 (1985).
GONZALEZ, M. A., A. H. MORANCHEL, S. DURAN, A. PICHARDO, J. L. MAGANA, B. PAINTER, A. FORREST, G. L. DRUSANO: Multiple-dose pharmacokinetics of ciprofloxacin administered intravenously to normal volunteers. Antimicrob. Ag. Chemother. *28:* 235–239 (1985).
HÖFFKEN, G., K. BORNER, P. D. GLATZEL, P. KOEPPE, H. LODE: Reduced enteral absorption of ciprofloxacin in the presence of antacids. Eur. J. Clin. Microbiol. *4:* 345 (1985).
HUDSON, S. J., H. R. INGHAM, M. H. SNOW: Treatment of Salmonella typhi carrier state with ciprofloxacin. Lancet *II:* 1047 (1985).
HUMPHREYS, H., E. MULVIHILL: Ciprofloxacin-resistant Staphylococcus aureus. Lancet *II:* 383 (1985).
KOTILAINEN, P., J. NIKOSKELAINEN, P. HUOVINEN: Emergence of ciprofloxacin-resistant coagulase-negative staphylococcal skin flora in immunocompromised patients receiving ciprofloxacin. J. Infect. Dis. *161:* 41–46 (1990).
LEDERGERBER, B., J. D. BETTEX, B. JOOS, M. FLEPP, R. LÜTHY: Effect of standard breakfast on drug absorption and multiple-dose pharmacokinetics of ciprofloxacin. Antimicrob. Ag. Chemother. *27:* 350–352 (1985).
MILLER, M. R., M. A. BRANSBY-ZACHARY, D. S. TOMPKINS, P. M. HAWKEY, R. MYLES GIBSON: Ciprofloxacin for Pseudomonas aeruginosa meningitis. Lancet *I:* 1325 (1986).
OPPENHEIM, B. A., J. W. HARTLEY, W. LEE, J. P. BURNIE: Outbreak of coagulase negative staphylococcus highly resistant to ciprofloxacin in a leukaemia unit. Br. Med. J. *299:* 294–297 (1989).
ORIEL, J. D.: Ciprofloxacin in the treatment of gonorrhoea and non-gonococcal urethritis. J. Antimicrob. Chemother. *18D:* 129–132 (1986).
PATTON, W. N., G. M. SMITH, M. J. LEYLAND, A. M. GEDDES: Multiple resistant Salmonella typhimurium septicaemia in an immunocompromised patient successfully treated with ciprofloxacin. J. Antimicrob. Chemother. *16:* 667 (1985).

Peloquin, C. A., T. J. Cumbo, D. E. Nix, M. F. Sands, J. J. Schentag: Evaluation of intravenous ciprofloxacin in patients with nosocomial lower respiratory tract infections. Impact of plasma concentrations, organism, minimum inhibitory concentration, and clinical condition on bacterial eradication. Arch. Intern. Med. *149:* 2269–2273 (1989).
Roberts, C. M., J. Batten, M. E. Hodsen: Ciprofloxacin resistant pseudomonas. Lancet *I:* 1442 (1985).
Rosenberg-Arska, M., A. W. Dekker, J. Verhoef: Ciprofloxacin for selective decontamination of the alimentary tract in patients with acute leukaemia during remission induction treatment: the effect on faecal flora. J. Infect. Dis. *152:* 104 (1985).
Shalit, I., R. B. Greenwood, M. I. Marks, J. A. Pederson, D. L. Frederick: Pharmacokinetics of single-dose oral ciprofloxacin in patients undergoing chronic ambulatory peritoneal dialysis. Antimicrob. Ag. Chemother. *30:* 152–156 (1986).
Smith, G. M., C. Cashmore, M. J. Leyland: Ciprofloxacin-resistant staphylococci. Lancet *II:* 949 (1985).
Smith, M. J., M. E. Hodson, J. C. Batten: Ciprofloxacin in cystic fibrosis. Lancet *I:* 1103 (1986).
Tegelberg-Stassen, M. J. A. M., J. C. S. van der Hoek, L. Mooi, J. H. T. Wagenvoort, T. van Joost, M. F. Michel, E. Stolz: Treatment of uncomplicated gonococcal urethritis in men with two doses of ciprofloxacin. Eur. J. Clin. Microbiol. *5:* 244–246 (1986).
Valainis, G., D. Thomas, G. Pankey: Penetration of ciprofloxacin into cerebrospinal fluid. Eur. J. Clin. Microbiol. *5:* 206–207 (1986).
Wolfson, J. S., D. C. Hooper: Bacterial resistance to quinolones: Mechanisms and clinical importance. Rev. Infect. Dis. *11* (Suppl. 5): 960 (1989).

(4) Enoxacin

Proprietary name: Comprecin.

Properties: Enoxacin is not a fluoquinolone but a napthyridine-carboxylic acid derivative with a piperacinyl group. Tablets contain the sesquihydrate.

Spectrum of activity: Enoxacin has a broad spectrum of activity similar to that of ciprofloxacin and ofloxacin, but a considerably weaker antibacterial activity, so that the proportion of resistant strains in a given bacterial species is usually greater. Enoxacin is always ineffective against streptococci (including pneumococci and enterococci), against listerias and gardnerellas as well as all anaerobes. Some resistant strains are found in Proteus rettgeri, providencia, Pseudomonas aeruginosa, Pseudomonas cepacia, Xanthomonas maltophilia, Acinetobacter species, enterobacter, Klebsiella species and arizona.

Resistance: Partial cross-resistance with the new fluoquinolones. Nalidixic acid-resistant bacteria may be sensitive to enoxacin. Secondary development of resistance is possible.

Pharmacokinetics: Enoxacin is incompletely absorbed after oral dosage. After 200 and 400 mg by mouth, mean peak serum levels of 1.2 and 3.1 mg/l respectively are found after 1–1.5 h. *Half-life:* 4–6 h. *Plasma-protein binding:* 40%. Relatively high salivary and sputum concentrations. Biliary concentrations some five times higher than serum levels. *Excretion* up to 60% unchanged in the urine. An as yet unknown proportion is excreted with the bile and faeces. Four metabolites may be demonstrated in the urine: oxo enoxacin (14%), acetyl enoxacin (0.4%), formyl enoxacin (0.3%) and amino enoxacin (0.3%), all of which have weak antibacterial activity.

Side-effects: Overall frequency 6.4%. Enoxacin, as a napthyridine-carboxylic acid derivative, gives rise to more central nervous side-effects than other new quinolones. They include dizziness, headache, agitation, somnolence, insomnia, fits, disturbances of vision, photophobia, peripheral neuropathies, confusional states, hallucinations, depression, psychotic reaction, unsteady gait and tremor. Impairment of reactions while driving or operating machinery is therefore possible. Other side-effects are gastro-intestinal disorders, allergic reactions, hypotension, tachycardia, muscle pain, joint pain, renal tubular necrosis, hypoglycaemia, tenovaginitis, disorders of smell and taste, phototoxicity (e. g. bullous eruptions at sites exposed to light), elevation of serum liver enzymes and bilirubin and changes in the peripheral blood count (anaemia, leukocytopenia and thrombocytopenia).

Interactions: Concurrent administration of enoxacin delays the elimination of theophylline and caffeine (from caffeine-containing drinks and analgesics) and increases the blood concentrations of these substances. Enoxacin apparently inhibits detoxification processes in the liver. Simultaneous intake of enoxacin and fenbufen can cause fits. Simultaneous administration of mineral antacids substantially reduces the absorption of enoxacin from the gastro-intestinal tract.

Indications: Because of the relatively high rate of central nervous side-effects, the indications for enoxacin (systemic infections with susceptible organisms) are considerably reduced.

Contra-indications: Epilepsy and pre-existing central nervous disease, severe liver and renal insufficiency, pregnancy, lactation, childhood and adolescence in the phase of growth (because of the joint changes in young experimental animals).

Recommended dose: 200–400 mg every 12 h for 7 to 14 days (no longer than four weeks).

Presentation: Tablets of 200 mg and 400 mg.

Summary: Because of its weaker activity and relatively high rate of central nervous side-effects, enoxacin should only be used when better tolerated derivatives are not available.

References

PRINCE, R. A., E. CASABAR, C. G. ADAIR, D. B. WEXLER, J. LETTIERI, J. E. KASIK: Effect of quinolone antimicrobials on theophylline pharmacokinetics. J. Clin. Pharmacol. 29: 650–654 (1989).
RANNIKKO, S., A.-S. MALMBORG: Enoxacin concentration in human prostatic tissue after oral administration. J. Antimicrob. Chemother. 17: 123 (1986).
ROGGE, M. C., W. R. SOLOMON, A. J. SEDMAN, P. G. WELLING, J. R. KOUP, J. G. WAGNER: The theophylline-enoxacin interaction: II. Changes in the disposition of theophylline and its metabolites during intermittent administration of enoxacin. Clin. Pharmacol. Ther. 46: 420–428 (1989).
SIMPSON, J. K., M. J. BRODIE: Convulsions related to enoxacin. Lancet II: 161 (1985).
SPELLER, D., R. WISE: Enoxacin – a laboratory and clinical assessment. J. Antimicrob. Chemother. 21 (Suppl. B): 1 (1988).
TSUEI, S. E., A. S. DARRAGH, I. BRICK: Pharmacokinetics and tolerance of enoxacin in healthy volunteers administered at a dosage of 400 mg twice daily for 14 days. Antimicrob. Ag. Chemother. 14: 71 (1984).
VAN DER AUWERA, P., J. C. STOLEAR, B. GEORGE, M. N. DUDLEY: Pharmacokinetics of enoxacin and its oxometabolite following intravenous administration to patients with different degrees of renal impairment. Antimicrob. Agents Chemother. 34: 1491–1497 (1990).
WIJNANDS, W. J. A., C. L. A. VAN HERWAARDEN, T. B. VREE: Enoxacin raises plasma theophylline concentrations. Lancet II: 108–109 (1984).
WIJNANDS, W. J. A., T. B. VREE, C. L. A. VAN HERWAARDEN: Enoxacin decreases the clearance of theophylline in man. Br. J. Clin. Pharmacol. 20: 583–588 (1985).

(5) Fleroxacin

Properties: A quinoline carboxylic acid derivative (developed by Roche) with three fluorine atoms in the quinolone nucleus (Fig. 53, p. 233). Not yet approved for use.

Spectrum of activity: Similar to that of ofloxacin and ciprofloxacin. Fleroxacin has a similar *in-vitro* activity to ofloxacin. A few strains of Pseudomonas aeruginosa, Serratia marcescens, Proteus rettgeri and enterobacter are resistant. The following species are all resistant: streptococci (including pneumococci and enterococci) and anaerobes (including Bacteroides species), Treponema pallidum, Gardnerella vaginalis, Nocardia asteroides, Listeria species and Mycobacterium avium-intracellulare.

Resistance: Almost complete cross-resistance with the new fluoquinolones and partial cross-resistance with the older quinolones (nalidixic acid group). Secondary resistance may develop *in vitro*, particularly with pseudomonas, serratia, klebsiella, staphylococci and enterococci.

Pharmacokinetics: Well absorbed when given orally. After 400 mg by mouth, mean peak serum concentrations of 4.2 mg/l occur after 1.5 h which fall to

0.6 mg/l after 24 h. After i.v. infusion of 100 mg over 20 minutes, peak concentrations of 2.8 mg/l at the end of infusion fall after 24 h to 0.1 mg/l. *Half-life:* 9.5 h. *Plasma-protein binding:* 23%. Good *tissue penetration. Excretion* up to 57% unchanged via the kidneys in 4 days (after oral administration) and up to 73% (after i.v. administration), also as metabolites (N-oxide and N-demethyl derivatives). Active urinary concentration 24 h after 400 mg orally remains above 25 mg/l.

Side-effects occur frequently with repeated dosage of 200–400 mg. The most common are gastro-intestinal disturbances (nausea, vomiting, diarrhoea) as well as headache and giddiness, and less commonly insomnia or skin rashes. Psychotic reactions rarely occur.

Interactions: As for ofloxacin and ciprofloxacin. The simultaneous administration of mineral antacids inhibits the absorption of fleroxacin.

Indications: Infections of the urinary tract, intestine and soft tissues with susceptible organisms (with the limitations already given for ofloxacin).

Contra-indications: Pregnancy, lactation, childhood, epilepsy. Caution with certain pre-existing CNS conditions. Do not use in streptococcal or pneumococcal infections (because of lack of activity).

Suggested dosage: 400 mg once daily by mouth or 100 mg to 200 mg i.v. (as a short infusion) for 7 to 10 days.

Summary: So far as can be assessed from clinical trials, fleroxacin is a highly active antibacterial agent with a broad spectrum and prolonged activity.

References

CLARKE, A. M., S. J. V. ZEMCOV: In vitro activity of the new 4-quinolone compound RO 23-6240. Eur. J. Clin. Microbiol. *6:* 161–164 (1987).
HIRAI, K., H. AOYAMA, M. HOSAKA, Y. OOMOSI, Y. NIWATA, S. SUZUE, T. IRIKURA: In vivo antibacterial activity of AM-833, a new quinolone derivative. Antimicrob. Ag. Chemother. *29:* 1059–1066 (1986).
KROPEC, A., F. DASCHNER: In vitro activity of fleroxacin and 6 other antimicrobials against Acinetobacter anitratus. Chemotherapy *35:* 360–362 (1989).
MANEK, N., J. M. ANDREWS, R. WISE: In vitro activity of RO 23-6240, a new difluoroquinolone derivative, compared with that of other antimicrobial agents. Antimicrob. Ag. Chemother. *30:* 330–332 (1986).
SINGLAS, E., A. LEROY, E. SULTAN: Disposition of Fleroxacin, a New Trifluoroquinolone, and Its Metabolites. Pharmacokinetics in Renal Failure and Influence of Haemodialysis. Clin. Pharmacokinet. *19:* 67–79 (1990).
WEIDEKAMM, E., R. PORTMANN, K. SUTER, C. PARTOS, D. DELL, P. W. LÜCKER: Single- and multiple-dose pharmacokinetics of fleroxacin, a trifluorinated quinolone, in humans. Antimicrob. Agents Chemother. *31:* 1909–1914 (1987).

(6) Pefloxacin

Spectrum of activity: Pefloxacin (Rhône-Poulenc, Nattermann) has weaker *in-vitro* activity than ciprofloxacin and ofloxacin but a similar spectrum. Some strains of pseudomonas, serratia, streptococci and staphylococci are resistant. Bacteroides species and fusobacteria are generally insensitive.

Pharmacokinetic data suggest good absorption from the gastro-intestinal tract. *Half-life:* 11 h. *Serum protein binding:* 20–30%. Pefloxacin is extensively metabolised in the body, mainly to piperacin N-oxide, N-demethyl derivatives and oxopiperacin. Only about 9% is *excreted* unchanged in the urine.

Side-effects occur frequently. CNS side effects are not uncommon. Prolonged treatment carries a risk of skin photosensitisation. Pefloxacin reduces the clearance of theophylline and is at present licensed for clinical use in France.

References

BOEREMA, J. B. J., R. PAUWELS, J. SCHEEPERS, W. CROMBACH: Efficacy and safety of pefloxacin in the treatment of patients with complicated urinary tract infections. J. Antimicrob. Chemother. *17:* 103 (1986).

CLARKE, A. M., S. J. V. ZEMCOV, M. E. CAMPBELL: In-vitro activity of pefloxacin compared to enoxacin, norfloxacin, gentamicin and new beta-lactams. J. Antimicrob. Chemother. *15:* 39 (1985).

DELLAMONICA, P., E. BERNARD, H. ETESSE, R. GARRAFFO: The diffusion of pefloxacin into bone and the treatment of osteomyelitis. J. Antimicrob. Chemother. *17:* 93 (1986).

DOW, J., J. CHAZAL, A. M. FRYDMAN et al.: Transfer kinetics of pefloxacin into cerebrospinal fluid after one hour i.v. infusion of 400 mg in man. J. Antimicrob. Chemother. *17:* 81 (1986).

FRYDMAN, A. M., Y. LE ROUX, M. A. LEFEBVRE et al.: Pharmacokinetics of pefloxacin after repeated intravenous and oral administration (400 mg bid) in young healthy volunteers. J. Antimicrob. Chemother. 17 *(Suppl. B):* 65 (1986).

LAUWERS, S., W. VINCKEN, A. NAESSENS, D. PIERARD: Efficacy and safety of pefloxacin in the treatment of severe infections in patients hospitalized in intensive care units. J. Antimicrob. Chemother. 17 *(Suppl. B):* 111–115 (1986).

LIGTVOET, E. E. J., T. WICKERHOFF-MINOGGIO: In-vitro activity of pefloxacin compared with six other quinolones. J. Antimicrob. Chemother. *16:* 485 (1985).

MAESEN, F. P. V., B. I. DAVIES, J. P. TEENGS: Pefloxacin in acute exacerbations of chronic bronchitis. J. Antimicrob. Chemother. *16:* 379 (1985).

MONTAY, G., J. BARIETY, C. JACQUOT et al.: Pharmacokinetics of the antibacterial pefloxacin in renal and hepatic disease. Chemioterapia 4 (2) *(Suppl.):* 501 (1985).

SALVANET, A., A. FISCH, C. LAFAIX et al.: Pefloxacin concentrations in human aqueous humor and lens. J. Antimicrob. Chemother. *18:* 199 (1986).

VACHON, F., M. WOLFF, B. REGNIER, C. DALBOSS, M. NKAM: Penetration of pefloxacin into cerebrospinal fluid of patients with meningitis. Antimicrob. Agents Chemother. *26:* 289–291 (1984).

(7) Lomefloxacin

Spectrum of activity: Lomefloxacin (Searle) is a difluoroquinolone (structural formula shown in Fig. 53, p. 233) first synthesised in Japan. Its *in-vitro* activity against gram-negative and gram-positive aerobic bacteria is generally weaker than that of ofloxacin.

Pharmacokinetics: Lomefloxacin is well absorbed from the gastro-intestinal tract (unaffected by food intake) and is *excreted* 70–80% unchanged in the urine. *Half-life:* 7–8 h. The principal metabolite is the glucuronide (up to 4.5% excreted in the urine and 0.8% in the bowel); other metabolites appear in small quantities (less than 0.1%).

Side-effects occur in 2–4% with daily doses of 200–600 mg, CNS side-effects in 1%. Lomefloxacin has no effect on the clearance of theophylline when given concurrently. Clinical trials are not yet complete.

References

BALDWIN, D. R., D. HONEYBOURNE, J. M. ANDREWS, J. P. ASHBY, R. WISE: Concentrations of oral lomefloxacin in serum and bronchial mucosa. Antimicrob. Agents Chemother. *34:* 1017–1019 (1990).

HIROSE, T.: In vitro and in vivo activity of NY-198, a new difluorinated quinolone. Antimicrob. Ag. Chemother. *31:* 854–859 (1987).

LEBEL, M., F. VALLEE, M. ST. LAURENT: Influence of lomefloxacin on the pharmacokinetics of theophylline. Antimicrob. Agents Chemother. *34:* 1254–1256 (1990).

LEROY, A., J. P. FILLASTRE, G. HUMBERT: Lomefloxacin pharmacokinetics in subjects with normal and impaired renal function. Antimicrob. Agents Chemother. *34:* 17–20 (1990).

SEGRETI, J., J. A. NELSON, L. J. GOODMAN, R. L. KAPLAN, G. M. TRENHOLME: In vitro activities of lomefloxacin and temafloxacin against pathogens causing diarrhea. Antimicrob. Ag. Chemother. *33:* 1385–1387 (1989).

(8) Temafloxacin

Proprietary name: Teflox.

Properties: A trifluorinated quinolone derivative similar to lomefloxacin with a slightly different antibacterial activity.

Spectrum of action: Active against almost all gram-positive and gram-negative bacteria. The in vitro activity against Streptococcus pneumoniae is equal or twice that of ciprofloxacin. The activity against Bacteroides species and other anaerobes is quite good. More than 90% of Bacteroides fragilis strains are sensitive. A variable number of Pseudomonas aeruginosa and serratia strains are resistant.

Pharmacokinetics: Well absorbed after oral dosage. Half-life: 7–8 h. Plasma protein binding: 26%.

Side-effects: Shortly after its introduction, temafloxacin was withdrawn worldwide on account of its side-effects. These include severe hypoglycaemia, hepatic failure, haemolytic anaemia, deterioration of renal function including uraemia, and severe, sometimes fatal, anaphylaxis. It would seem that distinct chemical variations in the structural formula of quinolones may be followed by severe side-effects which are not observed with other chemically related substances.

Summary: No longer available because of severe side-effects.

g) Nitroimidazoles

Proprietary names:
Metronidazole: Flagyl;
Tinidazole: Fasigyn;
Nimorazole: Nagoxin 500.

Properties: Nitroimidazoles are a group of heterocyclic compounds based on a 5-membered nucleus (Fig. 54) with certain similarities to the nitrofurans. They act by oxygen deprivation, which explains their activity against protozoa and anaerobic bacteria and also as radiosensitisers. All agents of this group may be carcinogenic in laboratory animals and are mutagenic in the Ames test, but have not so far been found to have such effects in humans.

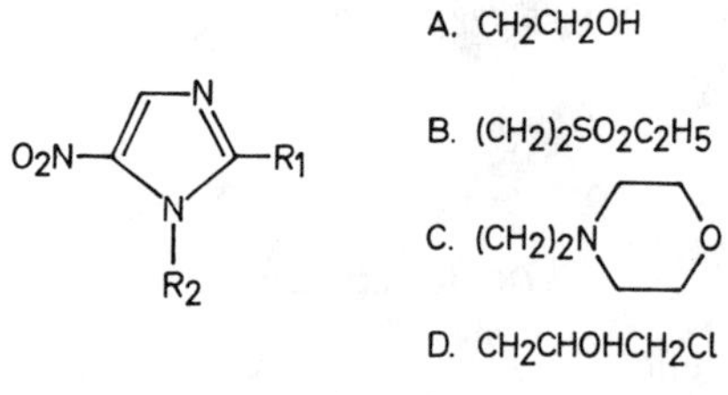

A. CH_2CH_2OH

B. $(CH_2)_2SO_2C_2H_5$

C. $(CH_2)_2N\underset{}{\diagup}O$

D. $CH_2CHOHCH_2Cl$

Fig. 54. Structures of metronidazole ($R_1 = CH_3$; $R_2 = A$); tinidazole ($R_1 = CH_3$; $R_2 = B$); nimorazole ($R_1 = H$; $R_2 = C$) and ornidazole ($R_1 = H$; $R_2 = D$).

Mode of action: Inhibition of nucleic acid synthesis of anaerobic bacteria. Strongly bactericidal.

Spectrum of action: Protozoa (Entamoeba histolytica, Trichomonas vaginalis, Giardia lamblia) are inhibited *in vitro* by metronidazole, tinidazole and nimorazole at low concentrations. These agents are active against all obligate anaerobic bacteria (clostridia and nonsporing anaerobes) except Propionibacterium and actinomyces.

Metronidazole and tinidazole are similar in their antibacterial activity, while nimorazole is less active. All aerobic and facultatively anaerobic bacteria are resistant.

Resistance: Primary resistance is very rare in sensitive species of anaerobes. Resistance or failure of therapy sometimes occurs with Trichomonas vaginalis and Entamoeba histolytica. There is complete cross-resistance among the nitroimidazoles, but no cross-resistance with antibiotics. Resistance does not develop during treatment.

Pharmacokinetics:
Well *absorbed* after oral administration. *Maximal serum concentrations* of 8 mg/l after 400 mg of metronidazole by mouth, 12 mg/l after 500 mg and 40 mg/l after 2 g and 40 mg/l with tinidazole. Peak serum concentrations of 16 mg/l are found after 1 g nimorazole.

Rectal application of metronidazole 500 mg gives peak serum concentrations of 4–5 mg/l after 3–8 h. *Intravaginal* administration of 200 and 500 mg metronidazole gives rise to serum concentrations between 0.4 and 1.0 mg/l.

Serum concentrations of 13–15 mg/l can be achieved after 500 mg of metronidazole i.v. by short infusion over 20 min. Repeated doses do not lead to accumulation. Mean serum concentrations of 15 and 32 mg/l are found at the end of i.v. infusion of 0.8 and 1.6 g tinidazole, respectively. *Half-life:* 7 h (metronidazole), 13 h (tinidazole), 10 h (nimorazole). *Plasma-protein binding:* 15% (metronidazole), 12% (tinidazole), 15% (nimorazole). Very good *tissue penetration* (particularly in the brain, liver, uterus, adipose tissue, skin, and abscess cavities). High concentrations in CSF, saliva, peritoneal fluid, vaginal secretions, amniotic fluid and breast milk. Metronidazole is extensively oxidised and conjugated in the liver to products with less antimicrobial activity. Tinidazole is less metabolised in the liver than metronidazole; the effective concentrations are therefore higher in the tissue and body fluids.

Excretion is mainly renal, both unchanged and as metabolites. Total urinary recovery: 30% (metronidazole), 15% (tinidazole), 55% (nimorazole). Metronidazole causes a reddish-brown discolouration of the urine.

Metronidazole is readily dialysed. About 10% of the metronidazole dose passes into the bile.

Side-effects: Dose-dependent, and apparently not as frequent after tinidazole as after metronidazole. Gastrointestinal upset in 3% (nausea, vomiting, diarrhoea). Some patients complain of an unpleasant metallic taste. The following symptoms sometimes occur during prolonged therapy and after high dosage: peripheral neuropathy (with paraesthesiae), central nervous disorders (dizziness, ataxia, clouding of consciousness, seizures etc.), glossitis, stomatitis, urticaria, rashes, itching, dysuria, cystitis, a sensation of pressure in the pelvis and reversible neutropenia. Thrombophlebitis may complicate i. v. administration. Potentiation of oral anticoagulants may occur. No increase in congenital abnormalities, premature deliveries or postnatal disorders has been observed after administration at different stages of pregnancy. However, because they are carcinogenic in animals, nitroimidazoles should be avoided in pregnancy and for long-term treatment unless their use is essential.

Interactions: The action of oral anticoagulants can be potentiated. The excretion of metronidazole may be accelerated by simultaneous administration of phenytoin or phenobarbitone as a result of liver enzyme induction. Cimetidine can prolong the half-life of metronidazole through delayed plasma clearance as a result of reduced liver enzyme activity.

Indications:
1. Drug of choice in trichomoniasis and vaginitis due to Gardnerella vaginalis (treat infected partner as well).
2. Amoebic dysentery (all types, and amoebic liver abscess).
3. Intestinal infections with Giardia lamblia and Balantidium coli.
4. Anaerobic bacterial infections including mixed infections with aerobic bacteria, e. g. septicaemia associated with thrombophlebitis, aspiration pneumonia, liver abscess, cerebral, pulmonary or pelvic abscesses, other intra-abdominal abscesses, peritonitis, pelvic infections, endometritis, puerperal sepsis, febrile abortion or gangrene. For mixed infections, always combine with a broad-spectrum antibiotic active against aerobes (e. g. an aminoglycoside or cephalosporin). In ulcerative stomatitis or gingivitis, peridontitis and gas gangrene, combine with benzylpenicillin.
5. Prophylaxis for major gynaecological and colon surgery and appendicectomy.
6. Sometimes effective in antibiotic-induced pseudomembranous enterocolitis (due to Clostridium difficile), if vancomycin cannot be given.
7. In Crohn's disease long-term treatment with metronidazole may be useful but peripheral neuropathy (usually reversible) occurs in 10–20% of cases.

Contra-indications: Active central nervous diseases, blood dyscrasias, 1st trimester of pregnancy. *Caution* in serious liver disease (reduce dosage). Avoid alcohol during treatment. Replace breast milk temporarily with cow's milk when mother is treated during lactation.

Administration and dosage:
For *amoebic dysentery* (all types): 800 mg 3 times a day (about 10 mg/kg 3 times a day in children) for 5–10 days after meals. A sequential course of diloxanide furoate, 500 mg 3 times a day is recommended for 10 days to eliminate luminal forms of the parasite.

For *trichomoniasis* and *giardiasis:* 250 mg 3 times a day (about 3 mg/kg 3 times a day for children) for 6 days, or a single dose for trichomoniasis with metronidazole, tinidazole or nimorazole: 2.0 g (4 tablets) in a single dose, preferably after meals. An alternative short oral course of metronidazole is 2 doses of 1 g, 6 hours apart, on the 1st day, followed by 1 g the next morning (total dose 3 g). Repeat after 4–6 weeks at the earliest. Simultaneous topical treatment with vaginal tablets, pessaries or vaginal gel is sometimes recommended but not essential. Stop treatment if ataxia or other signs of intolerance develop.

For *anaerobic infections* give by mouth, i. v. or rectally. Avoid rapid i. v. injection. Short i. v. infusion (in 20–30 min) required adequate dilution. Lower serum concentrations follow rectal administration. Oral dosage in adults: 400 mg metronidazole 3 times a day (or 0.5 g twice daily); 7 mg/kg 3 times a day for children, and half this dose in the newborn. For prophylaxis in gynaecological and colonic surgery, give a short course of 400 mg 3 times a day beginning on the day of operation. The same dose is used for i. v. administration (infuse 500 mg in 100 ml of solvent over 20 min). In gynaecological and abdominal surgical prophylaxis, give 0.5–1 g metronidazole i. v. or by suppository, or 400 mg by mouth, shortly before the operation, and continue the same dose 3 times a day for 24 hours. Longer courses should be regarded as treatment rather than prophylaxis. The dose need not be reduced in renal impairment.

Tinidazole is given orally for anaerobic infections in doses of 1 g once a day or 500 mg twice daily. The i. v. dose of tinidazole is 800 mg once a day. Nitroimidazoles should in general not be given for more than 10 days.

Preparations: Tablets and capsules of 250 mg and 400 mg (metronidazole), of 500 mg (nimorazole), of 1 g (tinidazole), suppositories (metronidazole) of 500 mg and 1 g, also vaginal tablets, suppositories or capsules (metronidazole), vials of 500 mg (metronidazole), of 800 mg (tinidazole).

Summary: A group of reliable chemotherapeutic agents in trichomoniasis, amoebic and anaerobic infections with a carcinogenic risk established in animal studies and occasional serious side-effects.

References

Alawattegama, A. B., B. M. Jones, G. R. Kinghorn et al.: Single dose versus seven-day metronidazole in Gardnerella vaginalis associated non-specific vaginitis. Lancet *1:* 1355 (1984).

Alper, M. M., N. Barwin, W. McLean, I. J. McGilveray, S. Sved: Systemic absorption of metronidazole by the vaginal route. Obstet. Gynecol. *65:* 781 (1985).

Alvarez, R. S., D. A. Richardson, A. E. Bent, D. R. Ostergard: Central nervous system toxicity related to prolonged metronidazole therapy. Am. J. Obstet. Gynecol. *145:* 640 (1983).

Andersson, K. E.: Pharmacokinetics of nitroimidazoles. Spectrum of adverse reactions. Scand. J. Infect. Dis. *Suppl. 26:* 60–67 (1981).

BAILES, J., J. WILLIS, C. PRIEBE, R. STRUB: Encephalopathy with metronidazole in a child. Amer. J. Dis. Child. *137:* 290 (1983).
BARKER, E. M., J. M. AITCHISON, J. S. CRIDLAND, L. W. BAKER: Rectal administration of metronidazole in severely ill patients. Brit. Med. J. *287:* 311 (1983).
BERGAN, T., O. LEINEBØ, T. BLOM-HAGEN, B. SALVESEN: Pharmacokinetics and bioavailability of metronidazole after tablets, suppositories, and intravenous administration. Scand. J. Gastroenterol. *19 (Suppl. 91):* 45–60 (1984).
BLAKE, P., W. E. BUTT: Ototoxicity of metronidazole. N. Z. Med. J. *97:* 241 (1984).
BOLTON, R. P.: Clostridium difficile-associated colitis after neomycin treated with metronidazole. Brit. Med. J. *2:* 1479 (1979).
BROGAN, O., P. A. GARNETT, R. BROWN: Bacteroides fragilis resistant to metronidazole, clindamycin and cefoxitin. J. Antimicrob. Chemother. *23:* 660–662 (1989).
CARMINE, A. A., R. N. BROGDEN, R. C. HEEL, T. M. SPEIGHT, G. S. AVERY: Tinidazole in anaerobic infections. A review of its antibacterial activity, pharmacological properties and therapeutic efficacy. Drugs *24:* 85–117 (1982).
CHAIKIN, P., K. B. ALTON, C. SAMPSON, H. S. WEINSTRAUB: Pharmacokinetics of tinidazole in male and female subjects. J. Clin. Pharmacol. *22:* 562–570 (1982).
CHARUEL, C., J. NACHBAUR, A. M. MONRO, D. DE PALOL: The pharmacokinetics of intravenous tinidazole in man. J. Antimicrob. Chemother. *8:* 343–346 (1981).
CHERRY, R. D., D. PORTNOY, D. S. DALY, D. G. KINNEAR, C. A. GORESKY: Metronidazole: an alternative therapy for antibiotic associated colitis. Gastroenterol. *82:* 849–851 (1982).
DANESHMEND, T. K., C. J. C. ROBERTS: Impaired elimination of metronidazole in decompensated chronic liver disease. Brit. Med. J. *288:* 405 (1984).
EARL, P., P. R. SISSON, H. R. INGHAM: Twelve-hourly dosage schedule for oral and intravenous metronidazole. J. Antimicrob. Chemother. *23:* 619–621 (1989).
EME, M. A., J. F. ACAR, F. W. GOLDSTEIN: Bacteroides fragilis resistant to metronidazole. J. Antimicrob. Chemother. *12:* 523 (1983).
FARRELL, G., L. ZALUZNY, J. BAIRD-LAMBERT et al.: Impaired elimination of metronidazole in decompensated chronic liver disease. Brit. Med. J. *287:* 1845 (1983).
FLUOVAT, B. L., C. IMBERT, D. M. DUBOIS, B. P. TEMPERVILLE, A. F. ROUX, G. C. CHEVALIER, G. HUMBERT: Pharmacokinetics of tinidazole in chronic renal failure and in patients on haemodialysis. Brit. J. Clin. Pharmacol. *15:* 735–741 (1983).
FRYTAK, S., C. G. MAERTEL, D. S. CHILDS: Neurology toxicity associated with high-dose metronidazole therapy. Ann. Intern. Med. *88:* 361–362 (1980).
GILAT, T., G. LEICHTMAN, G. DELPRE, J. ESHCHAR, S. BAR-MEIR, Z. FIREMAN: A comparison of metronidazole and sulfasalazine in the maintenance of remission in patients with ulcerative colitis. J. Clin. Gastroenterol. *11:* 392–395 (1989).
GUAY, D. R., R. C. MEATHERALL, H. BAXTER, W. R. JACYK, B. PENNER: Pharmacokinetics of metronidazole in patients undergoing continuous ambulatory peritoneal dialysis. Antimicrob. Ag. Chemother. *25:* 306–310 (1984).
GUPTE, S.: Phenobarbital and metabolism of metronidazole. New Engl. J. Med. *308:* 529 (1983).
HALLORAN, T. J.: Convulsions associated with high cumulative doses of metronidazole. Drug. Intel. Clin. Pharm. *16:* 409 (1982).
HIBBERD, A. D., R. J. NICOLL, W. A. MACBETH: Deafness is an adverse reaction to the prophylactic use of metronidazole. N. Z. Med. J. *97:* 128 (1984).
HOF, H., V. STICHT-GROH, K.-L. MÜLLER: Comparative in vitro activities of niridazole and metronidazole against anaerobic and microaerophilic bacteria. Antimicrob. Ag. Chemother. *22:* 332 (1982).
HUNT, P. S., A. J. L. DAVIDSON, J. ALDEN, S. CHENG: Bile and serum levels of tinidazole after single oral dose. Brit. J. Clin. Pharm. *13:* 233–234 (1982).

Jager-Roman, B., P. B. Doyle, J. Baird-Lambert, M. Caejlo, N. Buchanan: Pharmacokinetics and tissue distribution of metronidazole in the newborn infant. J. Pediat. *106:* 651–654 (1982).

Jerve, F., T. B. Berdal, P. Bohman et al.: Metronidazole in the treatment of non-specific vaginitis (NSV). Brit. J. Vener. Dis. *60:* 171 (1984).

Kulda, J., M. Vojtěchovská, J. Tachezy et al.: Metronidazole resistance of Trichomonas vaginalis as a cause of treatment failure in trichomoniasis. A case report. Brit. J. Vener. Dis. *58:* 394 (1982).

Kusumi, R. K., J. F. Plouffe, R. H. Wyatt, R. J. Fass: Central nervous system toxicity associated with metronidazole therapy. Ann. int. med. *93:* 59–61 (1980).

Kyrönseppä, H., T. Pettersson: Treatment of giardiasis: relative efficacy of metronidazole as compared with tinidazole. Scand. J. Infect. Dis. *13:* 311 (1981).

Ljungberg, B., I. Nilsson-Ehle, B. Ursing: Metronidazole: pharmacokinetic observations in severely ill patients. J. Antimicrob. Chemother. *14:* 275 (1984).

McEwen, J.: Hypersensitivity reactions to tinidazole (Fasigyn). Med. J. Aust. *1:* 498 (1983).

McWalter, P. W., D. R. Baird: Metronidazole-resistant anaerobes. Lancet *I:* 1220 (1983).

Mattila, J., P. T. Männistö, R. Mäntylä, S. Nykänen, U. Lamminsivu: Comparative pharmacokinetics of metronidazole and tinidazole as influenced by administration route. Antimicrob. Ag. Chemother. *23:* 721–725 (1983).

Mead, P. B., M. Gibson, J. J. Schentag, J. A. Ziemniak: Possible alteration of metronidazole metabolism by phenobarbital. New Engl. J. Med. *306:* 1490 (1982).

Packard, R. S.: Tinidazole: a review of clinical experience in anaerobic infections. J. Antimicrob. Chemother. *10 (Suppl. A):* 65 (1982).

Pehrson, P., E. Bengtsson: Treatment of non-invasive amoebiasis: a comparison between tinidazole and metronidazole. Ann. Trop. Med. Parasitol. *78:* 505 (1984).

Piot, P., E. Van Dyck, P. Godts: A placebo-controlled, double-blind comparison of tinidazole and triple sulfonamide cream for the treatment of nonspecific vaginitis. Amer. J. Obstet. Gynecol. *147:* 85 (1983).

Plotnick, B. N., I. Cohen, T. Tsang, T. Cullinane: Metronidazole-induced pancreatitis. Ann. Intern. Med. *103:* 891 (1985).

Ralph, E. D.: Clinical pharmacokinetics of metronidazole. Clin. Pharmacokin. *8:* 42–62 (1983).

Robson, R. A., R. R. Bailey, J. R. Sharma: Tinidazole pharmacokinetics in severe renal failure. Clin. Pharmacol. *9:* 88–94 (1984).

Roux, A. F., E. Moirot, B. Delhotal et al.: Metronidazole kinetics in patients with acute renal failure on dialysis: a cumulative study. Clin. Pharmacol. Ther. *36:* 363 (1984).

Scully, B. E.: Metronidazole. Med. Clin. North Am. *72:* 613 (1988).

Somogyi, A. A., C. B. Kong, F. W. Gurr et al.: Metronidazole pharmacokinetics in patients with acute renal failure. J. Antimicrob. Chemother. *13:* 183 (1984).

Speelman, P.: Single-dose tinidazole for the treatment of giardiasis. Antimicrob. Ag. Chemother. *27:* 227 (1985).

Sprott, M. S., H. R. Ingham, J. E. Hickman, P. R. Sisson: Metronidazole-resistant anaerobes. Lancet *I:* 1220 (1983).

Swedberg, J., J. F. Steiner, F. Deiss et al.: Comparison of single-dose vs. one-week course of metronidazole for symptomatic bacterial vaginosis. JAMA *254:* 1046 (1985).

Vutanen, J., H. Haataja, P. T. Männistö: Concentrations of metronidazole and tinidazole in male genital tissues. Antimicrob. Ag. Chemother. *28:* 812 (1985).

Vinge, E., K.-E. Andersson, G. Ando, E. Lunell: Biological availability and pharmacokinetics of tinidazole after single and repeated doses. Scand. J. Infect. Dis. *15:* 391 (1983).

Waitkins, S. A., D. J. Thomas: Isolation of Trichomonas vaginalis resistant to metronidazole. Lancet *II:* 590 (1981).

15. Antimycobacterial Agents

a) Isoniazid (INH)

Proprietary name: Rimifon.

Properties: Isonicotinic acid hydrazide, a water-soluble, synthetic chemotherapeutic agent, which is bactericidal to extra- and intracellular bacteria.

Mode of action: Inhibition of bacterial nucleic acid and mycotic acid synthesis. Bacteriostatic to tubercle bacilli at low concentrations, and bactericidal at 4 to 5 times higher concentrations, during the phase of active bacterial growth.

Spectrum of activity: Effective against Mycobacterium tuberculosis only, and not atypical mycobacteria (except some strains of M. kansasii), nor any other bacterial species.

Resistance: Primary resistance in M. tuberculosis is rare (1–4%), but resistance develops rapidly with single drug therapy. No cross-resistance with other antituberculous agents.

Pharmacokinetics:
Absorption occurs within 1–2 hours of an oral dose.
Metabolism: Human populations show genetically determined differences in the rate at which isoniazid is inactivated by acetylation. Rapid inactivators have the dominant genotype in homozygous or heterozygous form, whereas slow inactivators are homozygous recessives. Certain ethnic groups, particularly the Japanese and many Eskimos, are predominantly rapid inactivators. In others, e.g. Caucasians and Negroes, about half are slow inactivators. Rapid inactivators have lower blood concentrations, a shorter half-life and less frequent side effects such as neuritis. Isoniazid is partly metabolised in the body to acetyl-isoniazid to an extent which is determined genetically as above, but other metabolites such as isonicotinic acid, isonicotinuric acid, hydrazine and hydrazone derivatives are independent of genetic factors. All of these metabolites except the hydrazones are inactive.
Plasma concentrations after 200 mg by mouth are 2–3 mg/l after 1–2 h and 1.1 mg/l after 6 h in slow inactivators; after 300 mg orally they are 3–9 mg/l after 1–2 h and 1.4 mg/l after 6 h. These serum concentrations are 30–40% lower after 1 and 2 h in rapid inactivators, and this factor must be taken into account in the intermittent chemotherapy of tuberculosis. PAS is also acetylated and so the acetylation of isoniazid is reduced when PAS is given at the same time; correspondingly higher serum concentrations are then found.

Plasma protein binding: 20–30%. *Half-life:* 3 hours in slow inactivators and 1 hour in rapid inactivators. The half-life is prolonged in liver dysfunction. Only about 30–60% of the total dose of isoniazid remains active in the body.

Good *CSF penetration* with 50–80% of the serum concentration in meningitis. 50–80% of the serum concentration in pleural, peritoneal and synovial fluid. About 50% enters the fetal circulation. Good tissue penetration. Also penetrates areas of caseous necrosis and macrophages.

Excretion is predominantly through the kidneys by glomerular filtration, almost entirely as metabolites, and in smaller amounts with the faeces. Urinary concentrations of active isoniazid are 20–80 mg/l.

Side-effects (relatively rare with daily doses of up to 300 mg):

1. *Central nervous disorders and peripheral neuropathy* (dizziness, headaches, restlessness, psychological disorders, muscular fibrillation, cramps, paraesthesiae, retrobulbar neuritis). These occur more frequently with alcoholics, diabetics and slow inactivators and at higher dosage. Pyridoxine (vitamin B_6). 100–200 mg daily, can be given for the prophylaxis and treatment of isoniazid neuropathy. Drowsiness or incoordination often occur when barbiturates or diphenylhydantoin are given at the same time, because of delayed catabolism. Intolerance to alcohol is not uncommon.

2. *Gastrointestinal disorders and transient elevation of transaminases,* with hepatitis with or without jaundice in 1% of cases which can occasionally be fatal, particularly in people over 50. These are more frequent in combination with rifampicin than with ethambutol. The drug should be discontinued immediately at the first sign of hepatitis.

3. *Allergic rashes, fever and arthropathy.*

4. *Blood dyscrasias* (leukocytopenia, occasionally agranulocytosis, anaemia and thrombocytopenia).

5. *Bleeding tendency* due to damage to vessel walls, *cardiovascular disturbances, pellagra* and *acne.*

Interactions: The action of phenytoin may be potentiated by the simultaneous administration of isoniazid, as a result of delayed excretion. Carbamazepine concentrations can also be elevated during isoniazid treatment. Disulfiram activity (Antabuse effect) is potentiated by simultaneous isoniazid, so alcohol should be avoided because of intolerance.

Indications: The most important drug in the combined treatment of tuberculosis, in prophylaxis in contacts whose tuberculin test is positive or has converted (particularly in immunosuppressive therapy, prolonged corticosteroid treatment, leukaemia, and Hodgkin's disease) and in the chemoprophylaxis of contacts, particularly infants.

Isoniazid should never be used alone to treat clinical tuberculosis.

Contra-indications: Acute hepatitis. Use with caution in alcoholics, epileptics, diabetics and patients with chronic liver disease or renal insufficiency.

Administration: Usually by mouth. The i. v. route is rarely necessary.

Dosage: *Orally* 4–5 (–10) mg/kg a day, i. e. 200–300 (–600) mg for adults, 6 (–10) mg/kg for children, 5–10 mg/kg for infants, but only 5 mg/kg in 1 or more divided doses during the first month of life, on account of metabolic immaturity. With higher dosage, give supplementary pyridoxine (10–20 mg per 100 mg isoniazid). Liver function, blood count and neurological status should be monitored regularly.

Intravenous route: Slow injection of 2–5% solution. The single dose should not exceed 200 mg, and continuous intravenous infusion is preferable.

Intrathecal route (rarely necessary): 20–40 mg a day for adults, and 5–30 mg (about 1 mg/kg) for children.

Local instillation: About 300 mg every 2–4 days into the pleura, 50–100 mg into joints and 50–100 mg into the bladder. Take the quantity of locally instilled isoniazid into account when calculating the total dose.

Treatment by inhalation: 2 ml of 5% solution (= 100 mg) several times a day.

Preparations: 50, 100 and 200 mg tablets; a syrup containing 50 mg/5 ml, and 100 mg and 250 mg vials for injection.

Summary: A standard antituberculous agent which is quite well tolerated. Use only in combination with other antituberculous agents to avoid rapid development of resistance.

References

ALEXANDER, M. R., S. G. LOUIE, B. G. GUERNSEY: Isoniazid-associated hepatitis. Clin. Pharm. *1:* 148 (1982).
BERNSTEIN, R. E.: Isoniazid hepatotoxicity and acetylation during tuberculosis chemoprophylaxis. Amer. Rev. Respir. Dis. *121:* 429 (1980).
BISTRITZER, T., Z. BARZILAY, A. JONAS: Isoniazid-rifampicin-induced fulminant liver disease in an infant. J. Pediatr. *97:* 480 (1980).
BLOCK, S. H.: Carbamazepine-isoniazid interaction. Pediatrics *69:* 494 (1982).
CLAIBORNE, R. A., A. K. DUTT: Isoniazid-induced pure red cell aplasia. Amer. Rev. Respir. Dis. *131:* 947 (1985).
ELLARD, G. A.: The potential clinical significance of the isoniazid acetylator phenotype in the treatment of pulmonary tuberculosis. Tubercle *65:* 211 (1984).
GURUMURTHY, P., M. S. KRISHNAMURTHY, O. NAZARETH et al.: Lack of relationship between hepatotoxicity and acetylator phenotype in three thousand South Indian patients during treatment with isoniazid for tuberculosis. Am. Rev. Respir. Dis. *129:* 58 (1984).

Ishii, N., Y. Nishihara: Pellagra encephalopathy among tuberculous patients: its relation to isoniazid therapy. J. Neurol. Neurosurg. Psychiatry *48:* 628 (1985).
Lauterberg, B. H., C. V. Smith, E. L. Todd et al.: Pharmacokinetics of the toxic hydrazine metabolites formed from isoniazid in humans. J. Pharm. Exp. Ther. *235:* 566 (1985).
Livengood, J. R., T. G. Sigler, L. R. Foster et al.: Isoniazid-resistant tuberculosis. A community outbreak and report of a rifampicin prophylaxis failure. JAMA *253:* 2847 (1985).
Motion, S., M. J. Humphries, S. M. Gabriel: Severe "flu"-like symptoms due to isoniazid – a report of three cases. Tubercle *70:* 57–60 (1989).
O'Brien, R. J., M. W. Long, F. S. Cross et al.: Hepatotoxicity from isoniazid and rifampin among children treated for tuberculosis. Pediatrics *72:* 491 (1983).
Pellock, J. M., J. Howell, E. L. Kendig Jr. et al.: Pyridoxine deficiency in children treated with isoniazid. Chest *87:* 658 (1985).
Valsalan, V. C., G. L. Cooper: Carbamazepine intoxication caused by interaction with isoniazid. Brit. Med. J. *285:* 261 (1982).

b) Rifampicin

Proprietary names: Rifadin, Rimactane. Combined preparations (with isoniazid): Rifinah, Rimactazid; (with isoniazid and pyrazinamide): Rifater.

Description: Rifampicin (rifampin in the USA) is a semi-synthetic ansamycin antibiotic of the rifamycin group. It is soluble in organic solvents, and in water at acid pH, having a yellow-red colour. The ansamycins bear no relationship to other antibiotics.

Mode of action: Inhibition of bacterial RNA polymerase. Intensely bactericidal on proliferating bacteria including tubercle bacilli.

Spectrum of activity: Tubercle bacilli are very sensitive (minimal inhibitory concentration only 0.5 mg/l), as are gram-positive bacteria (staphylococci, streptococci, enterococci etc.), Bacteroides, gonococci and meningococci, Legionella pneumophila and Chlamydia trachomatis. Some atypical mycobacteria (M. kansasii, M. marinum, M. avium-intracellulare, M. scrofulaceum etc.) are moderately sensitive and gram-negative strains are relatively insensitive (except for Haemophilus influenzae, which is very sensitive). Rifampicin is effective in leprosy. Penicillin-resistant pneumococci are generally sensitive to rifampicin.

Resistance: Primary resistance in tubercle bacilli is rare (less than 1%). Resistance of the streptomycin type (one-step resistance) develops rapidly in staphylococci, gonococci, meningococci and other bacteria, but only after several weeks of single drug therapy in tubercle bacilli. No cross-resistance with other antituberculous agents.

Pharmacokinetics:
Absorption is good after oral intake. *Peak blood concentrations* occur after 2–4 hours. *Serum concentrations* after 600 mg by mouth are 7–14 mg/l at 2 h and 2 mg/l at 12 h. *Serum concentrations* at the end of 3-h i. v. infusions of 300 and 600 mg are 4 and 13 mg/l respectively. *Half-life:* 3 hours, which is shortened on continuous treatment, probably due to increased biliary excretion, and prolonged to 4–7 hours in liver disorders but unaffected by *renal failure*. Rifampicin does not accumulate. *Plasma protein binding:* 75 to 80%. This highly lipophilic antibiotic diffuses rapidly into the lungs, kidneys, adrenal glands and liver, where the concentration can even be higher than in the blood, depending on the time of administration. Rifampicin penetrates cells (e. g. leukocytes) as well as bronchial secretion, pleural and peritoneal fluid. Poor *CSF penetration* (0–11%), but better in meningitis (10–90%).

Excretion (after 900 mg orally) of about 40% in the bile and up to 30% in the urine, 30–50% of which is unchanged. The principal metabolite is desacetyl rifampicin, which also has antibacterial activity. The urinary recovery decreases with smaller doses, and a larger proportion is excreted in the bile, much of which is then reabsorbed in the intestines; this enterohepatic recirculation is partly responsible for the maintenance of therapeutic blood concentrations for 12 hours or more after each dose. Not eliminated by haemodialysis.

Side-effects: Increases in liver transaminases (aminotransferases) are found in about 5–20% of cases, although levels often return to normal in spite of continued treatment. Rifampicin therapy must be stopped immediately if the transaminases rise higher than 100 IU/litre or the serum bilirubin increases, since fatal acute hepatitis has been reported. Most patients will tolerate the resumption of rifampicin after an interval. This hepatotoxicity necessitates the regular monitoring of serum transaminases.

Other side-effects include gastrointestinal upset, cutaneous symptoms (pruritus and flushes with or without a rash) and transient leukocytopenia or thrombocytopenia. Central nervous disorders include drowsiness, ataxia, visual disturbances, muscle weakness, pain in the extremities and numbness. Rifampicin very occasionally causes renal failure, apparently as a result of hypersensitivity and shown as interstitial nephritis, acute tubular necrosis or severe cortical necrosis. This can result from the interruption and subsequent resumption of rifampicin therapy. The urine, saliva and other body secretions are coloured orange-red. Soft contact lenses will be discoloured, and patients should be warned of this side-effect before starting treatment.

Interactions: Rifampicin interferes with oral contraception with ovulation inhibitors and also with the activity of coumarin anticoagulants. Frequent coagulation tests are therefore necessary in patients on simultaneous long term dicoumarol treatment. Enzyme induction in the liver can shorten the metabolism of oral hypoglycaemic agents, digitalis derivatives, quinidine and corticosteroids. Regular methadone users may experience withdrawal symptoms because of increased hepatic metabolism of methadone. Simultaneous administration of hepatotoxic substances (e. g. ketoconazole) confers a higher risk of liver damage.

Indications: All stages of tuberculosis, including initial treatment in combination with isoniazid and ethambutol or streptomycin; infections with atypical mycobacteria; leprosy. Although activity on gram-positive cocci and neisseria is very good, the risk of rapid development of resistance is high in nontuberculous infections so treatment with rifampicin alone should generally be avoided. The drug is valuable, however, in combination with other agents (e. g. trimethoprim, vancomycin) to treat chronic or inaccessible infections with organisms resistant to other antibiotics, e. g. chronic infections of implanted heart valves or ventriculoperitoneal shunts with multi-resistant strains of Staphylococcus epidermidis. Rifampicin may be used in legionellosis in combination with erythromycin. Rifampicin is recommended for the prophylaxis of meningococcal infection in close contacts (household and saliva-exchange) of patients with meningococcal meningitis.

Contra-indications: Acute hepatitis, obstructive jaundice, other severe liver diseases, pregnancy (rule out pregnancy before starting treatment).

Caution when combined with hepatotoxic antituberculous drugs (prothionamide, pyrazinamide), in alcoholism, pre-existing liver disease and previous intolerance of rifampicin.

Administration and dosage: 10 mg/kg (generally 600 mg) in adults by mouth or i. v. infusion. 10 mg/kg daily in children aged 6 to 12 years but 15 mg/kg in 1–2 doses 1 h before meals in children up to 6 years. Use in the newborn only when unequivocally indicated (risk of haemorrhage), increasing the dose progressively (up to 10 mg/kg daily). Maximum dose in adults 750 mg (orally) and 600 mg (i. v.).

When treatment is resumed after long-term therapy, a progressively increasing dosage regime is recommended (initial dose 75 mg per day, increasing in stages of 75 mg per day up to the required dosage). Renal function should be carefully monitored.

For the chemoprophylaxis of haemophilus meningitis in infants and pre-school children up to the age of 4 years who are close contacts of cases, an oral dose of 10 mg/kg twice daily for 4 days is recommended. For prophylaxis of meningococcal infections give adults 600 mg and children 10 mg/kg every 12 h for 2 days.

Preparations: Capsules, coated tablets and tablets of 50 mg, 150 mg, 300 mg, 450 mg and 600 mg; syrup (20 mg/ml); ampoules of 300 mg and 600 mg.

Combined preparations:
Rifampicin 120 mg + isoniazid 50 mg + pyrazinamide 300 mg (Rifater),
Rifampicin 150 mg + isoniazid 100 mg (Rifinah 150),
Rifampicin 300 mg + isoniazid 150 mg (Rifinah 300),
Rifampicin 150 mg + isoniazid 100 mg (Rimactazid 150),
Rifampicin 300 mg + isoniazid 150 mg (Rimactazid 300).

Summary: Rifampicin is a very active oral first-line antituberculous agent which should always be used in combination with 1 or 2 other antituberculous agents (e. g. isoniazid and ethambutol) in order to prevent the development of secondary resistance. Rifampicin is not recommended for infections other than tuberculosis and leprosy except in severe or inaccessible infections by multiresistant staphylococci (always in combination with another antistaphylococcal agent).

References

ACOCELLA, G.: Pharmacokinetics and metabolism of rifampin in humans. Rev. Infect. Dis. 5 *(Suppl. 3):* 428 (1983).
BACIEWICZ, A. M., T. H. SELF, W. B. BEKEMEYER: Update on rifampin drug interactions. Arch. Intern. Med. *147:* 565 (1987).
COHN, J. R., D. L. FYE, J. M. SILLS, G. C. FRANCOS: Rifampicin-induced renal failure. Tubercle *66:* 289 (1985).
DANIELS, N. J., J. S. DOVER, R. K. SCHACHTER: Interaction between cyclosporin and rifampicin. Lancet *2:* 639 (1984).
GROSSET, J., S. LEVENTIS: Adverse effects of rifampin. Rev. Infect. Dis. 5 *(Suppl. 3):* 440 (1983).
GRÜNEBERG, R. N., A. M. EMMERSON, A. W. CREMER: Rifampicin for non-tuberculosis infections? Chemotherapy *31:* 324 (1985).
HACKBARTH, C. J., H. F. CHAMBERS, M. A. SANDE: Serum bactericidal activity of rifampin in combination with other antimicrobial agents against Staphylococcus aureus. Antimicrob. Ag. Chemother. *29:* 611 (1986).
HEIFETS, L. B.: Synergistic effects of rifampin, streptomycin and ethambutol on Mycobacterium intracellulare. Am. Rev. Respir. Dis. *125:* 43 (1982).
KAY, L., J. P. KAMPRANN, T. L. SVENDSEN et. al.: Influence of rifampin and isoniazid on the kinetics of phenytoin. Br. J. Clin. Pharmacol. *20:* 323 (1985).
KHALIL, S. A. K., L. K. EL-KHORDAGUI, Z. A. EL-GHOLMY: Effect of antacids on oral absorption of rifampicin. Int. J. Pharm. *20:* 99 (1984).
LOWY, F. D., D. S. CHANG, P. R. LASH: Synergy of combination of vancomycin, gentamicin, and rifampin against methicillin-resistant, coagulase-negative staphylococci. Antimicrob. Ag. Chemother. *23:* 932 (1983).
MARIETTE, X., M. T. MITJAVILA, J. P. MOULINIE, A. BUSSEL, J. C. BROUET, W. VAINCHENKER, J. P. FERMAND: Rifampicin-induced pure red cell aplasia. Am. J. Med. *87:* 459–460 (1989).
MURPHY, T. V., D. F. CHRANE, G. H. MCCRACKEN JR., J. D. NELSON: Rifampin prophylaxis vs. placebo for household contacts of children with Haemophilus influenzae type b disease. Am. J. Dis. Children. *137:* 627 (1983).
NICOLLE, L. E., B. POSTL, E. KOTELEWETZ et al.: Emergence of rifampin-resistant Haemophilus influenzae. Antimicrob. Ag. Chemother. *21:* 498 (1982).

Pezzia, W., J. W. Raleigh, M. C. Bailey et al.: Treatment of pulmonary disease due to Mycobacterium kansasii: recent experience with rifampin. Rev. Infect. Dis. *3:* 1035 (1981).

Powell-Jackson, P. R., A. P. Jamieson, B. J. Gray et. al.: Effect of rifampicin administration on theophylline pharmacokinetics in humans. Am. Rev. Respir. Dis. *131:* 939 (1985).

Raghupati Sarma, G., C. Immanuel, S. Kailasam et. al.: Rifampicin-induced release of hydrazine from isoniazid: a possible cause of hepatitis during treatment of tuberculosis with regimens containing isoniazid and rifampin. Am. Rev. Respir. Dis. *133:* 1072 (1986).

Skakun, N. P., V. V. Shamanko: Synergistic effect of rifampicin on hepatotoxicity of isoniazid. Antibiot. Med. Biotechnol. *30:* 185 (1985).

Varaldo, P. E., E. Debbia, G. C. Schito: In vitro activities of rifapentine and rifampin, alone and in combination with six other antibiotics, against methicillin-susceptible and methicillin-resistant staphylococci of different species. Antimicrob. Ag. Chemother. *27:* 615 (1985).

Wilkins, E. G., E. Hnizdo, A. Cope: Addisonian crisis induced by treatment with rifampicin. Tubercle *70:* 69–73 (1989).

c) Ethambutol

Proprietary names: Myambutol. Combined with isoniazid in various dose ratios as Mynah.

Description: A stable, synthetic, water-soluble, dextrorotatory ethylene diamine derivative.

Spectrum of activity: Bacteriostatic on proliferating, but not resting bacteria.

Active against Mycobacterium tuberculosis and many strains of Mycobacterium kansasii, M. avium-intracellulare, M. scrofulaceum and M. marinum, but not Mycobacterium fortuitum or Mycobacterium chelonei. Resistance develops slowly during therapy. No cross-resistance with other antituberculous agents. Primary resistance is found in about 4% of strains of M. tuberculosis.

Pharmacokinetics:
Absorption after oral intake: 70–80%, with maximum blood concentrations after 2 hours. *Serum concentrations* (after 25 mg/kg by mouth): 4.4 mg/l (2 h) and 2.3 mg/l (8 h). *Half-life:* 4–6 h. Concentrated in the erythrocytes which contain 2–3 times as much ethambutol as the plasma. Little *serum protein binding.* *Cerebrospinal fluid* concentrations of 1–2 mg/l are found in tuberculous meningitis (after 25 mg/kg daily by mouth).

Slow renal excretion of 70–80% of the dose, including 8–15% as inactive metabolites. About 20% passes out with the faeces.

Side-effects: Retrobulbar neuritis of the optic nerve, shown initially as disturbance of green vision followed by general weakness of vision, hemianopia and finally optic nerve atrophy. This effect is common at high doses but rare at doses of 15 mg/kg or less. These changes are initially reversible but regress slowly and are seldom irreversible. Their frequency at normal dosage is 0–6%. Peripheral neuropathy, central nervous disorders, allergic rashes, attacks of gout (due to increased uric acid) and transient disturbances of liver function are rare.

Indications: Combined treatment of pulmonary tuberculosis, and in infections caused by atypical mycobacteria or where the organisms are resistant to other antituberculous agents.

Contra-indications: Optic nerve atrophy or a history of retrobulbar neuritis. Reduce dose in renal failure.

Administration and dosage: The initial dose of 15 mg/kg once a day by mouth should always be combined with 1 or 2 other effective antituberculous agents. Higher doses (25 mg/kg) for up to 2 months may be given when treatment needs to be repeated, after which the daily dose should be reduced to 15 mg/kg. The dose by the i.m. or i.v. route is the same as by mouth. An ophthalmic examination should be performed before the start and then every 4 weeks during treatment, and should test colour vision, visual fields, visual acuity and the appearance of the fundus. A fundus check alone is not sufficient. Give the maintenance dose every 36 hours when the creatinine clearance is 10–50 ml/min, and every 48 hours with creatinine clearances of less than 10 ml/min.

Preparations: Tablets of 100 and 400 mg and ampoules of 200 and 400 mg and 1 g. A combined oral preparation with isoniazid is available in 4 dose ratios of ethambutol to isoniazid, namely 200 mg:100 mg (Mynah 200), 250 mg:100 mg (Mynah 250), 300 mg:100 mg (Mynah 300) and 365 mg:100 mg (Mynah 365).

Summary: An effective first-line antituberculous agent.

References

Gulliford, M., A. D. Mackay, K. Prowse: Cholestatic jaundice caused by ethambutol. Brit. Med. J. 292: 866 (1986).
Khanna, B. K. I., V. P. Gupta, M. P. Singh: Ethambutol-induced hyperuricemia. Tubercle 65: 195 (1984).
Pöso, H., L. Paulin, E. Brander: Specific inhibition of spermidine synthase from mycobacteria by ethambutol. Lancet 2: 1418 (1983).
Prasad, R., P. K. Mukerji: Ethambutol-induced thrombocytopenia. Tubercle 70: 211–212 (1989).

d) Streptomycin

Properties: Aminoglycoside (aminocyclitol), which is stable, readily soluble in water and marketed as the sulphate.

Mode of action: More actively bactericidal in the proliferative than in the resting phase of bacterial growth (in the presence of metabolic activity).

Range of action: Mycobacterium tuberculosis, brucella, Haemophilus ducreyi, Francisella tularensis and Yersinia pestis are usually sensitive. There is variable sensitivity (some strains being resistant) amongst Mycobacterium xenopi and M. ulcerans, streptococci, enterococci, staphylococci, Escherichia coli, Klebsiella, Proteus species, Pseudomonas aeruginosa, Actinomyces israeli and certain other species.
Other atypical mycobacteria, clostridia, bacteroides and rickettsiae are resistant.

Resistance: Primary resistance in strains of Mycobacterium tuberculosis is found with varying frequency (2–30%), but is rare in advanced countries. It is seen more often, however, in patients from developing countries where tuberculosis is common and often inadequately treated. Resistance can develop rapidly within a few days by mutation (one-step resistance). There is cross-resistance in tubercle bacilli between streptomycin on the one hand and kanamycin, viomycin and capreomycin on the other, but it is usually one-way, so that strains which have become resistant to streptomycin are generally still sensitive to these other drugs, but not the other way around.

Pharmacokinetics:
Virtually *not absorbed* by mouth.
Serum concentrations after i. m. injection of 500 mg are 14–30 mg/l after 1–2 h and 2–3 mg/l after 11–12 h; after 1 g, they are 20–45 mg/l after 1–2 h and 4–6 mg/l after 11–12 h (Fig. 55).
Half-life: 2½ hours; prolonged in renal failure and in the newborn. *Plasma protein binding:* 30%.
CSF penetration: Very poor (2–4% of serum concentrations, increased to 10–20% in acute meningitis).
Tissue diffusion: Adequate concentrations are attained in lung, muscle, uterus, intestinal mucosa, adrenals and lymph nodes. Diffusion into bone, brain and aqueous humor is poor. Increasing concentrations of 30–100% of peak plasma levels can be achieved on repeated dosing in pleural, peritoneal and synovial fluids. The breast milk has the same concentration as serum. 50% of the mother's serum concentrations are found in cord blood and amniotic fluid.
Excretion: 50–60% excreted in the urine, predominantly by glomerular filtration. Urinary concentrations after 500 mg i. m. are 200–1500 mg/l in the first

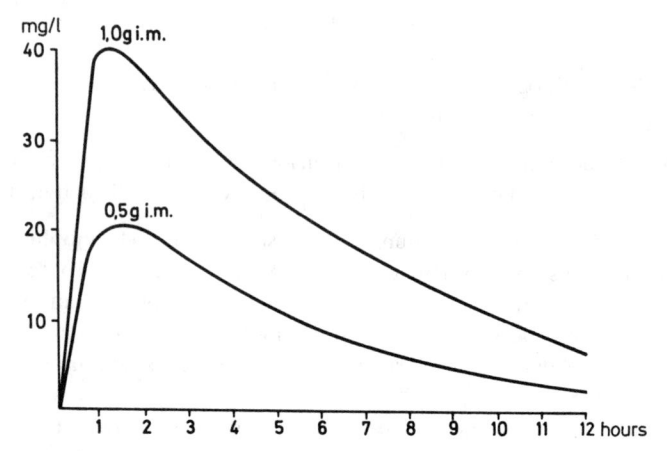

Fig. 55: Blood concentrations after a single i. m. injection of streptomycin.

6 hours. About 2% of the dose is excreted in the bile and faeces. Slowly haemodiatysable.

Side-effects:
1. *Neurotoxicity:* Vestibular damage can be caused by streptomycin in about 30% of cases, and cochlear damage by dihydrostreptomycin in about 26%. These toxic effects depend on the dose and length of treatment and are commoner when the daily dose of 1 g or the total dose of 60 g are exceeded. *Dihydrostreptomycin* should no longer be used because of its greater ototoxicity. In rare cases (about 6%) streptomycin may cause deafness. Renal, vestibular and auditory function should be monitored regularly throughout streptomycin therapy, preferably every 2 weeks. If audiometry is not possible, for example in small children, assay blood concentrations of streptomycin to detect accumulation due to impaired excretion, as shown by rising "trough" (pre-dose) concentrations. Do not exceed a maximum ("peak") concentration of 25 mg/l. These precautions also apply to combinations of streptomycin with pantothenic acid, which have the same neurotoxicity. The patient can only be protected from permanent damage by careful dosage, regular monitoring of oto- and neurological function, and the prompt cessation of streptomycin at the first signs of any disorder of balance or hearing. Streptomycin given during pregnancy may damage the hearing of the baby, and so should only be used then if there is no alternative.
2. *Nephrotoxicity* can be acute in overdose and is shown by an increased blood urea, proteinuria, microhaematuria and casts.

3. *Allergic reactions* are relatively common, as shown by eosinophilia and rashes but rarely as anaphylactic shock or exfoliative dermatitis. Nursing staff sometimes suffer from contact dermatitis.
4. *Immediate reactions* (perioral paraesthesia, blurred vision, dizziness, behavioural disturbances) are harmless and are probably caused by the release of histamine from tissue mast cells.
5. *Others:* Hepatotoxic effects, eye muscle damage, scotoma, aplastic or haemolytic anaemia, agranulocytosis, leukocytopenia and thrombocytopenia are extremely rare.
6. The *intraperitoneal injection* of streptomycin may lead to a dangerous neuromuscular blockade with respiratory arrest, which can also occur after i. m. injection prior to anaesthesia or in conjunction with a muscle relaxant. Patients with myasthenia gravis are at particular risk. Treat with artificial respiration and inject prostigmine (0.1 mg i. v. every 2 min up to a total dose of 1 mg) and calcium gluconate.

Indications: Combination with other antibiotics to treat tuberculosis. For endocarditis and brucellosis, gentamicin is a better combination partner.

Incorrect use: As a single agent in tuberculosis.

Contra-indications: Anuria, severe renal failure and pregnancy. Use with care in the elderly (reduce daily dose). Avoid dihydrostreptomycin. Do not combine streptomycin with capreomycin, gentamicin or other aminoglycosides, or rapidly acting diuretics such as ethacrynic acid or frusemide (Lasix), which are also ototoxic.

Administration:
Parenteral route: Generally by i. m. injection of streptomycin sulphate at concentrations which do not exceed 500 mg/ml, i. e. 1 g in 2 ml, but occasionally as a continuous i. v. infusion (concentration 1 mg/ml) delivered 1 (–2) g over 7–8 hours in order to achieve a constant high blood level. There is a theoretical risk of toxic peaks of concentration with i. v. injection, although infusion carries the risk of thrombophlebitis. Do not instil streptomycin into the peritoneum because of the risk of respiratory arrest.

Dosage: *I. m. route* (adults) 700 mg–1.5 g (15 mg/kg) a day; for children (3 months –12 years): 20–30 mg/kg/day with a maximum of 1 g; for infants aged up to 3 months: 10 mg/kg/day up to a maximum of 50 mg in 3 divided doses; 1 injection per day is sufficient for tuberculosis. The daily dose for patients over 50 should not exceed 500 mg. Duration of treatment: 1–2 months in tuberculosis, with a maximum total dosage of 30–60 g for adults, 15–20 g for children and 10 g for infants. Longer courses of treatment are permissible, provided regular audiometry and vestibular tests are performed and treatment is stopped at the

onset of any signs of inner ear damage, which is generally reversible at that stage. If renal insufficiency is not severe, prolong the dosage interval to:
48 h (creatinine clearance of 60 ml/min),
72 h (creatinine clearance of 40 ml/min),
96 h (creatinine clearance of 30 ml/min).

The following concentrations may be used for *intrapleural* and *intra-articular* instillation: 0.5–1 g in 20–25 ml (25–50 mg/ml), and less in children, depending on their age.

Intrathecal administration is irritant and can give rise to other side-effects; since the advent of newer antituberculous agents which penetrate the CSF well intrathecal streptomycin is now almost never necessary.

Preparations: Vials of 500 mg, 1 g.

Summary

Advantages: Bactericidal on tubercle bacilli when used in combination with other agents.

Disadvantages: Rapid development of resistance when used alone, neurotoxicity and risk of hypersensitivity.

Streptomycin should now be regarded as an agent for use in combination with others in tuberculosis only. Dihydrostreptomycin is still available in some countries (not Britain) but should no longer be used because of its toxicity.

References

FARBER, B. F., G. M. ELIOPOULOS, J. I. WARD et al.: Resistance to penicillin-streptomycin synergy among clinical isolates of viridans streptococci. Antimicrob. Ag. Chemother. *24:* 871 (1983).

SARKAR, S. K., S. D. PUROHIT, T. N. SHARMA et al.: Stevens-Johnson syndrome caused by streptomycin. Tubercle *63:* 137 (1982).

e) Thioamides (Ethionamide and Prothionamide)

Proprietary names: Prothionamide and ethionamide are no longer marketed in Britain.

Description: Ethionamide is an α-ethylthioisonicotinamide (a derivative of isonicotinic acid), and prothionamide is a propyl-2-thionicotinic acid amide; both are unstable, poorly soluble in water but readily soluble in dimethyl sulphoxide.

Mode of action: Bacteriostatic at therapeutic concentrations, but bactericidal at higher concentrations.

Spectrum of action: Tubercle bacilli, M. leprae and some atypical mycobacteria (e. g. M. kansasii).

Resistance develops rapidly. Complete cross-resistance between ethionamide and prothionamide. No cross-resistance with isoniazid.

Pharmacokinetics:
Absorption after oral intake is more rapid with prothionamide than with ethionamide; the *serum concentration* of prothionamide after 1 h is therefore almost twice as high as that of ethionamide (5.7 mg/l after 500 mg by mouth), but after 6 h it is only one third of the ethionamide concentration (0.9 mg/l). *Half-life:* 3 h. *Tissue* and *CSF penetration* are both good (30–60%), as is penetration into cells. Metabolism is almost complete (more than 95%). One of the numerous metabolites is sulphoxide, which has antituberculous properties itself.

Excretion: Primarily renal, but less than 1% in active form; the mean urinary concentration of active ethionamide after 500 mg by mouth is 10–20 mg/l.

Side-effects: Gastrointestinal disorders are less frequent with prothionamide than with ethionamide, and are less frequent after i. v. injection. Other side-effects include neurotoxic and psychic disturbances (headaches, dizziness, restlessness, sleep disturbances, peripheral neuropathy, depression, and convulsions in epileptics), acne and pellagra, photosensitisation of the skin, liver damage (particularly in diabetics), hypoglycaemia in diabetics, hypothyroidism, eosinophilia, leukocytopenia, gynaecomastia and menstrual disorders. Prophylaxis and treatment of these effects with pyridoxine (50–150 mg a day) is sometimes effective.

Indication: Used in tuberculosis in combination with other antituberculous agents, particularly when there is resistance to isoniazid, and in leprosy.

Contra-indications: Early pregnancy, severe liver damage, gastric complaints. Use with care in epilepsy and psychotic patients. Avoid alcohol. Avoid combination with isoniazid and cycloserine and wherever possible because of the potentiation of side-effects.

Dosage:
By mouth, give ethionamide and prothionamide in small doses initially and slowly increase to:

Adults	750 mg (–1 g)	
Children up to 4 y.	25 mg/kg	in 3–4 divided doses
Children 4–8 y.	20 mg/kg	
Children of 8 y. and above	15 mg/kg	

Every patient treated with prothionamide should have serum transaminases monitored to detect incipient hepatotoxicity.

Preparations: Tablets and coated tablets of 250 mg, and infusion packs of 500 mg.

Summary: Reliable antituberculous agents which diffuse well into tissues but which cause frequent side-effects and carry the risk of rapid development of bacterial resistance; use only in small doses, combined with other agents, as second-line drugs when others have failed or not been tolerated.

References

BAOHONG, J. I., C. JIAKUN, W. CHENMIN, X. GUANG: Hepatotoxicity of combined therapy with rifampicin and daily prothionamide for leprosy. Lepr. Rev. 55: 283 (1984).

CARTEL, J. L., Y. NAUDILLON, J. C. ARTUS, J. H. GROSSET: Hepatotoxicity of the daily combination of 5 mg/kg prothionamide plus 10 mg/kg rifampin. Int. J. Leprosy 53: 15 (1985).

DRUCKER, D., M. C. EGGO, I. E. SALIT, G. N. BURROW: Ethionamide-induced goitrous hypothyroidism. Ann. Intern. Med. 100: 837 (1984).

JENNER, P. J., G. A. ELLARD, P. J. K. GRUER, V. R. ABER: A comparison of the blood levels and urinary excretion of ethionamide and prothionamide in man. Antimicrob. Ag. Chemother. 13: 267 (1984).

f) Pyrazinamide

Proprietary name: Zinamide.

Description: Pyrazine carboxylic acid amide, a stable, moderately water-soluble chemotherapeutic agent.

Mode of action: Bactericidal on human but not bovine tubercle bacilli, nor usually on atypical mycobacteria. More active at acid pH, so particularly effective in caseous necrosis. Almost inactive at neutral pH. No cross-resistance with other antituberculous agents.

Pharmacokinetics:
Absorption: Maximum blood concentrations occur after 1–2 hours.
Serum concentrations (after a single oral dose of 1 g): 40–45 mg/l after 2 h and 10 mg/l after 15 h. *Half-life:* 6 h. Highly metabolised. Good *tissue* and *CSF penetration.*
3% *excreted* unaltered through the kidneys, the remainder as the weakly antibacterial compound pyrazinoic acid.

Side-effects: The risk of liver damage has been overestimated. Functional disorders of the liver were apparently mostly caused by the simultaneous administration of PAS. Besides jaundice, there may be gastrointestinal complaints, hyperuricaemia with attacks of gout, and hyperglycaemia. Photosensitisation may occur.

Interactions: Concurrent allopurinol can reduce uric acid excretion, and the simultaneous administration of an oral antidiabetic agent can further depress the blood sugar.

Indications: Initial therapy of caseous tuberculosis. Treatment for longer than 2 months is not recommended.

Contra-indications: Severe liver damage and gout. Reduce dose in renal impairment.

Administration and dosage: 1.5–2.5 g daily by mouth for *adults*, and 30 mg/kg a day for *children* in 2 or 3 divided doses. Check the serum transaminases every 2–3 weeks during treatment and stop therapy at the first sign of liver damage.

Preparations: Tablets of 500 mg.

Summary: A bactericidal antituberculous agent for initial chemotherapy (first-line drug).

References

PILHEU, J. A., M. C. DE SALVO, O. R. KOCH et al.: Effect of pyrazinamide on the liver of tuberculosis patients: electron microscopic study. Bull. Int. Union Tuberc. *59:* 115 (1984).

SALFINGER, M., A. J. CROWLE, L. B. RELLER: Pyrazinamide and pyrazinoic acid activity against tubercle bacilli in cultured human macrophages and in the BACTEC system. J. Infect. Dis. *162:* 201–207 (1990).

SARMA, G. R., G. S. ACHARYULU, M. KANNAPIRAN et al.: Role of rifampicin in arthralgia induced by pyrazinamide. Tubercle *64:* 93 (1983).

g) Capreomycin

Proprietary name: Capastat.

Description: An aminoglycoside. The sulphate is stable and water-soluble. Bacteriostatic on tubercle bacilli, but little action on other bacteria; generally less active than streptomycin *in vitro* and *in vivo*.

Resistance: Primary resistance is rare. Resistance develops quite rapidly during treatment, and there is partial cross-resistance with kanamycin.

Pharmacokinetics:
Not *absorbed* by mouth. *Maximum blood concentrations* occur 1–2 hours after i.m. injection. *Serum concentrations* after 1 g i.m. are 29 mg/l after 2 h and 4 mg/l after 10 h. *Half-life:* 5 hours. *Excretion* is about 50–70% in active form with the urine.

Side-effects: Ototoxicity is possibly somewhat less than with streptomycin and kanamycin, as is nephrotoxicity. Fever, rashes and eosinophilia can occur.

Indications: Treatment of tuberculosis with strains resistant to streptomycin. May also be used as initial therapy of recurrent tuberculosis.

Contra-indications: Severe renal insufficiency, pre-existing middle ear damage, pregnancy.

Dosage: 1 g a day for *adults*, 20 mg/kg a day for *children*, for 1–2 months, later 2–3 times a week. Regular audiometric and renal functions tests are necessary. Use only in combination with two other antituberculous agents, but not with streptomycin (additive toxicity). In moderate *renal impairment*, prolong the dose interval to 48 h (creatinine clearance 60 ml/min), to 72 h (creatinine clearance 40 ml/min) or to 96 h (creatinine clearance 30 ml/min).

Preparations: Vials of 1 g.

Summary: A very effective second-line antituberculous agent which carries a risk of ototoxicity. Of only minor importance today.

References

ANDREWS, R. H., P. A. JENKINS, J. MARKS, A. PINES, J. B. SELKON, A. R. SOMNER: Treatment of isoniazid-resistant pulmonary tuberculosis with ethambutol, rifampicin and capreomycin: A co-operative study in England and Wales: Tubercle *55:* 105 (1974).
MCCLATCHY, J. K., W. KANES, P. T. DAVIDSON, T. S. MOULDING: Cross-resistance in M. tuberculosis to kanamycin, capreomycin and viomycin. Tubercle *58:* 29 (1977).

h) Dapsone

Properties: A diaminodiphenyl sulphone. A crystalline powder insoluble in water. Inhibits folic acid synthesis in leprosy bacteria. Secondary resistance can occur after use as a single agent at low dosage for periods of years. It should therefore only be used in combination with rifampicin and/or clofazimine. Also useful for non-specific treatment of dermatitis herpetiformis. Its structural formula is shown in Fig. 56.

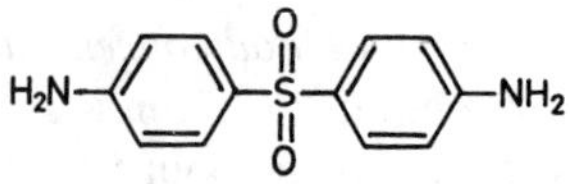

Fig. 56. Structural formula of dapsone

Pharmacokinetics: Well absorbed after oral administration with *maximal serum concentrations* after 4–8 h. The long *half-life* of 1–2 days and slow urinary excretion as water-soluble metabolites gives rise to almost constant blood levels and high tissue concentrations, particularly in affected skin.

Side-effects occur frequently. Regular blood counts are necessary because of the danger of haemolysis (particularly in G-6-PD deficiency), methaemoglobinaemia and blood dyscrasias. Gastro-intestinal disorders and allergic reactions occasionally occur. Peripheral neuropathy and renal damage are rare. Erythema nodosum leprosum occurs frequently and usually requires corticosteroids if dapsone treatment is to continue.

Interactions: Rifampicin reduces the blood levels of dapsone as a result of decreased plasma clearance. Pyrimethamine increases the danger of blood dyscrasia.

Dosage: Leprosy is treated by dapsone 100 mg daily by mouth, combined with rifampicin 600 mg once a month. Clofazimine (see page 276) may be considered as a third agent. Clofazimine may also be given in place of dapsone in sulphone-resistant leprosy. The duration of treatment varies according to the type of disease but is usually for many years and sometimes lifelong.

References

CARTEL, J.-L., J. MILLAN, C. C. GUELPA-LAURAS, J. H. GROSSET: Hepatitis in leprosy patients treated by a daily combination of dapsone, rifampin, and a thiomide. Int. J. Lepr. *51:* 461 (1983).
FOUCAULD, J., W. UPHOUSE, J. BERENBERG: Dapsone and aplastic anemia. Ann. Intern. Med. *102:* 139 (1985).
IMKAMP, F. M. J. H., R. ANDERSON, E. M. S. GATNER: Possible incompatibility of dapsone with clofazimine in the treatment of patients with erythema nodosum leprosum. Lepr. Rev. *53:* 148 (1982).
LEOUNG, G. S., J. MILLS, P. C. HOPEWELL et al.: Dapsone-trimethoprim for Pneumocystis carinii pneumonia in the acquired immunodeficiency syndrome. Ann. Intern. Med. *105:* 45 (1986).
LEVY, L.: Primary resistance to dapsone among untreated lepromatous patients in Bamako and Chingleput. Leprosy Rev. *54:* 177 (1983).
PELLIL, J. H. S.: Dapsone-induced haemolytic anaemia. Brit. J. Dermatol. *102:* 365 (1980).
POULSEN, A., B. HULTBERG, K. THOMASEN, G. L. WANTZING: Regression of Kaposi's sarcoma in AIDS after treatment with dapsone. Lancet *1:* 560 (1984).
WALDINGER, T. P., R. J. SIEGLE, W. WEBERT, J. J. VOORHEES: Dapsone induced peripheral neuropathy: case report and review. Arch. Dermatol. *120:* 356 (1984).
YAWALKAR, S. J., A. C. McDOUGALL, J. LANGUILLON, S. GHOSH, D. V. A. OPROMOLLA et al.: Once-monthly rifampicin plus daily dapsone in initial treatment of lepromatous leprosy. Lancet *1:* 1199 (1982).

i) Clofazimine

Proprietary name: Lamprene.

Properties: A phenazine dye with special activity against Mycobacterium leprae; it should only be given in combination with one or two other anti-leprosy drugs. Clofazimine may be used to prevent the emergence of secondary resistance during long-term treatment with dapsone.

Indications:
1. Prevention of secondary sulphone resistance in leprosy.
2. Prevention of lepra reactions in lepromatous and borderline leprosy.
3. Treatment of sulphone-resistant leprosy.
4. Treatment of lepra reactions (e.g. erythema nodosum).
5. Treatment of infections with susceptible atypical mycobacteria.

Contra-indications: Pregnancy, severe hepatic or renal failure.

Dosage and administration:
1. To prevent sulphone resistance and lepra reactions, 50–100 mg daily or 100 mg thrice weekly may be given by mouth during the first 4–6 months of long-term treatment with dapsone.
2. In sulphone-resistant leprosy, 100 mg should be taken daily by mouth in combination with rifampicin 600 mg daily during the first 2–3 months.
3. In lepra reactions 300 mg daily by mouth are recommended for the duration of the reaction for up to 3 months. As soon as the lepra reaction is under control, this dose should be reduced to a level which is barely suppressive.

The capsules should always be taken with a meal or with some milk. Reduce the dose if gastro-intestinal disorders arise. During long-term therapy and in the presence of pre-existing liver and kidney disease, hepatic and renal function should be monitored every 4 weeks.

Side-effects: Clofazimine is in general well tolerated. Red or brown-black discoloration of the skin and the leprosy lesions occurs frequently, particularly in areas exposed to the light in fair-skinned patients. Discoloration of the hair, the conjunctiva and tears, and of sweat, sputum, urine and faeces also occur. Less common side-effects are dry skin, ichthyosis, photosensitivity, acne-like eruptions and non-specific skin reactions. Nausea, vomiting, abdominal pain, diarrhoea, loss of appetite and loss of weight also occur not infrequently, particularly in the presence of concurrent amoebic or bacterial dysentery or when large doses are used for periods longer than 3 months.

References

ANDERSON, R.: Enhancement by clofazimine and inhibition by dapsone of production of prostaglandin E_2 by human polymorphonuclear leukocytes in vitro. Antimicrob. Ag. Chemother. 27: 257 (1985).
BROWNE, S. G., D. J. HARMAN, H. WAUDBY, A. C. MCDOUGALL: Clofazimine in the treatment of lepromatous leprosy in the United Kingdom. Int. J. Lepr. 49: 167 (1981).
CUNNINGHAM, C. A., D. N. FRIEDBERG, R. E. CARR: Clofazimine-induced generalized retinal degeneration. Retina 10: 131–134 (1990).
FARB, H., D. P. WEST, L. A. PEDVIS: Clofazimine in pregnancy complicated by leprosy. Obstet. Gynaecol. (USA) 59: 122 (1982).
JOB, C. K., L. YODER, R. R. JACOBSON, R. C. HASTINGS: Skin pigmentation from clofazimine therapy in leprosy patients: a reappraisal. J. Am. Acad. Dermatol. 23: 236–241 (1990).
KAUR, I., J. RAM, B. KUMAR et al.: Effects of clofazimine on eye in multibacillary leprosy. Indian. J. Lepr. 62: 87–90 (1990).
MERRET, M. N., R. W. KING, K. E. FARRELL, H. ZEIMER, E. GULI: Orange/black discolouration of the bowel (at laparotomy) due to clofazimine. Aust. N. Z. J. Surg. 60: 638–639 (1990).
OOMMEN, T.: Clofazimine-induced lymphoedema (letter). Lepr. Rev. 61: 289 (1990).
O'SULLIVAN, S., M. CORCORAN, M. BYRNE et al.: Absorption and analysis of clofazimine and its derivatives. Biochem. Soc. Trans. 18: 346–347 (1990).
PAVITHRAN, K.: Exfoliative dermatitis after clofazimine. Int. J. Leprosy 53: 645 (1985).
SCHAAD-LANYI, Z., W. DIETERLE, J.-P. DUBOIS, W. THEOBALD, W. VISCHER: Pharmacokinetics of clofazimine in healthy volunteers. Int. J. Leprosy 55, 1: 9–15 (1987).
VENKATESAN, K., A. MATHUR, B. K. GIRDHAR, V. P. BHARADWAJ: The effect of clofazimine on the pharmacokinetics of rifampicin and dapsone in leprosy. J. Antimicrob. Chemother. 18: 715–718 (1986).
WARNDORFF-VAN DIEPEN, T.: Clofazimine resistant leprosy, a case report. Int. J. Leprosy 50: 139 (1982).

j) Rifabutin

Properties: Rifabutin, an ansamycin, is a spiro-piperidyl derivative of rifamycin S whose *in-vitro* and therapeutic antituberculous activity is similar to that of rifampicin. Not available in Britain.

Spectrum of action: Ansamycin is active against Mycobacterium tuberculosis and M. leprae, including strains resistant to rifampicin. Ansamycin also inhibits Mycobacterium avium-intracellulare, M. kansasii, M. marinum and M. xenopi, as well as some strains of M. fortuitum and M. chelonei.

Pharmacokinetics: Mean serum concentrations of 0.5 mg/l are found in serum after ansamycin 300 mg orally. The tissue concentrations should, however, be considerably higher. Infections with M. avium-intracellulare in AIDS patients respond to ansamycin in 50–75% of cases.

Dosage: 150–300 mg daily per mouth.

References

HAWKINS, J. E., W. M. GROSS, F. S. VADNEY: Ansamycin (LM 427) activity against mycobacteria in vitro. Am. Rev. Respir. Dis. *129 (Suppl.):* 187 (1984).
HASTINGS, R. C., V. R. RICHARD, R. R. JACOBSON: Ansamycin activity against rifampicin-resistant Mycobacterium leprae. Lancet *1:* 1130 (1984).
HEIFETS, L. B., M. D. ISEMAN: Determination of in vitro susceptibility of mycobacteria to ansamycin. Am. Rev. Respir. Dis. *132:* 710 (1985).
PERUMAL, V. K., P. R. J. GANGADHARAM, L. B. HEIFETS et al.: Dynamic aspects of the in vitro chemotherapeutic activity of ansamycin (rifabutine) on Mycobacterium intracellulare. Am. Rev. Respir. Dis. *132:* 1278 (1985).
WOODLEY, CL., J. O. KILBURN: In vitro susceptibility of Mycobacterium avium complex and Mycobacterium tuberculosis to a spiro-piperidyl rifamycin. Am. Rev. Respir. Dis. *126:* 586 (1982).

16. Antiviral Agents

Antiviral agents should act selectively on virus-specific processes during viral replication without damaging the body's own cells. Antiviral agents can act at various points in the viral replication cycle (Fig. 57). Their activity also depends on the nature of the viral infection.

Three types of infection are recognised:

a) *Lytic infection,* in which the viral-infected cells die.

b) *Persistent infection,* in which viruses replicate in the cells but the cells survive.

c) *Latent infection,* in which viral replication becomes dormant (Fig. 58, p. 280).

In lytic viral infections (e.g. influenza) it is possible to prevent penetration of the virus into the cell (e.g. by amantadine). In persistent viral infections (e.g. AIDS) an antiviral agent (e.g. azidothymidine) can prevent viral replication but will not destroy viruses which are already present in the cells. In latent viral infections (e.g. in the course of herpes simplex) antiviral agents which inhibit viral replication (e.g. acyclovir) are ineffective during the latent period of the virus.

Of the currently available antiviral agents, amantadine acts on virus penetration, acyclovir and the other nucleoside analogues on viral replication and the interferons predominantly on the assembly and release of viruses (Table 25, p. 281).

a) Acyclovir

Proprietary name: Zovirax.

Properties: Acycloguanosine (a guanine derivative with an acyclic side chain). Active only against herpes viruses (herpes simplex and varicella zoster) but not, or only weakly, active against cytomegalovirus and Epstein-Barr virus. The poor activity against CMV and EBV is explained by the absence of viral thymidine kinase in these viruses. The structural formula is shown in Fig. 59, p. 282.

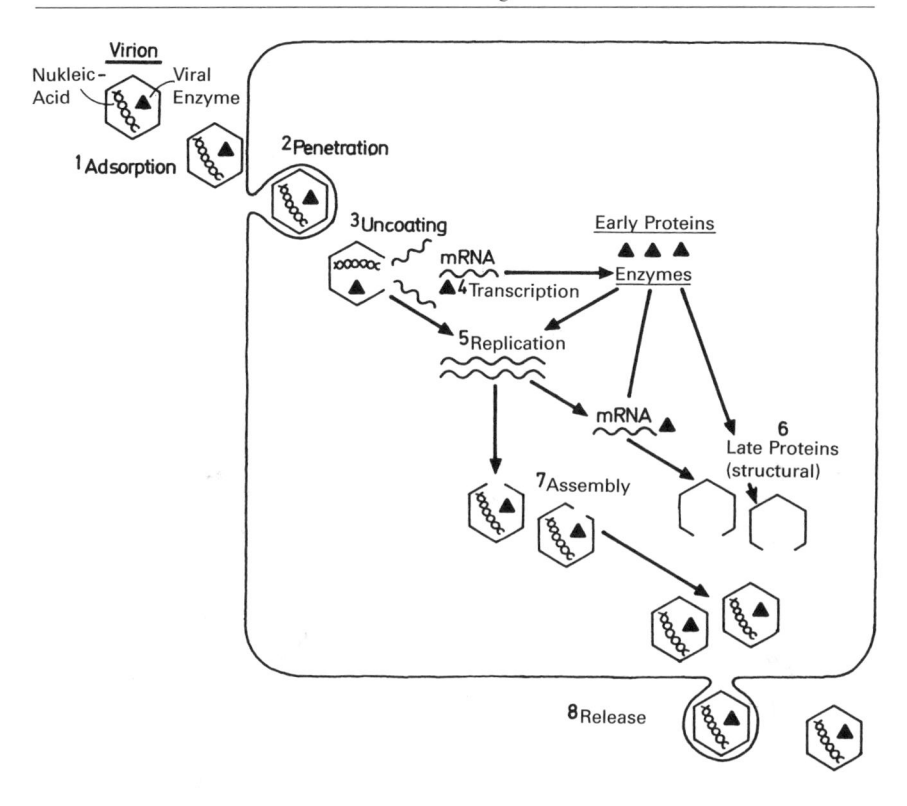

1. Adsorption of virion to cell membrane.
2. Penetration.
3. Uncoating (removal of the protein envelope).
4. Transcription of viral protein and early gene expression.
5. Replication and synthesis of DNA strands.
6. Late gene expression, transcription of messenger RNA and transfer of late protein synthesis.
7. Maturation and assembly.
8. Release of viral particles.

Fig. 57. Stages of viral replication in the cell [after BRYSON, Y. J.: Antiviral agents. In: FEIGIN, R. D., J. D. CHERRY (eds.): Textbook of Pediatric Infectious Diseases. Saunders, Philadelphia 1981].

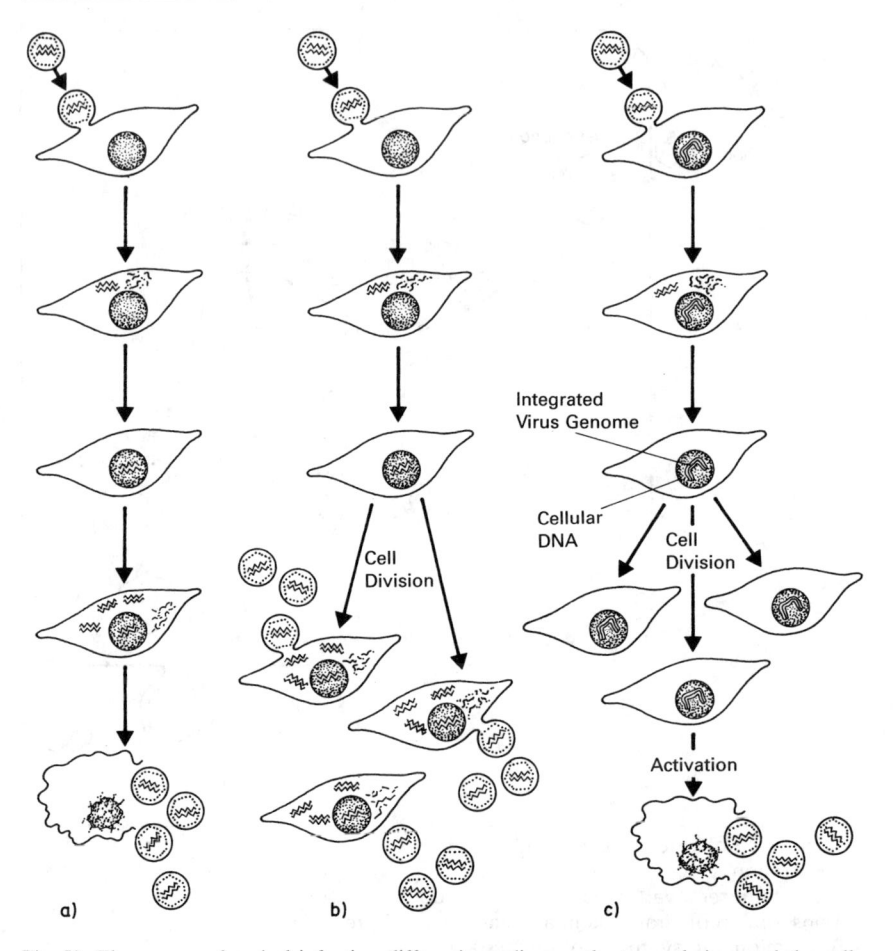

Fig. 58. The course of a viral infection differs depending on the type of virus and the cells involved.

a) *A lytic infection* eventually destroys the affected cells. After the virus has lost its protein coat within the cell, its genetic material takes over the metabolic apparatus of the cell in such a way that it produces viral proteins and nucleic acids, which are then assembled into new viral particles. The cell finally disintegrates and releases the new particles into the environment.

b) In a *persistent infection* the virus replicates but the cell survives and divides while releasing viral particles.

c) In a *latent infection* viral replication stops. The viral genome can be incorporated into the chromosomes of the cell. When the cell divides, viral material is copied at the same time and passed to the daughter cells. Under certain conditions (e. g. additional infection with another agent) the virus can suddenly be reactivated in a few cells.

Table 25. Mode and spectrum of action of antiviral agents. Uncoating = removal of the protein coat, VZV = varicella zoster virus, CMV = cytomegalovirus, RSV = respiratory syncytial virus, DDJ = Didesoxyinosine, DDC = Didesoxycytosine.

Effect on:	Drug	Inhibition of:
Penetration Uncoating	Amantadine Rimantadine	Influenza A
Replication	Idoxuridine Vidarabine Acyclovir Ganciclovir Azidothymidine, DDI, DDC Ribavirin	Herpes simplex Herpes simplex, VZV Herpes simplex, VZV CMV HIV RSV
Viral protein synthesis	Methisazone Interferon	Vaccinia, variola DNA and RNA viruses
Assembly, release	Interferon	RNA tumour viruses

Mode of action: After uptake into the infected cell, acyclovir is first transformed into acycloguanosine monophosphate by a viral thymidine kinase. The cell's own kinases produce the triphosphate from this monophosphate. This triphosphate is the active substance. Viral DNA polymerase, which catalyses the synthesis of viral DNA, attaches to the drug as though it were a normal nucleoside triphosphate (the natural DNA building unit) and hangs it on to the end of a growing DNA chain. One of the phosphate groups in acyclovir forms a bond with the 3'-hydroxyl group (OH) in the last sugar ring of the DNA chain, while both other phosphate residues are split off. Unlike a normal nucleoside, acyclovir itself possesses no sugar ring and therefore no 3'-hydroxyl group. Thus no further nucleotide can be added onto the chain. Acyclovir therefore acts as a chain terminator. Furthermore, the viral DNA polymerase which would normally catalyse the assembly of further chains remains firmly attached in the complex with the DNA and the drugs and is thus inactivated.

Acyclovir has no effect on latent viral infections, when there is no viral replication. Thus acyclovir has very little toxicity on uninfected body cells because it is only taken up by these cells and then converted into its active form in very small amounts; moreover, human DNA polymerase is not as sensitive as viral DNA polymerase to acyclovir.

Resistance: Rare strains of herpes simplex and varicella zoster have been found which are resistant *in-vitro* to acyclovir because they lack viral thymidine kinase. Such strains have also been isolated from patients during treatment, as yet without apparent clinical significance. Acyclovir-resistant herpes simplex viruses seem to be less pathogenic. They are usually sensitive to foscarnet and ganciclovir.

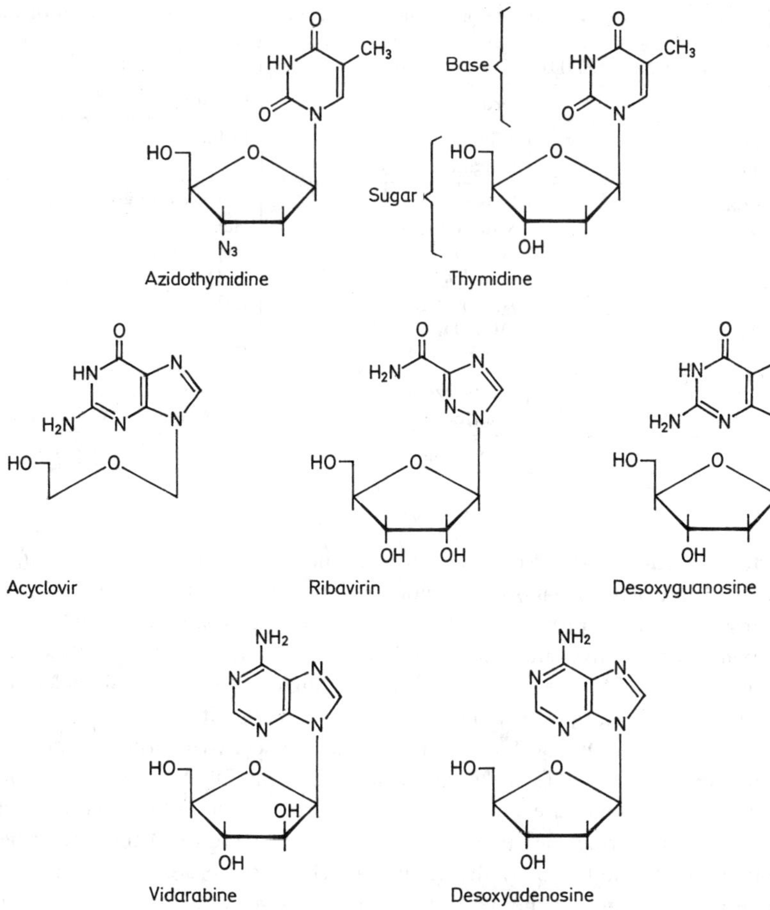

Fig. 59. Structural formulae of antiviral agents.

Pharmacokinetics: Acyclovir is only 20% absorbed by mouth. Peak serum concentrations after 200 mg and 400 mg orally are 0.6 mg/l and 0.2 mg/l respectively, and 10 mg/l at the end of an i.v. infusion of 5 mg/kg given over 1 h. *Half-life:* 2.5 h (prolonged fivefold in anuria). *Plasma protein binding:* 9–33%. *CSF concentrations* are 50% of the serum concentration. *Good tissue penetration* with high concentrations also in brain, uterus, vaginal mucosa and secretions.

Excretion is predominantly through the kidneys (by glomerular filtration and tubular secretion). 15% is excreted unchanged (orally), 75% unchanged (i.v.) and the remainder is excreted as the 9-carboxymethoxymethyl guanine metabolite.

Side-effects: Acyclovir is generally well tolerated. Oral administration gives rise in less than 3% to nausea and vomiting, and diarrhoea, headache, giddiness and skin rashes are rare. I.v. administration can cause phlebitis (in about 14% at the site of infusion), transient increase in serum creatinine, skin rashes or urticaria (4% each). Central nervous effects (somnolence, tremor, confusion, hallucinations, fits) occur in about 1% at higher dosages. Transient impairment of renal function (with elevated creatinine and occasional haematuria) are caused by crystallisation of acyclovir in the renal tubules and may be avoided by slow infusion of an adequately diluted solution and ample fluid intake. Acyclovir should not be injected rapidly i.v.

The skin cream, which contains propylene glycol and cetyl stearyl alcohol as additives, may cause burning, redness, desiccation and desquamation at the site of application. Prolonged use of the eye ointment may give rise to superficial inflammatory reactions of the lower lid and adjacent conjunctiva.

Interactions: Probenecid retards renal excretion and prolongs the *half-life* of acyclovir.

Indications:
Acyclovir i.v.:
1. Herpes simplex encephalitis.
2. Zoster, varicella and herpes simplex in HIV-infected patients.
3. Herpes simplex and varicella zoster infections in immunosuppressed patients (with leukaemia, lymphoma and organ transplants).
4. Severe primary genital herpes in non-immunosuppressed patients.
5. Herpes simplex infections in the newborn (poor prognosis).
6. Possible prophylaxis of varicella zoster infections in exposed patients after organ transplants (together with specific hyperimmune globulin).

Acyclovir orally:
1. Primary genital herpes or relapse.
2. Prophylaxis of herpes simplex infection after organ transplantation.
3. Treatment of persistent herpetic infections in AIDS.
4. Herpes zoster in non-immunosuppressed patients.

Acyclovir eye ointment:
1. Herpes simplex keratitis.
2. Corneal zoster.

Acyclovir skin cream: Palliative treatment of genital herpes and herpes labialis (though activity is unreliable). Local treatment alone of the skin with acyclovir is not sufficient in oncological patients with herpes zoster.

Contra-indications: Pregnancy, lactation. The skin cream should not be used in the eyes, the mouth or the vagina.

Administration and dosage: *As an i.v. infusion* (over 60 min) of 10 mg/kg 8-hourly for 10 days (in herpes encephalitis, varicella zoster infections in immunosuppressed patients and in all infections in the newborn) but 5 mg/kg every 8 hours for 5 days in all other infections (see above).

In impaired renal function, reduce the dose to:
5 mg/kg 12-hourly (creatinine clearance 25–50 ml/min)
5 mg/kg 24-hourly (creatinine clearance 10–25 ml/min)
2.5 mg/kg 24-hourly (creatinine clearance <10 ml/min)

As tablets: 200 mg (400 mg in immunosuppressed patients) 5 times a day for 5–10 days in adults and in children above the age of 3 years; 100 mg 5 times a day in children under 3 years. 200 mg four times daily may be sufficient for prophylaxis.

800 mg 5 times daily for 7 days may be given by mouth for herpes zoster in non-immunosuppressed patients.

Preparations: Tablets of 200 mg, vials of 250 mg, eye ointment, skin cream.

Summary: A well-tolerated antiviral agent with selective activity for severe herpes simplex and varicella zoster infections; also suitable for prophylaxis. Relapses may occur.

References

BALFOUR JR., H. H.: Acyclovir therapy for herpes zoster: advantages and adverse effects. J. Am. Med. Assoc. *255:* 387 (1986).
BALFOUR JR., H. H.: Intravenous acyclovir therapy for varicella in immunocompromised children. J. Pediatr. *104:* 134 (1984).
BEAN, B., D. AEPPLI: Adverse effects of high-dose intravenous acyclovir in ambulatory patients with acute herpes zoster. J. Infect. Dis. *151:* 362 (1985).
BIRON, K. K., J. A. FYFE, J. E. NOBLIN, G. B. ELION: Selection and preliminary characterization of acyclovir-resistant mutants of Varicella zoster virus. Amer. J. Med. *73 (Acyclovir Symposium):* 383 (1982).
COBO, I. M.: Oral acyclovir in the treatment of acute herpes zoster ophthalmicus. Ophthalmology *93:* 763 (1986).
DE MIRANDA, P., M. R. BLUM: Pharmacokinetics of acyclovir after intravenous and oral administration. J. Antimicrob. Chemother. *Suppl. B12:* 29 (1983).
DOUGLAS, J. M. et al.: A double-blind study of oral acyclovir for suppression of recurrences of genital herpes simplex virus infection. N. Engl. J. Med. *310:* 1551 (1984).
ENGLUND, J. A., et al.: Herpes simplex virus resistant to acyclovir. Ann. Intern. Med. *112:* 416 (1990).
FINN, R., M. A. SMITH: Oral acyclovir for herpes zoster. Lancet *2:* 575 (1984).
HANN, I. M., H. G. PRENTICE, H. A. BLACKLOCK et al.: Acyclovir prophylaxis against herpes virus infections in severely immunocompromised patients: randomised double blind trial. Brit. Med. J. *6:* 384 (1983).
HINTZ, M., J. D. CONNOR, S. A. SPECTOR et al.: Neonatal acyclovir pharmacokinetics in patients with herpes virus infections. Am. J. Med. *73 (1A):* 210 (1982).

KINGHORN, G. R., M. JEAVONS, M. ROWLAND et al.: Acyclovir prophylaxis of recurrent genital herpes: randomised placebo controlled crossover study. Genitourin. Med. *61:* 387 (1985).
LASKIN, O. L. et al.: Effects of probenecid on the pharmacokinetics and elimination of acyclovir in humans. Antimicrob. Ag. Chemother. *21:* 804 (1982).
LASKIN, O. L. et al.: Acyclovir kinetics in end-stage renal disease. Clin. Pharmacol. Ther. *31:* 594 (1982).
LJUNGMAN, P., M. N. ELLIS, R. C. HACKMAN, D. H. SHEPP, J. D. MEYERS: Acyclovir-resistant herpes simplex virus causing pneumonia after bone marrow transplantation. J. Infect. Dis. *162:* 244 (1990).
MCLAREN, C., M. S. CHEN, I. GHAZZOULI et al.: Drug resistance patterns of herpes simplex virus isolates from patients treated with acyclovir. Antimicrob. Ag. Chemother. *28:* 740 (1985).
MCKENDRICK, M. W., J. I. MCGILL, A. M. BELL et al.: Oral acyclovir for herpes zoster. Lancet *2:* 925 (1984).
NOVELLI, V. M. et al.: Acyclovir administered perorally in immunocompromised children with varicella-zoster infections. J. Infect. Dis. *149:* 478 (1984).
O'BRIEN, J. J., D. M. CAMPOLI-RICHARDS: Acyclovir. An updated review of its antiviral activity, pharmacokinetic properties, and therapeutic efficacy. Drugs *37:* 233 (1989).
OLIVER, N. M., F. COLLINS, J. VAN DER MEER, J. W. VAN'T WOUT: Biological and biochemical characterization of clinical isolates of herpes simplex virus type 2 resistant to acyclovir. Antimicrob. Agents Chemother. *33:* 635 (1989).
PERREN, T. J., et al.: Prevention of herpes zoster in patients by long-term oral acyclovir after allogeneic bone marrow transplantation. Am. J. Med. *85 (2A):* 99 (1988).
PETERSLUND, N. A., V. ESMANN, J. IPSEN et al.: Oral and intravenous acyclovir are equally effective in herpes zoster. J. Antimicrob. Chemother. *14:* 185 (1984).
ROBINSON, G. E., G. S. UNDERHILL, G. E. FORSTER et al.: Treatment with acyclovir of genital herpes simplex virus infection complicated by eczema herpeticum. Brit. J. Vener. Dis. *60:* 241 (1984).
RUHNEK-FORSBECK, M., E. SANDSTRÖM, B. ANDERSSON et al.: Treatment of recurrent genital herpes simplex infections with oral acyclovir. J. Antimicrob. Chemother. *16:* 621 (1985).
RUSSLER, S. K., M. A. TAPPER, D. R. CARRIGAN: Susceptibility of human herpesvirus 6 to acyclovir and ganciclovir. Lancet *2:* 382 (1989).
SCHALM, S. W., R. A. HEYTINK, H. R. VAN BURREN et al.: Acyclovir enhances the antiviral effect of interferon in chronic hepatitis B. Lancet *2:* 358 (1985).
SHEPP, D. H. et al.: Oral acyclovir therapy for mucocutaneous herpes simplex virus infection in immunocompromised recipients. Ann. Intern. Med. *102:* 783 (1985).
SKÖLDENBERG, B., M. FORSGREN, K. ALESTIG et al.: Acyclovir versus vidarabine in herpes simplex encephalitis. Randomised multicentre study in consecutive Swedish patients. Lancet *2:* 707 (1984).
SYLVESTER, R. K., W. B. OGDEN, C. A. DRAXLER, F. B. LEWIS: Vesicular eruption: a local complication of concentrated acyclovir infusions. J. Am. Med. Assoc. *255:* 385 (1986).
TOMSON, C. R., T. H. J. GOODSHIP, R. S. C. RODGER: Psychiatric side-effects of acyclovir in patients with chronic renal failure. Lancet *2:* 385 (1985).
WADE, J. C., J. D. MEYERS: Neurologic symptoms associated with parenteral acyclovir treatment after marrow transplantation. Ann. Intern. Med. *98:* 921 (1983).

b) Ganciclovir

Proprietary name: Cymevene (Syntex).

Properties: Ganciclovir is an acyclic nucleoside analogue of guanine. Its chemical formula is dihydroxypropoxymethylguanine (DHPG). Ganciclovir in its phosphorylated form inhibits the nucleic acid (DNA) synthesis of cytomegalovirus (CMV) in the infected cell. The antiviral activity of ganciclovir against CMV is some 8- to 20-fold greater than the closely related acyclovir, but activity against herpes simplex and varicella zoster virus is weaker. Ganciclovir is also active against Epstein-Barr virus. The vials contain ganciclovir sodium as a lyophilised powder.

Mode of action: Ganciclovir does not acquire antiviral activity until it has been phosphorylated (i.e. changed into the triphosphate) in virus-infected cells of the body kinases of the host cell. The resultant ganciclovir triphosphate, which resembles a genuine nucleoside, is bound to the viral DNA polymerase, which catalyses DNA synthesis and, after two phosphate groups have been split off, is attached as the monophosphate to an elongating DNA chain. Since, unlike a normal nucleotide, ganciclovir has no 3'-hydroxyl group, there is no site of attachment for the next nucleotide. The DNA chain is therefore unable to grow further. Another action of ganciclovir is that it binds long-term as a false nucleotide to viral polymerase, which is then no longer available for DNA synthesis. The good anti-CMV activity of ganciclovir is thus explained by the slower breakdown of phosphorylated ganciclovir in the viral-infected cells, so ganciclovir acts longer than acyclovir.

Pharmacokinetics: The mean serum concentrations at the end of a one-hour i.v. infusion of 5 mg/kg are 10 mg/l, 5 mg/l 1 h later, and 1.5 mg/l 7 h later. *Half-life:* about 4 h (up to 16 h in impaired renal function). *Plasma protein binding:* 1–2%; *excretion* predominantly unchanged in the kidneys.

Side-effects: Reversible neutropenia in 50%, thrombocytopenia (24%), anaemia (4%), rashes (7%), fever (6%), nausea, vomiting and diarrhoea (4%), muscle spasm and cognitive disorders (each 3%), headaches and psychoses (each 2%). Serum transaminases, alkaline phosphatase and creatinine may rise transiently. Ganciclovir is teratogenic in animal experiments and inhibits spermatogenesis, even causing testicular atrophy at high dosage. Fertility is suppressed in female animals. Such effects have not yet been reported in man. Ganciclovir can give rise to mutations in animal experiments.

Interactions: The haemotoxicity of ganciclovir can be increased when it is combined with cytotoxic agents. Azidothymidine has to be withdrawn during treatment with ganciclovir.

Indications: Life- and sight-threatening cytomegalovirus infections in immunosuppressed patients (in AIDS, malignancy and after transplantation). The best results (clinical improvement and reversion of cultures to negative) are found in CMV retinitis (80%) and CMV colitis (80%), while in CMV pneumonia, only 50% of cases improve clinically. The majority of patients relapse 2–14 weeks after the end of treatment, so that maintenance therapy is necessary until immunity returns to normal. Combination with CMV immunoglobulin seems advisable. In most patients, relapse responds well to further treatment.

Contra-indications: Severe neutropenia (<500 neutrophils/µl) and thrombocytopenia; pregnancy.

Administration and dosage: I.v. infusion of 5 mg/kg over 1 h every 12 h for 2–3 weeks. Stop treatment if the neutrophil count is less than 500/µl or thrombocyte count falls sharply.

As a maintenance dose, 5 mg/kg once daily i.v. is recommended until the immunodeficiency has improved.

In impaired renal function, give:
3 mg/kg every 12 hours (creatinine clearance 25–50 ml/min)
3 mg/kg every 24 hours (creatinine clearance 10–25 ml/min)
1.5 mg/kg every 24 hours (creatinine clearance <10 ml/min)

References

BACH, M. C., S. P. BAGWELL, N. P. KNAPP et al.: 9-(1,3-dihydroxy-2-propoxymethyl)-guanine for cytomegalovirus infections in patients with the acquired immunodeficiency syndrome. Ann. Intern. Med. *103:* 381 (1985).

CANTRILL, H. L., K. HENRY, N. H. MELROE, W. H. KNOBLOCH, R. C. RAMSAY, H. H. BALFOUR JR.: Treatment of cytomegalovirus retinitis with intravitreal ganciclovir. Long-term results. Ophthalmology *96:* 367 (1989).

CHACHOUA, A.: Ganciclovir in the treatment of cytomegalovirus gastrointestinal disease with AIDS. Ann. Intern. Med. *107:* 133 (1987).

Collaborative DHPG Treatment Study Group: Treatment of serious cytomegalovirus infections with 9-(1,3-dihydroxy-2-propoxymethyl)guanine in patients with AIDS and other immunodeficiencies. N. Engl. J. Med. *314:* 801–805 (1986).

D'ALESSANDRO, A. M., J. D. PIRSCH, R. J. STRATTA, H. W. SOLLINGER, M. KALAYOGLU, F. O. BELZER: Successful treatment of severe cytomegalovirus infections with ganciclovir and CMV hyperimmune globulin in liver transplant recipients. Transplant. Proc. *21:* 3560 (1989).

ERICE, A. et al.: Progressive disease due to ganciclovir-resistant cytomegalovirus in immuncompromised patients. N. Engl. J. Med. *320:* 289 (1989).

FAULDS, D., R. C. HEEL. Ganciclovir: A review of its antivitral activity, pharmacokinetic properties, and therapeutic efficacy in cytomegalovirus infections. Drugs *39:* 597 (1990).

FLETCHER, C., R. SAWCHUK, B. CHINNOCK et al.: Human pharmacokinetics of the antiviral drug DHPG. Clin. Pharmacol. Ther. *40:* 281 (1986).

GUDNASON, T., K. K. BELANI, H. H. BALFOUR JR.: Ganciclovir treatment of cytomegalovirus disease in immunocompromised children. Pediat. Infect. Dis. *8:* 436 (1989).

HENDERLY, D. E. et al.: Cytomegalovirus retinitis and response to therapy with ganciclovir. Ophthalmology *94:* 425 (1987).
KAULFERSCH, W., C. URBAN, C. HAUER et al.: Successful treatment of CMV-retinitis with ganciclovir after allogeneic marrow transplantation. Bone-Marrow Transplant *4:* 587 (1989).
LAKE, K. D. et al.: Ganciclovir pharmacokinetics during renal impairment. Antimicrob. Agents Chemother. *32:* 1899 (1988).
MAI, M., J. NERY, W. SUTKER, B. HUSBERG, G. KLINTMALM, T. GONWA: DHPG (gancyclovir) improves survival in CMV pneumonia. Transplant. Proc. *21:* 2263 (1989).
ROBINSON, M. R., C. TEITELBAUM, C. FINDLAY-TAYLOR: Thrombocytopenia and vitreous hemorrhage complicating ganciclovir treatment. Amer. J. Ophthal. *107:* 560 (1989).

c) Azidothymidine (Zidovudine, AZT)

Proprietary name: Retrovir.

Properties: Azidothymidine is an analogue of the DNA nucleoside thymidine (Fig. 59, p. 282). It is an antiviral agent which inhibits the reverse transcription of viral RNA into DNA during viral replication, thereby terminating the growth of the chain (Fig. 60).

Mechanism of action: After absorption azidothymidine is taken up by the cells of the body where it is activated through triple phosphorylation by the body's own cellular kinases. Azidothymidine triphosphate is deposited in reverse transcriptase, for which it has 100 times greater affinity than for cellular DNA polymerases. During transcription of the viral RNA into the viral DNA, which is thymidine-dependent, azidothymidine is accepted as thymidine by the reverse transcriptase and is incorporated into the DNA molecule. Thus viral DNA replication is interrupted.

Pharmacokinetics: Azidothymidine is 70% absorbed after oral intake. After repeated oral administration of 250 mg every 4 h, mean peak serum levels of 4.4 µmol/l are found. After repeated i.v. administration of 2.5 mg/kg every 4 h the mean peak serum levels are 4 µmol/l. *Half-life in serum:* 1 h; intracellular half-life much longer. *Plasma-protein binding* 34–38%. The *CSF levels* are 50% of the serum levels. *Excretion* predominantly in the kidneys (by glomerular filtration and tubular secretion), after i.v. administration up to 25% unchanged and up to 60% as the glucuronide.

Side-effects: Bone marrow depression is a regular effect of azidothymidine. Marked macrocytic anaemia usually occurs after 6 weeks of treatment but neutropenia after only 4 weeks of treatment. Changes in the blood count are more common in patients with AIDS than with ARC. The dose of azidothymidine must be reduced in severe anaemia and neutropenia. Blood transfusions are required relatively frequently. In this situation granulocyte colony stimulating factor

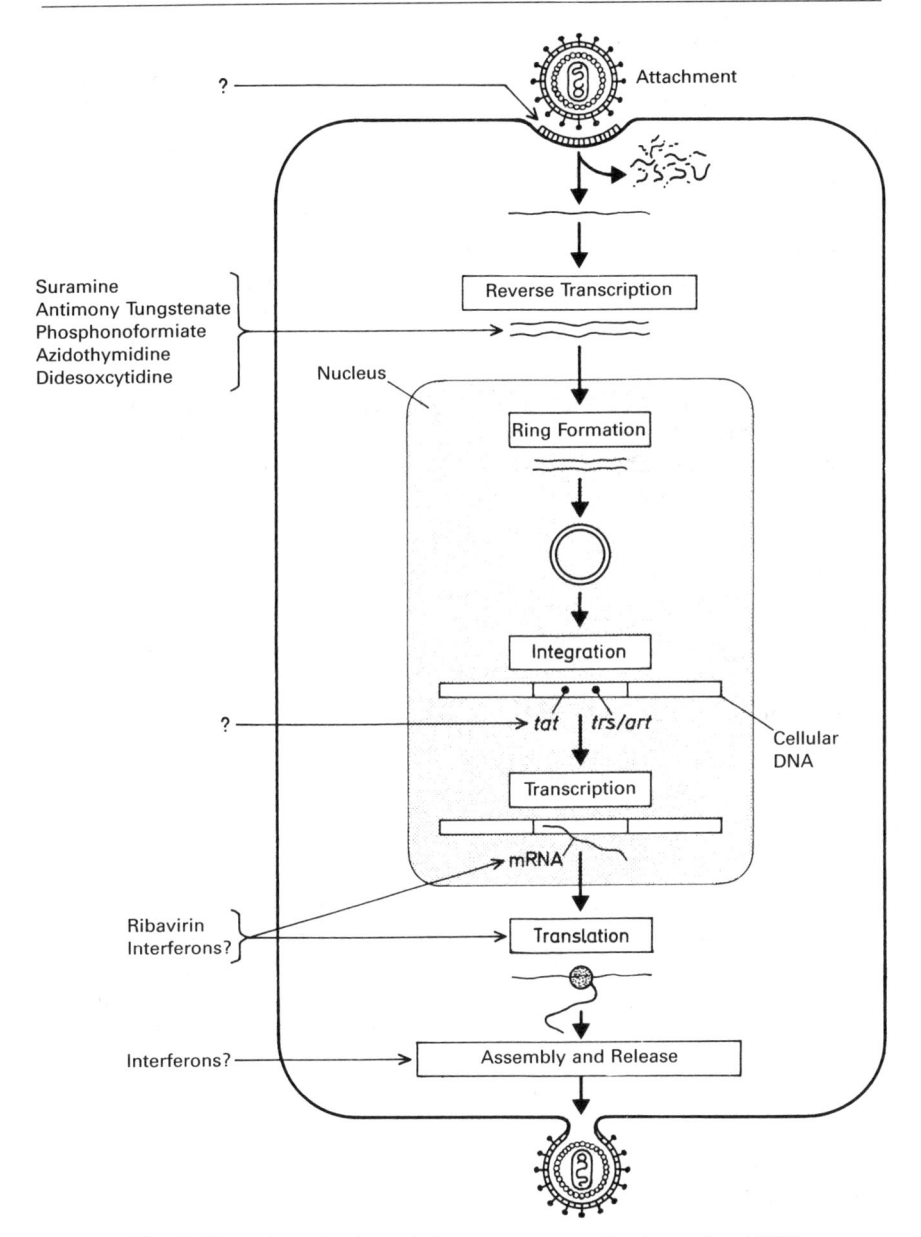

Fig. 60. Sites of attack of antiviral agents in the replication cycle of HIV.

(GCSF) and/or erythropoetin may be useful. Treatment may have to be interrupted for certain periods. Regular monitoring of the blood count during treatment is essential. Further side-effects are nausea, vomiting, abdominal pain, fever, myalgia, paraesthesiae, epileptiform fits and loss of weight. In CNS diseases, dramatic deterioration in the illness can occur during AZT treatment, forcing discontinuation of treatment.

Interactions: Concurrent administration of paracetamol may intensify the haemotoxicity of azidothymidine. Azidothymidine's side-effects may be increased by drugs which are glucuronidated in the liver or metabolised by other liver enzymes. These drugs include acetylsalicylic acid, morphine, indomethacin, ketoprofen, oxazepam, cimetidine and clofibrate. Potentially nephrotoxic or myelosuppressive drugs (e. g. ganciclovir) may increase the risk of azidothymidine side-effects. Alcohol intolerance occasionally occurs. Interactions with other drugs which are mainly metabolised by the liver (e.g. rifampicin, ketoconazole) are likely.

Indications: Severe manifestations of HIV infection [AIDS or ARC (AIDS related complex)], in particular:
1. when the T4-lymphocytes are less than $250/\mu l$,
2. clinical progression of HIV infection,
3. first manifestation of full blown AIDS.

Potential indications are inoculation with contaminated blood, neuro-AIDS, early infection without major clinical symptoms.

The criteria for selection for therapy are still somewhat controversial. It is possible that many patients have been treated much too late in the course. There is clearly no point in instituting AZT therapy in moribund AIDS patients. There is the argument that the use of the drug in earlier stages of the disease, particularly in patients who have clearly recently seroconverted, would be of more value. A contrary view is that the limited beneficial effect of AZT may be wasted if the drug is given at too early a stage of the disease. Studies of the use of AZT after accidental inoculation, e. g. by a contaminated i.v. cannula, have shown failures of protection. Large numbers of patients will need to be evaluated before the long term efficacy of AZT can be proven. Studies of combination therapy with DDI or DDC are also of interest. A large controlled study of the combination with acyclovir has shown no beneficial effects but an increase in side-effects.

The use of AZT in children seems justified only in controlled studies.

Contra-indications: Pregnancy, lactation, terminal AIDS, neutropenia (less than 750 neutrophils/μl), haemoglobin below 7.5 g/dl, liver or renal failure. Women should not become pregnant and men should not have unprotected intercourse during and after treatment. Reaction times while driving and during machine operation may be impaired.

Administration and dosage: Early experiences with AZT were obtained with high doses. The daily oral dose in adults has now been reduced to 200–600 (–1000) mg. When haemoglobin values are between 7.5 and 9 g/dl and neutrophil counts between 750 and 1,000 per µl, the normal individual dose should be reduced. Treatment should be stopped if these values fall further. Improvement in the blood count usually occurs after treatment has been stopped for 2 weeks, and treatment may then resume with a reduced daily dose. Erythropoetin and/or granulocyte colony stimulating factor (GCSF) may be given. Normal dosage may be resumed 2–4 weeks after improvement in the blood count. Duration of treatment varies with different individuals. An alternative is intermittent treatment (with 500–800 mg daily every 2nd month).

AZT can be administered as an i. v. infusion (60 min) in adequate dilution.

Preparations: Capsules of 100 mg and 250 mg; infusion bottles of 200 mg.

Summary: Clinical experience with azidothymidine is increasing. Azidothymidine is not curative but can give prolonged improvement in advanced stages of HIV infection. Azidothymidine usually leads initially to an increase in body weight, reduced frequency of opportunistic infection and improvement in quality of life. The incidence of oral candidiasis also decreases. In controlled studies the mortality was markedly reduced. Despite clear clinical improvement, pneumocystis pneumonia and toxoplasma infection may occur. The positive effect of AZT ceases after 12–18 months in most patients. If treatment with pyrimethamine and sulphonamides, ganciclovir or cytotoxic drugs becomes necessary, azidothymidine must be interrupted. Azidothymidine has no effect on Kaposi's sarcoma or lymphoma.

Azidothymidine is still the standard treatment in advanced stages of HIV infection.

References

Fischl, M. A., et al.: The safety and efficacy of zidovudine (AZT) in the treatment of subjects with mildly symptomatic human immunodeficiency virus type 1 (HIV) infections. Ann. Intern. Med. *112:* 727 (1990).

Fischl, M. A., D. D. Richman, M. H. Grieco et al.: The efficacy of 3'-azido-3'-deoxythymidine (azidothymidine) in the treatment of patients with AIDS and AIDS-related complex: a double-blind placebo-controlled trial. N. Engl. J. Med. *317:* 185–191 (1987).

Henderson, D. K., J. L. Gerberding: Prophylactic zidovudine after occupation exposure to the human immunodeficiency virus and interim analysis. J. Infect. Dis. *160:* 321 (1989).

Langtry, H. D., D. M. Campoli-Richard. Zidovudine: A review of its pharmacodynamics and pharmacokinetic properties, and therapeutic efficacy. Drugs *27:* 408 (1989).

Larder, B. A., G. Darby, D. D. Richman: HIV with reduced sensitivity to zidovudine *(AZT)* isolated during prolonged therapy. Science *243:* 1731 (1989).

Laskin, O. L., P. de Miranda, M. R. Blum: Azidothymidine steady-state pharmacokinetics in patients with AIDS and AIDS-related complex. J. Infect. Dis. *159:* 745 (1989).

LHAISSON, R. E., J.-P. ALLAIN, P. A. VOLBERDING: Significant changes in HIV antigen level in the serum of patients treated with azidothymidine. New Engl. J. Med. *315:* 1610–1611 (1986).
MITSUYA, H., K. J. WEINHOLD, P. A. FURMAN et al.: 3'-azido-3'-deoxythymidine (BW A509U): an antiviral agent that inhibits the infectivity and cytopathic effect of human T-lymphotropic virus type III/lymphadenopathy-associated virus in vitro. Proc. Nat. Acad. Sci. USA *82:* 7096–7100 (1985).
RICHMAN, D. D., M. A. FISCHL, M. H. GRIECO et al.: The toxicity of azidothymidine (AZT) in the treatment of patients with AIDS and AIDS-related complex: a double-blind. placebo-controlled trial. N. Engl. J. Med. *317:* 192–197 (1987).
TABURET, A.-M., et al.: Pharmacokinetics of zidovudine in patients with liver cirrhosis. Clin. Pharmacol. Ther. *47:* 731 (1990).
WARRIER, I., J. M. LUSHER: Retrovir therapy in hemophilic children with symptomatic human immunodeficiency virus infection: efficacy and toxicity. Am. J. Pediatr. Hematol. Oncol. *12:* 160–163 (1990).
YARCHOAN, R. et al.: Clinical pharmacology of 3'-azido-2,3'-dideoxythymidine (zidovudine) and related dideoxynucleosides. N. Engl. J. Med. *321:* 726 (1989).
YARCHOAN, R., S. BRODER: Development of antiretroviral therapy for the acquired immunodeficiency syndrome and related disorders. New Engl. J. Med. *316:* 557 (1987).
YARCHOAN, R., R. W. KLECKER, K. J. WEINHOLD et al.: Administration of 3'-azido-3'-deoxythymidine, an inhibitor of HTLV-III/LAV replication, to patients with AIDS or AIDS-related complex. Lancet *1:* 575–580 (1986).

d) Vidarabine (Adenine Arabinoside)

Proprietary name: Vira-A.

Properties: Vidarabine (Ara-A) is a purine nucleoside analogue which, after triple phosphorylation in the body cells, inhibits DNA polymerase and hence intracellular viral replication. Its effect on herpes simplex virus types 1 and 2 and varicella zoster virus is considerably greater than that on cytomegalovirus. Unlike acyclovir (see p. 278), no viral thymidine kinase is required for the phosphorylation of vidarabine in the body cells. Vidarabine is therefore also active against viruses which themselves form no thymidine kinase. The disadvantages are certain cytotoxic side-effects. The substance is closely related to cytosine arabinoside.

Pharmacokinetics: After i.v. infusion vidarabine is extensively metabolised in the liver to a metabolite (hypoxanthine arabinoside) which is less actively antiviral than the parent substance. *Half-life:* 4 h. *Excretion* predominantly via the urine (up to 50% as the metabolite and about 3% unchanged).

Side-effects: Nausea, vomiting and diarrhoea are frequently observed with i.v. infusion of 5–15 mg/kg/day for 5 to 15 days. At higher dosage, tremor, EEG changes, bone marrow suppression and loss of weight may occur and, with longer i.v. administration, polyneuropathy. In animal experiments vidarabine is teratogenic, mutagenic and oncogenic. Use of the eye cream may lead to lacrimation, burning, conjunctival redness and inflammatory changes in the cornea.

Indications: Vidarabine was for many years the only available chemotherapeutic agent for herpes encephalitis but acyclovir is clinically superior and has fewer side-effects. The increasing range of antiviral agents has made vidarabine obsolete, and the drug is now little used.

Contra-indications: Pregnancy.

References

BURDGE, D. R., A. W. CHOW, S. L. SACHS: Neurotoxic effects during vidarabine therapy for herpes zoster. Can. Med. Assoc. J. *132:* 392 (1985).
CRUMPACKER, C. S., L. E. SCHNIPPER, P. N. KOWALSKY, D. M. SHERMAN: Resistance of herpes simplex virus to adenine arabinoside and E-5-(2-bromovinyl)-2'-deoxyuridine: a physical analysis. J. Infect. Dis. *146:* 167 (1982).
LOK, A. S. F., L. A. WILSON, H. C. THOMAS: Neurotoxicity associated with adenine arabinoside monophosphate in the treatment of chronic hepatitis B virus infection. J. Antimicrob. Chemother. *14:* 93 (1984).
SHEPP, D. A., P. S. DANDLIKER, J. D. MEYERS: Treatment of varicella-zoster virus infection in severely immunocompromised patients: a randomized comparison of acyclovir and vidarabine. N. Engl. J. Med. *314:* 208 (1986).
VAN ETTA, L., J. BROWN, A. MASTRI, T. WILSON: Fatal vidarabine toxicity in a patient with normal renal function. JAMA *246:* 1703 (1981).
WHITLEY, R. J., C. A. ALFORD, M. S. HIRSCH et al.: Vidarabine versus acyclovir therapy in herpes simplex encephalitis. N. Engl. J. Med. *314:* 144 (1986).

e) Tribavirin (Ribavirin)

Proprietary name: Virazid (Great Britain). Virazole (USA).

Properties: A synthetic guanoside analogue (Fig. 59, p. 282). The ampoules contain the lyophilised powder, which is freely soluble in water and may be used as an aerosol when dissolved. Tribavirin has a relatively broad spectrum of activity and inhibits both DNA and RNA viruses in tissue culture, but has no activity against HIV. Its activity against RSV (respiratory syncytial virus) and against arenaviruses (which cause Lassa fever) are of clinical interest.

Mode of action: The mode of action is not precisely known. Ribavirin is phosphorylated after uptake into the body's cells and then inhibits a viral enzyme (inosine monophosphate dehydrogenase) which is necessary for the synthesis of guanosine triphosphate. This results in the depletion of the intracellular nucleotide pool. The phosphorylated ribavirin can also inhibit the attachment of a modified guanosine molecule to the newly formed viral mRNA during viral replication at the end of transcription (see Fig. 60, p. 289). The inhibition of replication of viral mRNA impairs the formation of viral protein and is thus virostatic. The transfer of human mRNA, on the other hand, is little affected.

Pharmacokinetics: A small fraction of ribavirin is absorbed from the mucous membranes after inhalation of the aerosol for 2.5 h or 20 h daily; the mean serum concentrations are 0.8 and 7 mol/l respectively, while the concentration in the tracheal secretion rises to many times the inhibitory concentration in tissue culture. *Half-life* in blood: 9 h. The tissue levels are not known. Ribavirin is, however, concentrated in the erythrocytes (*half-life:* 40 days). *Excretion* of the absorbed fraction is predominantly through the kidneys (unchanged and as the metabolite).

Side-effects: Administration of aerosol inhalations to severely ill infants with life-threatening underlying disease is a difficult procedure. Deterioration in lung function, apnoea and ventilator dependence can all occur during aerosol treatment, as can hypotension and cardiac arrest (possibly as a result of the underlying disease). Precipitates of tribavirin in the ventilatory apparatus may cause problems in mechanically ventilated infants. Other side-effects are skin reactions, conjunctivitis and a rise in blood reticulocytes as a result of haemolysis. Tribavirin is relatively well tolerated after systemic administration. Reversible anaemia can develop at high dosage. In animal experiments tribavirin is teratogenic and carcinogenic and can induce mutations. Testicular atrophy has been observed in animal experiments.

Interactions: Tribavirin must not be mixed with other drugs during inhalation. A small particle aerosol generator must be used for aerosol inhalation.

Indications: Treatment is reserved for severely ill children in the first year of life with bronchiolitis or pneumonia due to RSV infection, particularly in the presence of underlying diseases such as bronchopulmonary dysplasia and severe congenital heart defects. Rapid diagnostic methods for RSV infection are now available. Aerosol treatment with tribavirin should only be undertaken in hospital and with careful monitoring of pulmonary function. Arenavirus infections (Lassa, Junin, Machupo, LCM) are rare but important indications. The use of tribavirin for other virus infections (e.g. measles or hepatitis) is under evaluation. AIDS is apparently not affected.

Contra-indications: Pregnancy; mechanical ventilation.

Administration and dosage: Dissolve and dilute the tribavirin to a final concentration of 20 mg/ml according to the manufacturer's instructions. The aerosol is put into a specially designed nebuliser in an oxygen hood designed for infants and inhaled by the child for 12–18 h a day for 3 to 7 days. A face mask or oxygen tent may be used instead of the oxygen hood. An improvement in respiratory function, retraction, rhonchi and cough and an increase in the pO_2 are usually seen by the third day of treatment. Although RSV frequently disappears from the secretions during treatment, the virus may be demonstrated for several days after the inhalation has stopped. RSV is unlikely to develop resistance to ribavirin.

In Lassa fever and other arenavirus infections, tribavirin should be given i.v.: 1 g 4 times a day for 4 days, followed by 0.5 g 3 times a day for 6 days.

References

COSGROVE, M., H. R. JENKINS, P. H. ROWLANDSON, O. P. GRAY: Idiosyncratic reaction to nebulised ribavirin in an artificially ventilated neonate. J. Infect. *19:* 85 (1989).
EVERARD, M., A. D. MILNER, A. CLARK: Ribavirin and acute bronchiolitis in infancy. Brit. med. J. *298:* 323 (1989).
HALL, C. B., J. T. BCBRIDE, E. E. WALSH et al.: Aerosolized ribavirin treatment of infants with respiratory syncytial viral infection. A randomized double-blind study. New Engl. J. Med. *308:* 1443 (1983).
KNIGHT, V., B. E. GILBERT: Ribavirin aerosol treatment of influenza. Infect. Dis. Clin. North Am. *1:* 441 (1987).
Leading article: Ribavirin and respiratory syncytial virus. Lancet *1:* 362 (1986).
MCCLUNG, H. W., V. KNIGHT, B. E. GILBERT et al.: Ribavirin aerosol treatment of influenza B virus infection. JAMA *249:* 2671 (1983).
MCCORMICK, J. B., I. J. KING, P. A. WEBB et al.: Lassa fever. Effective therapy with ribavirin. New Engl. J. Med. *314:* 20 (1986).
PARONI, R., M. DEL PUPPO, C. BORGHI, C. R. SIRTORI, M. GALLI-KIENLE: Pharmacokinetics of ribavirin and urinary excretion of the major metabolite 1,2,4-triazole-3-carboxamide in normal volunteers. Int. J. Clin. Pharmacol. Ther. Toxicol. *27:* 302 (1989).
SHARLAND, M., N. WHITEHOUSE, S. QURESHI: Ribavirin in respiratory syncytial virus infection. Arch. Dis. Childh. *64:* 425 (1989).
TABER, L. H., V. KNIGHT, B. E. GILBERT et al.: Ribavirin aerosol treatment of bronchiolitis associated with respiratory syncytial virus infection in infants. Pediatrics *72:* 613 (1983).
WHITE, P. A., N. DUNNE: Ribavirin and acute bronchiolitis in infancy (letter). BMJ *298:* 752–753 (1989).
WILSON, S. Z., B. E. GILBERT, J. M. QUARLES et al.: Treatment of influenza A (H_1N_1) virus infection with ribavirin aerosol. Antimicrob. Ag. Chemother. *26:* 200 (1984).

f) Idoxuridine

Idoxuridine (5-iodo-2'-desoxyuridine) was the first antiviral agent to be used clinically against herpes simplex virus. It is a halogenated thymidine analogue and inhibits virus synthesis as a result of competitive antagonism of thymidine (5-methyl desoxyuridine) by the incorporation of altered nucleotide bases. Since it has a similar effect in non-infected cells and is rapidly broken down in the body, it is out of the question for general treatment. Systemic treatment in generalised herpes or herpes encephalitis is no longer justifiable on account of its unreliable activity and considerable side-effects. A skin ointment containing 0.2% idoxuridine (Virunguent) is available in some countries for the treatment of herpes simplex infections of the skin and transitional epithelium, but its use is unreliable because of poor solubility and unnecessary in most self-limiting infections. A solution containing 0.1% idoxuridine should be used several times daily on the affected parts of the skin.

In *cutaneous herpes* zoster and herpes simplex, a 5% idoxuridine solution in dimethyl sulphoxide (Herpid, Iduridin, Virudox) may be applied four times a day to the affected areas (side-effects: stinging on application). Idoxuridine fluid (Idoxene, Kerecid) is still used for the local treatment of *herpes simplex keratitis;* 1–2 drops are instilled into the affected cornea, initially hourly during the day and two hourly at night, and after improvement commences every 2 h daily and every 4 h at night, for 3 to 5 days. The eye ointment can be introduced every 4 h (about 5 times a day) into the conjunctival sac. More frequent use can give rise to irritation (pain, itching, oedema, photophobia and even small areas of superficial ulceration). Since acyclovir, vidarabine and trifluridine are considerably better tolerated on the cornea than idoxuridine, the latter is no longer recommended for treatment of keratitis.

Preparations: Eye drops (0.1%), eye ointment (0.1%), gel (0.3%) and a solution for sub-conjunctival injection (0.5%).

References

Collum, L. M. T., A. Benedict-Smith, I. R. Hillary: Randomized, double-blind trial of acyclovir and idoxuridine in dendritic corneal ulceration. Br. J. Ophthalmol. *64:* 766 (1980).
Coster, D. J. et al.: A comparison of acyclovir and idoxuridine as treatment for ulcerative herpetic keratitis. Br. J. Ophthalmol. *64:* 763 (1980).
Hasumi, K., T. Kobayashi, M. Ata: Topical idoxuridine for genital condyloma acuminatum. Lancet *1:* 968 (1984).

g) Trifluridine

Trifluridine (Trifluorothymidine) is a halogenated pyrimidine with a structure similar to that of idoxuridine and thymidine. It has greater and more rapid activity than idoxuridine in herpetic corneal ulcers and, on account of its toxicity, should only be used for the local treatment of herpes simplex keratitis.

Side-effects of mild conjunctival irritation and epithelial damage may occur. Trifluridine is available as eye drops and eye ointment.

References

De Koning, E. W. J., O. P. van Bijsterveld, K. Cantell: Kombinationstherapie der Keratitis dendritica mit Humanleukozyten-Interferon und Trifluorthymidin. Br. J. Ophthalmol. *66:* 509–512 (1982).
La Lau, C., L. A. Oosterhuis, J. Versteeg et al.: Multicenter trial of acyclovir and trifluorothymidine in herpetic keratitis. Amer. J. Med. *73 (Acyclovir Symposium):* 305 (1982).
Nesburn, A. B., G. H. Lowe 3rd, N. J. Lepoff, E. Maguen: Effect of topical trifluridine on Thygeson's superficial punctate keratitis. Ophthalmology *91:* 1188 (1984).
Shearer, D. R., W. M. Bourne: Severe ocular anterior segment ischemia after long-term trifluridine treatment for presumed herpetic keratitis. Amer. J. Ophthal. *109:* 346 (1990).

h) Amantadine

Proprietary names: Amantadine, Symmetrel.

Amantadine (1-amantadinamine hydrochloride) inhibits virus penetration into the cell and, when given promptly, has a prophylactic effect against influenza A_2 infection (but not against influenza B virus). The mechanism of action is still unclear but may involve inhibition of uncoating of the protein coat of influenza A viruses after their uptake into the cell. Whether amantadine is still effective in the first two days after influenza A_2 infection is still disputed. The drug is also used in the treatment of Parkinson's disease.

Pharmacokinetics: Amantadine is well absorbed after oral administration. The *maximum blood concentrations* are achieved after 4 h. The *half-life* is 15 h. The urinary recovery is 90% (unchanged).

Side-effects: Amantadine has considerable side-effects such as agitation, tremor, ataxia, lack of concentration, dulling of senses, depression, dryness of the mouth, disorders of speech and vision as well as heart failure, hypotension and urinary retention.

Interactions: The anticholinergic side-effects of amantadine are intensified by the simultaneous administration of anticholinergic drugs, and the central nervous effects by the concurrent use of sympathomimetic agents. Amantadine reduces the tolerance of alcohol.

Contra-indications: Pregnancy, lactation, glaucoma. Use with caution in patients with epilepsy and right-sided heart failure as well as those with renal disease. It should be used only as a prophylactic for influenza under specified conditions and with influenza immunisation. Adults should be given 200 mg orally per day in 1–2 doses, children aged 5–9 years 150 mg daily and children aged 1–5 years 50–100 mg daily for at least 10 days after exposure. If the patient is actively immunised at the onset of treatment, the treatment should continue until the onset of immunity after three weeks.

Tromantadine, a related chemical compound, may be used for the local treatment of herpes infections of the skin and eyes. Its activity is weak and it frequently gives rise to contact allergy.

References

Aoki, F. Y., D. S. Sitar: Amantadine kinetics in healthy elderly men: Implications for influenza prevention. Clin. Pharmacol. Ther. *37:* 137 (1985).
Dolin, R., R. C. Reichman, H. P. Madore et al.: A controlled trial of amantadine and rimantadine in the prophylaxis of influenza A infection. New Engl. J. Med. *307:* 580 (1982).
Hayden, F. G., J. M. Gwaltney Jr., R. L. Van de Castle et al.: Comparative toxicity of amantadine hydrochloride and rimantadine hydrochloride in healthy adults. Antimicrob. Ag. Chemother. *19:* 226 (1981).
Hayden, F. G., H. E. Hoffman: Comparative single dose pharmacokinetics of amantadine HCl and rimantadine HCl in young and elderly adults. Antimicrob. Ag. Chemother. *28:* 216 (1985).
Hayden, F. G., H. E. Hoffman, D. A. Spyker: Differences in side-effects of amantadine hydrochloride and rimantadine hydrochloride relate to differences in pharmacokinetics. Antimicrob. Ag. Chemother. *23:* 458 (1983).
Heider, H., B. Adamczyk, H. W. Presber et al.: Occurrence of amantadine- and rimantadine-resistant influenza A virus strains during the 1980 epidemic. Acta virol. *25:* 395 (1981).
Horadam, V. W. et al.: Pharmacokinetics of amantadine hydrochloride in subjects with normal and impaired renal function. Ann. Intern. Med. *94:* 454 (1981).
Millet, V. M., M. Dreisbach, Y. J. Bryson: Double-blind controlled study of central nervous system side-effects of amantadine, rimantadine, and chlorpheniramine. Antimicrob. Ag. Chemother. *21:* 1 (1982).
Payler, D. K., P. A. Purdham: Influenza A prophylaxis with amantadine in a boarding school. Lancet *1:* 502 (1984).
WHO Consultation Meeting, Vienna, 1983: Current status of amantadine and rimantadine as anti-influenza-A agents: Memorandum from a WHO Meeting. Bull. WHO *63:* 51 (1985).
Younkin, S. W., R. F. Betts, F. K. Roth, R. G. Douglas Jr.: Reduction in fever and symptoms in young adults with influenza A/Brazil/78 H1N1 infection after treatment with aspirin or amantadine. Antimicrob. Ag. Chemother. *23:* 577 (1983).

i) Interferons

Proprietary names: *Interferon α*: Intron A, Roferon A, Wellferon.
Interferon β: Fiblaferon

Properties: Interferons are naturally occurring species-specific glycoproteins formed in the body's cells; they have complex actions on cell function and

immunity. Their activities are *antiviral, antiproliferative* (inhibiting the proliferation of tumour cells) and *immunomodulatory* (affecting immunity and phagocytosis). The interferon formed by infected body cells protects the neighbouring cells and, by humoral mediation, cells at remote sites from the progressive viral infection. Interferons have a broad spectrum of antiviral activity, though adenoviruses are generally resistant. Independent of the mode of activity, interferons are protective against many viral species (in contrast to the specific activity of antibodies). This is due to the fact that interferons do not directly inhibit viruses but improve the host cellular defences. Three types of interferon are distinguished on the basis of their chemical structure:
1. Interferon α, which is obtained from blood leukocytes or from permanent lymphoblastoid cell lines,
2. Interferon β, which is produced by diploid fibroblast cultures,
3. Interferon γ, which is obtained from T-lymphocyte cultures.

As a result of modern gene technology, all types of interferon can be produced in large quantities and great purity. Their formation in the human body can be stimulated by viral or naturally occurring non-viral inducers (e.g. fungal and bacterial components). There are also synthetic inducers (e.g. polynucleotides such as Poly I:C) which, however, are usually toxic and are rapidly degraded before the onset of action. Interferon α principally increases the cytotoxic activity of the natural killer cells, which have a lytic effect on viral infected cells (without pre-existing sensitisation).

Interferon β, which is obtained naturally by the stimulation of human fibroblasts, does not attack the virus directly; its antiviral effect results from the stimulation of cellular defence mechanisms. Like interferon α, it increases the activity of the natural killer cells and also has an antiproliferative effect.

Interferon γ and other lymphokines affect the cytotoxic activity of thymus-dependent sensitised T lymphocytes directed against viral antigens on cell membranes.

Kinetics: After virus induction, 6–18 h elapse before interferon is released from the infected cells in the body. Its formation ceases after only a few hours. Minute quantities of interferon are sufficient to protect large numbers of cells from viral infection. Parenterally administered interferon can be demonstrated for only a few hours in the blood (*half-life:* 2–4 h; interferon γ only 24 min). Tissue antiviral activity lasts for 24 h, however. Peak serum levels of interferon α are achieved 5 to 8 hours after i.m. injection and 8 to 10 h after subcutaneous injection. Interferon β must be given i.v. (through prolonged infusion) if it is to remain active. *CSF penetration* is low. Interferon α is not absorbed when used locally, e.g. in the eye.

Side-effects: The frequency and severity of side-effects depends on the dose administered parenterally and the purity of the interferon preparation. Febrile reactions and rigors are common and clearly due to the drug. Nausea, vomiting and diarrhoea occur fairly often, as do headache and muscle pain. Transient changes in the blood count (neutropenia, thrombocytopenia, fall in reticulocytes and haemoglobin), prolongation of the partial thromboplastin time and an increase in serum liver enzymes can all occur. Hypotension and hyperventilation are rare. When interferon α is used prophylactically in the nose, nosebleeds and drying of the mucous membranes may occur. When interferon α eye drops are used, no side-effects are observed.

Interactions: I.v. interferon may possibly potentiate the action of oral anticoagulants.

Potential uses: The parenteral administration of interferon α has so far only been generally recommended for the treatment of hairy-cell leukaemia. Interferon α also has some activity against Kaposi's sarcoma. Interferon α has been used in clinical trials to combat cytomegalovirus infection in renal transplant recipients, and been found to reduce the period of viraemia and viral excretion. In chronic active hepatitis B, the Dane DNA polymerase can be reduced by interferon α and the hepatitis B core antigenaemia declines.

The **topical use of interferon α** in the eye in epithelial herpetic keratitis (keratitis dendritica) can accelerate resolution and reduce complication. It is not sufficient alone, however, but must always be given with other antiviral chemotherapeutic agents, such as trifluorothymidine or acyclovir, or combined with epithelial abrasion. Prophylaxis in the healthy eye is ineffective because the loosening of the epithelium and consequent increase in permeability caused by the disease is essential for the penetration of interferon into the basal cells of the corneal epithelium.

Interferon β is recommended by its manufacturers for the treatment of severe viral infections (e.g. viral encephalitis, generalised herpes zoster and varicella in immunosuppressed patients). The most favourable effect (impairment of the progress of the disease and shortening of the course) is most likely to be achieved in the early stage of the infection.

Simultaneous acyclovir should not be withheld, however. Interferon β can also be used locally in the eye to treat herpes keratitis (always with another antiviral agent such as trifluoridine). Interferon β has been used for the treatment of primary and metastatic nasopharyngeal carcinoma (after the completion of radiotherapy).

Interferon γ has a predominantly immunomodulatory action; its clinical relevance is still unclear.

Contra-indications: Pregnancy (for parenteral use); also hypersensitivity to human proteins. Through their immunostimulatory action interferons may counteract therapeutic immunosuppression.

Administration and dosage: Interferon β can be given by chronic i. v. infusion of 0.5×10^6 IU/kg for 3–10 days. The partial thromboplastin time and the thrombocyte and leukocyte counts should be determined regularly during therapy. Concurrent anticoagulants (e.g. heparin) must be avoided.

Interferon-α-2 eyedrops are applied twice daily to the affected eye (one drop at intervals of 10 min). The eye drops should not be given at the same time as local antiviral agents, but about 30 minutes beforehand. Such focal use in the eye, which serves to protect uninfected cells, must always be combined with a basic treatment, such as local antiviral chemotherapy or thermoabrasion of the cornea. Treatment should continue for 6 days.

References

DAVIS, G. L., et al.: Treatment of chronic hepatitis C with recombinant interferon alpha. N. Engl. J. Med. *321:* 1501 (1989).
DE KONING, E. W. J., O. P. VAN BUSTERVELD: Combination therapy for dendritic keratitis with acyclovir and alpha interferon. Arch. Ophthalmol. *101:* 1866 (1983).
DIBISCEGLIE, A. M., et al.: Recombinant interferon alfa therapy for chronic hepatitis C. A. randomized, double-blind, placebo-controlled trial. N. Engl. J. Med. *321:* 1506 (1989).
DOUGLAS, R. M., B. W. MOORE, H. B. MILES et al.: Prophylactic efficacy of intranasal alpha-2-interferon against rhinovirus infections in the family setting. N. Engl. J. Med. *314:* 65 (1986).
FRASCA, D., L. ADORINI, S. LANDOLFO, G. DORIO: Enhancing effect of interferon-γ on helper T cell activity and IL2 production. J. Immunol. *134:* 3907 (1985).
HAYDEN, F. G., J. K. ALBRECHT, D. I. KAISER, J. M. GWALTNEY: Prevention of natural colds by contact prophylaxis with intranasal alpha-2-interferon. N. Engl. J. Med. *314:* 71 (1986).
HO, M.: Interferon for the treatment of infections. Annu. Rev. Med. *38:* 51 (1987).
KRIGEL, R. I., C. M. ODAJUYK, L. J. LAUBENSTEIN et al.: Therapeutic trial of interferon-γ in patients with epidemic Kaposi's sarcoma. J. Biol. Resp. Modif. *4:* 358 (1985).
PERRILLO, R. P., et al.: A randomized, controlled trial of interferon alpha-2b alone and after prednisone withdrawal for the treatment of chronic hepatitis B. N. Engl. J. Med. *323:* 295 (1990).
SACKS, S. L. et al.: Antiviral treatment of chronic hepatitis B virus infection: Pharmacokinetics and side-effects of interferon and adenine arabinoside alone and in combination. Antimicrob. Ag. Chemother. *21:* 93 (1982).
SCHONFELD, A. et al.: Intramuscular human interferon-β injections in treatment of Condylomata acuminata. Lancet 1038–1042 (1984).
SCULLARD, G. H., R. B. POLLARD, J. L. SMITH et al.: Antiviral treatment of chronic hepatitis B virus infection. I. Changes in viral markers with interferon combined with adenine arabinoside. J. Infect. Dis. *143:* 772 (1981).
TROFATTER, K. F., JR.: Interferon. Obstet. Gynecol. Clin. North Am. *14:* 569 (1987).

j) Immunoglobulins

Immunoglobulins should only be used in the prevention of virus infections when specifically indicated. Varicella-zoster immunoglobulin should be considered when a mother was exposed to **varicella zoster** virus within the last 5 days before delivery and had no prior history of varicella infection. Varicella-zoster immunoglobulin (0.1 ml/kg) is injected i.m. If contact occurred earlier (in the last 3 weeks before delivery) the newborn baby can be treated with acyclovir, which should prevent the often fatal neonatal varicella. In the event of exposure after birth, the newborn baby is no longer at such great risk, and 0.6 ml/kg of normal human immunoglobulin should then be used.

Hepatitis B hyperimmune globulin (given at the same time as active immunisation) is necessary to protect the newborn baby of an HB_s-Ag-positive mother. For family exposure to a hepatitis B viral carrier, seronegative family members may be immunised actively against hepatitis B. Some protection from exposure to hepatitis A or C virus can be obtained with normal human immunoglobulin.

HIV infection in children may be attenuated by high doses of normal human immunoglobulin (200 ml i.v. every 2 weeks) during the stage of the lymphadenopathy syndrome. The mechanism of action is unclear (possibly immunomodulation). In adults this effect has not been clearly demonstrated. For the immunoprophylaxis of **other viral infections,** see Table 26.

Table 26. Passive immunisation with polyvalent gamma globulin (normal human immunoglobulin) or specific hyperimmune globulin for the prevention of viral infections. BW = body weight.

Passive immunisation against:	Dosage (ml/kg BW) of:	
	Normal human immunoglobulin (i.m.)	Specific hyperimmune globulin (i.m.)
Measles	0.2–0.4	0.25
Varicella	0.2–1.0	0.25 U/kg
Rubella (in pregnant women)	20 ml (total)*	0.2
Mumps	1.0	0.2
Hepatitis A	0.05	–
Hepatitis B	–	0.05
Hepatitis C	0.05	–
Rabies	–	20 U/kg
Cytomegalovirus	–	0,2

* When exposure to rubella occurred >7 days previously: 50 ml (total) +15 ml of rubella hyperimmune globulin (simultaneously).

References

Centers for Disease Control: Varicella-zoster immune globulin for the prevention of chickenpox: recommendations of the immunization practices advisory commitee. Am. Intern. Med. *100:* 859 (1984).

PARYANI, S. G., A. M. ARVIN, C. M. KOROPCHAK: Comparison of varicella-zoster antibody titers in patients given intravenous immune serum globulin or varicella-zoster immune globulin. J. Pediat. *105:* 200 (1984).

PERRILLO, R. P., C. R. CAMPBELL, S. STRONG: Immune globulin and hepatitis B immune globulin: prophylactic measures for intimate contacts exposed to acute type B hepatitis. Arch. Intern. Med. *144:* 81 (1984).

SMALLWOOD, L. A., E. TABOR, J. S. FINLAYSON: Antibodies to hepatitis A virus in immune serum globulin. J. Med. Virol. *7:* 21 (1981).

WINSTON, D. J., W. G. HO, C. H. LIN: Intravenous immune globulin for modification of cytomegalovirus infections associated with bone marrow transplantation. Preliminary results of a controlled trial. Am. J. Med. *76 (3A):* 128 (1984).

WONG, V. C., H. M. H. IP, H. W. REESINK: Prevention of the HBs-Ag carrier state in newborn infants of mothers who are chronic carriers of HBsAg and HBcAg by administration of hepatitis-B vaccine and hepatitis-B immunoglobulin. Lancet *1:* 921 (1984).

C. Treatment of Infections and Infectious Diseases

1. Infections with Facultative Pathogenic Bacteria

Most antibiotics are used for the treatment of infections with facultative pathogens. These organisms occur naturally as part of the normal commensal flora at some sites in the body and as colonising flora at others. It is only when, under abnormal conditions, they obtain access to organs or tissues where they are not normally found that true infection arises. The rules for treatment of these infections differ from those applied to classical infectious diseases. For example, clinically similar infections of an organ such as the gall-bladder or urinary bladder can be caused by a number of different bacteria.

About one-third of all infections of this type are caused by a mixture of species. Infections of some organs (e. g. pyelonephritis) are associated with a typical range of causative organisms. For example, Escherichia coli is the principal pathogen in acute pyelonephritis and is found more frequently than Proteus mirabilis or enterococci; pyelonephritis is very seldom caused by staphylococci.

Most infections are endogenous, that is, caused by invasion of organisms from the patient's own bacterial flora. They are much less commonly due to pathogens from the inanimate environment. Person-to-person transfer of bacterial infection is exceptional, and is undoubtedly due in part to prior interchange of skin and mucous membrane bacteria between persons who live in close physical contact. The selection pressure exerted by certain antibiotics plays an important part in infections with facultative pathogens. Individual species can vary in their pathogenicity and certain strains within a single species can be particularly virulent. Staphylococci, members of the Enterobacteriaceae and Pseudomonas have variable antibiotic susceptibilities. Wherever possible, therefore, treatment of infections involving these organisms should be based on laboratory reporting of appropriate antibiotic sensitivities.

a) Infections Caused by Enterobacteriaceae

Escherichia coli, klebsiella, enterobacter and *proteus* are normally present in the human intestine. If they gain access to other organs, they can cause serious infections such as pyelonephritis, cholecystitis or cholangitis, wound infections, septicaemia and meningitis. Such infections are therefore generally *endogenous,* that is, infection by the body's own flora of an organ which is functionally impaired by, for example, congenital abnormality, stones, or impaired defence mechanisms. Apparatus such as inhalers, humidifiers, and anaesthetic equipment can be a source of *exogenous* infection. A knowledge of likely pathogenic species and their antibiotic sensitivity is necessary for effective therapy, since bacteria acquired in this way from a hospital environment vary considerably in their sensitivity to antibiotics, and many are multiresistant.

In order to facilitate assessment of the differences in antibiotic sensitivity pattern of individual bacterial species, Tables 27 and 28 summarise the minimal inhibitory concentrations found in ≤50% and 90% of a series of hospital isolates. The results are presented for three groups of antibiotics. The first group is composed of ampicillin, three acylaminopenicillins (mezlocillin, azlocillin and piperacillin) and temocillin. The second group comprises cephalothin, cefuroxime, cefoxitin and cefotiam, while the third group contains the newer cephalosporins (cefotaxime, ceftriaxone, ceftizoxime, latamoxef, cefotetan, cefoperazone and ceftazidime). The results of these three groups are compared with those for imipenem.

Tables 27 and 28. Differences in the *in vitro* activity of β-lactam antibiotics against various gram-negative bacilli (author's series of isolates from patients in the University Children's Hospital, Kiel, Germany). MIC_{50} = minimal inhibitory concentration in 50% of strains. n = number of strains.

Table 27

Antibiotic	Escherichia coli MIC		Klebsiella pneumoniae MIC		Enterobacter aerogenes MIC		Proteus vulgaris MIC	
	50%	90%	50%	90%	50%	90%	50%	90%
Ampicillin	3.1	200	100	>200	>200	>200	25	50
Mezlocillin	1.6	50	6.2	>200	3.1	12.5	0.8	3.1
Azlocillin	6.2	200	100	>200	25	>200	3.1	50
Piperacillin	1.6	50	6.2	200	1.6	6.2	0.4	0.8
Temocillin	1.6	1.6	3.1	6.2	3.1	6.2	1.6	6.2
Cephalothin	3.1	6.2	6.2	50	>200	>200	>200	>200
Cefuroxime	3.1	3.1	3.1	6.2	12.5	50	200	>200
Cefoxitin	3.1	3.1	3.1	6.2	50	200	6.2	12.5
Cefotiam	0.1	0.4	0.2	0.4	0.4	1.6	25	50
Cefotaxime	0.05	0.1	0.05	0.1	0.2	0.8	<0.05	0.05
Ceftriaxone	0.02	0.1	<0.05	0.1	0.2	0.8	<0.05	0.05
Ceftizoxime	0.02	0.1	0.02	0.05	0.2	0.8	0.05	0.1
Latamoxef	0.1	0.1	0.1	0.5	0.1	0.2	<0.02	0.2
Cefotetan	0.1	0.1	0.8	0.2	0.2	0.5	>200	>200
Cefoperazone	0.1	1.6	0.2	6.2	0.2	0.8	<0.8	1.6
Ceftazidime	0.1	0.2	0.1	0.4	0.2	0.4	<0.05	0.1
Imipenem	0.1	0.2	0.4	1.6	0.4	0.8	1.6	6.2

1. Infections with Facultative Pathogenic Bacteria

Table 28

Antibiotic	Citrobacter freundii MIC		Serratia marcescens MIC		Pseudomonas aeruginosa MIC	
	50%	90%	50%	90%	50%	90%
Ampicillin	6.2	>200	>200	>200	>200	>200
Mezlocillin	3.1	100	3.1	12.5	50	200
Azlocillin	6.2	>200	>200	>200	12.5	100
Piperacillin	1.6	50	1.6	12.5	6.2	12.5
Temocillin	3.1	6.2	3.1	6.2	>200	>200
Cephalothin	50	>200	>200	>200	>200	>200
Cefuroxime	12.5	100	50	100	>200	>200
Cefoxitin	50	200	12.5	25	>200	>200
Cefotiam	50	>200	100	>200	>200	>200
Cefotaxime	0.4	25	0.2	12.5	25	100
Ceftriaxone	0.4	25	0.2	25	25	100
Ceftizoxime	0.4	100	0.4	25	50	200
Latamoxef	0.1	3.1	0.2	12.5	25	50
Cefotetan	0.2	0.4	0.2	0.4	>200	>200
Cefoperazone	0.8	12.5	0.4	12.5	6.2	12.5
Ceftazidime	0.4	25	0.2	12.5	1.6	6.2
Imipenem	0.4	0.4	1.6	3.2	0.8	1.6

In the **ampicillin group,** mezlocillin and piperacillin are more effective on the basis of both MIC 50% and 90% against Escherichia coli than ampicillin and azlocillin. The same is true with Klebsiella pneumoniae and Enterobacter aerogenes. Ampicillin is not generally active against Proteus vulgaris, and mezlocillin and piperacillin are more active than azlocillin. Citrobacter freundii is generally more sensitive to piperacillin than to the other acylaminopenicillins. Some strains of Serratia marcescens are susceptible to piperacillin and mezlocillin but not to azlocillin and ampicillin.

There are no major differences against Escherichia coli in the **basic and intermediate cephalosporin groups,** apart from the greater effect of cefotiam. Cefuroxime and cefoxitin have similar activity against Klebsiella pneumoniae, while cephalothin is frequently ineffective; cefotiam is the most active of the intermediate cephalosporins. Cephalothin and cefoxitin are not usually effective against Enterobacter aerogenes; cefuroxime has some activity, and here, too, cefotiam is the best. Cefoxitin is superior to the other three against Proteus vulgaris. Citrobacter freundii is generally more sensitive to cefuroxime, while Serratia marcescens is more frequently inhibited by cefoxitin. Pseudomonas is always resistant to cephalothin, cefuroxime, cefoxitin and cefotiam.

In the **cefotaxime group,** ceftriaxone and ceftizoxime have the greatest activity against Escherichia coli. The minimal inhibitory concentrations of the other agents in this group are considerably lower than in the ampicillin and basic cephalosporin groups. All members of this group have similar activity against Klebsiella pneumoniae. At 6.2 mg/l, however, the MIC_{90} of cefoperazone is much higher than that of the other drugs. Enterobacter aerogenes is inhibited by all drugs of the cefotaxime group in concentrations under 1 mg/l. Proteus vulgaris is most sensitive to cefotaxime, ceftriaxone and ceftazidime and less so to cefoperazone. The MIC_{50} for all drugs of this group against Citrobacter freundii and Serratia marcescens is low, while the MIC_{90} varies between 12.5 and 25 mg/l (but is 100 mg/l for ceftizoxime against Citrobacter). Only latamoxef has a lower MIC_{90} against Citrobacter freundii. Pseudomonas aeruginosa is inhibited best by ceftazidime, followed by cefoperazone. Cefotaxime, ceftriaxone and latamoxef are less active against pseudomonas, and ceftizoxime is inactive. These studies suggest that only a few species show therapeutically important differences in sensitivity, namely pseudomonas, Serratia marcescens and Citrobacter freundii. Cefotaxime, ceftriaxone and cefoperazone are reported to be frequently ineffective against Enterobacter cloacae, while latamoxef is more active.

A **comparison of the activity** of these three groups shows members of the cefotaxime group to be the most active against most bacterial species. Since even these new agents have important gaps in their spectrum, however, life-threatening infections where the causative organisms are unknown should always be treated by a combination of antibiotics, to include an agent with reliable activity against pseudomonas and/or anaerobes.

As seen in Tables 27, penicillin treatment of **Escherichia coli infections** must be based on sensitivity testing because no penicillin is predictably effective. Some 30–40% of hospital strains of Escherichia coli produce β-lactamase and so are resistant to ampicillin, and often to mezlocillin and piperacillin also. As with the staphylococci, a separation has developed between sensitive and multi-resistant strains. The newer aminoglycosides and β-lactamase-stable cephalosporins, on the other hand, are almost always active against Escherichia coli, as are aztreonam, imipenem, the new quinolones and ticarcillin/clavulanate. The frequency of cotrimaxole-resistant strains has increased recently.

Klebsiella pneumoniae, Enterobacter aerogenes and **Enterobacter cloacae** are quite resistant to a number of antibiotics. Because they produce β-lactamase, they are usually resistant to ampicillin, and sometimes to mezlocillin and piperacillin, but temocillin and mecillinam are nearly always active. Co-amoxiclav is active against β-lactam-producing klebsiellae. Klebsiellae are mostly sensitive to parenteral cephalosporins. Enterobacter aerogenes is almost always inhibited by agents in the cefotaxime group, aztreonam, imipenem, temocillin and mecillinam. Enterobacter cloacae, on the other hand, is often resistant to the penicillins and most of the cephalosporins, whilst aztreonam, imipenem and the new quinolones (norfloxacin, ofloxacin and ciprofloxacin) are active. In recent years Enterobacter cloacae has become an important organism in the hospital environment. These bacteria are often selected by treatment with newer cephalosporins such as cefoxitin or cefotaxime. Although frequently isolated, they rarely cause serious infections. Enterobacter cloacae is generally resistant to most β-lactams but sensitive to other antibiotics such as tetracycline, co-trimoxazole, aminoglycosides and fluoquinolones. The rate of resistance of members of the Klebsiella/ Enterobacter group to aminoglycosides is low.

Proteus species (particularly Proteus mirabilis) are frequently found in urinary infections. Indole-positive species of proteus (e. g. Proteus vulgaris) often occur as secondary pathogens in the presence of chronic necrotic lesions such as decubitus and crural ulcers and necrotising tumours. Proteus mirabilis *(indole-negative)* is susceptible to ampicillin and cefazolin. *Indole-positive* species of proteus are generally not sensitive to ampicillin and the older parenteral cephalosporins (Tab. 29), whilst cefoxitin, cefotaxime, ceftriaxone, aztreonam, imipenem and the new quinolones are almost always effective. All species of proteus are susceptible to temocillin and mecillinam. Co-amoxiclav is only active against otherwise resistant species of Proteus when the resistance is due to bacterial β-lactamase production. Co-trimoxazole inhibits almost all strains of Proteus mirabilis, as well as most indole-positive strains, but not providencia. Norfloxacin,

Table 29. Comparative antibacterial activity of various cephalosporins against Proteus vulgaris (86 strains) in serial dilution tests. MIC_{50} and MIC_{90} = minimum inhibitory concentrations (mg/l) for ≤50% and 90% of the strains, respectively.

Antibiotic	Proteus vulgaris	
	MIC_{50}	MIC_{90}
Cephalothin	>200	>200
Cefuroxime	200	>200
Cefazolin	100	>200
Cefamandole	100	200
Cefotiam	25	50
Cefoxitin	6.2	12.5
Cefoperazone	0.8	1.6
Cefotetan	0.2	0.4
Latamoxef	0.2	0.2
Ceftazidime	0.05	0.1
Cefotaxime	0.01	0.05
Ceftriaxone	0.01	0.05

ciprofloxacin and the other new quinolones are almost always active against all species of proteus.

Of the urinary disinfectants nalidixic acid is frequently effective but nitrofurantoin rarely so, because it is inactive at the alkaline pH which results from the production of ammonia by the cleavage of urea by urease elaborated by Proteus spp.

Less common members of the Enterobacteriaceae: Multiresistant "coliforms" such as hafnia, erwinia, citrobacter etc. are occasionally encountered; their sensitivity to antibiotics varies considerably. Citrobacters are often selected by cefoxitin treatment; their pathogenicity is low. Newer quinolones and imipenem are almost always effective, as are often mecillinam and aztreonam.

b) Serratia marcescens Infections

Occurrence and importance: Serratia marcescens is an opportunistic bacterium which is normally non-pathogenic but can cause infection in patients with lowered resistance. Some strains of Serratia marcescens form a red pigment and are easily recognised; most significant clinical isolates are non-pigmented, however. Serratia marcescens is sometimes found in the intestinal flora of healthy patients, on the perineal skin and in the urethra. Urinary catheterisation, particularly when long-term, gives Serratia access to the bladder, causing severe infections which are difficult to treat. Such infections are particularly common in patients with a paraplegic bladder. Serratia marcescens bacteraemia is frequently caused by infection of a venous catheter (see Serratia septicaemia, p. 339). Necrotising pneumonia with Serratia marcescens is only found in patients with severe primary disease (chronic underlying lung or renal disease) and after treatment with corticosteroids or immunosuppressants. The bacteria can also enter the lungs during inhalation treatment and cause infection.

Resistance and antibiotic therapy: Serratia marcescens is resistant to most antibiotics and chemotherapeutic agents. Some strains are inhibited by co-trimoxazole, piperacillin, mezlocillin, temocillin and mecillinam. Cefotaxime, aztreonam, imipenem, amikacin and the new 4-quinolones are generally effective. In recent years, the percentage of gentamicin-resistant strains has increased. A single antibiotic is likely to be effective against fully sensitive strains, but combinations are usually necessary for more resistant isolates. Strains formerly called Enterobacter liquefaciens are now classified as Serratia and are also resistant to most antibiotics.

c) Pseudomonas Infections

Occurrence and relevance: Pseudomonas aeruginosa is found in wound and urinary infections and less commonly in pneumonia, septicaemia, skin diseases, ophthalmic and foreign body infections. These bacteria are important causes of infection because of their resistance to many antibiotics, their ability to produce toxin and their transmissibility. Control of the spread of pseudomonas is a problem in many hospitals. Pseudomonas aeruginosa is a major cause of secondary bacterial infection in patients with bone-marrow suppression. Pseudomonas is very common in the hospital environment, resistant to many disinfectants, and easily spread, particularly in surgical wards. Common reservoirs where the organism may be found are sinks, wash-basins, waste-bins, urinals and catheters. A small percentage of patients excrete Pseudomonas aeruginosa in the faeces. Pseudomonas occasionally occurs in hospital food, especially salads. Its spread in hospital should therefore be controlled by appropriate hygienic measures (asepsis, antisepsis, careful hand-washing, disinfection or sterilisation of apparatus, isolation etc.). Chemoprophylaxis with antibiotics is of no value. Infections should be treated with an antibiotic appropriate to the site of infection and susceptibility (see Table 30).

Table 30. Activity of important antibiotics against 433 strains of Pseudomonas aeruginosa (after E. PEREA, University of Seville Hospitals, Spain).

Antibiotic	Pseudomonas aeruginosa	
	MIC_{50}	MIC_{90}
Azlocillin	4	64
Cefoperazone	4	16
Cefotaxime	16	128
Cefsulodin	4	8
Ceftazidime	2	4
Ceftriaxone	16	128
Imipenem	2	4
Latamoxef	8	128
Piperacillin	4	64
Ticarcillin	8	64
Ciprofloxacin	0.25	0.5
Ofloxacin	1	4
Amikacin	4	16
Gentamicin	4	16
Netilmicin	8	64
Sisomicin	1	8
Tobramicin	1	8

MIC_{50} and MIC_{90} are the minimal inhibitory concentrations (mg/l) against ⩽50% and 90% of tested strains respectively.

Resistance rate and antibiotic therapy: Even though the number of active substances has recently increased, all are likely to encounter some resistant strains. Gentamicin has good anti-pseudomonal activity (resistance rate: 0–8%), but that of tobramycin is slightly better. Amikacin, and to a lesser extent netilmicin, are active against many gentamicin-resistant strains of pseudomonas.

Infections with pseudomonas are relatively difficult to treat. Aminoglycosides are almost entirely excreted unchanged by the kidneys and, although urinary infections will usually respond to an aminoglycoside alone, systemic and soft tissue infections should be treated with a combination of, for example, azlocillin and tobramycin. Carbenicillin and ticarcillin have been largely superceded by azlocillin and piperacillin, which are 4–8 times more active, may be given in lower dosage and contain less sodium. Since clavulanic acid does not generally inhibit the β-lactamase of pseudomonas, ticarcillin/clavulanate (Timentin) has no advantage as a single agent in the treatment of β-lactamase-producing Pseudomonas aeruginosa. Up to 5% of hospital isolates of pseudomonas are resistant to azlocillin and piperacillin.

New cephalosporins with anti-pseudomonal activity have increased the number of therapeutic options. Cefsulodin, a narrow-spectrum agent, may be useful in specific treatment where there is azlocillin resistance or penicillin allergy. Ceftazidime has the best antipseudomonal activity of the cephalosporins. Aztreonam and imipenem are also very effective. Of the new quinolones, ciprofloxacin has the greatest antipseudomonal activity, and ofloxacin and norfloxacin are also useful in urinary infections caused by pseudomonas. Resistant strains are, however, not infrequently found in chronic infections.

Polymyxins (colistin and polymyxin B) have poor tissue diffusion and unreliable activity, and should only be used topically. Povidone iodine, silver compounds (Flamazine), and occasionally neomycin or framycetin may also be used locally. Other pseudomonas (P. cepacia, P. maltophilia, P. putida and P. fluorescens) are increasingly found as causes of wound infections, septicaemia and urinary infections. Some of these species are multiresistant, particularly P. cepacia, and may be selected by treatment with penicillins and cephalosporins.

d) Haemophilus influenzae Infections

Occurrence and importance: In adults, and particularly the elderly, Haemophilus influenzae is a cause of acute exacerbations of chronic bronchitis. In young children, Haemophilus influenzae is a common cause of otitis media and sinusitis and the commonest cause of acute epiglottitis. Septicaemia (sometimes with the Waterhouse-Friderichsen syndrome), meningitis and osteomyelitis (sometimes associated with immunodeficiency) are particularly dangerous in children. In young children and the elderly, Haemophilus influenzae can also cause bronchopneumonia (and lobar pneumonia in children). Haemophilus endocarditis, pericarditis and arthritis are rare. Purulent and catarrhal conjunctivitis can be caused by Haemophilus influenzae.

Resistance rate: As seen in Table 31, only a small proportion of Haemophilus strains are resistant to tetracycline, co-trimoxazole and chloramphenicol. Ampicillin resistance is generally increasing and in some parts of the USA has already reached 30%. In Spain a resistance rate of up to 60% has been reported. Normal laboratory methods may fail to detected ampicillin resistance. Most strains of haemophilus are moderately sensitive to erythromycin and roxithromycin but resistant to josamycin. Of the cephalosporins, cefazolin, cefazedone, cefoxitin, cephalexin, cefadroxil and cephradine are always ineffective, whereas cefotaxime, cefuroxime, cefotiam, cefaclor, cefixime and cefpodoxime include ampicillin-resistant strains in their spectrum. Imipenem and the new quinolones (ofloxacin, ciprofloxacin) are always effective.

Table 31. Minimal inhibitory concentrations (MIC) of susceptible strains of Haemophilus influenzae and the frequency of resistance to various antibiotics.

Antibiotic	MIC (mg/l)	Frequency of resistance (%)
Ampicillin	0.1	(1–) 5–10 (–30)
Chloramphenicol	1–2	<1 (–50)
Tetracycline	6.2	5–10 (–50)
Doxycycline	1.6	5–10 (–50)
Erythromycin	0.1–12.5	50
Josamycin	6.2–100	100
Cefalexin	25	100
Cefaclor	3.1	0
Cefuroxime	0.8	0
Cefotaxime	0.02	0
Imipenem	1.0	0
Trimethoprim	0.1	1–2 (–60)
Ciprofloxacin	0.01	0
Ofloxacin	0.05	0

Choice of antibiotic: The most active agents are the broad spectrum cephalosporins of the cefotaxime group and the newer quinolones (ofloxacin, ciprofloxacin), and these are the antibiotics of choice in severe haemophilus infections. When imipenem is used as "best guess" therapy or for the treatment of mixed infections, it is likely to have good activity against haemophilus. In children, who should not be given quinolones, oral treatment with co-amoxiclav (amoxycillin/clavulanate) or cefixime, cefaclor or cefuroxime axetil may be used. Mild haemophilus infections in which treatment may possibly fail because of the emergence of bacterial resistance (e.g. in suppurative bronchitis) may be subsequently treated with doxycycline or co-trimoxazole. Erythromycin is no longer recommended because of its poor activity against haemophilus.

References

POWELL, M.: Chemotherapy for Infections caused by Haemophilus influenzae: current problems and future prospects. J. Antimicrob. Chemother. *27:* 3–7 (1991).

e) Staphylococcal Infections

Occurrence and importance: Severe infections with **Staphylococcus aureus** are commoner in hospital patients with impaired resistance than in outpatients. Infants and the elderly are at particular risk. Staphylococci are said to cause about 40% of pneumonia cases, 20–40% of septicaemias and 30–90% of wound infections, although these rates vary with different hospitals and patient groups.

Resistance: While only 30–50% of staphylococci acquired in the community are resistant to benzylpenicillin and other non-penicillinase-stable penicillins, the frequency of resistance in hospital isolates is 60–80% (see Tab. 32). There are penicillin-tolerant staphylococci against which this antibiotic is bacteriostatic only, even at high concentration. Tolerant strains may appear sensitive *in vitro*, but infections fail to respond to treatment. In such cases rifampicin, clindamycin, vancomycin and fosfomycin, preferably in combination, are usually effective. Penicillin-tolerant staphylococci are rare at present in Europe.

The proportion of staphylococcal isolates resistant to penicillinase-stable penicillins (e.g. methicillin) and cephalosporins is small. Such isolates are commonly designated MRSA (methicillin-resistant S. aureus); epidemic strains are EMRSA (epidemic MRSA). Isolation with undue frequency from hospital patients suggests a special epidemiological situation such as the spread of a particular phage-type of staphylococcus. Differences in the anti-staphylococcal activity of new cephalosporins are shown in Table 33.

Even methicillin-resistant strains can be sensitive *in vitro* to other β-lactam antibiotics, although β-lactams are not generally advised in such cases. Methicillin-resistant staphylococci are generally sensitive to fusidic acid and vancomycin, and can often be treated with fosfomycin or rifampicin as well. New quinolones have adequate anti-staphylococcal activity, usually less than their activity against gram-negative bacilli; occasional resistant strains are found or may emerge during treatment.

The rate of resistance varies between 5 and 30% with erythromycin and between 1 and 12% with clindamycin. Staphylococci resistant to vancomycin are very uncommon. Staphylococci resistant to teicoplanin and fusidic acid are also uncommon. On the other hand, 7–50% are resistant to chloramphenicol, 35–67% to tetracycline, and 10–30% now to neomycin and gentamicin in some hospitals.

1. Infections with Facultative Pathogenic Bacteria

Table 32. Resistance of Staphylococcus aureus to various antibiotics.

Antibiotic	Frequency of resistance of Staphylococcus aureus (in %)
Benzylpenicillin[1]	(50–) 60–75 (–80)
Penicillinase-stable penicillins[2]	0–2 (–15)
Cefazolin	0–2 (–15)
Cefotaxime	0–2 (–15)
Imipenem	0–2 (–15)
Erythromycin	5–15 (–30)
Clindamycin	1–5 (–12)
Co-trimoxazole	2–12
Chloramphenicol	(7–) 10–20 (–50)
Tetracycline	35–45 (–67)
Neomycin	10–20 (–30)
Gentamicin	0–10 (–30)
Vancomycin	<1
Fusidic acid	0–2
Ofloxacin, ciprofloxacin	<1

[1]Including phenoxymethylpenicillin, ampicillin, amoxycillin, azlo-, mezlo-, piperacillin, mecillinam etc.
[2]Including methicillin, oxacillin, dicloxacillin, flucloxacillin.

Table 33. Activity of new cephalosporins against Staphylococcus aureus in comparison with cephalothin. GM = geometric mean minimal inhibitory concentrations (mg/l), MIC_{50} and MIC_{90} = minimal inhibitory concentrations (mg/l) against ≤50% and 90% of tested strains.

Antibiotic	GM	MIC_{50}	MIC_{90}
Cephalothin	0.2	0.1	0.4
Cefamandole	0.2	0.2	0.8
Cefotiam	1.4	0.4	0.8
Cefoxitin	1.6	1.6	3.1
Cefotaxime	2.0	1.6	3.1
Ceftizoxime	4.0	1.6	3.1
Ceftriaxone	4.1	3.1	6.2
Cefoperazone	3.8	3.1	6.2
Ceftazidime	6.8	4.0	8.0
Latamoxef	10.0	8.0	16.0

Staphylococcus epidermidis is normally found on the skin and mucous membranes and may be sensitive. However, infections of intravenous catheters, implanted foreign bodies, Spitz-Holter valves, the urinary tract and abnormal heart valves occur, and some strains are resistant to a number of antibiotics, including methicillin. The elimination of staphylococci from infected foreign bodies, even when sensitive to the antibiotic used, is hindered by bacterial slime formation. The most effective antibiotic combination is usually vancomycin + rifampicin.

Unlike methicillin-resistant strains of Staphylococcus aureus, those of Staphylococcus epidermidis are mostly sensitive to cephalosporins. Many strains are multiresistant, however. Staphylococcus saprophyticus, which occurs in acute urinary infections in young, sexually active women, is generally sensitive to benzylpenicillin.

Choice of antibiotic: Because of their good tolerance and low resistance rate, penicillinase-stable penicillins have been the drugs of choice. Oral di- or flucloxacillin (2–3 g a day) can be given for mild staphylococcal infections, and parenteral flucloxacillin (5–10 g a day) or a cephalosporin for severe infections. Alternatives are oral cephalexin or clindamycin. Treatment should not be stopped too early because of the risk of abscess formation or relapse; 4–6 weeks of therapy may be necessary in severe infections. If the isolates are sensitive to benzylpenicillin, this agent (or oral phenoxymethylpenicillin) is preferred because of its greater antibacterial activity. Patients allergic to penicillin should receive erythromycin or a cephalosporin. Where the patient fails to respond to a β-lactam antibiotics, treatment should be changed promptly to another antibiotic or combination (e. g. vancomycin, clindamycin, vancomycin + rifampicin, fosfomycin + clindamycin). Newer quinolones (e. g. ofloxacin, ciprofloxacin) are also effective against methicillin-resistant staphylococci, but should be given only for short periods because of the risk of developing resistance. Certain second-line antibiotics such as fusidic acid, which is well tolerated, can be used in skin and bone infections but secondary resistance can develop rapidly when fusidic acid is used as a single agent. Vancomycin is recommended in cases of resistance or allergy to cephalosporins, but should not be given to patients with poor renal function because of the risk of ototoxicity. Broad-spectrum antibiotics such as tetracycline, ampicillin, azlocillin, mezlocillin and co-trimoxazole are often ineffective against staphylococcal infections.

References

Chandrasekar, P. H., J. A. Sluchak: Newer agents against methicillin and/or gentamicin-resistant and -susceptible staphylococci. Chemotherapy 35: 333 (1989).

Maple, P. A., J. M. Hamilton-Miller, W. Brumfitt: World-wide antibiotic resistance in methicillin-resistant Staphylococcus aureus. Lancet I: 537 (1989).

f) Streptococcal and Pneumococcal Infections

Streptococcus pyogenes infections: Streptococcus pyogenes, that is, β-haemolytic streptococci of Lancefield Group A, are still of considerable importance as the cause of streptococcal sore throat, erysipelas and impetigo, although streptococci of groups B (Streptococcus agalactiae), C and G can also cause sore throat. Wound infections and puerperal sepsis are rare nowadays, though they can be fulminant. Glomerulonephritis and rheumatic fever can both arise as complications of pyogenic streptococcal infection.

Streptococcus pyogenes infections should always be treated with antibiotics, preferably with *penicillin*. Sore throat, erysipelas, impetigo and mild wound infections respond well to oral phenoxymethylpenicillin. Streptococcal septicaemia and severe wound infections should be treated with high doses of intravenous benzylpenicillin, which is still more active than any other penicillin or cephalosporin against Streptococcus pyogenes; penicillin resistance has not yet been reported. Alternative antibiotics are only necessary in patients with penicillin allergy, when erythromycin or sometimes cephalosporins should be considered. Co-trimoxazole does not eradicate streptococci satisfactorily from tissue infection.

Viridans streptococci, which typically cause subacute bacterial endocarditis, and **anaerobic streptococci** (peptostreptococci), which cause infections of the uterine adnexa, diverticulitis, cerebral abscess and dental sepsis, are almost always sensitive to penicillin. Strains with reduced sensitivity (MIC 1 mg/l instead of 0.01 mg/l) are only very occasionally found in subacute bacterial endocarditis. Streptococcus milleri, an uncommon species of viridans streptococcus, is more pathogenic and can cause septicaemia and abscesses, particularly of liver and brain. Streptococcus milleri is always sensitive to penicillin.

Pneumococci (Streptococcus pneumoniae) have until now been very sensitive to benzylpenicillin. Multiresistant strains occurred for the first time in epidemic fashion in South Africa in 1977 and were resistant to penicillin, cephalosporins, lincomycin, erythromycin, chloramphenicol and tetracyclines. Penicillin-resistant pneumococci have recently also been reported from Mexico, Australia, the USA and Great Britain, and may well become important in the future. Between 2.5 and 50% of strains of streptococci (generally about 10%) and 4–20% of pneumococci are resistant to tetracycline. Erythromycin- and clindamycin-resistant strains occur only occasionally. The new quinolones have relatively poor activity against pneumococci. Strains with primary resistance are occasionally found.

Group B streptococci (Streptococcus agalactiae) are an important cause of neonatal septicaemia and meningitis. The infection arises before birth as a result of premature rupture of the membranes, or from the birth canal during parturition, and leads to severe septicaemia of either early or late onset which should be treated urgently with benzylpenicillin. The early-onset type appears within 24 hours of birth, and the late form often after 2–4 weeks. Group B streptococci are carried in the vagina of many healthy women and can cause urinary infection at any age.

An increasing number of cases are being reported of group B streptococci causing septicaemia and other infections in immunocompromised and normal adults. The relatively poor activity of the penicillins and marked synergy with the aminoglycosides are the basis for treatment with benzylpenicillin and gentamicin in combination.

The **enterococci** (Enterococcus faecalis and Enterococcus faecium) and other group D streptococci are exceptional among streptococci in not being inhibited by moderate doses of benzylpenicillin. Enterococci are, however, mostly sensitive to ampicillin, mezlocillin and piperacillin but not, or only very slightly, to cephalosporins. The new cephalosporins such as cefoxitin, cefotaxime and ceftazidime are not active against enterococci, which are frequently selected by their use. The most active β-lactam against enterococci is mezlocillin. The bactericidal activity of all penicillins is weak and killing is slow; increasing the concentration can further impair bacterial killing (the Eagle effect). Aminoglycosides alone are virtually inactive against enterococci, but in combination with a penicillin show marked synergy and a rapid bactericidal effect. Severe enterococcal infections such as endocarditis must therefore be treated with a combination of agents such as ampicillin plus gentamicin, or high doses of penicillin plus gentamicin.

In patients allergic to ampicillin, imipenem, ofloxacin or ciprofloxacin are possible alternative treatments; urinary infections can also be treated with norfloxacin. In endocarditis, i. v. vancomycin is a good alternative when the organism has been shown to be sensitive. 30–55% of enterococci are resistant to tetracyclines.

References

BERGHASH, S. R., G. M. DUNNY: Emergence of multiple beta-lactam-resistance phenotype in group B streptococci of bovine origin. J. Infect. Dis. *151:* 494 (1985).
CASAL, J.: Antimicrobial susceptibility of Streptococcus pneumoniae: serotype distribution of penicillin-resistant strains in Spain. Antimicrob. Ag. Chemother. *22:* 222 (1982).
Centers for Disease Control: Isolation of multiply antibiotic-resistant pneumococci – New York. Morb. Mortal. Wkly. Rep. *34:* 545 (1985).
DENIS, F. A., B. D. GREENWOOD, J. L. REY, M. PRINCE-DAVID, S. MBOUP, N. LLOYD-EVANS, K. WILLIAMS, I. BENBACHIR, N. EL NDAGHRI, D. HANSMAN, V. OMANGA, K. KRUBWA, M. DUCHASSIN, J. PERRIN: Etude multicentrique des serotypes de pneumocoques en Afrique. Bull. WHO *61:* 661–669 (1983).
KLUGMAN, K., H. J. KOORNHOF, V. KUHNLE et al.: Meningitis and pneumonia due to novel multiply resistant pneumococci. Brit. Med. J. *292:* 730 (1986).
LATORRE, C., T. JUNCOSA, I. SANFELIU: Antibiotic resistance and serotypes of 100 Streptococcus pneumoniae strains isolated in a children's hospital in Barcelona, Spain. Antimicrob. Ag. Chemother. *28:* 357 (1985).

Liu, H. H., A. Tomasz: Penicillin tolerance in multiply drug-resistant natural isolates of Streptococcus pneumoniae. J. Infect. Dis. *152:* 365 (1985).
Rauch, A. M., M. O'Ryan, R. Van, L. K. Pickering: Invasive disease due to multiply resistant Streptococcus pneumoniae in a Houston, Tex. day-care center. Am. J. Des. Child. *144:* 923–927 (1990).

g) Anaerobic Infections

Frequency: The anaerobic gram-positive *sporing bacilli* such as Clostridium perfringens, which causes gas gangrene, should be differentiated from the *non-sporing anaerobes,* the most important of which are listed in Table 34.

Bacteroides species are the most common anaerobic pathogens (80–90%, of which Bacteroides fragilis is found in more than half of all anaerobic infections). Other pathogens include Peptostreptococcus species (anaerobic streptococci) and Peptococcus species (anaerobic staphylococci). Infections with fusobacteria, Veillonella, Propionibacterium, Campylobacter and Actinomyces are less common. The frequency of organisms in particular clinical infections often depends on the proximity of the infected organ to the mouth, intestinal or vaginal mucosa, where these anaerobes are regularly found in large numbers (in the colon, 300–1000 anaerobes to 1 aerobe). Bacteroides fragilis, which is normally found in the intestine, is a more common pathogen in abdominal and genital infections than in the lower respiratory tract. Where anaerobes cause lung infection, Bacteroides melaninogenicus is the commonest species involved.

Half of all infections with gram-negative anaerobic rods are mixed with facultatively anaerobic bacteria such as Escherichia coli and Klebsiella pneumoniae, and some 35% are multiple infections caused by 2–7 different anaerobes, including clostridia. These frequencies should be borne in mind, in view of the difficulties of culture and differentiation of anaerobes in the average clinical laboratory. Full bacteriological reports may require at least 2–3 days, and the clinician who suspects anaerobic infection on clinical grounds generally has to

Table 34. The most important non-sporing anaerobes (facultative pathogens).

Gram stain	Cocci	Bacilli
Negative	Veillonella	Bacteroides fragilis Bacteroides melaninogenicus Fusobacterium necrophorum Campylobacter spp.
Positive	Peptococcus Peptostreptococcus	Actinomyces israeli Propionibacterium acnes Eubacterium spp.

start treatment much earlier, based on his "best guess" of the most effective antibiotic combination to cover the likely aerobic and anaerobic bacteria involved.

Illnesses: Non-sporing anaerobes cause infection in the upper and lower respiratory tracts, the gastrointestinal and female genital tract. They can also cause endocarditis, septicaemia, and abscesses in organs such as the brain and liver. Certain clinical features such as pus with a foul, offensive odour are typical. Anaerobes colonise areas where the oxidation/reduction potential is reduced, as in parts of the body remote from active capillary perfusion such as the intestinal lumen, the vagina, tonsillar crypts and nasal sinuses. Aerobic bacteria use up oxygen and so improve the environment for anaerobes. Tissue injury can predispose to anaerobic infection by interrupting the capillary blood circulation, as occurs in surgical operations, arteriosclerosis, malignant tumours and chemical necrosis. The oxidation-reduction potential is reduced, a process often aided by multiple infection with O_2-consuming bacteria (e. g. Escherichia coli), which encourages the multiplication of anaerobic species with varying oxygen sensitivity. Some clostridia, for example, are much more sensitive to oxygen than Campylobacter fetus.

Anaerobic infection is often associated with localised thrombosis and thrombophlebitis, particularly in the pelvis. The exact cause is unknown, but could be the production of a bacterial heparinase or possibly an endotoxic effect. Infected emboli can give rise to small or large metastatic infarcts in the liver, lungs, brain and other organs, forming anaerobic abscesses. Severe cases of septicaemia due to gram-negative anaerobes often develop disseminated intravascular coagulation (consumption coagulopathy). Infections with non-sporing anaerobes are most often found in:

1. *Lower respiratory tract:* Single or multiple lung abscesses, diffuse pulmonary infiltrates or necrotising pneumonia with cavitation can develop as a consequence of either inhalation of oro-pharyngeal secretions or of embolism from anaerobic infections in the abdomen or pelvis. The anaerobes usually found are Bacteroides melaninogenicus, fusobacteria, peptococci, peptostreptococci and veillonella (often in association with staphylococci). Empyema may develop as a complication.

2. *Gastrointestinal tract:* Ulcers and tumours in the gastrointestinal tract form the portals of entry for aerobic and anaerobic bacteria, which can cause local or diffuse peritonitis, intra-abdominal abscesses and liver abscesses, sometimes with septicaemia. The commonest anaerobic causes are Bacteroides fragilis and Clostridium perfringens.

3. *Female genital tract:* Anaerobic septicaemia is a not uncommon complication of septic abortion and chorioamnionitis. Anaerobic salpingitis can also develop in the non-pregnant patient, for example as a complication of gynaecological operations. The anaerobes most frequently isolated are peptostreptococci,

peptococci, Bacteroides species and clostridia. Mixed infections are common. Gonorrhoea and chlamydial infections must be excluded.
4. *Endocarditis:* Endocarditis caused by anaerobes is very rare. Embolic complications of anaerobic endocarditis are frequent. The primary focus is generally inflammation of the oropharynx or gastrointestinal tract. Acute and subacute endocarditis can be caused by Bacteroides fragilis, fusobacteria and Clostridium perfringens. Propionibacterium acnes, a normal skin resident, has been shown to cause endocarditis in a number of patients after the insertion of a prosthetic aortic valve.
5. *Central nervous system:* Cerebral abscesses due to anaerobes can arise from sinusitis or mastoiditis and generally lead to an epidural abscess and meningitis; they may also be metastatic, caused by infected emboli from a lung infection or endocarditis. Because of the reduced O_2 saturation of the arterial blood, anaerobic cerebral abscesses have a greater association with congenital cardiac defects with a right-left shunt than with any other heart defect.

For accounts of gas gangrene, see p. 497; for tetanus, see p. 496; for botulism, see p. 407 and for pseudomembranous enterocolitis, see p. 406.

Anaerobic culture and antibiotic sensitivity determination: Successful anaerobic culture depends on rapid transport of the specimen under anaerobic conditions to the laboratory and appropriate culture thereafter. Once anaerobes have been isolated, differentiation of subspecies (other than clostridia) is normally only undertaken by a reference laboratory. Slow growth and difficulties in evaluating anaerobic culture can delay the final result. Where the clinical features suggest mixed or anaerobic infection, the culture of a single anaerobe, or of aerobic bacteria only, does not exclude the possibility that further anaerobes are present. A gram-stained smear of the material submitted should always be examined thoroughly, because anaerobic bacteria may be seen microscopically even if they fail to grow. Direct gas chromatography of pus is also a useful, rapid indicator of the presence of anaerobic organisms.

Antibiotic sensitivity testing by the conventional disc method may give erroneous results when used for slow-growing anaerobes. Measurement of the minimal inhibitory concentration by tube dilution also gives variable results according to the technique used. The composition, pH and thickness of the culture medium, the bacterial inoculum and the incubation period must all be strictly standardised to achieve valid results. Bacteroides fragilis in particular can only be regarded as sensitive when the antibiotic concerned is completely stable to the β-lactamases of Bacteroides fragilis. In practice, cases where there is clinical suspicion of mixed or anaerobic infection are started on a combination of antibiotics which reliably covers Bacteroides fragilis as well as coexistent flora, such as a broad-spectrum bactericidal antibiotic + clindamycin or metronidazole.

Choice of antibiotic: Since anaerobic infections are almost always due to a mixture of pathogens, treatment should always cover the range of typical aerobic as well as anaerobic micro-organisms. In respiratory tract infections, a mixture of any or all of the peptococci, peptostreptococci, aerobic streptococci and penicillin-sensitive gram-negative anaerobes (particularly Bacteroides melaninogenicus) is usually present. High doses of benzylpenicillin are generally the best in this situation. Benzylpenicillin is also active against the clostridia which can be present in mixed infections. If staphylococci are possibly involved in mixed infections, clindamycin is preferable. Mixed infections with Bacteroides fragilis, gram-negative bacilli and streptococci are common in infections of the abdomen, female genital tract and in arteriosclerotic gangrene; combinations such as cefotaxime + metronidazole or clindamycin + mezlocillin are useful here.

Imipenem is the only antibiotic at present which combines an extremely broad spectrum of action with excellent activity against staphylococci, gram-negative bacilli and anaerobes. It may therefore be considered as a single agent to treat anaerobic infections. The methoxycephalosporins (cefoxitin, cefotetan, latamoxef and flomoxef) are also active against Bacteroides fragilis and its usual accompanying flora. Chloramphenicol and rifampicin may be kept in reserve for anaerobic infections; they should only be considered as components of an antibiotic combination. The quinolones cannot be relied upon as single agents in the treatment of anaerobic infections; their activity against the Enterobacteriaceae makes them suitable components in a combination (e.g. ciprofloxacin + metronidazole).

Since penicillin-sensitive species of Bacteroides are involved in anaerobic infections of the respiratory tract, reliable activity against Bacteroides is essential. Such activity is often shown by benzylpenicillin, which is well tolerated, may be used at high dosage and is therefore the treatment of choice in infections with Bacteroides melaninogenicus. Benzylpenicillin is also effective against most other anaerobes, including streptococci and clostridia.

The commonest cause of anaerobic infections in the lower half of the body and of septicaemia is Bacteroides fragilis, against which penicillin is ineffective. Clindamycin is then the most active agent, and also has the best activity against other anaerobic species. Clindamycin therefore remains the antibiotic of choice for anaerobic infections, despite the risk of pseudomembranous enterocolitis. Alternatives are metronidazole, which is almost as active, other nitroimidazoles, cefmetazole, flomoxef and cefotetan. Azlocillin, mezlocillin, piperacillin and cefotaxime are not sufficiently stable to the β-lactamases of Bacteroides fragilis.

Tetracyclines and erythromycin are not usually effective against Bacteroides fragilis. The frequency of resistance in Bacteroides fragilis is less than 3% with clindamycin and chloramphenicol, more than 60% with tetracyclines and more than 90% with benzylpenicillin.

Of the *other anaerobic gram-negative bacilli*, fusobacteria are the most sensitive to penicillin and are usually sensitive also to metronidazole, chloramphenicol, the tetracyclines and clindamycin, although occasional strains can be completely resistant to all these agents. Erythromycin has little activity against fusobacteria.

Anaerobic gram-positive cocci (Peptococcus, Peptostreptococcus) are almost always sensitive to clindamycin, penicillin and cephalothin but are often resistant to tetracycline (30–40%) and erythromycin (10–20%). With a few exceptions, metronidazole is also effective.

Of the *anaerobic gram-positive bacilli,* Actinomyces israeli is the most sensitive to penicillin but less sensitive to other agents and generally resistant to metronidazole (see p. 253). The most active antibiotic against Clostridium perfringens is benzylpenicillin, followed in decreasing order of sensitivity by clindamycin, metronidazole, vancomycin, erythromycin and chloramphenicol. 20–30% of strains are resistant to the tetracyclines. Other Clostridium species (e.g. Clostridium ramosum) have variable resistance to penicillin, the tetracyclines, erythromycin and clindamycin, while metronidazole, vancomycin and chloramphenicol are always active. Clostridium difficile (see p. 406) is very sensitive to vancomycin but only weakly sensitive to metronidazole. The only cephalosporin with activity against these organisms is flomoxef. Most other antibiotics are ineffective.

References

CHUHURAL, G. J. JR., et al.: Susceptibility of the Bacteroides fragilis group in the United States: Analysis by site of infection. Antimicrob. Agents Chemother. *32:* 717 (1988).

HILL, G. B., O. M. AYERS: Antimicrobial susceptibilities of anaerobic bacteria isolated from female genital tract infections. Antimicrob. Ag. Chemother. *27:* 324 (1985).

STVRT, B., and S. L. GORBACH: Recent developments in the understanding of the pathogenesis and treatment of anaerobic infections. N. Engl. J. Med. *321:* 298 (1989).

TALLY, F. P., G. J. CUCHURAL, N. V. JACOBUS et al.: National study of the susceptibility of the Bacteroides fragilis group in the United States. Antimicrob. Ag. Chemother. *28:* 675 (1985).

TALLY, F. P., S. L. GORBACH: Therapy of mixed anaerobic-aerobic infections: Lessons from studies of intra-abdominal sepsis. Am. J. Med. *78 (6A):* 145 (1985).

2. Septicaemia

Definition of septicaemia: Septicaemia is generalised bacterial infection in which bacteria are released continuously or intermittently from a primary focus of infection into the blood stream, giving rise to a severe illness, including the formation of infected metastases in other organs. The portal of entry of the infective agent, e.g. an infected wound, can itself be the initial septic focus from which bacteria repeatedly enter the blood stream; once this site has closed or resolved, the septicaemia can continue to arise from a metastatic focus which may be difficult to find. Transient bacteraemia associated with minor, localised infections or after tonsillectomy or dental extraction does not cause severe symptoms and foci of infection do not develop in other organs except in certain abnormal situations (e. g. rheumatic damage to heart valves; prosthetic implants in the vascular or central nervous systems).

Septicaemias can be **classified** according to the species of causative organism and to the portal of entry or initial septicaemic focus (e. g. tonsillitis, urinary infection, cholangitis, cholecystitis, septic abortion, umbilical infection etc.). The initial focus of cryptogenic septicaemia is, by definition, unknown. Bacterial endocarditis and septicaemia associated with foreign bodies are special forms of this infection.

The **clinical diagnosis** of septicaemia (based on intermittent fever, rigors, splenomegaly, demonstration of the initial and metastatic septic foci) is sometimes difficult because specific symptoms may be lacking in patients with impaired resistance (leukaemia, carcinomatosis, premature and newborn babies), patients in intensive care units and where prior antibiotic treatment has been given. Blood cultures should always be obtained where septicaemia is suspected to enable a bacteriological diagnosis to be made and specific chemotherapy to be given.

Important investigations:
1. *Blood cultures* repeated at intervals of 4–6 hours, if possible before antibiotics are given. Blood is best cultured during a rigor but should not only be taken during peaks of temperature, since septicaemia can be afebrile under some circumstances, e. g. in the newborn and elderly. Each bottle of a set of 2 bottles containing suitable liquid media for aerobic and anaerobic culture is inoculated aseptically at the bedside with and without ventilation (for aerobic and anaerobic organisms), and sent to the laboratory. Blood should not be sent in plain specimen tubes because sensitive organisms can die in transit and time may be lost while the specimen is awaiting culture in the laboratory. Blood should be taken by venepuncture after careful skin disinfection with tincture of iodine or 70% isopropyl alcohol. Blood samples should be drawn through indwelling venous catheters only when a catheter infection is suspected, and then cultures from a peripheral vein should be examined in parallel. Blood should be cultured routinely under both aerobic and anaerobic conditions. Improved isolation rates are obtainable from modern, automated methods such as Bactec®.
2. The *latex agglutination test* for the demonstration of antigen in serum, urine and possibly also CSF is sometimes positive when septicaemia is suspected with meningococci, pneumococci, group B streptococci, Haemophilus influenzae (type b), Candida albicans and Cryptococcus neoformans; false positive and false negative results sometimes occur. This test can also detect the cause of the septicaemia several days after treatment has begun.
3. *Bacteriological culture* of pus, cerebrospinal fluid, sputum, urine or aspiration of the septic focus or its metastases. If there is likely to be a delay before the

specimens reach the bacteriological laboratory, purulent CSF or aspirated pus can also be inoculated into 2 broth culture bottles and precultured overnight in the hospital, if transport to the laboratory has to wait until the following day. If this procedure is followed, part of the specimen should also be sent in a sterile container or on a swab in transport medium for microscopic examination, for the recognition of contamination and mixed infections, and for the inoculation of special culture media.
4. *Sensitivity testing* of possible pathogens provides a basis for the choice of antibiotic and the dosage required.
5. *Treatment should, where necessary, be monitored* by further blood cultures, particularly if there is any clinical evidence of relapse, a change in mixed infection or re-infection with a different organism.

General rules for the treatment of septicaemia:
1. If treatment is to be successful, the *initial septic focus must be cleared*, if necessary by drainage of pus or by operation.
2. Antibiotics must *be given for a sufficient period at adequate dosage*, since relapse is commoner when treatment is too short or the dose is too small. Bactericidal antibiotics are generally preferable although even they cannot completely protect against relapse. Parenteral antibiotics can usefully be followed by an oral agent. If a relapse occurs despite good therapy, the possibility of intercurrent resistance should be considered. Relapses are mostly caused by reinfection with a different pathogen or persistence of sensitive organisms in inaccessible sites, such as large collections of pus or an infected foreign body.
3. The *choice of antibiotic* should be guided by the causative organism, the clinical picture and the antibiotic sensitivity pattern. Penicillins and cephalosporins are usually the most suitable antibiotics since they can be given in large doses without particular risk. Benzylpenicillin in large doses is the antibiotic of choice in septicaemia due to streptococci, pneumococci and meningococci (Table 35). *Antibiotic combinations* which increase bactericidal activity are recommended for infections with less sensitive or poorly accessible bacteria. Broad-spectrum combinations are useful for "best-guess" initial therapy. This concept has been achieved in combinations such as cefoxitin + azlocillin, cefuroxime + azlocillin, and cefotaxime + azlocillin. Combinations of azlocillin or piperacillin with cefotaxime have the advantage of an overlapping spectrum which gives a double cover effect. Certain combinations of antibiotics can be useful even when synergy cannot be demonstrated in vitro. Azlocillin or piperacillin may also be combined with another cephalosporin. The spectrum of these combinations can be extended by an aminoglycoside, metronidazole or clindamycin. Ciprofloxacin + azlocillin (or piperacillin) and ciprofloxacin + gentamicin are also rational combinations. When there is a strong suspicion of a staphylococcal cause,

vancomycin may be included in the combination (but not given at the same time as gentamicin). Although imipenem includes the entire spectrum of important pathogens, its activity against pseudomonas can still be usefully enhanced by combination with an aminoglycoside.

Table 35. Daily dose in septicaemia.

Antibiotic	Adults	Children	Preferred route and dose-interval
Benzylpenicillin	12–18 g	300 mg/kg, infants: 600 mg/kg	I. v. injection or short i. v. infusion every 6 hours
Ampicillin Flucloxacillin Dicloxacillin Oxacillin	6–10 (–20) g	150 (–400) mg/kg	Short i. v. infusion or slow injection every 6–8 hours
Azlocillin Mezlocillin Piperacillin	6–15 (–20) g	200–300 mg/kg	Short i. v. infusion or slow i. v. injection every 6–8 h
Ticarcillin	15–20 g	200–300 mg/kg	Short i. v. infusion or slow i. v. injection every 6–8 h
Cefazolin Cefoxitin Cefuroxime Cefotaxime (and other i. v. cephalosporins)	6 g	150 mg/kg	Short i. v. infusion or slow i. v. injection every 6–8 h
Ceftriaxone	2–4 g	30–60 mg/kg	Short i. v. infusion every 12 h
Imipenem	1.5–3 g	50 mg/kg	I. v. infusion every 6–8 h
Aztreonam	8 g	120 mg/kg	Short i. v. infusion or slow i. v. injection every 6–8 h
Gentamicin Tobramycin Netilmicin	240–320 mg	3–5 mg/kg	Every 8–12 h i. m. or i. v.
Amikacin	1 g	10–15 mg/kg	Every 8–12 h i. m. or i. v.
Vancomycin	2 g	40 mg/kg	Short i. v. infusion every 12 h
Clindamycin	1.2–1.8 g	20–30 mg/kg	Short i. v. infusion every 6 h
Ciprofloxacin	0.4 g	–	Short i. v. infusion (30–60 min) every 12 h
Metronidazole	1.5–2 g	20–30 mg/kg	Short i. v. infusion every 6–8 h

Inappropriate combinations include the simultaneous use of a β-lactam antibiotic with a bacteriostatic agent (e. g. chloramphenicol, tetracycline or erythromycin), since this inhibits the bactericidal effect of the penicillin or cephalosporin, which only occurs in the actively dividing bacteria. Care must be taken when using antibiotics together that similar side-effects of two agents do not summate. The pharmacokinetics and possible interactions of the antibiotic components must also be taken into account.

4. Patients treated with large doses of antibiotics should be carefully observed for *side-effects*, since generalised septicaemia can impair renal function and hence delay the excretion of the antibiotic. High doses of the sodium salts of certain antibiotics (e. g. ticarcillin, fosfomycin) can cause hypernatraemia and hypokalaemia. Neurotoxicity (convulsions) can occur after daily doses of more than 12 g of benzylpenicillin, particularly when excretion is impaired, or with meningitis, when the permeability of the blood-CSF barrier is increased.

5. *Supplementary measures:* Treatment of shock, blood transfusion, correction of acidosis, fluid therapy, restoration of electrolyte balance and surgical measures.

6. *Failure of treatment* may be attributed to inadequate dosage, a change in infecting organism, an increase in bacterial resistance, relapse due to persistent forms, failure to eradicate the initial focus of infection, anatomical inaccessibility of the organisms (e. g. in an abscess cavity), an incorrect choice of antibiotics or even the Münchhausen syndrome.

Frequency of causes of septicaemia (Table 36): At one time, streptococci and pneumococci were the commonest causes of septicaemia, but staphylococci and gram-negative intestinal bacteria such as Escherichia coli, klebsiella, Enterobacter, proteus, Pseudomonas aeruginosa and bacteroides now predominate. Meningococci occur either sporadically or in epidemics. Other organisms, such as

Table 36. Percentage frequency of causes of septicaemia in a study by the Paul-Ehrlich Society (PEG, Rosenthal, Deutsche medizinische Wochenschrift 1986) and in the Centre for Internal Medicine of the University of Frankfurt/M., Germany (1986).

Causative organism	PES	CIM
Staphylococcus aureus	19.9	25
Staphylococcus epidermidis	10.4	6
Enterococci	5.5	9
Pneumococci	2.5	3
Candida species	1.9	2
Escherichia coli	22.0	21
Pseudomonas aeruginosa	4.8	6
Klebsiella species	5.9	4
Enterobacter species	4.6	4
Others	22.5	20

Haemophilus influenzae, clostridia, Bacteroides fragilis, salmonella, Pasteurella multocida, gonococci, aeromonas, campylobacter and Serratia marcescens are uncommon. Saprophytic bacteria (coagulase-negative staphylococci, Acinetobacter species, diphtheroids, aerobic spore-bearing bacilli) and yeasts can give rise to septicaemia under certain conditions, such as the implantation of synthetic prostheses in cardiac operations or after shunt operations (Spitz-Holter valve, Scribner shunt).

a) Initial Therapy (Pathogen Unknown)

If the patient has a severe infection and the causative organism is not yet known, initial treatment must be guided by the clinical features. The choice of antibiotic must be based on the possible portals of entry, septic foci, the presence of underlying diseases which impair resistance and the development of septic shock or renal failure. *Bactericidal antibiotics are preferable.* Combinations of antibiotics are generally needed to extend the spectrum of activity and increase the likelihood of clinical efficacy. The best initial treatments available currently are based on β-lactamase-stable cephalosporins such as cefotaxime. They can be supplemented by an aminoglycoside and/or by metronidazole if necessary. If, in addition to enterobacteria, Pseudomonas aeruginosa is a likely pathogen, a combination of ceftazidime with azlocillin or piperacillin is a sound first choice, possibly with tobramycin also.

If infection with multiresistant organisms is suspected in immunosuppressed patients already treated with antibiotics in hospital, the combination of imipenem + gentamicin (possibly also + clindamycin) may be indicated. Ciprofloxacin i. v. should also be considered in adults. Such very broad spectrum regimes cover virtually all bacterial causes of septicaemia but are ineffective against fungi.

Every type of clinical septicaemia has a typical range of possible causes which should be taken into account in the initial treatment.

Septicaemia associated with infections of the normal **urinary tract** is commonly caused by Escherichia coli and other enterobacteria and may be treated with β-lactamase-stable cephalosporins or mezlocillin. More resistant gram-negative rods (proteus, pseudomonas, serratia, klebsiella and enterobacter) are often found after urological operations in patients with chronic indwelling catheters and where there are congenital, neurological or other urinary abnormalities.

Initial treatment is best with combinations such as cefotaxime or mezlocillin + gentamicin. This initial treatment should be reviewed as soon as antibiotic sensitivities are available.

The causative organisms of **biliary septicaemia** cannot be reliably obtained by culture of the duodenal contents; blood culture should always be performed.

Escherichia coli, other enterobacteria, micro-aerophilic and anaerobic streptococci are the commonest causes. Bacteroides, clostridia and pseudomonas are found less frequently.

Mezlocillin, piperacillin and cefotaxime are probably the most suitable agents for *initial treatment* since they have an adequate spectrum of activity, high serum, tissue and biliary concentrations, no loss of activity in bile, and their use is well supported by clinical trials. The tetracyclines were once the drugs of choice, but should no longer be given in severe biliary infections because of the widespread resistance amongst enterobacteria. Mechanical factors sustaining cholangitis or cholecystitis, such as gall stones, must be removed by operation or papillotomy. Septic complications after endoscopic retrograde cannulation of the pancreatic duct (ERCP) are often caused by pseudomonas. Cefazolin, cefazedone or ampicillin are useful in infections of the bile ducts without cholestasis. The combination of a β-lactam antibiotic with an aminoglycoside is often valuable. Its broad spectrum and pharmacokinetic properties would suggest that ciprofloxacin should be suitable, but experience in biliary infection with this agent is still scanty.

Postoperative septicaemia, which often originates in infected wounds, is commonly caused by penicillin-resistant staphylococci. Mixed infections with gram-negative bacteria are not uncommon, particularly in abdominal wounds. A cephalosporin with good activity against staphylococci (e.g. cefazolin, cefazedone) may be given as *initial treatment,* possibly in combination with an aminoglycoside. Severe postoperative sepsis has a high mortality rate and so requires a broad-spectrum combination or treatment with imipenem.

Wound infections after intestinal or gynaecological operations are generally mixed, due to enterobacteria, Bacteroides fragilis and anaerobic streptococci. Initial treatment must be effective against enterobacteria and anaerobes such as bacteroides. This spectrum of pathogens is usually covered by a combination of cefotaxime + metronidazole, or ciprofloxacin + clindamycin. In severe infections where an aminoglycoside is used, a combination of ampicillin or an acylaminopenicillin, gentamicin and metronidazole is generally effective.

Septicaemia after minor skin lesions (with lymphangitis): Mainly caused by staphylococci, sometimes streptococci and occasionally mixed infections including anaerobes. *Treatment* with cefazolin or cefuroxime i.v., clindamycin can also be used.

Septicaemia in patients with bone-marrow suppression (e.g. leukaemia or agranulocytosis) may be caused by a number of micro-organisms, including Pseudomonas aeruginosa, Escherichia coli, klebsiella, proteus and staphylococci, although a range of other organisms may also be involved.

Intervention therapy, which should be started immediately, must take account not only of preceding antibiotic therapy, but also of the clinical symptoms and possible portals of entry. Intervention therapy in patients with solid tumours with a brief period of granulocytopenia may differ from that used in patients with leukaemia. When the period of granulocytopenia is short, a less intensive treatment with, for example, a cephalosporin or piperacillin, will usually be sufficient. Ofloxacin, ciprofloxacin and imipenem would also be suitable. Patients with prolonged periods of granulocytopenia, however, require very broad-spectrum intervention therapy which includes all the relevant organisms.

Of the many possible variations, there are four basic patterns, namely
1. Broad-spectrum cephalosporin + acylaminopenicillin.
2. Acylaminopenicillin + aminoglycoside.
3. Broad-spectrum cephalosporin + aminoglycoside.
4. Cephalosporin + acylaminopenicillin + aminoglycoside.

The superiority of any one of these 4 patterns is not yet established. There would seem to be merit, therefore, in adopting the recommendations from the study carried out by the Paul Ehrlich Society (see Fig. 65, p. 607), according to which treatment begins with a combination of two β-lactam antibiotics or of a β-lactam antibiotic with an aminoglycoside. Patients whose temperature has returned to normal in 3–4 days are counted as responders and the same treatment is then continued for a further 4–8 days. Where the temperature remains elevated after 3–4 days (non-responders), treatment is changed to other antibiotics or to antifungal agents. This intervention therapy is likely in future to make greater use of imipenem and the new quinolones, but their definitive role is not yet established.

Septic abortion and puerperal sepsis (see p. 448): The commonest causes are bacteroides, followed by Escherichia coli, staphylococci, aerobic and anaerobic streptococci, clostridia etc., often in mixed infections. A cervical swab for gram stain and culture (aerobic and anaerobic) and blood cultures should be taken before starting treatment.

Treatment with high doses of antibiotics should cover the broad range of causative bacteria which may be involved. Suitable agents for use singly are cefoxitin, cefotetan, latamoxef, imipenem and flomoxef. Alternatively, combinations including mezlocillin, cefotaxime, metronidazole or clindamycin may be used. Where necessary, retained products of conception should be removed by curettage, and in extreme cases emergency hysterectomy may be needed. Active measures should be taken to treat shock.

Septicaemia complicating severe tonisillitis or tonsillar abscess is generally caused by bacteroides, staphylococci or haemolytic streptococci and very rarely by gram-negative bacteria.

Treatment: A parenteral cephalosporin such as cefoxitin i.v., if necessary combined with an aminoglycoside. Intravenous clindamycin, benzylpenicillin or flucloxacillin may also be used. If septic thrombosis develops in the jugular vein, ligature may be necessary.

Foreign body septicaemia originates from an infected foreign body such as a prosthetic heart valve, a Spitz-Holter valve, a Scribner shunt or an indwelling venous catheter. Bacteraemia is considerably more frequently associated with central venous catheters than with peripheral lines. The risk of septicaemia is much greater in neutropenic patients, when veins are inflamed or thrombosed, and when the same venous catheter is used for a long period without being changed. Other complications are also associated with venous catheters, such as thrombophlebitis, cellulitis, mural right-sided endocarditis, infection of prosthetic implants and septic embolism and infarction (e. g. pulmonary infarction).

The causative agents are mainly saprophytic skin organisms, the commonest being staphylococci (70–80%) with gram-negative bacilli (10–20%) and fungi (1–5%) occurring less frequently. These organisms can originate from the skin of the patient or attendant staff. The contamination of total parenteral nutrition fluids by candida is a particularly serious risk, and other fungi such as aspergillus, Torulopsis glabrata and mucor are occasionally found. Aqueous infusion fluids are not uncommonly contaminated with klebsiella, enterobacter, serratia, Pseudomonas cepacia and Citrobacter freundii.

The diagnosis of venous catheter septicaemia can be difficult. Culture of blood from the venous catheter and the peripheral circulation both qualitatively and quantitatively is of value since blood from the venous catheter usually contains at least 10 times as many bacteria as that obtained by peripheral venepuncture (>2000 organisms/ml). Quantitative blood culture is best performed by the pour-plate method in which 1 ml of blood is thoroughly mixed with 9 ml of molten agar in a sterile petri dish. An assessment of bacterial quantity is also sometimes possible by use of Micrognost blood culture bottles (Roche Diagnostics), which have slides coated with nutrient media attached to removable caps. The slides should be flooded immediately after inoculation with the blood. The identical organisms can sometimes be recovered from the infusion container, and from the site of entry and the tip of the venous catheter. When fungal septicaemia is suspected, it is better to culture arterial blood since venous blood often contains no fungi.

Treatment: The best means of curing the patient is by removing the venous catheter under broad-spectrum antibiotic cover with a combination such as cefotaxime + piperacillin + gentamicin. A more active antistaphylococcal agent such as cefotiam, cefamandole or flucloxacillin may be used in place of cefotaxime. A proven infection with Pseudomonas aeruginosa is best treated with tobramycin + azlocillin, and a staphylococcal infection with vancomycin + rifampicin. A combination is also advisable for fungal infection (e. g. amphotericin B + flucytosine).

There is some dispute about whether infection of an intravascular foreign body should initially be treated with antibiotics alone. The chances of success are poor when thrombophlebitis has become established or when a fungal or pseudomonas infection is present. In a proportion of cases, treatment with effective antibiotics leads to persistent absence of bacteria from the bloodstream. Frequently the blood culture is negative during the antibiotic treatment only, and fever recurs after treatment stops, with the same organisms reappearing. When the foreign body cannot be removed (e.g. prosthetic heart valves), long-term suppression of infection with active oral agents may be necessary.

Infusion bacteraemia: Contaminated infusion solutions can lead to marked febrile reactions, sometimes with severe shock. Since the contaminated bottle can be clear, the empty bottle should always be cultured afterwards. The bacteraemia resulting from contaminated infusion fluids is sometimes transient and can often be treated with antibiotics without needing to change the catheter.

Treatment with a cephalosporin or an acylaminopenicillin is advised, even if spontaneous improvement is usual. Similar reactions and septicaemic illnesses can be evoked by stored blood and blood products.

Neonatal septicaemia can vary greatly in its presentation and clinical features. It can develop *in utero* (e.g. listeria), during birth (Escherichia coli, pseudomonas, group B streptococci etc.) and post-partum (staphylococci and other organisms). Prompt, early *treatment* is essential when infection is first suspected (once blood and CSF have been collected for culture). When septicaemia of intrauterine origin is suspected following premature rupture of the membranes, a blood culture of placental blood obtained by puncture of a placental vessel from the exterior should always be obtained. When the amniotic fluid is infected, this blood culture yields the same organisms as are obtained from the first passage of meconium and from the deep ear swab immediately after birth. When blood cultures in premature rupture of the membranes are positive, antibiotic treatment should be started immediately even in the absence of clinical features of septicaemia, since these usually follow 1–2 days later. Because of the serious prognosis, a combination of antibiotics is usually given, based on the likely causes of infection but modified to take account of the physiological impairment of drug metabolism and excretion at this age (see p. 612).

Treatment should be well tolerated, cover a broad spectrum of bacteria, and include resistant staphylococci. Some useful combinations for initial treatment are a cephalosporin together with an acylaminopenicillin, e.g. cefotaxime + piperacillin. These combinations can be complemented by vancomycin (if multiresistant staphylococci occur frequently) or by an aminoglycoside (gentamicin or amikacin).

b) Directed Therapy (Pathogen Known)

Staphylococcus aureus septicaemia: The bacteraemia is usually continuous and originates from skin infections (sometimes with lymphangitis), wound or umbilical infections, thrombophlebitis, mastoiditis, parotitis or pneumonia. It is relatively common in heroin addicts and in intravascular foreign body infections. Septic metastatic foci commonly occur in the kidneys, bone marrow, joints, brain and meninges, lungs, endocardium etc.

The tendency to abscess formation and to inadequate treatment is associated with a considerable relapse rate; a prolonged course of antibiotics, preferably as a combination of a β-lactam antibiotic with fusidic acid, should be given.

Treatment: Benzylpenicillin may be given for sensitive staphylococci in a dose of 7.2–12 g daily for adults and older children and 1.8–6 g for the newborn and infants, in several short i. v. infusion. Combination with fusidic acid is advisable.

For penicillin-resistant staphylococci, use flucloxacillin, 6–12 g a day in 3–4 short i. v. infusions or slow i. v. injections for adults and 150–400 mg/kg for children; cefazolin (6 g a day for adults) is an alternative. 3 g of fusidic acid a day may be added.

In cases of penicillin allergy, use cefazolin, cefazedone, cefuroxime or cefamandole, 6–8 g a day for adults, 200 mg/kg for children, in 3–4 short i. v. infusions or slow i. v. injections. Erythromycin or clindamycin should be considered where cross-hypersensitivity between penicillins and cephalosporins is suspected.

In patients with cephalosporin allergy or with methicillin-resistant staphylococci, consider vancomycin as a daily dose of 2 g in adults or 40 mg/kg in children, divided into two short i. v. infusions. Avoid vancomycin in renal failure because of the increased risk of ototoxicity.

Length of treatment: 4–6 weeks, or even longer, may be necessary. Reduce dosage when improvement is established, but continue parenteral administration. Surgical intervention (drainage of abscesses and the removal of infected foreign bodies etc.) may also be necessary.

Fosfomycin, rifampicin, clindamycin and imipenem should be kept in reserve for staphylococcal septicaemia resistant to the above antibotics.

Staphylococcus epidermidis septicaemia: Septicaemia with coagulase-negative staphylococci has recently become more common. Intravenous foreign bodies (intravenous catheters, dialysis shunts etc.) have been the main portals of entry. Occasional cases develop endocarditis. The diagnosis can only be made when the same strain is isolated on a number of occasions from blood culture. Multiresistant strains which include resistance to methicillin are quite frequent.

Treatment must be based on antibiotic sensitivities, e. g. with flucloxacillin or a parenteral cephalosporin + gentamicin. Methicillin-resistant strains are not treatable with penicillins or cephalosporins, even if apparently sensitive *in vitro*. In many cases the combination of vancomycin plus rifampicin is effective. The infected foreign body should, if possible, be removed. If this is not possible, the only solution is suppressive treatment with a well tolerated oral agent chosen on the basis of antibiotic sensitivities. Thus, suppressive therapy with cephalexin or clindamycin may be indicated for an infected prosthetic heart valve.

Group A streptococcal septicaemia is relatively uncommon nowadays, but can still be fulminating and must always be treated very seriously. Portals of entry are provided by infections of the skin, wounds, the female reproductive tract or the upper respiratory tract. Fulminant infections which progress rapidly and affect a number of sites in the body occur regularly.

Treatment: Benzylpenicillin 3–6 (–12) g/day for adults in several short i.v. infusions or injections; 0.6–3 g/day over 1–2 weeks in small children and the newborn. When clinical recovery is well established, treatment may be changed to phenoxymethylpenicillin, 0.75–1.5 g a day for 2 weeks. Alternatives (in cases of penicillin allergy) are a parenteral cephalosporin (see Table 44), clindamycin (1.2–1.8 g a day) or vancomycin.

Pneumococcal septicaemia may be a complication of pneumonia but is sometimes seen in patients with impaired resistance (e.g. after splenectomy), as a complication of sinusitis, or with no recognisable portal of entry. The disease can progress rapidly with septic shock and occasionally meningitis.

Treatment: Large doses of benzylpenicillin, as for Group A streptococcal septicaemia. Use imipenem, rifampicin or vancomycin where strains are resistant to penicillin (still very uncommon in north-western Europe).

Group B streptococcal septicaemia is particularly a disease of the newborn where it is seen in two forms, one of early onset acquired in utero and manifest in the first 24–48 hours of life, and one of late onset, presumably acquired at birth or soon after but presenting after an interval of a few weeks. The disease can be fulminating and the prognosis is often poor. It is occasionally found in adults with impaired resistance.

Prompt *treatment* with benzylpenicillin in combination with gentamicin gives the best results, though parenteral cephalosporins and broad-spectrum penicillins also eliminate group B streptococci effectively.

Septicaemia with other streptococci: Viridans or non-haemolytic streptococci of other groups are not uncommonly isolated in blood cultures from patients without endocarditis.

They can be a sign of bacteraemia without septicaemia, and can also arise from colonic carcinoma or mixed anaerobic infection. Apart from the enterococci, such streptococci are almost always sensitive to penicillin but treatment should often take the possible presence of other organisms into account, as part of a gut-related mixed infection from which streptococci have been the only component to be isolated. Streptococcus milleri typically gives rise to septicaemia with a tendency to abscess formation.

Treatment with benzylpenicillin + metronidazole is often, therefore, better than penicillin alone.

Enterococcal septicaemia is rare. The portal of entry is usually through the intestinal or urogenital tract, occasionally through extensive burns. Septicaemic metastases are uncommon. Often associated with bacterial endocarditis (see p. 345), and sometimes as part of a mixed infection with enterobacteria and Bacteroides.

Treatment: Ampicillin, 6–10 (–20) g a day for adults and older children; 150–400 mg/kg for young children, divided into 4 short i. v. infusions or slow i. v. injections. The bactericidal activity of ampicillin is greatly enhanced by combination with gentamicin.

Vancomycin i. v. should be given to patients who are allergic to penicillin. The cephalosporins as a group have very poor activity against enterococci; imipenem is very active.

Meningococcal septicaemia: The portal of entry is the nasopharynx and the septicaemia is usually accompanied by meningitis or arthritis and rarely by endocarditis; the most severe (the Waterhouse-Friderichsen syndrome) is commonest in children and was almost always fatal. Meningococci can occasionally be demonstrated in stained blood smears as gram-negative kidney-shaped diplococci.

Treatment: Benzylpenicillin in a daily dose of 12–18 g in adults, 0.3 g/kg in younger children and 0.6 g/kg in the newborn, in 4–6 short i. v. infusions or slow i. v. injections. Combination with other antibiotics is not necessary. Treatment should continue until the patient's clinical improvement is well established and the ESR has returned to normal. The initial high doses of penicillin may be reduced once improvement has started. Meningococci are nowadays often resistant to sulphonamides, which are therefore no longer reliable.

Chloramphenicol should be given to patients with penicillin allergy, or a strong history of epileptiform convulsions, in an adult dose of 3 (–4) g a day (50–80 mg/kg for children) orally or i. v.

Prophylaxis is advisable for close (usually household) contacts. Give rifampicin 10 mg/kg (children up to 12 y.) or 600 mg (adults) every 12 h for 2 days. Primary rifampicin resistance has been reported. Ofloxacin and ciprofloxacin are alternatives to rifampicin (see p. 243).

The **Waterhouse-Friderichsen syndrome** occurs in meningococcal and other forms of septicaemia and is expressed as profound shock, loss of water and electrolytes, internal and external bleeding and a consumption coagulopathy with thrombocytopenia and a deficiency of fibrinogen, prothrombin and factors V and VII.

Treatment consists not only of large doses of penicillin but also of expanding the plasma volume, correcting the electrolyte imbalance, heparin (to prevent further clotting abnormalities), the possible administration of antithrombin III or streptokinase to activate fibrinolysis, and fresh blood transfusions to replace the lack of clotting factors. The role of prednisone is controversial since it may favour the development of a consumption coagulopathy.

Escherichia coli septicaemia is the commonest form of septicaemia in the newborn and young infant. It is also found as a complication of urinary infection or cholangitis in children and adults and often gives rise to septic shock, which carries a high mortality rate.

Treatment: Cefotaxime is likely to be effective against almost all infections caused by Escherichia coli (for dosage, see Table 35). Ampicillin, which is often given, is much less active than cefotaxime and is inactive against β-lactamase producing strains. It is unwise in serious cases to rely for β-lactamase stability solely on a clavulanate-potentiated penicillin such as co-amoxiclav (amoxycillin/ clavulanate [Augmentin]) or ticarcillin/clavulanate. If a penicillin is required, mezlocillin or piperacillin should be used instead of ampicillin, possibly in combination with gentamicin to increase the bactericidal effect. Other alternatives are aztreonam, imipenem and ciprofloxacin, against which resistance is extremely uncommon. The duration of treatment is governed by the clinical response.

In **septic shock,** the most important measure is the rapid institution of bactericidal antibiotic therapy in high dosage, preferably with β-lactam antibiotics. The view that bactericidal antibiotics can intensify septic shock is obviously incorrect. Other supportive measures which are recommended include prednisone, volume replacement, correction of acidosis, digitalisation, oxygen and haemodialysis if renal failure develops. If an aminoglycoside is used, serum concentrations must be monitored frequently because of the labile renal function.

Treatment: Shock lung must be adequately treated with mechanical ventilation if necessary. Fluid balance should be carefully controlled by monitoring central venous and pulmonary arterial pressure and urinary output. Dopamine and dobutamine have a positive inotropic effect on the heart and increase the blood pressure. Adrenaline, noradrenaline and other peripheral vasoconstrictors are contraindicated. Prednisone can be useful. In disseminated intravascular coagulation, treatment with antithrombin III etc. is necessary at the appropriate stage. The use of anti-endotoxins (monoclonal) or anti TNF (monoclonal, pentoxyfyllin) is still investigational.

When signs of shock are severe and associated with a rash like that of scarlet fever, conjunctivitis and enanthemata, staphylococcal toxic shock syndrome should be suspected. In this condition, bacteraemia seldom occurs but the staphylococci can be isolated from the vagina, from wounds or from abscesses see p. 451).

2. Septicaemia

Klebsiella and Enterobacter septicaemia occur not uncommonly in hospitals. Initial foci include pneumonia, infections of wounds, the urinary tract or venous catheter sites and cholangitis. Septic shock is common and antibiotic treatment must be guided by sensitivity testing because antibiotic resistance is usually present.

Treatment: Cefotaxime and similar cephalosporins have the greatest activity against klebsiella. Enterobacter aerogenes is regularly inhibited by the newer cephalosporins. Most strains of Enterobacter cloacae, however, are resistant to all penicillins and most cephalosporins, but are almost always sensitive to imipenem and ciprofloxacin. A few klebsiellas and enterobacters are resistant to the aminoglycosides. Klebsiella or enterobacter septicaemia is best treated with a combination of a newer cephalosporin and an aminoglycoside, which is often synergistic. Most penicillins (ampicillin, ticarcillin) are inactive against klebsiella, though mezlocillin and piperacillin have some activity against a few strains of Klebsiella pneumoniae. Fixed combinations with β-lactam antagonists (e. g. co-amoxiclav, ticarcillin/clavulanate) should not be relied upon as single agents in septicaemia with these organisms.

Serratia marcescens septicaemia is increasingly found in intensive care units and usually arises from infections of the urinary or respiratory tracts or of venous catheter sites.

Treatment is difficult because strains are often resistant. Cefotaxime or a similar cephalosporin are usually the best, alone or in combination with an aminoglycoside such as amikacin. Mezlocillin or piperacillin, imipenem, aztreonam or a new quinolone (e. g. ciprofloxacin) are alternatives.

Dosage: see Table 35.

Proteus septicaemia: Common foci are infections of the urinary, intestinal or biliary tracts, the middle ear or infected areas of necrosis. Often gives rise to septic shock. Treat according to the species of proteus and the antibiotic sensitivity pattern.

Treatment: The treatment of proteus septicaemia has to take the probability of mixed infection into account. Because of its much greater activity against all species of proteus, cefotaxime has now replaced ampicillin, which used to be a first choice. Mezlocillin, piperacillin and ticarcillin/clavulanate are alternatives, but should always be given in combination with gentamicin. Imipenem, ciprofloxacin and aztreonam are always effective.

Dosage: see Table 35.

Pseudomonas septicaemia usually originates from infections of the urinary tract, burns or wounds and is a life-threatening septic complication of leukaemia. Septic shock is frequent, metastatic foci can occur in various organs, and treatment is difficult because of the limited range of sensitivities of the organism.

The *treatment of choice* is a combination of a fully active β-lactam antibiotic with high doses of an aminoglycoside, e.g. of azlocillin (15 g daily) with tobramycin (240–320 mg daily). Alternative β-lactams are ceftazidime, cefsulodin, piperacillin, piperacillin/tazobactam, aztreonam and imipenem; alternative aminoglycosides are gentamicin, netilmicin and amikacin. The initial treatment may need to be corrected when sensitivities become available. Ciprofloxacin is an alternative when resistance to the β-lactam or aminoglycoside is encountered, and can also be used for subsequent oral treatment.

Haemophilus septicaemia: The initial focus is usually the nasopharynx or respiratory tract and septicaemia with this organism is often associated with meningitis, septic arthritis, endocarditis (generally subacute) and acute epiglottitis. Predominantly seen in young children.

Treatment: The treatment of choice used to be intravenous ampicillin in high dosage, but strains which are resistant to ampicillin are becoming commoner. Intravenous chloramphenicol is an effective alternative, although resistance to chloramphenicol is also occasionally found. Cefotaxime and other broad-spectrum cephalosporins are much more active than ampicillin and are stable to β-lactamase. Other alternatives are cefuroxime or cefamandole. Dosage: see Table 35. A new quinolone such as ciprofloxacin may be considered in adults.

Clostridium septicaemia is caused by Clostridium perfringens (the causative organism of gas gangrene) or other clostridia and arises from wound, intestinal or puerperal infections, particularly after abdominal operations, abortions and in patients with bone-marrow insufficiency. Acute haemolysis with jaundice and disseminated intravascular coagulation are frequent complications.

Treatment: Benzylpenicillin, 6–12 g a day parenterally is the treatment of choice, and other antibiotics such as cefoxitin, tetracyclines and metronidazole are only recommended in patients with penicillin allergy. Treatment with hyperbaric oxygen in a special chamber is an important, though still somewhat controversial, adjunct to treatment, but is only available in a few specialized centres. The value of antitoxin against Clostridium perfringens is doubtful.

Bacteroides septicaemia may be acute or chronic, with a primary focus in the genital tract, nasopharynx or intestinal tract. Subacute endocarditis is uncommon, but abscesses with foul smelling pus are characteristic. Often associated with anaerobic streptococci, enterococci or Escherichia coli.

Treatment: Since sensitivity testing of bacteroides is technically difficult and time-consuming, initial treatment should be with clindamycin i.v., metronidazole i.v. or cefoxitin. These agents are reliably effective against all species of bacteroides including B. fragilis, which is not susceptible to penicillin although other species of bacteroides and anaerobic streptococci, which are often associated, generally are. Imipenem, rifampicin, latamoxef, cefotetan, azlo- and mezlocillin, piperacillin and tinidazole are often effective alternatives, but other penicillins, cephalosporins or aminoglycosides are not indicated in infections caused by bacteroides.

Melioidosis is caused by Pseudomonas pseudomallei, occurs mainly in southern Asia and Central and South America and presents acutely as septicaemia with profuse diarrhoea or subacutely and chronically with abscesses, particularly of the skin and bones, or a prolonged pneumonia with cavitation. The mortality rate is high.

Treatment: Tetracyclines or chloramphenicol in high dosage. Initial treatment should always be combined with co-trimoxazole. Gentamicin is ineffective. Abscesses should be drained where necessary.

Occasional bacterial causes of septicaemia: Gonococci (treat with penicillin or cefotaxime if resistant), Listeria monocytogenes (ampicillin), Pasteurella multocida (penicillin or tetracycline), Campylobacter fetus (gentamicin + erythromycin or clindamycin), aeromonas (co-trimoxazole), salmonella (see p. 502).

Fungal septicaemia occurs not infrequently in patients whose resistance to infection is impaired by immunological deficiencies, malignancies, cortisone treatment or venous catheter infections. Important causes of disseminated fungal sepsis are Candida species, aspergillus, Coccidioides immitis, Mucor species, Torulopsis glabrata and Histoplasma capsulatum.

Treatment: Amphotericin B i.v. with the addition of flucytosine if in vitro sensitivity can be shown. Flucytosine is always inactive against histoplasmosis and coccidioidomycosis (see p. 209) but ketoconazole or itraconazole may be effective.

References

BENEZRA, D., et al.: Prospective study of infections in indwelling central venous catheters using quantitative blood cultures. Am. J. Med. *85:* 495 (1988).
BRYAN, C. S., F. JOHN Jr., S. M. PAI, T. L. AUSTIN: Gentamicin vs. cefotaxime for therapy of neonatal sepsis. Relationship to drug resistance. Am. J. Dis. Child. *139:* 1086 (1985).
CASTOR, B., J. URSING, M. ABERG, N. PALSSON: Infected wounds and repeated septicemia in a case of factitious illness. Scand. J. Infect. Dis. *22:* 227–232 (1990).
DUGDALE, D. C., P. G. RAMSEY: Staphylococcus aureus bacteremia in patients with Hickman catheters. Am. J. Med. *89:* 137–141 (1990).
JACOBS, M. B., M. YEAGER: Thrombotic and infectious complications of Hickman-Broviac catheters. Arch. Intern. Med. *144:* 1597 (1984).
MORRISON, R. E., et al.: Melioidosis: A reminder. Am. J. Med. *84:* 965 (1988).
RUPAR, D. G., K. D. HERZOG, M. C. FISHER, S. S. LONG: Prolonged Bacteremia with catheter related central venous thrombosis. Am. J. Dis. Child. *144:* 879–882 (1990).
SIMON, C., H. SCHRÖDER, C. BEYER, T. ZERBST: Neonatal Sepsis in an Intensive Care Unit and Results of Treatment. Infection *19:* 146–149 (1991).

So, S. Y., P. Y. Chau, Y. K. Leung, W. K. Lam, D. Y. C. Yu: Successful treatment of melioidosis caused by a multiresistant strain in an immunocompromised host with third-generation cephalosporins. Am. Rev. Respir. Dis. *127:* 650–654 (1983).

Sprung, C. L. et al.: The effects of high-dose corticosteroids in patients with septic shock. A prospective, controlled study. N. Engl. J. Med. *311:* 1137 (1984).

3. Bacterial Endocarditis

Frequency of bacterial causes: Viridans and non-haemolytic streptococci 65–85%, enterococci 5–15% staphylococci 5–15%, non-bacteraemic forms 5–10%, haemophilus 1–2% and gram-negative intestinal bacteria 2–6%. Staphylococci and gram-negative intestinal bacteria are usually associated with acute endocarditis and streptococci with subacute endocarditis (the classical endocarditis lenta). Almost all microbial species can occasionally cause endocarditis (Haemophilus influenzae, H. aphrophilus, Cardiobacterium hominis, gonococci, pneumococci, campylobacter, listeria, Erysipelothrix rhusiopathiae, brucella, Bacteroides species, fusobacteria, candida and other fungal species, Coxiella burnetii etc.). Endocarditis in heroin addicts is often caused by staphylococci, gram-negative bacilli and fungi. A series of septic emboli can give rise to pneumonia. Endocarditis can also occur in immunocompromised patients as a result of bacteraemia or fungaemia arising from an indwelling venous catheter.

Acute ulcerative endocarditis (septic endocarditis), which is generally caused by Staphylococcus aureus, can attack and rapidly destroy normal heart valves. Septic metastases may develop in the brain, meninges, kidneys or on the skin.

Subacute bacterial endocarditis, classically described as endocarditis lenta, is usually caused by viridans or non-haemolytic streptococci or enterococci and occasionally by Staphylococcus epidermidis, haemophilus or fungi. It virtually always affects a diseased or congenitally abnormal valve, usually after old rheumatic heart disease. The mitral and aortic valves are the most commonly involved. Cases of pure mitral stenosis are rarely affected. The clinical features are changing heart murmurs, fever, high ESR (except for polycythaemia in cyanotic heart disease), symptoms of focal nephritis, splenomegaly and small skin haemorrhages. There is often a recent history of dental extraction, tonsillectomy, abdominal surgery or intestinal disease. If there is a thick fibrinous exudate on the infected valves or if the causative organisms are very fastidious and difficult to grow in liquid media, cultures can sometimes fail to yield an isolate. This "abacteraemic" form can then be difficult to differentiate the condition from rheumatic endocarditis or lupus erythematosus. Culture-negative endocarditis is uncommon with good blood culture technique; it is usually attributable to antecedent antibiotic treatment but, if relevant coxiella infection should also be excluded by serological tests. Echocardiograms are very useful for the localisation of valvular or mural vegetations and for the diagnosis of valve perforation.

Endocarditis after open heart surgery can occur in early or late forms. The early form (in the first 2 months of life) is usually associated with *Staphylococcus epidermidis* and diphtheroid corynebacteria, and occasionally with gram-negative bacilli and fungi (Candida, Aspergillus). The latter are particularly unfavourable in infections of prosthetic valves and Teflon patch prostheses. The late form is usually caused by staphylococci and streptococci. Typical signs of endocarditis are often absent. Several positive cultures are necessary to make the diagnosis. In the early form the causative organisms enter the blood-stream either during the operation or soon afterwards (e. g. through contamination of venous catheters, endotracheal tubes or drainage tubes). In the late form, neglect of antibiotics for the prophylaxis of endocarditis (see below) in dental or similar procedures can be the cause. The early form has a poorer prognosis than the late form, particularly when the aortic valve is affected, and is frequently combined with myocardial abscess, valve rupture of purulent pericarditis. If no bacteria or fungi can be isolated from culture (in about 5–15%), it can be difficult to distinguish the condition from a post-cardiotomy syndrome, from pulmonary embolism, or from transfusion-associated cytomegalovirus infection. When antibiotics are used to treat endocarditis after a cardiac operation, an early re-operation to replace the prosthetic valve is usually unavoidable. Two, and preferably three, antibiotics should be given for at least six weeks and often longer. Before culture of the causative organism, initial treatment with a combination of vancomycin, gentamicin and ampicillin is recommended. Where replacement of the valve is not possible, treatment with rifampicin plus vancomycin may be tried.

Bacteriological diagnosis: Antibiotic treatment of acute septic endocarditis should not begin until at least 2 sets of blood cultures have been taken at short intervals; if subacute endocarditis is suspected 3–5 blood cultures should be taken at intervals of 4–6 hours. The prognosis depends on the availability of an isolate. Because a number of causative organisms of endocarditis are difficult to culture, a reliable general blood culture technique is essential, using liquid or biphasic media which support aerobic and anerobic bacteria as well as fungi. A suitable blood culture technique is described on p. 326. When testing antibiotic sensitivities of staphylococci, it is important not to misread methicillin resistance as susceptibility; a heavy bacterial inoculum and incubation at 30° C for 3 days is important to avoid this error.

The treatment of endocarditis is governed by *rules* similar to those for the treatment of septicaemia (see p. 327), but with different doses and varying duration of treatment. Because of the risk of secondary bacteraemia, with infection of the damaged valve, peripheral or central venous catheters to administer treatment should be avoided if possible. While bacteriostatic drugs can be effective in other forms of septicaemia, bacterial endocarditis can only be eradicated by a bactericidal agent. Corticosteroids and anticoagulants are contraindicated because of the risk of valve perforation or embolic disease.

The *efficacy of antibiotic treatment* may be *predicted* by determining (a) the minimal inhibitory concentration (MIC) and minimal bactericidal concentration (MBC) of the antibiotics used against the patient's isolate; (b) the presence or absence of synergy in the antibiotic combination used against the patient's isolate, or (c) the bactericidal activity of the patient's serum during treatment against his own isolate.

Treatment can be considered *satisfactory* when dilutions of at least 1 in 4 are completely bactericidal to the patient's isolate and this index, which is easily determined in a hospital bacteriology laboratory, correlates well with the clinical outcome of treatment.

Criteria of successful treatment: Defervescence, return to normal ESR, resolution of clinical symptoms, absence of fever after discontinuation of antibiotics and subsequent negative blood cultures. Treatment at full antibiotic dosage should continue for 4–6 weeks or until the ESR returns to normal. Longer courses of treatment are necessary for endocarditis after the insertion of a prosthetic heart valve, and the prognosis is poor. Blood concentrations should be carefully monitored when potentially ototoxic antibiotics (e. g. gentamicin) are used and when renal failure is suspected. Blood should be taken immediately prior to an injection, when the serum concentrations should be less than 1 mg/l if no accumulation of the aminoglycoside has occurred.

Surgical replacement of the diseased valve should be considered early if the causative organism is resistant to bactericidal therapy, or if signs of valve perforation develop.

Streptococcal endocarditis is mostly subacute (*endocarditis lenta*) and due to viridans and non-haemolytic streptococci; an acute form due to haemolytic streptococci or pneumococci is rare. Benzylpenicillin is the drug of choice at a dosage related to the sensitivity of the isolate, in combination with gentamicin at standard dosage (240 mg daily in patients with normal renal function).

Standard treatment (also applicable to less sensitive strains of streptococci with minimal inhibitory concentrations *in vitro* of 0.6–1.2 mg/l of penicillin):

12–18 g of benzylpenicillin sodium in 4–6 short i. v. infusions, and possibly as a large dose of procaine penicillin i. m. at night. The addition of an aminoglycoside (formerly streptomycin, now gentamicin, 80 mg i. m. 2–3 times a day) is of proven value with the lower doses of penicillin used formerly, and is essential when the sensitivity to penicillin is poor. Treatment should last for 4–6 weeks, if possible until the ESR has returned completely to normal. Blood cultures taken at intervals during treatment should be negative.

Where the *streptococci* are *very sensitive* to penicillin (MIC less than 0.06 mg/l), the dose of penicillin can be reduced to 3–6 g per day.

In patients *allergic to penicillin,* combine cefazolin i.v. in high dosage with gentamicin, having ruled out cross-allergy. Vancomycin and clindamycin are alternative treatments.

Enterococcal endocarditis is generally subacute but occasionally acute and is difficult to treat because of antibiotic resistance. Occurrence in women is usually after febrile abortion or during a urinary infection.

Treatment: Ampicillin or amoxycillin, 10–20 g a day in 2–3 short infusions or slow i.v. injections (for 6–8 weeks); combination with gentamicin (80 mg i.m. or i.v. 3 times a day) is essential to overcome the Eagle effect (see p. 584) and to achieve bactericidal activity through synergy. The failure to treat with this synergistic combination amounts to clinical malpractice. Mezlocillin is a more active alternative to ampicillin.

Vancomycin in combination with imipenem or gentamicin may be used as an alternative to ampicillin in cases of allergy or resistance.

Endocarditis caused by Streptococcus bovis (also in Lancefield group D but not a true enterococcus) is often associated with carcinoma of the colon and is more responsive to antibiotics than enterococcal endocarditis.

Treatment: Benzylpenicillin (18–24 g a day) + gentamicin.

Endocarditis with Staphylococcus aureus or S. epidermidis: If the organism is *sensitive to penicillin,* give benzylpenicillin, 12–24 g a day, as 4 short infusions or slow i.v. injections.

Against *penicillin-resistant* organisms, give flucloxacillin, 12–15 g in 4 short infusions or slow i.v. injections combined with gentamicin (80 mg i.m. 3 times a day). If staphylococcal endocarditis is suspected from the outset, the best treatment is vancomycin 1 g twice a day (see p. 176), combined with rifampicin (0.3 g 3 times a day by mouth). An alternative is clindamycin (0.6 g 3 times a day).

Allergy to penicillin: treat with cefazolin i.v. in high dose (rule out cross-allergy), possibly in combination with vancomycin or gentamicin.

Long-term treatment is necessary; when improvement is sufficient for oral antibiotics to be given, continue with flucloxacillin or phenoxymethylpenicillin by mouth, according to sensitivities. If antibiotic treatment of post-cardiotomy endocarditis fails, a further operation should be considered which should remove residual foci of infection, particularly if mycotic vegetations are still present.

Endocarditis due to gram-negative bacteria carries a poor prognosis, is little affected by antibiotics and maximum dosage is always necessary (see Table 35). In general, a combination of a β-lactam antibiotic with an aminoglycoside should be given, according to antibiotic sensitivities. Experience with imipenem and ciprofloxacin is still scanty, but both agents are promising.

Escherichia coli: Cefotaxime (or possibly mezlocillin) + gentamicin.

Klebsiella pneumoniae: Cefotaxime + gentamicin; possibly also imipenem + gentamicin.

Enterobacter species: According to antibiotic sensitivity testing, cefotaxime, ceftriaxone or imipenem + gentamicin.

Pseudomonas aeruginosa: Azlocillin + tobramycin, possibly also piperacillin, cefsulodin, ceftazidime or imipenem in combination with amikacin. Surgical removal of the infected heart valve is often necessary.

Proteus mirabilis: Cefotaxime + gentamicin, or alternatively ampicillin + gentamicin.

Other Proteus species: Cefotaxime + an aminoglycoside. Mezlocillin, piperacillin, imipenem or ciprofloxacin in combination with an aminoglycoside may also be considered.

Salmonellae: Cefotaxime + an aminoglycoside, or alternatively imipenem or ciprofloxacin + an aminoglycoside.

Serratia: Cefotaxime (or ceftazidime) + an aminoglycoside, or alternatively mezlocillin, piperacillin, imipenem or ciprofloxacin in combination with an aminoglycoside (e.g. amikacin), according to the antibiotic sensitivity pattern.

Haemophilus species: Cefotaxime + an aminoglycoside should replace the former treatment with ampicillin + an aminoglycoside.

Campylobacter endocarditis: Occurs in both healthy and damaged heart valves. The organism is isolated from anaerobic blood culture and treatment should be with gentamicin i.m. + clindamycin i.v. for at least 4 weeks.

Fungal endocarditis: Occurs in heroin addicts, after cardiac operations and in patients with prolonged indwelling venous catheters. Candida or aspergillus may be involved and can sometimes only be cultured from arterial blood.

Candida endocarditis: Give amphotericin B in increasing dosage up to 1 mg/kg/day (see p. 193), in combination with flucytosine (if *in vitro* activity has been proven). The efficacy of fluconazole, itraconazole and ketoconazole in fungal endocarditis is uncertain (no fungicidal effect!). Surgical removal of the infected valve, with prosthetic replacement, is usually essential, as is the operative removal of large septic emboli.

Q-fever endocarditis: Coxiella burnetii cannot be isolated from blood culture. A provisional diagnosis is made in the absence of other bacterial causes of the endocarditis, but with a positive C. burneti CFT and a supporting clinical picture. *Treatment* may be attempted with doxycycline (200 mg per day) for ½–1 year, possibly in combination with co-trimoxazole or rifampicin, but often fails to sterilise the valve. Valve replacement may be necessary.

Initial treatment before culture results are available: When there is a strong clinical suspicion of *acute* endocarditis, the patient should be treated promptly with a combination of vancomycin + cefotaxime, which should be modified appropriately when culture results become available. When the clinical course is *subacute* and the sensitive organism has not been identified, combine penicillin with gentamicin as in "abacteraemic" endocarditis (see below).

Culture-negative or "abacteraemic" endocarditis: If cultures of several blood samples using satisfactory culture methods remain sterile in a patient not pretreated with antibiotics and with a typical clinical picture of subacute endocarditis, a diagnosis of culture-negative or "abacteraemic" endocarditis can be assumed, and the patient should be treated with benzylpenicillin 24 g a day, + gentamicin 240 mg a day. A high level of C-reactive protein (CRP) in serum is supportive evidence of bacterial infection. If a clinical response fails to occur within 48–72 hours, a causative organism resistant to penicillin and gentamicin (Q-fever, chlamydiae, haemophilus) should be suspected. Since haemophilus infections are commoner, cefotaxime should be tried first and, if the patient fails to respond, changed to doxycycline i. v., which is active against Q-fever and chlamydias.

Endocarditis in heroin addicts: Staphylococci cause the majority (approx. 50%) of infections and enterobacteria about 20%. Pseudomonas, streptococci, enterococci, candida and mixed infections are less common. The endocarditis is usually acute and often affects the right side of heart with multiple pulmonary infiltrates. Heart murmurs are sometimes absent. Left heart involvement suggests a poor prognosis. Severe neurological signs frequently develop, caused by metastatic foci of infection. Because of the poor prognosis, *antibiotic treatment should be started as soon as possible* after taking the initial blood cultures, with combination such as cefotaxime + azlocillin + gentamicin. The antibiotic regime should be modified according to the results of sensitivity testing. Candida endocarditis requires surgical removal of the valve and treatment with amphotericin B + flucytosine (if the isolate is sensitive to the latter).

All forms of bacterial endocarditis can extensively **damage the affected heart valves** and give rise to uncontrollable heart failure, correctable only by urgent valve replacement. When endocarditis follows open heart surgery, the infected prosthetic valve may itself need replacement but a trial of intensive bactericidal antibiotic therapy may be worthwhile before operative removal.

Prevention of endocarditis: The development of bacterial endocarditis can be prevented by prophylactic antibiotics. Patients with rheumatic heart disease or congenital heart defects or who have had cardiac surgery or a previous attack of bacterial endocarditis are at particular risk when they undergo dental extractions, tonsillectomy, urogenital or intestinal operations, endoscopy or abscess drainage, and these procedures should be covered by antibiotic prophylaxis. Two doses of antibiotic are normally given, the first 1 h before the procedure and the second 6 h after its completion. A different prophylactic regime is used perioperatively in cardiac operations (see below).

For dental procedures under local anaesthesia, including patients with a prosthetic heart valve but not those who have had endocarditis before, give oral amoxycillin 3 g 1 h before the procedure, or, *if penicillin allergic,* either oral erythromycin 1.5 g 1 h before the procedure, then 500 mg 6 h later, or oral clindamycin 600 mg 1 h before the procedure. Patients who have had endocarditis should receive amoxycillin plus gentamicin, as under general anaesthesia.

For dental procedures under general anaesthesia in patients at no special risk, give either amoxycillin 1 g i. m. before induction, then oral amoxycillin 500 mg 6 h later, or oral amoxycillin 3 g 4 h before induction, then oral amoxycillin as soon as possible after the procedure, or oral amoxycillin 3 g plus oral probenecid 4 h before the procedure.

For patients at special risk (patients with a prosthetic heart valve or who have had endocarditis previously), give amoxycillin 1 g i. m. plus gentamicin 1.5 mg/kg i. m. immediately before induction, then oral amoxycillin 500 mg 6 h later; such patients who are penicillin allergic should be given vancomycin 1 g i. v. over 60 min, then gentamicin 1.5 mg/kg i. v. before induction.

For genito-urinary and colonic procedures, give amoxycillin 1 g i. m. plus gentamicin 1.5 mg/kg i. m. immediately before induction, then amoxycillin 500 mg orally or i. m. 6 h later. If penicillin-allergic, give vancomycin 1 g i. v. over 60 min, then gentamicin 1.5 mg/kg i. v. immediately before induction; metronidazole may also be added.

For drainage of a collection of pus caused by Staphylococcus aureus (e. g. an abscess), give flucloxacillin or dicloxacillin 1 g 1 h before and 6 h after the procedure. Use cefazolin or vancomycin i. v. in penicillin allergy.

Perioperative prophylaxis in cardic operations: In cardiac operations and diagnostic procedures in the heart and great vessels, there is a particular danger of staphylococcal endocarditis. Perioperative prophylaxis with cefazolin i. v. (or with another cephalosporin), possibly complemented with gentamicin, for several days is essential.

References

BACKES, R. J., W. R. WILSON, J. E. GERACI: Group B streptococcal infective endocarditis. Arch. Intern. Med. *145:* 693 (1985).

BARST, R. J., A. S. PRINCE, H. C. NEU: Aspergillus endocarditis in children: case report and review of the literature. Pediatrics *68:* 73 (1981).

BAYER, A. S., K. LAM: Efficacy of vancomycin plus rifampin in experimental aortic valve endocarditis due to methicillin-resistant Staphylococcus aureus: In vitro – in vivo correlations. J. Infect. Dis. *151:* 157 (1985).

BESNIER, J. M., C. LEPORT, A. BURE, J. L. VILDE: Vacomycin-aminoglycoside combinations in therapy of endocarditis caused by Enterococcus species and Streptococcus bovis. Eur. J. Clin. Microbiol. Infect. Dis. *9:* 130–133 (1990).

BISNO, A. L., et al.: Antimicrobial treatment of infective endocarditis due to viridans streptococci, enterococci, and staphylococci. J.A.M.A. *261:* 1471 (1989).

BODNAR, E., D. HORSTKOTTE, A. BODNAR (eds): Infective Endocarditis. ICR Publishers Pinner 1991.

DURACK, D. T.: Prophylaxis of Infective Endocarditis. In G. L. Mandell, R. G. Douglas, Jr., and J. E. BENNETT (eds.): Principles and Practice of Infectious Diseases (3rd ed.). New York: Churchill Livingstone, 1990. Pp. 716–721.

DWORKIN, R. J., B. L. LEE, M. A. SANDE, H. F. CHAMBERS: Treatment of right-sided Staphylococcus aureus endocarditis in intravenous drug users with ciprofloxacin and rifampicin. Lancet 2: 1071–1073 (1989).
FINCH, R. G., D. C. SHANSON, W. A. LITTER, R. HOFFENBERG (Eds): Infective Endocarditis. Academic Press, London 1988.
HOLLIMAN, R., E. SMYTH: Gentamicin-resistant enterococci and endocarditis. Postgrad. M. J. 65: 390–393 (1989).
JULANDER, I., et al.: Haemophilus parainfluenzae: An uncommon cause of septicemia endocarditis. Scand. J. infect. Dis. 12: 85 (1980).
KAATZ, G. W., S. M. SEO, N. J. DORMAN, S. A. LERNER: Emergence of teicoplanin resistance during therapy of Staphylococcus aureus endocarditis. J. Infect. Dis. 162: 103–108 (1990).
LAUFER, D., P. D. LEW, I. OBERHANSLI, J. N. COX, M. LONGSON: Chronic Q-fever endocarditis with massive splenomegaly in childhood. J. Pediatr. 108: 535–539 (1986).
MACFARLANE, T. W., D. A. MCGOWAN, K. HUNTER, D. MACKENZIE: Prophylaxis for infective endocarditis: antibiotic sensitivity of dental plaque. J. Clin. Pathol. 36: 459 (1983).
SHULMAN, S., D. P. AMREN, A. L. BISNO, A. S. DAJANI, D. T. DURACK, M. A. GERBER, E. L. KAPLAN, H. D. MILLARD, W. E. SANDERS, R. H. SCHWARTZ, C. WATANAKUNAKORN: Prevention of bacterial endocarditis. A statement for health professionals by the Committee of rheumatic fever and infective endocarditis of the council on cardiovascular diseases in the young of the American heart association. Circulation 70: 1123A–1127A (1984).
SHULMAN, S. T., D. P. AMREN, A. L. BISNO et al.: Prevention of bacterial endocarditis. Pediatrics 75: 603 (1985).
SIMMONS, N. A., R. A. CAWSON, S. J. EYKYN et al.: Prophylaxis of endocarditis. Lancet 1: 127 (1986).
SIMMONS, N. A., R. A. CAWSON, S. J. EYKYN et al.: Prophylaxis of endocarditis. Lancet 1: 1267 (1986).
SMALL, P. M., H. F. CHAMBERS: Vancomycin for Staphylococcus aureus endocarditis in intravenous drug users. Antimicrob. Ag. Chemother. 34: 1227–1231 (1990).
THAUVIN, C., F. LECOMTE, I. LE BOETE et al.: Efficacy of ciprofloxacin alone and in combination with azlocillin in experimental endocarditis due to Pseudomonas aeruginosa. Infection 17: 31–34 (1989).
TUAZON, C. U., V. GILL, F. GILL: Streptococcal endocarditis: single vs. combination antibiotic therapy and the role of various species. Rev. Infect. Dis. 8: 54 (1986).
WESSEL, A., C. SIMON, D. REGENSBURGER: Bacterial and fungal infection after cardiac surgery. Eur. J. Pediatr. 146: 31 (1987).
Working Party of the British Society for Antimicrobial Chemotherapy: Antibiotic prophylaxis of infective endocarditis. Lancet 1: 88 (1990).
YEBRA, M., J. ORTIGOSA, F. ALBARRAN, M. G. CRESPO: Ciprofloxacin in a case of Q fever endocarditis (letter). N. Engl. J. Med. 323: 614 (1990).

4. Bacterial Pericarditis

Pericarditis has a number of causes and forms, namely

1. **Purulent pericarditis:** Staphylococcus aureus and Haemophilus influenzae (type b) have displaced pneumococci and other streptococci of various types as the commonest causes of purulent pericarditis. Meningococci, gonococci, anaerobes, salmonellae, enterobacteria and pseudomonas are now rarely found in this

condition. *Staphylococcal pericarditis* usually arises haematogenously from pneumonia with empyema, acute osteomyelitis, a soft-tissue abscess or after open-heart operations, and sometimes in the course of staphylococcal endocarditis. Its features include severe shock, and the condition is often fatal. *Haemophilus pericarditis* can arise as a complication of pleuropneumonia or meningitis with this organism and is more common in infants and young children. Purulent pericarditis complicates some 5% of cases of *meningococcal septicaemia* in young adults, becoming apparent on or after the third day of the disease and generally following a less severe course than that of staphylococcal and haemophilus pericarditis. *Anaerobes* may be suspected if pericarditis develops as a complication of a lung abscess, an intra-abdominal infection or a deep wound infection. Purulent pericarditis can also be caused by *fungi,* and complicate tuberculosis and amoebiasis.

Treatment: Because of the wide range of possible causes, a full microbiological examination (including anaerobes and fungi) of the pericardial fluid is essential, as are serological tests for syphilis, rickettsiae and chlamydiae, in order that *specific treatment* can be started (as for septicaemia and endocarditis). *Non-specific treatment* with broad-spectrum antibiotics effective against the commonest bacterial causes (staphylococci, pneumococci, other streptococci, haemophilus, meningococci, gonococci and anaerobes) may be started initially. Suitable combinations are likely to include a broad-spectrum cephalosporin plus clindamcyin or metronidazole (in adequate dosage). In patients who are immunosuppressed or who have just undergone cardiac operations, an aminoglycoside (gentamicin or tobramycin) should be added because of the possibility of infection with pseudomonas and enterobacteria. If fungi are demonstrated, treatment with amphotericin B is necessary.

Open or closed drainage is necessary from the outset, and regular tests of clinical progress by ultrasound are important. Supportive measures include oxygen, treatment of shock, isoprenaline etc. *Constrictive pericarditis* which may arise from the eighth day, must be treated by pericardiectomy. Treatment with the most appropriate antibiotics found on sensitivity testing should be continued intravenously for at least 3–4 weeks.

2. **Tuberculous pericarditis:** Nowadays rare in Western Europe, it can arise as a complication of pulmonary or miliary tuberculosis. The onset is gradual, with malaise, fever, anorexia, night sweats and typical symptoms of pericarditis. The pericardial effusion may be serous or purulent. The diagnosis is supported by a positive tuberculin test, the demonstration of the organism in pericardial fluid and by histological examination. Antituberculous *treatment* (p. 523) is effective but often fails to prevent constrictive pericarditis.

3. **Rheumatic pericarditis** (see p. 493) is treated with benzylpenicillin, with the addition of prednisone and possibly acetylsalicylic acid. Pericarditis in *rheumatoid arthritis* and systemic *lupus erythematosus* does not require antibiotic treatment.

The *post-cardiotomy syndrome* with a pericardial and often a pleural effusion is not bacterial, but usually autoimmune or viral (e. g. cytomegalovirus) in origin. *Uraemic pericarditis* should not be treated with antibiotics, and can also give rise to constrictive pericarditis.

4. **Viral pericarditis,** which is relatively common, is usually due to infection with coxsackie B virus or less commonly adenovirus, EB virus, varicella virus and others. Massive pericardial effusions are rare. The course is often protracted (3–4 weeks), but generally less severe. Cardiac tamponade and constrictive pericarditis are the exception. *Treatment* with bed-rest and analgesics is usually sufficient, and the pericarditis may recur. In serous pericarditis, the possibility of infection with Mycoplasma pneumoniae or Chlamydia psittaci (ornithosis) should be considered and, if confirmed, treated with doxycycline.

5. CNS Infections
a) Meningitis

Meningitis is best **classified** according to its cause, which may be *viral, bacterial, fungal or protozoal*. Although the distinction between lymphocytic and purulent meningitis is important, it is not invariably related to aetiology, because not all cases of lymphocytic meningitis are caused by viruses (tuberculous, cryptococcal and leptospiral meningitis, and the phase of resolution of purulent meningitis); not all cases of purulent meningitis are bacterial (a polymorphonuclear leucocytic exudate can predominate at the beginning of an echo- or coxsackievirus meningitis). At the onset of bacterial meningitis the cell count may be low, rising first during the course of the disease, despite treatment. The distinction between serous meningitis, with a clear CSF and a cell count of less than 300/µl, and purulent meningitis with cloudy CSF and a cell count greater than 300/µl is also not an entirely reliable guide to the cause.

Viruses are frequently associated with serous meningitis but so, on occasion, are bacteria and fungi (Borrelia burgdorferi, Mycobacterium tuberculosis, Treponema pallidum, Campylobacter, Leptospira). On the other hand, cloudy CSF is not always an index of bacterial meningitis, since quite high cell counts of around 3000/µl are found in certain viral infections (e. g. mumps meningitis, echovirus meningitis), making the CSF slightly opaque. In purulent bacterial meningitis, and occasionally in viral meningitis also, the lactate dehydrogenase (LDH) and lactic acid content of the CSF are greatly increased. The serum CRP (C-reactive protein) can still be negative at the onset of purulent meningitis and is often negative in serous meningitis of bacterial origin, so that CRP alone is of little value in distinguishing bacterial from viral meningitis. Non-infectious causes such as leukaemia, irritation from adjacent lesions (sympathetic meningitis in sinusitis, otitis, mastoiditis, brain abscess), brain tumour etc. should also be considered. When clinical signs of meningitis are present, other causes such as a subarachnoid haemorrhage, cervical spine syndrome and encephalitis have to be ruled out.

A lumbar puncture should be performed whenever meningitis is suspected, and if possible before beginning antibiotic treatment. Antibiotics should not, however, be delayed in cases presenting with a purpuric rash typical of meningococcal sepsis, in whom the infection may be fulminant and prompt antibiotic therapy lifesaving. The cell count should be performed as soon as possible after CSF collection, at which time methylene blue, gram and giemsa preparations are made for the demonstration of bacteria (Table 37) and differentiation of cells. At the onset of purulent meningitis in small children, there are sometimes few cells at first, but many bacteria. In meningococcal meningitis, the bacteria are often only found in the deposit after centrifugation of the CSF. The rapid identification of meningococcal, pneumococcal, group B streptococcal and haemophilus antigen in CSF is now possible using a simple latex agglutination technique which can readily be performed in every hospital laboratory. A negative result does not, however, exclude a bacterial cause.

When pneumococci are present in the CSF smear they are often very numerous. They are lanceolate gram-positive diplococci, often extracellular and surrounded by a mucous capsule. Meningococci are predominantly intracellular in the cytoplasm of polymorphonuclear leucocytes; they are gram-negative, kidneyshaped diplococci and are often only present in small numbers in the CSF. Haemophilus influenzae is a fine gram-negative extracellular rod of varying size (pleomorphism); in some cases it resembles a cocco-bacillus, and in others it is a

Table 37. Microscopic diagnosis of the most important types of bacterial meningitis.

Morphology	Location	Gram stain	Number	Pathogen
Lanceolate diplococci, often with capsules	extracellular	positive	numerous	pneumococci
Kidney-shaped diplococci	intracellular	negative	scanty to very scanty	meningococci
Large, thick rods	extracellular	negative	scanty to numerous	enterobacteria (Escherichia coli, Proteus)
Delicate, often pleomorphic rods	extracellular	negative	scanty to numerous	Haemophilus influenzae
Rods, often short	often intracellular	positive	scanty	Listeria monocytogenes

long and spindly gram-negative bacillus. Other causes of meningitis are only broadly classifiable as gram-negative or gram-positive rods or cocci by microscopic examination, although Listeria monocytogenes is typically found as scanty, partly intracellular, short gram-positive rods.

Regardless of the microscopical findings, a bacterial culture should always be made. Where the CSF cell count is below 1000/µl, the centrifuged deposit should be stained by the Ziehl-Neelsen method and acid-fast bacilli sought. The CSF from serous meningitis should be refrigerated overnight and examined for a spider web clot of suspected tuberculosis the next day. If found, the clot is examined for acid-fast bacilli microscopically after heat-fixation and staining by the Ziehl-Neelsen method. Where gram-positive or gram-negative cocci or bacilli are seen, a rapid direct sensitivity test with the appropriate antibiotics can be performed with an inoculum from the spun deposit and read within 8–12 hours.

A blood culture should always be taken before treatment, since it is often positive in haematogenous meningitis, sometimes when the CSF is still negative. The patient should be examined for the likely focus of infection, such as sinusitis, otitis media, lobar pneumonia, skull fracture etc., if necessary in consultation with an ophthalmologist, an otorhinolaryngologist or a chest physician. A chest x-ray is useful in pneumococcal meningitis (concomitant lobar pneumonia or bronchiectasis) and in tuberculous meningitis. A low CSF sugar with a predominantly lymphocytic picture is very suggestive of tuberculous meningitis. Where the CSF is serous but the cell count increased, viral culture should be performed on CSF, a throat swab and faeces, and serum samples taken in the acute phase and 10–14 days later may be usefully tested for a rise in specific antibody titres.

Antibiotic treatment should be started as a matter of urgency, since any delay may prejudice the chance of a complete cure. Early fatalities during the first 24 hours of treatment are generally due not to failure of antibiotics but to the effects of an already well-established meningitis or to a fulminant infection with particularly virulent organisms. The clinical outcome may well depend on the rapidity with which the patient can be admitted to hospital, the CSF examined and treatment commenced. Where possible, the patient should not be given an antibiotic before the lumbar puncture has been performed because of the danger of failure to culture the causative organism and test antibiotic sensitivities. If the transport of the patient to hospital is likely to take more than 2 hours, however, an antibiotic may be given as immediate treatment before lumbar puncture, such as cefotaxime 2 g slowly i. v. or i. m. for adults and 100 mg/kg for small children. This course may be life-saving in fulminant meningococcal septicaemia and meningitis, which is readily recognisable by a spreading purpuric rash in a shocked patient with worsening meningism and a deteriorating level of consciousness.

The CSF usually becomes sterile after 24 hours of successful treatment, and a further lumbar puncture is useful at this time.

The **frequency of different causes of meningitis** depends on the patient's age, background, underlying disease and geographical situation. While meningococci are the commonest single bacterial cause of meningitis in adults and older children (about 40–50%, or 25% overall), pneumococci are twice as common as causes of meningitis in adults (about 40%) as in children. Meningitis due to Haemophilus influenzae, on the other hand, accounts for about 20% of cases in unvaccinated children and only 1% in adults. Meningitis due to enterobacteria (Escherichia coli, klebsiella etc.) and group B streptococci predominates in the newborn and young infants. Other bacterial causes of meningitis (salmonellae, staphyloccoci, streptococci, listeria, Pseudomonas aeruginosa, Klebsiella pneumoniae, Enterobacter aerogenes, proteus etc.) are rare in younger adults. In the elderly, pneumococci commonly cause meningitis, listeria and enterobacteria occasionally, while meningococci are rare. The culture of skin organisms such as Staphylococcus epidermidis, corynebacteria and aerobic spore-bearing bacilli must be evaluated critically, since they may well be contaminants unless the patient has an indwelling Spitz-Holter valve or a CSF rhinorrhoea. Mixed infections sometimes occur in otogenic meningitis.

The **CSF penetration** of the antibiotics given is a key factor in successful treatment. The percentage of the serum concentration of various antimicrobials to enter the CSF of normal individuals is about 50% for certain sulphonamides, 30–50% for chloramphenicol, 30% for minocycline, about 10% for the other tetracyclines and less than 1% for penicillins and cephalosporins. Some antibiotics diffuse better through infected meninges into the CSF than they do in healthy persons. Effective CSF concentrations are obtained more rapidly after i.v. injection than after oral or i.m. administration. In meningitis, high doses of benzylpenicillin (6–12 g/day) produce effective concentrations against meningo- and pneumococci in the CSF. Adequate tissue concentrations are just as important as the CSF levels. The choice of antibiotic and its proper dosage are, therefore, more important for successful treatment than intrathecal administration, the effect of which may be unreliable.

Meningitis is *not* suitable for clinical trial of new antibiotics. It is unethical to use inadequately tested antibiotics in bacterial meningitis until animal experiments have clearly shown adequate CSF penetration and efficacy in experimental meningitis and the clinical effectiveness of the agent in less serious infections in man is well established.

Other aspects of treatment: Intensive care, treatment of respiratory distress, tracheotomy in patients with prolonged unconsciousness, mechanical ventilation and regular aspiration of respiratory secretions, treatment of shock, maintenance of fluid and electrolyte balance, parenteral or nasogastric nutrition etc. Unconscious patients should receive antacids through a nasogastric tube to prevent stress ulcers. Cerebral oedema should be treated with dexamethasone i.v. (10 mg initially, then 4 mg every 6 h), and with frusemide, if necessary with mechanical hyperventilation and barbiturates. Repeated lumbar puncture may be needed to relieve pressure, and is useful to monitor treatment, since an increase in the CSF cell count may indicate failure of treatment or a change of infecting agent. Epileptiform convulsions may arise as a result of penicillin overdosage, and a maximum of 12 g of benzylpenicillin a day in adults or 7.2 g a day in children should be given in the acute phase of meningitis, when the permeability of the blood-CSF barrier is increased. Convulsions caused by penicillin overdosage can be controlled with diazepam (Valium) or barbiturate, and the penicillin may have to be discontinued temporarily. If a brain abscess is suspected, a computerized axial tomogram (CT scan) should be obtained as soon as possible, in order to guide any neurosurgical intervention. Once antibiotic treatment has started, antrotomy may be performed in cases of definite otogenic meningitis, and sinus irrigation where sinusitis is the initial focus.

Failure of antibiotic treatment where the CSF continues to yield positive cultures, the cell count increases or fever continues can have a number of causes, including choice of the wrong antibiotic, underdosage, re-infection with a new microorganism, persistence of a local focus of infection (cerebral abscess, subdural abscess, cranial osteomyelitis, sinusitis, mastoiditis, otitis etc.), purulent metastases in the brain, subdural haemorrhage, loculated residual foci of meningitis, relapse after premature discontinuation of antibiotics, and metastatic abscesses in other organs (e.g. endocarditis). Persistent fever is sometimes caused by an allergy to drugs (drug fever) and may be associated with eosinophilia and a skin rash. In haemophilus meningitis, fever can persist for 1–3 weeks despite elimination of the causative organism. A rise in temperature and vomiting in the newborn and children are often caused by a developing hydrocephalus, which should be treated by the insertion of a shunt. Purulent meningitis can cause subdural effusion in children, especially with pneumococcal infection, which can be detected by echoencephalography and computerized tomography.

The appropriate antibiotic, given in the correct **dosage** (see Table 38) by the best route (always parenteral initially and i.v. if possible) for a sufficiently long period are all important in obtaining optimal blood, tissue and CSF concentrations, which should be bactericidal where possible. When penicillins are used, they should be continued in high dosage even when the meningitis is healing, because decreasing CSF penetration in a resolving meningitis may otherwise lead to relapse. Chloramphenicol, which penetrates into CSF better, can be used as an alternative to penicillin, provided the bacterial isolate is sensitive. Chloramphenicol also has the advantage of being well absorbed by mouth and the benefits of its use are still considered by many paediatricians to outweigh the very rare but serious risk of blood dyscrasia.

Table 38. Dosage of parenteral agents used to treat meningitis.

Antibiotic	Daily dose for children	Daily dose for adults
Benzylpenicillin	(Maximum dose 7.2 g) 600 mg/kg (newborn and infant) 300 mg/kg (older children)	6–12 g
Ampicillin Flucloxacillin (and other isoxazolylpenicillins)	100 mg/kg (newborn) 200–300 mg/kg (children)	10 (–20) g
Azlocillin Mezlocillin Piperacillin	100 mg/kg (newborn) 300 mg/kg (older children)	15–20 g
Cefotaxime	100 mg/kg (newborn) 150 mg/kg (older children)	8–12 g
Chloramphenicol	25 mg/kg (newborn in the 1st and 2nd week) 50 mg/kg (3rd–4th week) 80–100 mg/kg (infants) 50–80 mg/kg (older children)	3 (–4) g
Gentamicin (only in combinations)	6 mg/kg	5 mg/kg

The value of *cephalosporins* in meningitis varies according to the individual compounds. The earlier cephalosporins and some of the newer ones are unsuitable for the treatment of meningitis. Of the broad-spectrum cephalosporins, the greatest experience is with cefotaxime, which is indicated in infections by otherwise resistant enterobacteria and Haemophilus influenzae. Other new cephalosporins and β-lactam antibiotics and the new quinolones should only be used to treat meningitis when careful clinical trials have established their effectiveness for this indication.

α) Initial Therapy (Pathogen Unknown)

Initial treatment must be started without delay and is based on the CSF findings and the clinical situation. When pneumococci or meningococci are *seen by direct microscopy* and the latex agglutination test with CSF, serum or urine is positive, benzylpenicillin is the drug of choice. If no organisms are seen or if, in a young child, gram-negative bacilli are detected microscopically, the cause may be Haemophilus influenzae; the specific latex agglutination test is usually positive. Cefotaxime is now the treatment of choice and preferable to chloramphenicol or ampicillin.

Where direct microscopy fails to show organisms *in adults*, listeria is occasionally a cause; ampicillin, which is also effective against meningococci and pneumococci, is then the best initial therapy though chloramphenicol may also be used.

Many organisms can cause meningitis in *the first two months of life*, and a combination of cefotaxime, piperacillin and gentamicin in adequate dosage (see Table 38) has generally proved to be satisfactory initial treatment.

β) Directed Chemotherapy (Pathogen Known)

Meningococcal meningitis is almost always haematogenous in origin. Meningococcal antigen can now be demonstrated rapidly using the latex agglutination test, which is also positive in patients in whom treatment has already been started. CSF should be cultured in the usual manner; where there is no diagnostic bacteriological laboratory on site and delay in transit may occur, the CSF may be inoculated into a commercial kit blood culture bottle and incubated pending transmission.

Benzylpenicillin in large doses is the antibiotic of choice (12 g a day for adults, 300 mg/kg/day for children and 600 mg/kg/day for the newborn) in short i.v. infusions every 6–8 hours until improvement (at least 3 days after defervescence) followed by a reduced dose (3–6 g) for 7–10 days. Resistance of meningococci to penicillin has been reported in Britain, Spain and South Africa and, while still uncommon, could rapidly increase.

In patients *allergic to penicillin* give cefotaxime or ceftriaxone (having excluded cross-allergy) or chloramphenicol in the dosage shown in Table 38. Treatment with a sulphonamide alone is no longer reliable because of the prevalence of sulphonamide-resistant strains of meningococci.

Treatment of the *Waterhouse-Friderichsen syndrome* is described on p. 337.

For *prophylaxis* in close household contacts use rifampicin 600 mg in adults, 10 mg/kg in children aged 1–2 years, and 5 mg/kg in children under one year old, all twice a day for 2 days. Minocycline, which used to be recommended, is no longer used because of the frequent side-effect of giddiness. The efficacy of sulphonamides, penicillins and cephalosporins is unreliable. A single dose of ciprofloxacin has been shown to reduce nasopharyngeal carriage rates in contacts by 97%.

Pneumococcal meningitis is haematogenous in origin or spreads directly from the paranasal sinuses, mastoid, a cerebral abscess or skull fracture; examination by an otorhinolaryngologist may be helpful, as may surgery after antibiotic treatment. The rapid demonstration of pneumococcal antigen in the CSF, serum or urine by latex agglutination is important in the differentiation from other gram-positive organisms.

Treatment: Benzylpenicillin in large dosage (12 g a day for adults, 300 mg/kg for children and 600 mg/kg for the newborn) given as a short i. v. infusion every 6 hours. Duration of treatment: at least 10 days at full dosage (Table 39). Meningitis caused by penicillin-resistant pneumococci which were also resistant to chloramphenicol has been reported in South Africa; the only reliably effective antimicrobial treatment was vancomycin i. v. (adults 2 g daily, children 50 mg/kg). Rifampicin and imipenem are active *in vitro,* but there is little clinical experience with these agents at present.

Chloramphenicol is the best alternative in patients *allergic* to penicillin; it also penetrates CSF well, even if the meninges are not inflamed. Cefotaxime may also be used (rule out cross-allergy). Additional intrathecal penicillin is not necessary.

Table 39. Duration of therapy for different causes of meningitis.

Cause of meningitis	Duration of therapy (days)
Meningococci	7–10
Pneumococci	10–14
Haemophilus	10–14
Staphylococci	14–21 or longer (depending on other processes)
Listeria	28–42
Gram-negative intestinal bacteria	10–14 (after CSF becomes sterile)

Haemophilus influenzae meningitis is of haematogenous, otogenic or rhinogenic origin, is much commoner in children than in adults, and can carry a poor prognosis. It is mainly caused by serotype b, in which case the rapid latex agglutination test for the demonstration of antigen in CSF, serum or urine is usually positive, even after treatment has begun.

Treatment: Chloramphenicol or ampicillin have until recently been the drugs of choice. The testing of ampicillin sensitivity is unreliable since not all resistant strains produce β-lactamase *in vitro* and some resistant strains can appear sensitive. The number of strains resistant to chloramphenicol, and sometimes to both antibiotics, has increased and cefotaxime has therefore become the most reliable treatment of haemophilus meningitis and is very active at low concentrations. Haemophilus *prophylaxis* is now advised for children under 4 years who have been in close contact with the patient. Oral rifampicin 20 mg/kg per day should be given for 4 days.

Escherichia coli meningitis may have few, ill-defined signs in infants, which are easily overlooked. The prognosis is poor. It is rare in adults, in whom it is usually found after head injuries or neurosurgical operations, and occasionally found after urogenital surgery.

Treatment: When plump gram-negative rods are seen on direct microscopy of the CSF deposit, an antibiotic combination in high dosage should be given before culture and antibiotic sensitivities are available because the disease is life-threatening.

Cefotaxime is now more successful than traditional treatment with chloramphenicol, mezlocillin or ampicillin in combination with gentamicin (for dosage, see Table 38). Intrathecal instillation of gentamicin is no longer necessary when a highly active cephalosporin is used for treatment. Treatment is continued for 10–14 days after the CSF has become sterile.

Listeria meningitis is generally intrauterine in origin in premature and full-term neonates, although it can occur in later childhood and occasionally in adults, usually when resistance is lowered by some underlying disease. It is always haematogenous and develops into a purulent or serous meningitis.

Treatment: Ampicillin i. v., 10 g a day for adults (200–300 mg/kg for children) in 3–4 single doses, possibly in combination with gentamicin.

Minocycline may be used in cases of allergy to penicillin (200 mg a day for adults, 4 mg/kg a day for children in combination with gentamicin.

Large doses of benzylpenicillin (12 g), piperacillin and chloramphenicol have also been given successfully.

Duration of treatment: until the CSF has returned to normal, and generally for at least 4–6 weeks. Cephalosporins are ineffective.

Staphylococcal meningitis: Occurs during staphylococcal septicaemia or endocarditis of otogenic, rhinogenic or post-traumatic origin. Staphylococcal meningitis may accompany a septic focal encephalitis or a brain abscess, and the initial focus should be sought. Staphylococci are the usual causes of septicaemia and meningitis associated with shunts (after hydrocephalus operations) and are sometimes combined with ventriculitis. If the shunt is the only part of the system to be infected, it can be rendered sterile by injecting 10 mg vancomycin intrathecally into the cranial or distal arm. In most cases, however the infected shunt has to be removed for the infection to be eradicated. Failure of treatment is relatively common.

Treatment: Benzylpenicillin + flucloxacillin i. v. initially (dosage: see Table 38), until antibiotic sensitivities are available. Benzylpenicillin i. v. may be given for sensitive staphylococci, and flucloxacillin i. v. for penicillin-resistant staphylococci. For methicillin-resistant staphylococci use fosfomycin + rifampicin or imipenem + rifampicin. Although vancomycin is reliably effective against all staphylococci, it penetrates CSF poorly (for dosage, see Table 35, p. 328).

Cefuroxime i. v. is an alternative in patients *allergic to penicillin,* since it achieves better CSF concentrations than many other cephalosporins. The dose is 8–12 g a day for adults and 200 mg/kg for children in 3–4 short infusions. High-dose antibiotic therapy should be maintained for 3–4 weeks, and followed by a further 3–4 weeks of flucloxacillin, cephradine, clindamycin or erythromycin (according to sensitivity testing) to prevent relapse.

Group B streptococcal meningitis is relatively common in the newborn and young infant. Non-capsulated gram-positive diplococci are seen in the CSF deposit. The latex agglutination test is positive in CSF and serum.

Treatment: Benzylpenicillin in high dosage. Since some strains of group B streptococci are penicillin-tolerant (i.e. are not killed by penicillin), combination with gentamicin is recommended.

Enterococcal meningitis is rare, and is an occasional complication of enterococcal endocarditis. The initial focus must be eradicated.

Treatment: Ampicillin i.v. + gentamicin (dosage: Table 38). Minocycline i.v. in cases with allergy to penicillin or resistance to ampicillin, 0.2 g a day for adults, and 4 mg/kg for children.

Duration of treatment: 2–4 weeks, followed by minocycline for 2–3 weeks to prevent relapse.

Pseudomonas aeruginosa meningitis generally arises by direct inoculation, not uncommonly after diagnostic, therapeutic or surgical procedures. Spread is sometimes direct from the ear and sometimes haematogenous as part of a pseudomonas septicaemia.

Treatment: Azlocillin or piperacillin i.v. in combination with tobramycin (dosage: Table 38); ceftazidime, imipenem, ciprofloxacin or amikacin in case of resistance to other agents. An additional intrathecal instillation of gentamicin (5 mg in adults and 0.5–1 mg in children) may be necessary for at least 2–3 days.

Duration of treatment: until the CSF returns to normal.

Salmonella meningitis is a rare complication of typhoid or paratyphoid fever or salmonella gastro-enteritis, particularly in children.

Treatment of choice: Chloramphenicol (dosage: Table 38, p. 356), although cefotaxime (8–12 g i.v. daily) has given good results in localised salmonella infections and in meningitis due to Escherichia coli. Because of the risk of relapse, treatment should be followed with a further course of oral chloramphenicol or, if the total recommended dose has been exceeded or early signs of marrow depression are seen, with amoxycillin, cefotaxime or co-trimoxazole. Combination initially with gentamicin is advisable, since salmonella meningitis is difficult to overcome effectively.

Duration of treatment: at least 3 weeks, preferably longer.

Meningitis due to Klebsiella or Enterobacter is rare (except in the newborn and young infant), and difficult to treat effectively because of the frequent and variable antibiotic resistance of these organisms.

Treatment: Because of the poor prognosis, combined treatment with effective drugs on the basis of tested antibiotic sensitivities is essential, preferably with a combination of a β-lactamase-stable cephalosporin (e.g. cefotaxime against klebsiella, latamoxef or imipenem in high dosage against enterobacter) with gentamicin or amikacin. Sensitive strains may be treated with mezlocillin or piperacillin, in combination with an aminoglycoside. Ciprofloxacin may also be considered in adults.

Proteus meningitis: *Treatment* according to the species of proteus and the antibiotic sensitivity pattern. Cefotaxime, ampicillin or mezlocillin in combination with gentamicin are recommended. Chloramphenicol may be used if the isolate is sensitive, and ciprofloxacin may be considered in adults.

Borreliosis (Lyme disease): Meningitis or meningoencephalitis due to Borrelia burgdorferi can arise 2–11 weeks after a tick bite. The bite, which in 60% of cases has gone unnoticed, gives rise in half the cases to cutaneous erythema migrans, which resolves after a few weeks. In the meningitis which follows later, fever is usually mild or absent. Cranial nerve palsies are frequent. The CSF is not turbid and contains predominantly lymphocytes. The causative organism can only rarely be demonstrated. The serum CRP and IgG are generally normal. Specific IgM antibodies are initially absent from the serum but can be demonstrated later. Borreliosis should always be considered when subacute serous meningitis is accompanied by cranial nerve palsies or polyradiculitis, or when a myocarditis with AV block or an arthritis develops at the same time.

This often ambiguous disease resolves with high doses of benzylpenicillin i.v. Adults should be given 12 g and young children 180 mg/kg daily. Treatment should be continued for at least 14 days. Treatment of the early form (erythema migrans), even though it would resolve spontaneously, is nowadays strongly recommended in order to prevent as far as possible the neurological and other late features (arthritis, acrodermatitis atrophicans) of this infection. Treatment for 10 to 21 days with doxycycline 0.2 g daily, phenoxymethylpenicillin 1.8 g daily, ceftriaxone 2 g daily or erythromycin 1 g daily are all suitable.

Campylobacter meningitis is rare, occurring generally in the newborn, occasionally crossing the placenta. The clinical picture is of septicaemia, sometimes accompanied by mucous and blood-stained diarrhoea and associated with encephalitis, generally in the newborn. The CSF may be grossly clear, but with a moderate increase in cells and gram-negative curved rods in a stained smear. Culture should be performed anaerobically on special culture media, incubated for several days.

Treatment: Parenteral chloramphenicol at a dosage related to age (Table 38) for 1–2 weeks, preferably in combination with gentamicin.

Fungal meningitis (Candida albicans, Cryptococcus neoformans, and very occasionally Aspergillus fumigatus): CSF culture on Sabouraud's agar is often only positive after prolonged incubation (up to 10 days). Cryptococcus can only be seen microscopically after staining with India ink. A latex agglutination test is available for the detection of antigen in CSF or serum, and an ELISA method for Aspergillus fumigatus. *Treatment* should be attempted with amphotericin B i.v. in combination with flucytosine (dosage: p. 193 and p. 210), supplemented by intrathecal instillation of amphotericin B. Prednisone (10 mg) is first instilled by the intralumbar (or in young infants the intraventricular route) and followed by slow instillation of amphotericin B (0.5 mg) diluted with CSF in the syringe. This dose is repeated after 2–3 days. Candida albicans and Cryptococcus neoformans should always be tested against flucytosine *in vitro* since resistant strains occur. If the meningitis is associated with a Spitz-Holter or other valve implant, this foreign body must be removed.

Fluconazole (see p. 204), a new azole compound, is suitable for treatment of CNS infections by cryptococcus or candida.

Amoebic meningo-encephalitis: Various pathogens are causative; infection is usually seen in persons who have spent time in tropical countries. *Naegleria fowleri* is transmitted by water from ponds, lakes, unchlorinated swimming baths and occasionally tap water and penetrates the nasal mucosa, probably through the cribriform plate. The meningitis is acute and usually fatal, and motile amoebae may be seen microscopically in uncentrifuged purulent CSF which has not been cooled. The organism may be cultured. *Treatment* is with amphotericin B, possibly in combination with rifampicin.

Acanthamoeba species is spread by the blood stream in immunosuppressed patients and gives rise to a granulomatous encephalitis with a low-grade accompanying lymphocytic meningitis. The causative organism may be shown in brain biopsy but not in the CSF.

Treatment with sulphonamide and flucytosine may be tried.

Serous meningitis: For the treatment of tuberculosis, see p. 513; for syphilis, p. 484; for leptospirosis, p. 510.

Herpes meningo-encephalitis: This rare but dangerous condition is now treatable with acyclovir if started early. Acyclovir is more effective than vidarabine, which was previously recommended but is poorly tolerated. Herpes encephalitis can occur at any age and in association with both primary and recurrent infections. There is a focal, necrotising encephalitis which principally affects the frontal and temporal lobes. After a prodromal febrile illness lasting 1–7 days (with or without vesicles on the skin or mucous membranes), central nervous symptoms develop, often initially with convulsions, then altered consciousness, speech disorders, ataxia, disorders of thought etc. The CSF contains 50–2,000 cells per µl, initially predominantly neutrophils but later lymphocytes and, in 80% of cases, erythrocytes also. The virus can hardly ever be cultured from the CSF. The EEG shows unilateral or bilateral periodic focal peaks on a background of very slow activity (not pathognomonic). The CT scan is often still normal initially and foci of increased density with oedema and haemorrhage, particularly in the temporal region, are frequently not demonstrable until later. Seroconversion occurs in blood and CSF in primary infections, but is often gradual and delayed. A rise in the specific IgM titre in blood and CSF of at least fourfold is typical of recurrent infection.

Herpes encephalitis should be suspected in cases of serous meningitis in which:
1. symptoms of encephalitis (including cerebral nerve palsies, disorders of speech or convulsions) develop, or
2. a constant focus is demonstrable in the EEG or CT-scan.

Because of the poor prognosis, the results of CSF and blood tests should not be awaited, but intravenous acyclovir on well-founded clinical suspicion initiated immediately. The dose is 10 mg/kg (or 250 mg/m^2 body surface) 3 times a day. The drug is well tolerated. Full recovery is possible if treatment is started in the first few days of the illness. Acyclovir is not effective in encephalitis caused by other viruses, except for varicella.

Partially treated purulent meningitis in which no pathogen has been identified but which shows signs of improvement should be treated further with the same antibiotic, i.e. benzylpenicillin, ampicillin, or cefotaxime, provided it is without risk. Treatment should otherwise be continued with cefotaxime. When clinical progress is unsatisfactory, chloramphenicol may be considered. Despite treatment, the latex agglutination test for meningococci, pneumococci and Haemophilus influenzae often remains positive in the CSF for several days.

Culture-negative purulent meningitis: An acute meningitis which has not already been treated, where there is no indication of an otogenic or rhinogenic origin and from which no bacterial pathogen has been isolated, has, in adults, most probably been caused by meningococci, which may not survive transport to the laboratory. Such cases should be treated with large doses of benzylpenicillin. Metastatic foci on the skin and a purpuric rash suggest meningococcal infection. Chloramphenicol or cefotaxime in combination with gentamicin are preferable in cases of suspected otogenic or rhinogenic meningitis. Meningococcal infections are rare in infants older than 3 months; cefotaxime is preferable in infants because of the relatively greater incidence of meningitis with Haemophilus influenzae at this age.

References

ANDRÍOLE, V. T. Lyme disease and other spirochetal diseases. Rev. Infect. Dis. *11* (Suppl. 6): S1433–S1525 (1989).
ASENSI, F., D. PEREZ-TAMARIT, M. C. OTERO et al.: Imipenem cilastatin therapy in a child with meningitis caused by a multiple resistant pneumococcus (letter). Pediatr. Infect. Dis. J. *8:* 895 (1989).
ASMAR, B. I., M. C. THIRUMOORTHI, J. A. BUCKLEY et al.: Cefotaxime diffusion into cerebrospinal fluid of children with meningitis. Antimicrob. Ag. Chemother. *28:* 138 (1985).
BENACH, J. L., E. M. BOSLER, J. P. HANRAHAN et al.: Spirochetes isolated from the blood of two patients with Lyme disease. New Engl. J. Med. *308:* 740 (1983).
CHERUBIN, C. E., J. LEFROCK: Cefotaxime in the treatment of meningitis. Infection *13 (Suppl. 1):* 68 (1985).
DATTWYLER, R. J. et al. Ceftriaxone as effective therapy in refractory Lyme disease. J. Infect. Dis. *155:* 1322 (1987).
DATTWYLER, R. J. et al.: Treatment of late Lyme borreliosis – randomized comparison of ceftriaxone and penicillin. Lancet *1:* 1191 (1988).
DOTEVALL, L., and L. HAGBERG: Penetration of doxycycline into cerebrospinal fluid in patients treated for suspected Lyme neuroborreliosis. Antimicrob. Agents Chemother. *33:* 1078 (1989).
VAN ESSO, E., D. FONTANALS, S. URIZ: Neisseria meningitidis strains with decreased susceptibility to penicillin. Paediatr. Infect. Dis. *6:* 438 (1987).
GOOSSENS, H., G. HENOCQUE, L. KREMP et al.: Nosocomial outbreak of Campylobacter jejuni meningitis in newborn infants. Lancet *2:* 146 (1986).
JACOBS, R. F., T. G. WELLS, R. W. STEELE, T. YAMAUCHI: A prospective randomized comparison of cefotaxime vs ampicillin and chloramphenicol for bacterial meningitis in children. J. Pediatr. *107:* 129 (1985).
LAPOINTE, J. R., C. BELIVEAU, L. CHICOINE, J. H. JONCAS: A comparison of ampicillin-cefotaxime and ampicillin-chloramphenicol in childhood bacterial meningitis: an experience in 55 patients. J. Antimicrob. Chemother. *14 (Suppl. B):* 167 (1984).
Leading Article: Herpes simplex encephalitis. Lancet *ii:* 535 (1986).
LECOUR, H., A. SEARA, A. M. MIRANDA, J. CORDEIRO: Cetotaxime in pneumococcal meningitis. Infection *13 (Suppl. 1):* 73 (1985).
MOROOKA, T., T. ODA, H. SHIGEOKA: In vitro evaluation of antibiotics for treatment of meningitis caused by Campylobacter fetus subspecies fetus. Pediatr. Infect. Dis. J. *8:* 653–654 (1989).
MURPHY, T. V., G. H. MCCRACKEN JR., T. C. ZWEIGHAFT, E. J. HANSEN: Emergence of rifampin-resistant Haemophilus influenzae after prophylaxis. J. Pediatr. *99:* 406 (1981).
NAQVI, S. H., M. A. MAXWELL, L. M. DUNKLE: Cefotaxime therapy of neonatal gramnegative bacillary meningitis. Pediatr. Infect. Dis. *4:* 499 (1985).
PELTOLA, H., M. ANTTILA, O. V. RENKONEN: Randomised comparison of chloramphenicol, ampicillin, cefotaxime and ceftriaxone for childhood bacterial meningitis. Finnish Study Group. Lancet *1:* 1281–1287 (1989).
PLOTKIN, S. A. et al.: Meningitis in infants and children. Pediatrics *81:* 904 (1988).
ROWLEY, A. H. et al. Rapid detection of herpes simplex virus DNA in cerebrospinal fluid of patients with herpes simplex encephalitis. Lancet *335:* 440 (1990).
SAEZ-NIETO, J. A., D. FONTANALS, J. GARCIA DE JALON: Isolation of Neisseria meningitidis strains with increase of penicillin minimal inhibitory concentrations. Epid. Inf. *99:* 463 (1987).

SCHELD, W. M., R. J. WHITLEY, D. T. DURACK: Infections of the Central Nervous System. Raven Press, New York 1991.
SMEGO JR., R. A., J. R. PERFECT, D. T. DURACK: Combined therapy with amphotericin B and 5-fluorocytosine for Candida meningitis. Rev. Infect. Dis. *6:* 791 (1984).
STANEK, G.: Lyme borreliosis. Zentralblatt für Bakteriologie, Suppl. *18:* 1989.
STEERE, A. C.: Lyme disease. N. Engl. J. Med. *321:* 586–596 (1989).
STEERE, A. C., A. R. PACHNER, S. E. MALAWISTA: Neurological abnormalities of Lyme disease: successful treatment with high-dose intravenous penicillin. Ann. Intern. Med. *99:* 767 (1983).
SUTCLIFFE, E. M.: Penicillin-insensitive meningococci in the UK. Lancet *I:* 657–658 (1988).
THONG, Y. H.: Chemotherapy for primary amebic meningoencephalitis. New Engl. J. Med. *306:* 1295 (1982).
TUNKEL, A. R., B. WISPELWEY, W. M. SCHELD: Bacterial meningitis: Recent advances in pathophysiology and treatment. Ann. Intern. Med. *112:* 610 (1990).

b) Cerebral Abscess

Cerebral abscess can be otogenic, traumatic or haematogenous. The origin is usually the ear (mastoiditis) or less frequently the sinuses (sinusitis) or a boil in the nose or on the lip (with septic thrombophlebitis) or a skull fracture. Haematogenous spread can occur in the presence of bronchiectasis, lung abscesses, skin infections, bacterial endocarditis, and with congenital heart defects with a right-to-left shunt. Cerebral abscess as a complication of purulent meningitis is rare. Fever, leucocytosis and a raised ESR may all be absent. Localise by computerised axial tomography. Rupture of a cerebral abscess into a ventricle or the subarachnoid space is a dangerous complication.

Aetiology: Staphylococcus aureus, bacteroides, anaerobic streptococci, and in otogenic cerebral abscesses often Escherichia coli, proteus, klebsiella etc. Less common causes: Nocardia asteroides (sometimes with pulmonary nocardiosis), Entamoeba histolytica (often with simultaneous pulmonary and hepatic involvement, see p. 407), Toxoplasma gondii (e. g. in AIDS), fungi (in oncological patients and those with AIDS or after bone-marrow transplantation).

Treatment: Possibly a neurosurgical operation at the optimal time (when the abscess persists despite antibiotics), eradication of the initial focus, and prolonged antibiotic therapy in high dosage (as for purulent meningitis, see p. 356).

Most cases of cerebral abscess have to be treated without knowledge of the causative agent. Benzylpenicillin is the most effective agent against anaerobic streptococci and sensitive staphylococci, but a high dosage of 12–24 g is necessary on account of poor penetration into the abscess. Metronidazole has proved to be an excellent chemotherapeutic agent in brain abscess in recent years, with the advantages of very good penetration into the brain tissue and abscess as well as good activity against anaerobes. The combination of benzylpenicillin (12–24 g) + metronidazole (1.5–2 g daily) is usually appropriate. When penicillin-resistant staphylococci are isolated, flucloxacillin i. v. (adults 10 g, children 300–400 mg/kg daily), clindamycin, fosfomycin, cefazolin or fusidic acid (in combination with a second antistaphylococcal agent) are indicated. Cefotaxime or latamoxef may also be indicated in otogenic cerebral abscess, preferably in combination with metronidazole because of the frequency of mixed infections. Ofloxacin penetrates brain tissue well, but there are as yet no reports of its use in cerebral abscess. Increased intracranial pressure as a result of cerebral oedema should be treated appropriately (e. g. with frusemide and dexamethasone i. v.). Toxoplasmosis, which can complicate AIDS, should be treated with pyrimethamine and a sulphonamide (see p. 556); operative drainage is contraindicated.

c) Subdural Empyema

Subdural empyema should be considered in every case of purulent meningitis with a sterile CSF which presents with frontal sinusitis and develops hemiparesis, hemiplegia or aphasia. The diagnosis is confirmed by computerised axial tomography. A subdural empyema can also originate from sphenoidal sinusitis, mastoiditis or osteomyelitis of the roof of the skull, or develop during the course of purulent meningitis. The causative organisms are usually aerobic and anaerobic streptococci or staphylococci, and less frequently gram-negative rods (Escherichia coli, proteus, klebsiella, pseudomonas). The empyema should be drained and initially treated with benzylpenicillin + metronidazole or cefotaxime + metronidazole, changing to specific agents such as clindamycin when the bacteriological culture and sensitivities become available.

An *epidural abscess* requires intensive antibiotic therapy and removal of the focus from which it originated, as for cerebral abscess.

References

BARSOUM, A. H., H. C. LEWIS, K. L. CONNILLE: Nonoperative treatment of multiple brain abscesses. Surg. Neurol *16:* 283–287 (1981).
BOOM, W. H., C. V. TNAZON: Successful treatment of multiple brain abscesses with antibiotics alone. Rev. Infect. Dis. *7:* 189–199 (1985).
FONG, K. M., E. M. SENEVIRATNE, J. G. MCCORMACK: Mucor cerebral abscess associated with intravenous drug abuse. Aus. N. Z. J. Med. *20:* 74–77 (1990).
KAMIN, M., D. BIDDLE: Conservative management of focal intracerebral infection. Neurology *31:* 103–106 (1981).
DE LOUVOIS, J.: Antimicrobial chemotherapy in the treatment of brain abscess. J. Antimicrob. Chemother *12:* 205 (1983).
MANCINI, J., M. CHOUX, N. PINSARD: A cerebral abscess due to Listeria monocytogenes in a 15-month-old infant. Ann. Pediatr. Paris. *37:* 299–302 (1990).
OUTIN, H. D., J. MERRER, M. MOLHO et al.: Solitary listerial abscess of the brain stem. Cure with antibiotic treatment. Rev. Neurol. Paris *145:* 153–156 (1989).
SCHLIAMSER, S. E., K. BACKMAN, S. R. NORRBY: Intracranial abscesses in adults: An analysis of 54 consecutive cases. Scand. J. Infect. Dis. *20:* 1, 1988.
YANG, S. Y.: Brain abscess: a review of 400 cases. J. Neurosurg. *55:* 794–799 (1981).

6. Respiratory Infections

Upper respiratory infections are *viral* in origin in more than 90% of cases. Antibiotics are indicated only if a bacterial cause has been found, the illness is severe, or if a primary viral infection has given rise to bacterial superinfection. Antibiotics are also useful for the prevention of bacterial complications of influenza in patients with severe underlying chest disease.

A bacterial cause is suggested by:
1. purulent secretions or suppuration from an inflamed mucosa,
2. peripheral granulocytosis,
3. predominance of a potential pathogen in cultures taken from a patient who is not receiving antibiotics,
4. painful regional lymphadenitis,
5. no connection with a known viral epidemic.

Viral infections are generally characterised by serous rhinitis, bilateral catarrhal conjunctivitis, non-suppurative pharyngitis, vesiculation, swelling of lymphoid follicles, herpangina, tracheitis with a dry cough (particularly with influenza), generalised lymphadenopathy, a non-specific rash, myalgia, a normal peripheral white cell count, or an epidemiological connection with a known outbreak of viral infection. Respiratory infections of bacterial and viral origin cannot reliably be distinguished by clinical or haematological findings.

Bacterial infections of the lower respiratory tract are almost always associated with some disorder of the normal mechanisms of resistance (ciliary activity, mucous secretion, alveolar phagocytosis, cough reflex, IgA, IgG, IgE, lysozyme, white cell function etc.). This protective system can be disrupted by viral infection, chemical or physical damage, aspiration, pressure of a foreign body etc. The lower respiratory mucosa is normally sterile. Pathogens must be distinguished from commensal mouth bacteria when expectorated sputum is examined, which is often difficult and can give rise to misinterpretation of culture results. Once antibiotics have been given, considerable changes can occur in the mouth and pharyngeal flora, which may further complicate the picture. If the sputum is macroscopically purulent, microscopic examination of a gram-stained fleck of pus may help the interpretation of culture results, although there are pitfalls for the overconfident here, in that pneumococci are often indistinguishable from heavy oral contamination with commensal viridans streptococci on direct microscopic examination. The causative organisms of purulent bronchitis in children (pneumococci, haemophilus, branhamella) can often be cultured in pure growth from a deep nasal swab collected with the aid of a fine swab stick.

a) Rhinitis

If purulent rhinitis persists for more than 2–3 weeks, the possibility of paranasal sinusitis should be investigated. Although rhinitis of the newborn is often caused by staphylococci, the possibility of gonorrhoea and congenital syphilis must be ruled out. Purulent rhinitis in infants is occasionally caused by pneumococci and group A streptococci.

Antibacterial therapy of purulent rhinitis is necessary when complications such as purulent sinusitis arise and antibiotic treatment depends on the pathogen isolated. Treatment with phenoxymethylpenicillin (active against pneumococci and Streptococcus pyogenes) may be given or, if that fails, with flucloxacillin, which is active against penicillin-resistant staphylococci. Treatment of nasal diphtheria is as for pharyngeal diphtheria (p. 370).

b) Tonsillitis, Pharyngitis

Lacunar, follicular and catarrhal tonsillitis are generally caused by Streptococcus pyogenes (β-haemolytic streptococci of Lancefield group A) or viruses. A tonsillar exudate is not pathognomonic of streptococcal infection and may be absent, so a throat swab should always be cultured on media selective for haemolytic streptococci. Streptococcal antigen can be detected directly in the throat swab by a rapid test, albeit with a 10–15% false-negative rate. Purulent sore throat can also be caused by haemolytic streptococci of groups B, C or G. A marked granulocytosis and increased blood CRP are evidence in favour of streptococcal sore throat, as are pain on pressure of the superficial cervical lymph nodes. Leucocytopenia usually rules out a diagnosis of streptococcal tonsillitis. Asymptomatic streptococcal carriers usually have only few colonies on culture and do not show a rise in antistreptolysin O titre.

Treatment: Phenoxymethylpenicillin in normal dosage for 10–14 days, and a minimum of 7 days; this is important not only to prevent complications, particularly rheumatic fever, but also to eradicate streptococci from the throat, for a proportion will still have positive cultures after ten days of therapy and require a further course. In the USA benzathine penicillin (540 mg) is often given as a single intramuscular injection which is effective for 10 days. Sulphonamides, co-trimoxazole and the quinolones are inferior to penicillin because some streptococci are resistant and activity is lower. Tetracyclines should not be given because they are not bactericidal, they carry a much greater risk of side-effects, and many streptococcal strains are resistant. Ampicillin should also be avoided because it is less active than benzylpenicillin, and is associated with a cutaneous allergy, particularly in patients with glandular fever and similar disorder. Penicillin lozenges (not available in Britain) should never be given because of the risk of allergy and topical treatment with antiseptics is ineffective and does not prevent the serious complications of streptococcal infection. Infectious mononucleosis should be suspected in younger patients who do not respond to penicillin within 48 hours.

Penicillin allergy: Erythromycin by mouth, 1 g a day for adults, 30 mg/kg a day for children, or an oral cephalosporin. When resistant to erythromycin, which is very uncommon, Streptococcus pyogenes is not eradicated from the oropharynx by treatment. Although treatment of *streptococcal carriers* with penicillin is sometimes recommended, this fails to eradicate group A streptococci in a proportion of cases.

Vincent's angina is uncommon, and classically presents as a greasy ulcer, usually on the tip of the tonsil and often unilateral with no fever. It is more commonly associated with gingival sepsis. Fusospirochaetosis is probably not a disease in itself, but possible underlying diseases should be considered. *Treatment* with benzylpenicillin is normally adequate.

Chronic tonsillitis: The tonsils are inflamed, fissured and difficult to move, with a purulent exudate and pain on peritonsillar pressure. Some patients have an increased antistreptolysin O titre. Where clinically indicated, tonsillectomy should be performed under antibiotic cover with penicillin in normal dosage orally or i. m. from a few hours before surgery to 48–72 hours afterwards.

Pharyngitis is usually viral in origin, so antibiotics are not required. Phenoxymethylpenicillin should be given on suspicion of streptococcal pharyngitis, which is not uncommon, and treatment is as for lacunar tonsillitis (see above). Gonococcal pharyngitis (see p. 490) is best treated with large doses of benzylpenicillin or, when resistant, by cefuroxime or cefotaxime.

c) Peritonsillar or Retropharyngeal Abscess, Ludwig's Angina

Causative organisms: Mixed infections with aerobic and anaerobic streptococci, staphylococci, bacteroides etc.

Treatment: Clindamycin orally or i. v., 1.2 g a day, or flucloxacillin 6 g a day. Benzylpenicillin is a less suitable alternative since not all the bacteria involved are susceptible. Cefoxitin or imipenem may also be used in severe infections, since they have good activity against anaerobes. Needle aspiration and drainage of the pus or superficial incision is necessary; tonsillectomy may be necessary for peritonsillar abscess to remove the risk of recurrence. The pus should be examined microscopically and cultured both aerobically and anaerobically. A rare complication is jugular vein thrombosis with septicaemia and the vein may require ligation.

d) Diphtheria

Tonsillar and pharyngeal diphtheria are characterised by a grey, adherent membrane on the throat and tonsils which may spread to the soft palate. Fever is moderate and may be absent; some patients develop shock and a peripheral leucocytosis. At least three swabs should be taken from beneath the pseudomembrane, examined microscopically for suspicious gram-positive bacilli and stained to show metachromatic granules. Culture should include a medium containing potassium tellurite. The nose, ear, conjunctiva, larynx and wounds can also be affected. Because of childhood immunisation, diphtheria is now very uncommon in Western Europe and the USA but should be considered in patients from countries where routine immunisation is not practised. Glandular fever should always be excluded (blood film, Paul Bunnell test etc.).

Treatment: When diphtheria is suspected, give diphtheria antitoxin, 30,000–50,000 units as an i.v. infusion over 1 h, and 60,000–120,000 units in severe infections, always after prior intradermal skin test with an 1:100 dilution in physiological saline. Benzylpenicillin 0.72–1.44 g is given simultaneously and continued for 10 days. Give further antitoxin on each of the next 2 days; steroids may be used in severe cases. The patient may require intubation or even tracheotomy. Patients allergic to penicillin should receive erythromycin (40 mg/kg daily) for 10 days. Strict bed rest is essential because of the risk of myocarditis, and an electrocardiogram should be regularly checked. Three nasal and throat swabs should be negative three days after completion of treatment. Carriers and excretors should be treated with erythromycin in doses up to 2 g a day for adults and 40 mg/kg/day for children for 2 weeks.

e) Infectious Mononucleosis (Glandular Fever)

This condition is characterised by a moderate or high, usually prolonged fever, sometimes accompanied by a whitish, removable membrane on the swollen tonsils. There is generalised lymphadenopathy and splenomegaly (with risk of splenic rupture). The peripheral blood count is characteristic with more than 50% mononuclear cells, of which more than 10% are atypical lymphocytes. The monospot (modified Paul-Bunnell) test is usually positive in the acute phase of the infection, though it may be negative at the outset. IgM antibodies to the Epstein-Barr virus can be demonstrated in the serum although they disappear soon after recovery, whereas IgG antibodies persist. This is a common infection in young people.

Treatment: Because glandular fever is a viral infection, *antibiotics are contraindicated* unless group A streptococci are cultured. The use of antibiotics, particularly ampicillin, in glandular fever is associated with allergic skin rashes (p. 41). Corticosteroids may be useful if severe pharyngotonsillar oedema threatens to obstruct the airway. Bed rest is desirable during the acute phase of the illness.

f) Candida Stomatitis (Oral Thrush)

A whitish, removable membrane is present on the oral mucosa in the absence of fever. Thrush is usually secondary to an underlying disease (e. g. diabetes mellitus), immunodeficiency (e. g. AIDS) or broad-spectrum antibiotic treatment. Yeasts may be visualised microscopically in a smear of material stained with methylene blue or gram, and cultured.

Treatment is generally *topical,* with nystatin, miconazole, clotrimazole, natamycin or amphotericin B as lozenges, a mouthwash or an oral gel, and may need to be prolonged because of the risk of relapse. *Systemic* treatment is now available with fluconazole, 100 mg in adults and 2 mg/kg in children, once a day with food until one week after symptoms have resolved and cultures have become negative (not longer than 2 weeks). An alternative for systemic treatment is itraconazole (p. 202).

g) Acute Necrotising Gingivitis

This is a mixed fusospirillary infection, usually originating in the interdental papillae. Necrosis develops rapidly. The condition often occurs in young adults with predisposing underlying diseases such as AIDS. The causative organisms are always susceptible to penicillin and the condition responds well to phenoxymethylpenicillin or to metronidazole.

h) Secondary Throat Infections

Throat infections may arise as a consequence of bone marrow suppression, e. g. leukaemia, agranulocytosis, when they are usually mixed (aerobic and anaerobic streptococci, fusobacteria, spirillae, Bacteroides, enterobacteria, Pseudomonas etc.). The causative organism can change rapidly. The important measure is to treat the underlying disease effectively. Where agranulocytosis is drug-induced, the likely causative agent should be stopped at once. Very broad-spectrum antibiotic therapy, where possible in bactericidal combinations (p. 606) is recommended until the bone marrow recovers.

i) Laryngitis and Acute Epiglottitis

Laryngitis is usually associated with acute tracheitis in adults (hoarseness and a barking cough), generally as a result of viral infections (measles, influenza or parainfluenza) and rarely as a primary or secondary bacterial infection (Haemophilus influenzae, streptococci, pneumococci or staphylococci).

The presentation in children is more commonly as an *acute epiglottitis,* with a rapid onset, marked inspiratory stridor but no barking cough; these infections are usually due to Haemophilus influenzae and may be fatal unless intubation or tracheotomy is performed. The organism is readily cultured from the blood and may also be detected by latex agglutination of the serum. *Subglottic laryngitis* in children is generally viral in origin, with a gradual onset and no pain on swallowing. The symptoms are less severe and the illness usually responds to conservative treatment. Expiratory and inspiratory stridor is characteristic of acute laryngo-tracheo-bronchitis in the newborn and small infants. The laryngitis is usually caused by viruses but other causes of croup, especially acute epiglottitis and diphtheria, must always be considered since they demand urgent treatment, including antibiotics.

Symptoms of *laryngeal diphtheria* include hoarseness, a barking cough, inspiratory stridor where there is marked membrane development, dyspnoea, and jugular retraction. Chronic hoarseness can be caused by tuberculosis, syphilis or a carcinoma, and all require special treatment.

Treatment of acute laryngitis: Inhalation of steam and mucolytic agents, antitussives, and mild sedation. An attempt may be made to relieve swelling with calcium i.v. and prednisone. Acute epiglottitis in children (seldom in adults) demands urgent hospital admission for intubation or tracheotomy, and immediate antibacterial treatment with cefotaxime or chloramphenicol.

Treatment of laryngeal diphtheria: See p. 370.

j) Acute Bronchitis

Almost always viral (influenza, parainfluenza and other viruses), which often lead to secondary bacterial infections, particularly with pneumococci or Haemophilus influenzae. Superinfection with staphylococci, streptococci, bacteroides, meningococci, Branhamella catarrhalis, klebsiella and pseudomonas occasionally follows. Viral infections are likely when there is a dry cough (tracheitis), hoarseness, pharyngitis and a watery nasal discharge. Purulent sputum is suggestive of secondary bacterial infection.

A primary bacterial bronchitis can be caused by Bordetella pertussis (see p. 509), Branhamella catarrhalis, Mycoplasma pneumoniae (which does not necessarily cause pneumonia), Chlamydia psittaci and Chlamydia trachomatis, often with a pertussis-like cough, as well as Haemophilus influenzae in pre-school children. Any cough which persists for longer than 2 weeks in older children and young adults is suggestive of Mycoplasma pneumoniae infection.

Antibiotic treatment for patients at high risk (infants, the elderly, and patients with lowered resistance because of underlying systemic or lung disease): Erythromycin or amoxycillin, alternatively co-amoxiclav, cefuroxime axetil, cefaclor or cefixime, all of which are active against pneumococci, Haemophilus influenzae and Branhamella catarrhalis. When pneumococci are cultured, give phenoxymethylpenicillin; other pathogens are treated according to the bacterial isolate and its antibiotic sensitivity pattern. Unlike cephalexin and cephradine, cefaclor, cefixime and cefuroxime axetil in adequate dosage (see p. 591) have good activity against Haemophilus influenzae, even when resistant to ampicillin and erythromycin. Erythromycin is effective in bronchitis due to Mycoplasma pneumoniae, Branhamella catarrhalis and Chlamydia trachomatis. If the cough and purulent sputum persist and the sputum quantity is not reduced, further cultures, tuberculin testing and chest x-rays should be performed. For the technique of sputum examination, see p. 377.

k) Chronic Bronchitis

This disease is commonest in the elderly and smokers. Chronic bronchitis is a non-specific condition, characterised by chronic, recurrent cough with sputum production and very often combined with emphysema and bronchial obstruction. Acute exacerbations are due to bacterial superinfection. The long-term sequelae can be severe respiratory insufficiency and cor pulmonale. Recurrent bronchopneumonia and lung abscesses are much less common. Haemophilus influenzae and pneumococci are the commonest causes of acute exacerbations of chronic bronchitis. Staphylococci, Branhamella catarrhalis, klebsiella, and Pseudomonas aeruginosa are relatively rare. Chronic bronchial irritation and epithelial damage impair the mechanism of bacterial elimination from the bronchial tree, so the bronchi are constantly colonised with bacteria.

Some causes of chronic bronchitis specific to children are immunodeficiency, α_1-antitrypsin deficiency, progressive septic granulomatosis, cystic fibrosis (mucoviscidosis) and foreign body aspiration.

Technique of sputum examination: The most important test is inspection of sputum for macroscopic purulence. Sputum should be examined microscopically and by culture and, where necessary, cytologically as well. The antibiotic sensitivities of potential pathogens are determined. A fresh, deeply expectorated sputum collected after rising in the morning and cleaning the teeth, but before breakfast, is the best material for routine examination. Particles of purulent sputum are removed and rinsed in physiological saline to wash out as many oral bacteria as possible. Then direct smears are made for microscopical analysis and various media fractionally inoculated. Direct microscopic findings should include semiquantitative information. Sputum may be obtained at any time in the hospital patient by deep expectoration with the aid of physiotherapy, and transtracheal aspiration or even direct lung puncture have been used in some centres. Fibreoptic bronchoscopy for uncontaminated sputum collection is less traumatic and is especially useful in treatment failures.

Antibiotic treatment is of limited value because the functional and anatomical abnormalities are already present, but antibiotics are sometimes effective in suppressing acute exacerbations. Therapy is usually "best guess". The patient should never be given the same antibiotic used to treat the previous episode of infection. Long-term treatment during the winter with regular changes of antibiotic may reduce the frequency of exacerbations and is based on tetracycline, amoxycillin and co-trimoxazole, which act against Haemophilus influenzae and pneumococci and can be given for long periods. However, 4–20% of pneumococci and 5–10% of Haemophilus influenzae strains are resistant to tetracycline; strains resistant to ampicillin and erythromycin are also found. Cefaclor, cefixime, cefuroxime axetil and co-amoxiclav remain effective in such cases. The role of the new quinolones in chronic bronchitis is still unclear. The penicillins penetrate relatively poorly into sputum, so large doses have to be given. Relatively high sputum concentrations are obtained with minocycline, erythromycin, cefaclor and co-trimoxazole. Because of the risk of bone-marrow suppression, chloramphenicol, which used to be given frequently, is no longer recommended.

Intermittent therapy is important for acute exacerbations with purulent sputum, increasing cough and fever, which are treated for 1–2 weeks with oral amoxycillin (1.5 g/day), co-amoxiclav (0.375–0.75 g/day), doxycycline (0.2 g/day) or co-trimoxazole. The prompt commencement of treatment is very important. Co-operative patients should keep a suitable antibiotic at home in order to start treatment as soon as purulent sputum reappears.

Long-term treatment has now largely fallen out of favour. In a few cases, long-term treatment may still be useful during the winter months to prevent acute attacks and control the progression of obstructive bronchitis. Antibiotics used in this way in alternating fashion are doxycycline (100 mg daily), minocycline (200 mg daily), co-trimoxazole (2 tablets twice daily), amoxycillin by mouth (1.5 g daily), and the ampicillin esters. Phenoxymethylpenicillin and sulphonamides are less active against Haemophilus influenzae and are therefore inferior to the aminopenicillins.

Treatment is successful when the sputum loses its purulence and diminishes in quantity, and breathing and lung function improve.

The clinical picture can be improved considerably by supportive therapy including cessation of smoking, drugs which reduce bronchospasm or secretion, postural drainage of the bronchi (Trendelenburg's position), respiratory physiotherapy, inhalation of antibiotics through a modern nebuliser, digitalisation in cardiac insufficiency or a change in climate. In severe acute exacerbations, aspiration drainage of the respiratory tract, intubation, mechanical ventilation, rehydration or aminophylline i.v. may be necessary. Persistent atelectasis may require bronchoscopy and treatment of pneumonia. Improvement can also be achieved with aerosols of broncholytics, secretolytics, detergents, saline and other means. At the beginning of winter, the patient should be vaccinated against the current or anticipated strain of influenza because of his increased risk.

l) Bronchiolitis

Only occurs in infants and small children. *Pathogens:* Respiratory syncytial and other viruses, sometimes with bacterial superinfection (Haemophilus, staphylococci). *Severely ill infants:* In the USA, infants with severe RSV infection are treated with aerosolised tribavirin (p. 293), which is technically difficult. Secondary infection is treated with cefuroxime or cefamandole i.v. or oral cefaclor. Supportive treatment with oxygen, humidification of respired air, digitalis, prednisone, controlled fluid and electrolyte treatment and mechanical ventilation are all important.

m) Bronchiectasis

Usually a mixed bacterial infection with pneumococci and Haemophilus influenzae. Other organisms (staphylococci, gram-negative rods, pseudomonas, anaerobes) and mixed infections are commoner than in chronic bronchitis.

The initial *antibiotic treatment* of acute exacerbations is directed against the main organisms (pneumococci, haemophilus). Co-trimoxazole, mino- or doxycycline, cefaclor, cefixime or co-amoxiclav are given for at least 5–7 days. Severe cases may be treated for a few days with ceftazidime, ceftriaxone or cefotaxime i.v., particularly if earlier sputum cultures have yielded pseudomonas or other multiresistant organisms which have been considered clinically significant in that situation. Antibiotics such as cefaclor, co-amoxiclav or a new quinolone are otherwise directed against the bacteria isolated, if considered significant. The infecting agents change frequently, so the sputum should be regularly examined bacteriologically. As antibiotics often penetrate bronchiectatic pus poorly, systemic treatment can be supplemented by antibiotic inhalations such as neomycin (200 mg/ml), polymyxin B or gentamicin (10 mg/ml), thiamphenicol (see p. 133), bacitracin (250 units/ml) or tyrothricin (1 mg/ml) 2–3 times a day. As with chronic bronchitis, long-term treatment with doxy- or minocycline or co-trimoxazole is useful in severe cases. Antibiotics are only of limited value in bronchiectasis and other measures such as mucolytics, postural drainage and possibly lobectomy, when the bronchiectasis is localised, also play a part.

n) Cystic Fibrosis (Mucoviscidosis)

Patients with cystic fibrosis are threatened by severe, recurrent chest infections which are caused by Haemophilus influenzae, staphylococci, Pseudomonas aeruginosa, P. cepacia, Xanthomonas maltophilia and other bacteria. Antibiotics can generally be given intermittently as required, alternating between tobramycin or amikacin, azlo- or mezlocillin, piperacillin, ticarcillin/clavulanic acid, co-amoxiclav, a broad-spectrum cephalosporin, co-trimoxazole or a new quinolone such as ciprofloxacin (used with caution in patients aged under 16). Staphylococcal infection is effectively treated with flucloxacillin plus fusidic acid. Long-term treatment is sometimes necessary in severe cases. Chronic infection with pseudomonas is often not eradicable. Cystic fibrosis with lung involvement can be alleviated by intensive inhalation therapy as well as by bronchial drainage. After inhalation of a mucolytic drug, the patient inhales a topical antibiotic using an inhaler of good quality (see above). Many inhalers are heavily contaminated with pseudomonas and re-usable ones should be carefully cleaned and sterilised regularly.

Cystic fibrotics now often reach adult life. Many have chronic pseudomonas chest infections and extensive changes in their chest x-rays. The infection with pseudomonas cannot be eradicated, even with otherwise effective drugs, but clinical improvement often follows anti-pseudomonal treatment with intermittent parenteral antibiotics, e. g. ceftazidime + tobramycin for 10–14 days. Short courses of a quinolone (e. g. ofloxacin or ciprofloxacin) can also be effective, but such courses should not exceed 2–3 weeks because of the risk of secondary bacterial resistance, which can also emerge as a result of repeated short courses of a quinolone. Alternatives are piperacillin, azlocillin or ticarcillin/clavulanate with tobramycin, aztreonam or imipenem.

o) Pneumonia

The **main forms** are *bronchopneumonia* (especially in babies and the elderly), *lobar pneumonia* and *interstitial pneumonia* (the pneumonia of viral type which occurs in mycoplasma infections, ornithosis and Q-fever). *Genuine viral pneumonia* without bacterial involvement is rare and associated usually with influenza, parainfluenza, adenoviruses, respiratory syncytial viruses and varicella;

its x-ray changes are those of an interstitial pneumonia. Correlation between a particular form of pneumonia and a given pathogen is closest in primary pneumonias. The clinical picture of the more frequent secondary pneumonias is changed considerably by the primary disease and factors which lower resistance (e. g. cystic fibrosis, mitral valve disease, heart failure, pulmonary oedema, caustic gas inhalation and prolonged mechanical ventilation, aspiration, alcoholism, pulmonary infarction etc.).

Particular forms of pneumonia:
Pneumonia with abscess formation (due to staphylococci, Klebsiella pneumoniae, anaerobes).
Haematogenous pneumonia (septic pulmonary metastases).
Pneumonia complicating infectious diseases (whooping cough, measles, chicken-pox, influenza, actinomycosis, nocardiosis, brucellosis, tularaemia, plague, anthrax, typhoid fever etc.).
Chronic or recurrent pneumonia (often superimposed on a bronchial carcinoma).
Caseous pneumonia (tuberculosis).
Fungal pneumonia (Candidosis, aspergillosis, cryptococcosis, histoplasmosis).
Postoperative pneumonia (see p. 436).
Perinatal pneumonia (due to aspiration of infected amniotic fluid or atelectasis).
Pneumocystis carinii pneumonia (in babies from the second to the six month of life, but commoner in adults and older children with severe immune deficiency or malnutrition), sometimes occurring simultaneously with pulmonary cytomegalovirus infection. These infections often complicate the acquired immunodeficiency syndrome (AIDS).

Diagnosis: Wherever possible, a well-collected sputum sample should be carefully examined by microscopy and culture. The sample is best obtained by deep expectoration with the aid of physiotherapy, by fibre-optic bronchoscopy or by transtracheal aspiration (TTA) so that material from the lower respiratory tract is reliably obtained. The character of the sputum gives important information. A gram-stained direct smear of the sputum may show the causative organism as a single morphological type in association with abundant polymorphonuclear neutrophils. The presence of large numbers of epithelial cells suggests that any culture will be oral flora of no pathogenic significance. If a sputum sample is not forthcoming, a deep nasal swab using a thin swab stick can be obtained in children; its culture frequently reflects the bronchial flora. Since pneumococci and haemophilus do not survive for long on swabs, a bacterial transport medium should be used. The cultural result of the nasal swab only provides a pointer, never a firm diagnosis.

In pneumococcal, haemophilus, candida and cryptococcal pneumonia, rapid antigen detection by latex agglutination can be performed in serum and urine;

rapid latex tests are also available for group B streptococcal and meningococcal infection. When a pneumonia which is resistant to therapy and of unclear aetiology persists, fibre-optic bronchoscopy is justified in order to obtain deep bronchial secretions for culture, even though they are often contaminated with oral flora. Special cultures of these secretions can be set up for legionella, anaerobes, Pneumocystis carinii and fungi. Chlamydia trachomatis can cause pneumonia in infants and in oncology patients, Chlamydia pneumoniae in all age groups. Chlamydial antigen can be demonstrated in pharyngeal secretions by direct immunofluorescence (MicroTrak, Syva), by ELISA or by culture in certain cell lines.

Transtracheal aspiration (TTA) can be used in adults to obtain secretions from the lower respiratory tract. The culture of mycoplasmas, chlamydiae and rickettsias is difficult, and special transport media must be used to transmit the specimen to the special laboratory. If tuberculosis is suspected, a Ziehl-Neelsen stain of a sputum smear or laryngeal swab should be examined. Blood culture yields the organism in 30% of cases of pneumococcal pneumonia, but rarely in other types of bacterial pneumonia. Needle lung biopsy may be used to demonstrate pneumococci, group A streptococci (Streptococcus pyogenes) and Haemophilus influenzae type b by direct latex agglutination and by culture.

Frequent bacterial causes of pneumonia are pneumococci and staphylococci. Klebsiella pneumoniae, Branhamella, Haemophilus influenzae, Chlamydia pneumoniae, meningococci, Pseudomonas aeruginosa and bacteroides are less common (Table 40). Haemophilus influenzae is commoner in younger children, and Mycoplasma pneumoniae in older children. The range of pathogens varies considerably according to the clinical situation. Gram-negative rods (pseudomonas, klebsiella) are commoner in patients with a tracheotomy or on mechanical ventilation and in leukaemics; these organisms also colonise tracheotomy sites and endotracheal tubes, particularly if the patient is receiving antibiotics, and should only be regarded as causes of pneumonia in such patients if the tracheal secretion is clearly purulent and there are confirmatory radiological changes. Group B streptococci and enterobacteria also cause pneumonia in the newborn, mostly as a result of aspiration of infected amniotic fluid.

Because gram-negative rods are often part of the oral flora, particularly when the patient has received certain antibiotics, the diagnosis of gram-negative pneumonia from sputum culture is difficult. Viridans streptococci, non-pathogenic neisseriae and Bacteroides species are normally found in the mouth and therefore also in the sputum, as occasionally are pneumococci, staphylococci, Haemophilus influenzae and Candida species, though generally in smaller quantities. Klebsiella, Escherichia coli and pseudomonas are rarely present in the sputum of the normal patient. Treatment with ampicillin, certain other broad-spectrum antibiotics and also with large doses of benzylpenicillin causes selection of gram-negative bacilli in the oral cavity which has no relevance in patients not suffering from a serious

Table 40. Causes of different clinical forms of pneumonia.

Clinical form	Principal causes	Occasional causes
Lobar pneumonia, segmental pneumonia	Pneumococci	Klebsiella, streptococci, legionella, meningococci
Post-influenzal pneumonia	Staphylococci, pneumococci	Haemophilus, streptococci
Suppurative bronchopneumonia	Staphylococci, bacteroides	Klebsiella, pseudomonas
Aspiration pneumonia	Bacteroides, anaerobic steptococci	Staphylococci, pneumococci etc.
Postoperative pneumonia	Staphylococci	Pneumococci, streptococci, klebsiella
Primary interstitial pneumonia	Mycoplasma, chlamydia	Psittacosis (ornithosis), Q-fever, legionella
Pneumonia during prolonged mechanical ventilation	Pseudomonas, klebsiella	Proteus, staphylococci, candida
Pneumonia in AIDS patients	Pneumocystis carinii	Mycobacterium tuberculosis, atypical mycobacteria, fungi, cytomegalovirus etc.
Secondary pneumonia in immunodeficient patients without prior antibiotic treatment	Staphylococci, klebsiella, pneumococci, bacteroides	Escherichia coli, serratia etc.
Secondary pneumonia during antibiotic therapy	Any facultative pathogen, particularly those affected by standard antibiotic therapy, often including multiresistant strains of pseudomonas, klebsiella, staphylococcus, and serratia	

underlying disease. The selection of gram-negative bacilli can, however, play an important epidemiological role as a reservoir of potential pathogens in a group of severely ill patients, for example in an intensive care unit.

A **serological diagnosis** of some causes of pneumonia can be made by the demonstration of a rising titre of specific antibodies in the patient's blood:

Chlamydia psittaci:	CFT
Chlamydia pneumoniae:	immunofluorescence
Chlamydia trachomatis:	immunofluorescence, ELISA
Mycoplasma pneumoniae:	EIA (IgM antibodies)
Legionellosis:	immunofluorescence, EIA
Coxiella burnetii (Q-fever):	ELISA, CFT
Influenza, parainfluenza virus:	ELISA, CFT
Respiratory syncytial virus:	EIA
Cytomegalovirus:	ELISA, RIA
Toxoplasma gondii:	immunofluorescence (IgM antibodies)

Serological methods such as the enzyme-linked immunosorbent assay (ELISA) and specific microscopical immunofluorescence are now superceding the complement fixation test (CFT) in many centres since they are more specific, more economical of expensive reagents and readily automated when performed in batches of larger numbers of tests. Since various forms of pneumonia can occur in all stages of HIV infection, an HIV antibody test is an important basic investigation in the differential diagnosis of pneumonia.

The blood count in bacterial pneumonias usually shows a polymorph neutrophilia with a marked left shift; viral pneumonias tend to show a left shift without neutrophilia. The ESR is raised in almost all types of pneumonia. The serum CRP (C-reactive protein) is raised in most bacterial pneumonias, but not in pneumonia due to mycoplasma, Chlamydia pneumoniae, C. psittaci or C. trachomatis. Whilst the CRP remains low in most viral infections, it can rise just as with bacterial infections for some types of viral infection (e. g. adenovirus infection). When there are characteristic radiological findings, a specific history such as contact with birds, tuberculin conversion, contact with cases of influenza or high risk of HIV infection, together with relevant associated signs (e. g. purulent sputum, conjunctivitis, skin rash, myalgia etc.) may suggest a particular pathogen for which specific tests can be carried out. If, for technical reasons, the clinical diagnosis is not confirmed by bacteriological, virological or serological tests, the response to a given treatment can sometimes confirm a working diagnosis. In certain forms of viral pneumonia (e. g. influenza, parainfluenza, RSV, CMV), the virus may be cultured from a throat swab or other specimen. The delay before results are available makes this procedure retrospective in the individual patient, though often valuable in identifying causes of epidemics.

Principles of treatment: Antibiotic treatment should always be as appropriate as possible and based on relevant culture results and antibiotic sensitivities. A direct smear of the sputum stained by Gram's method or the result of a latex agglutination test on serum may give a guide to initial treatment in primary pneumonias. In secondary pneumonia, a bacterial diagnosis from culture of expectorated sputum is almost impossible because many pathogens of pneumonia are found in the mouth flora of hospital patients. Endobronchial aspirates through a fibre-optic bronchoscope and transtracheal aspirates (TTA) are more reliable, and direct microscopy gives a better guide to the likely cause in urgent cases. In patients with a tracheotomy or on long-term mechanical ventilation, the trachea is usually colonised by gram-negative bacilli. This is not necessarily a sign of pneumonia or the risk of pneumonia.

A suitable antibiotic is initially given parenterally in relatively large doses, which may be reduced and, where appropriate, given orally when the patient becomes convalescent. Bactericidal antibiotics are theoretically better, but are not essential. Pneumonias due to gram-negative bacilli should if possible be treated with a combination of a modern aminoglycoside and a β-lactam antibiotic (e. g. cefotaxime or piperacillin). The duration of treatment depends on the clinical and radiological findings and should be of adequate length, particularly where there is evidence of abscess formation.

Good general, cardiac and circulatory care, fluid balance, oxygen treatment, fresh air for children, drainage in bronchial obstruction, sedation, inhalations etc. are also important. Severe pneumonias are best managed in hospital, and cases of respiratory failure should be treated in a well-equipped intensive care unit. Pooled normal human immunoglobulin should only be given to patients with hypogammaglobulinaemia. Corticosteroids are justified only in exceptional cases (septic shock). The choice of antibiotics in pneumonia may be based on guidance given in Tables 41 and 42.

α) Best-guess Therapy

Microbiological confirmation of the diagnosis is only possible in a minority of cases of pneumonia. Treatment must therefore be guided principally by clinical criteria, to which the recommendations for intervention therapy (see p. 606) apply. If there is no response to the initial treatment, the antibiotic cover should be broadened (see Table 41).

1. **Primary community-acquired pneumonia** in previously healthy individuals is usually caused (if bacterial) by pneumococci or staphylococci (of which 50% or fewer are nowadays susceptible to penicillin).

   Treatment should first be tried with benzylpenicillin or cefazolin (which is also active against penicillin-resistant staphylococci) in high dosage (e. g. 2.4–6 g of benzylpenicillin twice daily) for the first few days until defervescence, then changing to 0.6–1.2 g of phenoxymethylpenicillin. If the fever persists for more than 48 h, interstitial pneumonia (due to mycoplasma, chlamydia or coxiella) should be suspected and treatment changed to doxycycline. Should the fever fail to respond within a further 48 h, possible causes are resistant staphylococci, legionella, klebsiellae or other gram-negative bacilli, and further treatment should be guided by the bacteriological results which will have become available in the interim (see below).

   The failure of beta-lactam antibiotics in afebrile pneumonias affecting infants in the first six months of life is likely to be due to Chlamydia trachomatis infection, which should be treated with erythromycin (50 mg/kg per day). Legionellosis is best treated with the combination of erythromycin + rifampicin.

2. **Primary interstitial pneumonia:** Clear sputum, absence of leukocytosis, a high fever, relative bradycardia and widespread, diffuse opacities on chest X-ray are all suggestive of mycoplasma pneumonia, infection by Chlamydia pneumoniae, psittacosis/ornithosis or Q-fever. Treatment is with doxycycline. In immuno-

Table 41. Treatment of pneumonia of unknown cause ("best-guess" antibiotic).

Clinical presentation	"Best-guess" antibiotic	Alternative antibiotics
Lobar pneumonia, segmental pneumonia	Benzylpenicillin	Cefazolin, cefuroxime, erythromycin
Post-influenzal pneumonia	Cefuroxime	Flucloxacillin + fusidic acid, cefotiam, cefazolin
Primary interstitial pneumonia	Doxycycline	Ofloxacin, ciprofloxacin (in adults), erythromycin (in children)
Suppurative pneumonia, aspiration pneumonia, post-operative pneumonia	Imipenem	Clindamycin + gentamicin, clindamycin + cefotaxime, cefoxitin + gentamicin
Pneumonia during prolonged mechanical ventilation	Ceftazidime + gentamicin	Cefotaxime + azlocillin or piperacillin + gentamicin
Secondary pneumonia (in hospital, without prior antibiotics)	Cefotiam	Cefotaxime + clindamycin
Secondary pneumonia (under antibiotic therapy)	Imipenem, cefotaxime + gentamicin	Ceftazidime, piperacillin, rifampicin, vancomycin, ciprofloxacin (in rational combination)
Pneumonia in AIDS patients (interstitial)	Co-trimoxazole (in large doses)	Pentamidine (parenteral), trimetrexate (investigational)
Pneumonia in AIDS patients (segmental)	Cefazolin, cefuroxime	Cefotaxime + rifampicin

suppressed patients, pneumocystis, cytomegalovirus, herpes or varicella pneumonia may also be present (see p. 283 for treatment of varicella with acyclovir).

3. **Secondary pneumonia in immunodeficient patients,** usually arising in hospital (e.g. postoperatively, in patients with underlying diseases which depress immunity, or after pulmonary infarction): The causative organisms are often resistant hospital flora (staphylococci, klebsiella etc.), mostly in mixed infections with Haemophilus influenzae, pneumococci, bacteroides, but rarely legionella.

Treatment if no prior therapy has been given is with high doses of cefotiam or cefotaxime (in a daily dose of 6 g in adults and 100 mg/kg in children), possibly in combination with the anti-staphylococcal and anti-anaerobic agent clindamycin. In secondary pneumonia which has arisen during antibiotic therapy, the antibiotics chosen must differ fundamentally from those previously used. The best choice is very broad-spectrum treatment with imipenem or cefotaxime +

gentamicin. Other agents may need to be added to close gaps in the range of activity in the combination chosen. Thus even unusual combinations such as cefotaxime + vancomycin + gentamicin may be logical here.

The trachea and bronchi of patients undergoing mechanical ventilation usually become colonised with bacteria. It may not be possible to decide whether bacteria isolated from the trachea are the cause of a concomitant pneumonia. Treatment in such cases must be with a combination which is also active against pseudomonas, e.g. cefotaxime (6 g a day) + azlocillin (6–8 g a day). If antibiotic treatment fails, fungal or pneumocystis pneumonia, and even tuberculosis, should be considered.

4. **Bronchopneumonia in chronic bronchitis** is usually a mixed infection with pneumococci, Haemophilus influenzae, staphylococci or gram-negative bacteria. When bacteriological results are not available, treat with a broad-spectrum antibiotic which has not been used recently for long-term treatment (e.g. cefuroxime or cefotiam), and change on the basis of antibiotic sensitivity testing when available.

5. **Aspiration pneumonia** can occur in patients who are unconscious, have disorders of swallowing, poisoning, post-operatively, in obstructions due to bronchial carcinoma etc. Abscess formation, possibly with pleural empyema, can also occur. The infections are almost always mixed with anaerobes (fusobacteria, bacteroides, peptostreptococci, and peptococci), sometimes with aerobic organisms (staphylococci, pseudomonas and enterobacteria). The sputum is foul and offensive.

Bacteriological culture of sputum is unhelpful because of contamination with oral flora and bronchoscopy or transtracheal aspiration are advisable.

Treatment: Imipenem, which is also effective against anaerobes, possibly in combination with gentamicin, which is particularly useful in mixed infections with enterobacteria and pseudomonas. Suitable alternatives are clindamycin i.v. or metronidazole i.v. + cefotaxime i.v. or cefoxitin + gentamicin.

6. **Influenza pneumonia** can appear in epidemics of influenza and tracheobronchitis and in severe cases is usually a superinfection with staphylococci, pneumococci and haemophilus.

Initial treatment should be with cefuroxime, flucloxacillin plus fusidic acid or cefotiam.

7. **Pneumonia of the newborn** often originates in areas of atelectasis or after aspiration of infected amniotic fluid (gram-negative bacilli, group B streptococci, mixed infections). Young infants are also predisposed to staphylococcal pneumonia.

Treatment: Parenteral cefotaxime + piperacillin or an intermediate cephalosporin (e.g. cefuroxime) + gentamicin.

8. **Pneumonia in the first 6 months of life** accompanied by an eosinophilia is usually due to Chlamydia trachomatis. *Drug of choice:* erythromycin.

β) Directed Therapy

Pneumococcal pneumonia: The pneumococcus is still the commonest cause of primary pneumonia, which can be lobar or segmental. Pneumococci are found in the sputum and blood culture and the latex agglutination test in serum and urine is often positive, even after treatment has begun. A secondary pneumococcal pneumonia can also occur in the compromised host.

Treatment: The drug of choice is still benzylpenicillin, since resistant pneumococci remain extremely uncommon. Benzylpenicillin 2.4–6 g is given parenterally as an i.v. infusion or i.m. for the first 2 days of the illness or until defervescence (usually within 48 h), followed by phenoxymethylpenicillin 0.6–1.2 g a day for at least 2 weeks. Cefazolin or erythromycin may be used in penicillin-allergic patients (Table 42). Imipenem is indicated in penicillin resistance. Tetracyclines are unreliable because resistant pneumococci are often found.

Pneumonia due to other streptococci: Group A streptococci are uncommon causes of pneumonia, associated with abscess formation and pleural empyema.

Table 42. Treatment of pneumonia of known bacterial cause (subject to sensitivity test).

Bacterial cause	Treatment of choice	Alternatives
Pneumococci, streptococci, staphylococci (non-penicillinase-producers), meningococci	Benzylpenicillin	Cefazolin, erythromycin
Staphylococci (penicillinase-producers)	Flucloxacillin + fusidic acid	Cefazolin, clindamycin, vancomycin, teicoplanin
Klebsiella pneumoniae	Cefotaxime + gentamicin	Imipenem, ciprofloxacin
Pseudomonas aeruginosa	Azlocillin + tobramycin	Cefsulodin, piperacillin, ceftazidime, amikacin, imipenem, aztreonam, ciprofloxacin
Haemophilus influenzae	Cefotaxime	Co-amoxiclav, cefuroxime, cefotiam
Bacteroides species	Metronidazole	Cefoxitin, clindamycin, imipenem
Mycoplasma pneumoniae, Chlamydia psittaci, Coxiella burnetii	Doxycycline	Erythromycin (mycoplasma only), rifampicin
Legionella pneumophila	Erythromycin	Rifampicin
Chlamydia trachomatis	Erythromycin	Doxycycline
Pneumocystis carinii	Co-trimoxazole (in high dosage)	Dapsone + trimethoprim, pentamidine, trimetrexate

Group B streptococci are relatively common causes of congenital pneumonia and may be detected by a rapid latex agglutination test on serum, urine or pleural pus.

Treatment: Benzylpenicillin, or cefazolin, cefuroxime or cefotaxime in patients with penicillin allergy (dosage as for pneumococcal pneumonia). Penicillin + gentamicin is a synergistic combination in group B streptococcal pneumonia.

Staphylococcal pneumonia commonly causes multiple abscesses of the lungs and often pyothorax, pneumothorax or septicaemia. Occurs particularly in young infants (often with pneumatoceles), in patients with impaired immunity or underlying diseases such as cystic fibrosis, thrombophlebitis associated with venous catheters, heroin addiction and after operations and influenza.

Penicillin-resistant staphylococcal infections should be treated with a penicillinase-stable penicillin, preferably flucloxacillin i. v. (5–10 g a day for adults, 100–200 mg/kg for children), possibly in combination with fusidic acid. After defervescence and clinical improvement, continue flucloxacillin or dicloxacillin by mouth (2–3 g a day for adults, 100 mg/kg for children) for several weeks if necessary, until the lung changes have completely resolved (high risk of relapse). An alternative treatment is oral clindamycin (900 mg daily).

Penicillin-sensitive staphylococcal pneumonia should be treated in the same way as pneumococcal pneumonia, but for a longer period.

In patients *allergic to penicillin* give cefazolin or cefazedone, 4–6 g a day for adults. Clindamycin, vancomycin or teicoplanin may also be effective against methicillin-resistant strains or in the rare cases of allergy to cephalosporins.

Klebsiella pneumonia (Friedländer's pneumonia) is a rare cause of primary lobar pneumonia, but commoner as a secondary infection in patients with severe underlying disease. Often found in alcoholics, producing a viscous, blood-stained mucopurulent sputum. The infection usually becomes chronic and has a high mortality.

Treatment is difficult and antibiotics should always be given in combination, such as cefotaxime (6 g a day) + gentamicin (240–480 mg a day). Imipenem or ciprofloxacin in high dosage are good alternatives.

Fever subsides slowly during treatment, which should be continued for at least one week after defervescence because of the risk of relapse.

Pseudomonas pneumonia is always secondary, particularly in cystic fibrosis, leukaemia, and mechanical ventilation. The prognosis is poor and frequently associated with pulmonary microabscesses.

Treatment: Azlocillin (6–15 g a day in 3 divided doses) + tobramycin (240 mg daily). Alternatives are piperacillin, cefsulodin, ceftazidime, aztreonam, imipenem, ofloxacin or ciprofloxacin.

Difficult to cure, and long courses of treatment are often necessary. The simultaneous intratracheal instillation of an aminoglycoside may be useful in intubated or tracheotomised patients.

Serratia pneumonia is rare, and may arise from contaminated ventilators or humidifiers. Patients affected almost always have impaired resistance or severe underlying disease.

Treatment: According to antibiotic sensitivity testing, preferably ceftazidime or cefotaxime i. v. (6 g daily), in combination with gentamicin or amikacin. Mezlocillin or piperacillin may be used if the isolate is sensitive. Imipenem is almost always effective.

Haemophilus influenzae pneumonia: Rare. Found most commonly in elderly patients with chronic bronchitis and in children under 5 years of age. Lobar or bronchial pneumonia, sometimes accompanied by pleural effusion. Latex agglutination positive (serum or pleural fluid) only in infections with type b strains.

Treatment: Initially with cefotaxime i. v., 4–6 g in adults in 3 divided doses followed by oral cefaclor, 2 g a day for adults, for 3–4 weeks. Sensitive strains may be treated with ampicillin or amoxycillin. Doxycycline, co-amoxiclav and co-trimoxazole are also suitable for the follow-up treatment of sensitive strains.

Whooping cough pneumonia: Particularly dangerous in young infants and generally associated with superinfection by staphylococci or other bacteria, although primary Bordetella infection of the lungs can also occur. A β-lactamase-stable cephalosporin such as cefuroxime or cefotaxime, 60 mg/kg a day, is now preferred; it is also active against Bordetella pertussis.

Fungal pneumonia: Associated with Candida albicans, invasive aspergillosis, mucormycosis or cryptococcosis. Diagnosis is difficult because of the chronic course and frequent occurrence in patients with agranulocytosis, leukaemia, or tumor. The presence of fungi in the sputum is not in itself evidence of a pulmonary mycosis, nor justification for treatment with amphotericin B, which has severe side effects. The demonstration of fungi in tracheal or bronchial secretions obtained by transtracheal aspiration or bronchoscopy, in pleural pus or in blood culture is more convincing, particularly when accompanied by radiological evidence of infiltration or cavitation. A specific latex agglutination test for serum antigen detection may be positive in candida, aspergillus and cryptococcal infection.

Treatment: Amphotericin B (see p. 193 for dosage) in combination with flucytosine (see p. 210) for several weeks, supplemented by inhalation of nystatin or amphotericin B with a modern inhaler. Alternatives: fluconazole or itraconazole orally. Aspergilloma will not respond to chemotherapy and must be removed surgically, eventually with local instillation of amphotericin B.

Histoplasmosis occurs mainly in the USA as a fairly innocuous primary pulmonary infection or as an allergic histoplasmosis reinfection (no specific treatment necessary). For fulminant allergic pneumonia (after the inhalation of large quantities of spores), give a short course of prednisone + amphotericin B in high doses. Chronic cavitating pulmonary histoplasmosis or disseminated histoplasmosis in immunosuppressed patients, which often begins in the lungs, should be treated with amphotericin B or ketoconazole for 2–4 weeks and treated surgically where necessary.

Pneumonia due to rare pathogens (Pseudomonas pseudomallei, see p. 578, Achromobacter, Enterobacter, Proteus etc.): *Treatment* according to antibiotic sensitivities as for septicaemia with the same organism. For legionellosis, see p. 388; for anthrax, see p. 499; actinomycosis: see p. 512; typhoid fever: see p. 502; for tularaemia, see p. 508.

Primary interstitial pneumonia may be caused by Chlamydia psittaci (psittacosis, ornithosis), Chlamydia pneumoniae, Chlamydia trachomatis, Coxiella burnetii (Q-fever), or Mycoplasma pneumoniae. These organisms were formerly classified with the viruses because of their small size, but can be grown on inanimate media (except for chlamydiae) and inhibited by antibiotics and so are biologically bacteria. *Diagnosis* is made on clinical and serological grounds. Doxycycline (0.2 g daily) is the drug of choice and should be started without delay when interstitial pneumonia is suspected on the grounds of severe headache, high fever, relative bradycardia, perihilar opacities with fan-like shadowing or ground-glass opacities on the x-ray, and absence of leukocytosis.

Duration of treatment: 14 days. If there is no response to tetracycline, other causes should be sought. Erythromycin and rifampicin are also effective against Mycoplasma pneumoniae, Legionella pneumophila, Chlamydia pneumoniae and Chlamydia trachomatis. Ofloxacin or ciprofloxacin may also be used in adults. Pneumocystis pneumonia should also be considered as a possible cause.

Pneumocystis carinii pneumonia is an interstitial pneumonia which may produce a plasma cell response and occurs particularly with leukaemia (often in the terminal stage) and other causes of immunosuppression, both iatrogenic, e. g. after renal transplantation, and acquired, e. g. the acquired immunodeficiency syndrome (AIDS). It also occurs in premature and newborn babies and malnourished children, often together with cytomegalovirus pneumonia. Symptoms are progressive tachypnoea and a dry cough, but no chest signs on auscultation. X-ray changes, where present, are mostly bilateral and sometimes focal. There is a high mortality rate, though spontaneous resolution occasionally occurs.

Diagnosis is based on needle lung biopsy or bronchial lavage, stained by silver impregnation. The microscopic demonstration of the organisms in tissue obtained by transbronchial lung biopsy or bronchopulmonary lavage is more reliable. Pneumocystis cannot be cultured routinely and sputum examination is unhelpful. Serum antibody detection is unreliable.

Treatment is with very high doses of co-trimoxazole (20 mg/kg trimethoprim and 100 mg/kg of sulphamethoxazole daily, i. e. four times the normal daily dose).

In patients in whom only the i. v. route of administration is available, a daily dose of 15 mg/kg of trimethoprim and 75 mg/kg of sulphamethoxazole should be given. In patients at high risk and in whom other causes of pneumonia have been excluded, treatment with co-trimoxazole is justified on clinical suspicion alone, if lung biopsy is not to be performed. Treatment with pentamidine 4 mg/kg i. m. once daily for 7–10 days has considerable side-effects (rise in blood urea, megaloblastic bone marrow changes); in addition, aerosolised pentamidine may be inhaled. Alternatives are dapsone + trimethoprim and trimetrexate + folinic acid (see p. 537).

CMV infection of the lungs: CMV infection, which may co-exist with pneumocystis pneumonia, should be considered in every case of progressive interstitial pneumonia in an immunosuppressed patient, particularly after bone-marrow transplantation and in AIDS. Without treatment, the mortality is very high. The aetiological diagnosis is difficult and requires open lung biopsy (with typical histology and positive culture). Direct detection of CMV antigen in bronchoalveolar lavage is possible by DNA assay after PCR amplification and in lung tissue by DNA hybridization techniques. Combined therapy is possible with ganciclovir (see p. 286) and anti-CMV immunoglobulin. Patients who respond may relapse after treatment is stopped.

Varicella pneumonia: This occurs almost exclusively in adults (particularly if immunosuppressed) who have severe, progressive varicella, and is fatal in 10–30% of cases. It can be difficult to distinguish from generalised zoster and generalised herpes with pulmonary involvement. Treatment is with acyclovir 10 mg/kg i. v. 3 times a day for 10 days. Zoster immune globulin (ZIG) may be given to prevent relapse.

RSV pneumonia: A life-threatening pneumonia can be caused by RSV in infants, particularly in those with congenital cardiac defects, and is treated in the USA with tribavirin inhalation (see p. 293). RS viral antigen can be demonstrated rapidly by EIA in nasal or pharyngeal mucus. Clinical experience with ribavirin is still scanty.

p) Legionellosis

The **causative organism,** Legionella pneumophila, is a gram-negative bacillus which is difficult to culture, relatively slow-growing, and found in tanked and piped water, particularly hot-water supplies. Infection takes place when a spray of contaminated water is inhaled (from a shower or air-conditioning plant), particularly in large buildings (hotels, hospitals). Person-to-person spread has not been described. The incubation period is 2–14 days. The legionellae only multiply intracellularly (in alveolar macrophages), giving rise to a predominantly lobar (intra-alveolar) pneumonia without involvement of the bronchi, and sometimes accompanied by a pleural effusion. The frequency of legionella as a cause of pneumonias is 5–15% in adults and about 1% in children. The disease can occur at any age, but particularly affects elderly people with previously damaged lungs (e. g. through smoking), immunosuppressed patients receiving corticosteroids or cytotoxic drugs, and patients with renal transplants. Infection gives rise to disease in only 5% of exposed people. The disease can occur epidemically or sporadically (with regional clusters). A milder form (without pneumonia) is known as *Pontiac fever*, with influenza-like symptoms (dry cough, chest pain, pharyngitis and malaise).

Typical symptoms are shortness of breath and a cough with scanty sputum which often contains blood and pus cells but few extracellular bacteria. Other features are diarrhoea, vomiting and severe abdominal pain as well as signs of encephalopathy (impaired consciousness, confusion, fits, ataxia) with normal CSF findings. Disorders of renal function and a rise in serum transaminases often occur. Prior treatment with a penicillin, cephalosporin or aminoglycoside has always been ineffective.

The chest X-ray shows bilateral pulmonary infiltration. Hypoxia and peripheral leukocytosis are often found, as are proteinuria and leukocyturia. Possible complications are renal or cerebral abscess, myocarditis, pericarditis or peritonitis.

The **diagnosis** must initially be made clinically. The causative organism can be cultured from sputum and sometimes also from a pleural aspirate and from the blood (after incubation of the cultures for several days). Antigen detection in expectorated macrophages by an immunofluorescent antibody can be used as a rapid test. Specific IgM antibodies are often not demonstrable until after several weeks. Rapid clinical improvement typically occurs after starting treatment with erythromycin, although the fever does not settle completely until after 5–7 days and the radiological appearances resolve only slowly.

Treatment is with erythromycin, which is initially given i. v. in severe illness in a daily dose of 3–4 g in adults and 60 mg/kg in children, changing to 2 g orally (30 mg/kg in children) after defervescence. Treatment should be continued for at least 3 weeks, and 4–6 weeks or longer in immunosuppressed patients, because of the danger of relapse. In severe infections and in immunosuppressed patients erythromycin is combined in the first week with rifampicin (0.6 g 2–3 times a day or 6 mg/kg 3 times a day). The new quinolones (ofloxacin and ciprofloxacin) are effective alternatives. Doxycycline and co-trimoxazole are unreliable. Any cytotoxic therapy should be interrupted if possible. Mechanical ventilation may be necessary if hypoxia is severe. Treatment has reduced the mortality in otherwise compromised patients from 80% formerly to below 20%. The *prevention* of further infections may require the disinfection of the water supply of a building or a residential area.

q) Lung Abscess

Primary lung abscesses develop in the course of a pneumonia or septicaemia (with multiple abscesses). The most common *bacterial causes* are staphylococci, anaerobic streptococci, Bacteroides species and occasionally Klebsiella pneumoniae and Pseudomonas aeruginosa. **Secondary lung abscesses** often develop in the lung as a result of bronchial obstruction due to a bronchogenic carcinoma or the aspiration of a foreign body (in paralysis of swallowing, coma or alcoholism). An abscess or necrotising lung infection can also develop in a pulmonary infarct or an infected lung cyst. These infections are usually mixed, with both aerobic and anaerobic bacteria. Sputum culture is usually unhelpful because the pathogens of lung abscesses are often constituents of the normal mouth flora. A transtracheal aspiration or bronchoscopy should be performed early to obtain pus for bacteriological examination. If there is also a pleural empyema, the causative organism may be isolated from a pleural aspirate. If the abscess drains into a bronchus, large amounts of pus are coughed up with an offensive smell in anaerobic infections. Other cavitating lesions such as tuberculosis, melioidosis, actinomycosis, nocardiosis, amoebiasis, echinococcus cysts and fungal infections (histoplasmosis, coccidioidomycosis) should be ruled out in the differential diagnosis. Pneumatoceles arising from infantile staphylococcal pneumonia should not be confused with lung abscesses.

Treatment: Because the abscesses are almost always due to mixed infection, treatment should cover all the common causative agents of lung abscess (staphylococci, anaerobic streptococci, bacteroides, enterobacteria), even if only one species has been isolated. Clindamycin i. v. (1.2 g a day) + gentamicin i. m. or i. v. (0.32 g a day) have been commonly used and include all the likely components of a mixed infection. Imipenem (3–4 g a day) is a good alternative which includes the same range of organisms as this combination. The combination of cefotaxime + clindamycin or metronidazole is also effective against almost all the likely pathogens. Benzylpenicillin in large doses (12 g a day) is active against anaerobic streptococci as well as non-penicillinase-producing staphylococci and sensitive strains of bacteroides. When penicillin-resistant staphylococci have been isolated, flucloxacillin or cefazolin are also indicated. For anaerobic infections, metronidazole may be added. Any antibiotics must be given in large doses because of the difficulty of achieving adequate concentrations in lung abscesses. Prolonged treatment is usually necessary before the abscess cavity disappears.

Improvement is shown by defervescence, reduction in sputum volume and foetid smell, disappearance of pathogens from the sputum and radiological shrinkage of the abscess cavity. Drainage of the abscess into a bronchus will accelerate a cure. Aspirated foreign bodies underlying an abscess-forming pneumonia have to be removed by endoscopy. Recurrent abscess-forming pneumonia in the same segment may be a sign of bronchial carcinoma. If conservative treatment for at least 8 weeks has resulted in no improvement, surgery should be considered (resection of a segment, or lobectomy).

r) Empyema

Usually develops at the same time as, or following, pneumonia, and associated often with pneumothorax. In infants, almost always the result of rupture of a lung abscess, for which pleural drainage is essential. In adults, generally associated with aspiration pneumonia, or as a progression of the infection. Sometimes associated with a subphrenic abscess or amoebic liver abscess. Pulmonary tuberculosis is nowadays a rare cause of empyema. A malignant cause (mesothelioma, pulmonary or breast carcinoma, lymphoma etc.) can be excluded by cytological differentiation of the aspirate.

When empyema is clinically suspected, try to obtain a sample for bacteriological testing by needle aspiration of the pus; the prognosis is much better when a known cause can be treated. In pleural empyema the LDH content of the pus is usually above 1,500 units/l and the protein content above 35 g/l, whereas these values are less in exudates. Foul-smelling pus is a sign of mixed anaerobic infection. In addition to staphylococci, pneumococci, aerobic and anaerobic streptococci, bacteroides, Pseudomonas aeruginosa, Klebsiella pneumoniae and other organisms are sometimes isolated. Latex agglutination for pneumococci, group B streptococci and haemophilus in serum or pleural pus remains positive for several days after antibiotic treatment has started. A pleural exudate results not infrequently from mycoplasma infection, in which case no bacterial growth occurs in standard culture. In such cases, tuberculosis should also be ruled out (by tuberculin testing, culture and pleural biopsy). Fungal colonisation of a pleural cavity with an exudate occasionally occurs in cryptococcal infection and mucormycosis of the lungs.

Since the causative organisms are easily seen and cultured in the pus, **antibiotic treatment** can be given in a targetted fashion, as for pneumonia where the pathogen is known (see p. 384). When mycoplasma infection has been demonstrated serologically, oral erythromycin is indicated. In less serious cases, antibiotic treatment can be supplemented by local measures such as drainage, irrigation, or instillation of substances into the cavity. In pyopneumothorax, viscous pus or loculated empyema, prompt drainage is essential if serious atelectasis or a residual empyema are to be prevented. Modern drainage bottles can be attached to the patient's body, permitting more freedom of movement and thus improving pulmonary ventilation. The following antibiotics may be instilled in the concentrations below into the pleural cavity although such instillation is not usually necessary with systemic therapy:

Gentamicin	1%	Amphotericin B	0.001%
Amikacin	0.2–1%	Flucytosine	0.005%
Oxacillin	1%	Streptomycin	2.5%

Because of the possibility of absorption, the prescribed daily dosage should not be exceeded.

In some cases, surgical measures such as rib resection or decortication are necessary.

References

ACAR, J. E.: Therapy for lower respiratory tract infections with imipenem/cilastatin: a review of worldwide experience. Rev. Infect. Dis. 7: 513 (1985).
BARTLETT, J. G., P. O'KEEFE, F. P. TALLY et al.: Bacteriology of hospital-acquired pneumonia. Arch. Intern. Med. 146: 868 (1986).
BAUERNFEIND, A., B. PRZYKLENK, C. MATTHIAS, R. M. BERTELE, K. HARMS: Selection of antibiotics for treatment and prophylaxis of staphyloccal infections in cystic fibrosis patients. Infection 18: 126 (1990).
CHANG, M. J., C. MOHLA: Ten-minute detection of group A streptococci in pediatric throat swabs. J. Clin. Microbiol. 21: 258 (1985).
CHAU, P. Y., W. S. NG, Y. K. LEUNG, S. LOLEKHA: In vitro susceptibility of strains of Pseudomonas pseudomallei isolated in Thailand and Hong Kong to some newer betalactam antibiotics and quinolone derivatives. J. Infect. Dis. 153: 167–170 (1986).
CORBERY, K. J., J. M. LUCE, and A. B. MONTGOMERY: Aerosolized pentamidine for treatment and prophylaxis of Pneumocystis carinii pneumonia: An update. Respir. Care 33: 676 (1988).
CROIZE, J., J. P. ROBERT, P. LE NOC: In vitro effect of various antibiotics: beta lactams, aminoglycosides and fluoroquinolones alone and in combination against P. aeruginosa isolated from patients with mucoviscidosis. Pathol. Biol. Paris 37: 573–577 (1989).
DOWLING, J. N., D. A. MCDEVITT, A. W. PASCULLE: Isolation and preliminary characterization of erythromycin-resistant variants of Legionella micdadei and Legionella pneumophila. Antimicrob. Ag. Chemother. 27: 272 (1985).
FALLON, R. J., W. M. BROWN: In-vitro sensitivity of legionellas, meningococci and mycoplasmas to ciprofloxacin and enoxacin. J. Antimicrob. Chemother. 15: 787 (1985).
GOLD, R. et al.: Controlled trial of ceftazidime vs. ticarcillin and tobramycin in the treatment of acute respiratory exacerbations in patients with cystic fibrosis. Pediatr. Infect. Dis. 4: 172 (1985).
GREENWOOD, D., A. LAVERICK: Activities of newer quinolones against Legionella group organisms. Lancet 2: 279 (1983).
GRENIER, B.: Use of the new quinolones in cystic fibrosis. Rev. Infect. Dis. 11 (Suppl. 5): S1245 (1989).
KAPLAN, E. L.: Benzathine penicillin G for treatment of group A streptococcal pharyngitis: a reappraisal in 1985. Ped. Infect. Dis. 4: 592 (1985).
KRILOV, L. R., J. L. BLUMER, R. C. STERN et al.: Imipenem/cilastatin in acute pulmonary exacerbations of cystic fibrosis. Rev. Infect. Dis. 7: 482 (1985).
KROBER, M. S., J. W. BASS, G. N. MICHELS: Streptococcal pharyngitis. Placebo-controlled double-blind evaluation of clinical response to penicillin therapy. J.A.M.A. 253: 1271 (1985).

Kurz, R. W. et al.: Failure of treatment of Legionella pneumonia with ciprofloxacin (letter). J. Antimicrob. Chemother. *22:* 389, 1988.
Levison, M. E., C. T. Mansura, B. Lorber et al.: Clindamycin compared with penicillin for the treatment of anaerobic lung abscess. Annals Int. Med. *98:* 466 (1983).
Lode, H., E. Wiley, P. Olschewski: Prospective randomized clinical trials of new quinolones versus beta-lactam antibiotics in lower respiratory tract infections. Scand. J. Infect. Dis. Suppl. *68:* 50–55 (1990).
Mandel, J. H.: Pharyngeal infections. Causes, findings, and management. Postgrad. Med. *77:* 187 (1985).
Meyer, R. D.: Legionella infections: a review of five years of research. Rev. Infect. Dis. *5:* 258 (1985).
Pennington, J. E.: Respiratory Infections: Diagnosis and Management. Raven Press, New York 1989.
Randolph, M. F. et al.: Effect of antibiotic therapy on the clinical course of streptococcal pharyngitis. J. Pediatr. *106:* 870 (1985).
Rolfe, M.: A study of Legionnaire's disease in Zambia. Ann. Trop. Med. Parasitol. *80:* 425–428 (1986).
Rudin, J. E., T. L. Evans, E. J. Wing: Failure of erythromycin in treatment of Legionella micdadei pneumonia. Amer. J. Med. *76:* 318 (1984).
Sande, M. A., L. D. Hudson, R. K. Root: Respiratory Infections. Churchill Livingstone, London 1986.
Scully, B. E., C. N. Ores, A. S. Prince, H. C. Neu: Treatment of lower respiratory tract infections due to Pseudomonas aeruginosa in patients with cystic fibrosis. Rev. Infect. Dis. *7 (Suppl. 4):* 669 (1985).
Siegel, S. E., L. J. Wolff, R. L. Baehner, D. Hammond: Treatment of Pneumocystis carinii pneumonitis. A comparative trial of sulfamethoxazole-trimethoprim vs pentamidine in pediatric patients with cancer: report from the Children's Cancer Study Group. Am. J. Dis. Child. *138:* 1051–1054 (1984).
Sienko, D. G. et al.: Q fever. A call to heighten our index of suspicion. Arch. Intern. Med. *148:* 609 (1988).
Singh, M., A. Saidali, A. Bakhtiar, L. S. Arya: Diphtheria in Afghanistan – a review of 155 cases. J. Trop. Med. Hyg. *88:* 373–376 (1985).
Unertl, K. E., F. P. Lenhart, H. Forst et al.: Ciprofloxacin in the treatment of legionellosis in critically ill patients including those cases unresponsive to erythromycin. Am. J. Med. *87:* 128S–131S (1989).

7. Infections of the Gastrointestinal Tract

a) Gastritis and Peptic Ulcer

Helicobacter pylori (formerly Campylobacter pyloridis, then Campylobacter pylori) is clearly involved in the pathogenesis of antral gastritis and duodenal ulceration. The ability of this organism to form a cytotoxin and to secrete a protease whose substrate includes the protective mucin layer plays a role in this. The organism can be demonstrated in the floor of the ulcer and in the mucous membrane in a large percentage of cases. When Helicobacter pylori is demonstrated histologically and by culture in a biopsy of the antral mucosa, a histologically confirmed antral gastritis is almost always present, whereas Helicobacter pylori seldom occurs in individuals without gastritis. When gastritis was induced experimentally in volunteers, H. pylori could only be cultured from gastric juice in 20% of those in whom it was culturable from a biopsy. The direct demonstration of urease activity in biopsy material can also be used in the diagnosis.

Helicobacter pylori is generally susceptible to erythromycin, tetracyclines, clindamycin, quinolones, metronidazole and tinidazole, but is resistant to trimethoprim and vancomycin. The optimal treatment (drug, dose, duration of therapy) of infection with Helicobacter pylori is still unclear. Relapse is frequent. The long-recognised beneficial effects of bismuth-containing antacids seems to be based on their inhibitory action on Helicobacter pylori. The best results at present are achieved with a combination of a bismuth preparation, metronidazole + amoxycillin. Duration of treatment: at least 4 weeks. Erythromycin is usually ineffective.

References

Axon, A. T.: Campylobacter pylori-therapy review. Scand. J. Gastroenterol. Suppl. *160:* 35–38 (1989).

Bonamico, M., A. Medici, C. Chiesa et al.: Treatment of Campylobacter gastritis in young children. J. Pediatr. *115:* 833–834 (1989).

Forsmark, C. E., C. M. Wilcox, J. P. Collo: Ciprofloxacin in the treatment of Helicobacter pylori in patients with gastritis and peptic ulcer. J. Infect. Dis. *162:* 998–999 (1990).

Glupczynski, Y., M. Labbe, A. Berette, M. Delmee, V. Aresani, C. Bruck: Treatment failure of ofloxacin in Campylobacter pylori infection. Lancet *I:* 1096 (1987).

Goodwin, C. S., J. A. Armstrong, B. J. Marshall: Campylobacter pyloridis, gastritis, and peptic ulceration. J. Clin. Pathol. *39:* 353 (1986).

Hirschl, A. M., E. Hentschel, K. Schutze et al.: The efficacy of antimicrobial treatment in Campylobacter pylori-associated gastritis and duodenal ulcer. Scand. J. Gastroenterol. Suppl. *142:* 76 (1988).

Lambert, T., F. Mégraud, G. Gerbaud, P. Courvalin: Susceptibility of Campylobacter pyloridis to 20 antimicrobial agents. Antimicrob. Agents Chemother. *30:* 510 (1986).

McNulty, C. A.: Bismuth subsalicylate in the treatment of gastritis due to Campylobcter pylori. Rev. Infect. Dis. *12* Suppl. 1: 94–98 (1990).

McNulty, C. A. M., J. Dent, R. Wise: Susceptibility of clinical isolates of Campylobacter pyloridis to 11 antimicrobial agents. Antimicrob. Ag. Chemother. *28:* 837 (1985).

McNulty, C. A. M., J. C. Gearty, B. Crump, M. Davis, I. A. Donovan, V. Melikian, D. M. Lister, R. Wise: Campylobacter pyloridis and associated gastritis; investigator-blind, placebo-controlled trial of bismuth salicylate and erythromycin ethylsuccinate. Br. Med. J. *293:* 645 (1986).

Oderda, G., D. Vaira, J. Holton, C. Ainley, F. Altare, N. Ansaldi: Amoxycillin plus tinidazole for Campylobacter pylori gastritis in children: assessment by serum IgG antibody, pepsinogen I, and gastrin levels. Lancet *I:* 690 (1989).

b) Enteritis

General introduction: A person falls ill with bacterial enteritis (gastro-enteritis, enteric infection) as a result of the interplay between a number of factors which include the infecting bacterial dose, the virulence of the causative pathogen and the general resistance to infection of that patient as host to the disease. Enteric pathogens which are sufficiently virulent to cause diarrhoeal disease after a very small infecting dose include shigellae, amoebae and giardia; these organisms can spread by several routes including person-to-person contact, direct faecal-oral transmission, and by ingestion of faecally-contaminated water or food (e.g. salads, raw vegetables).

Bacterial food-poisoning, on the other hand, implies multiplication of the organisms in the food before ingestion. Thus bacteria of lesser virulence can cause food poisoning because very large numbers of organisms (many millions per gram of food) or their pre-formed toxin are ingested. Bacteria which cause food poisoning multiply in a contaminated food vehicle, such as meat, sauce, eggs, mayonnaise, or in a prepared dish which incorporates such contaminated ingredients, before it is consumed. Such a situation may arise as a consequence of poor food hygiene or incorrect catering practice (e.g. cross-contamination, unsatisfactory time/temperature control during cooking, or cross-contamination or incorrect handling after cooking and before consumption).

An intermediate category, *food-borne infection,* is sometimes used to describe diarrhoeal disease which is transmitted principally by the ingestion of contaminated food or water but where significant multiplication in the vehicle has not occurred. The causative bacteria (e.g. campylobacter) may be recoverable only with difficulty from the food vehicle (e.g. unpasteurised milk). The distinction between food poisoning and food-borne infection is somewhat artificial and has given rise in countries such as Britain to confusion over whether there is a legal requirement to notify as food poisoning to the public health authorities food-borne diarrhoeal disease such as campylobacter enteritis. Some food-borne infections (e.g. listeriosis, hepatitis A) do not cause enteric infection, but give rise to other systemic illness (septicaemia and meningitis, hepatitis).

Other factors such as age (rotavirus infection), malnutrition (cholera), a surgical procedure (partial gastrectomy, blind loop etc.), lack of gastric acidity, ingestion of antacids and severe generalised disease can increase a person's susceptibility to diarrhoeal disease. Certain causes of gastroenteritis are commoner in immunosuppressed patients (see Table 43).

Pathogenesis: Two main forms of gastroenteritis may be distinguished according to the way in which they affect the intestinal tract (see Table 44). In the first, *entero-invasive disease* **(dysentery type),** the organisms invade the intestinal wall and cause severe inflammation and often ulceration, resulting in blood and mucus

Table 43. Principal causes of gastroenteritis and their associations.

Food poisoning	Immunosuppression	Travel	Play groups
Staphylococcus aureus	Salmonellae	Escherichia coli (enterotoxigenic)	Rotavirus
Clostridium perfringens	Cytomegalovirus	Salmonellae	Shigellae
Salmonellae	Clostridium difficile	Yersinia	Giardia lamblia
Campylobacter jejuni	Mycobacterium avium-intracellulare	Campylobacter	Cryptosporidium
Yersinia enterocolitica	Cryptosporidium	Giardia lamblia	
Clostridium botulinum	Isospora belli	Vibrio cholerae	
Bacillus cereus	Strongyloides		
Vibrio parahaemolyticus			
Aeromonas			
Plesiomonas			

Table 44. Enteric infection.

	Invasive	Non-invasive
Pathogenesis	Mucosal invasion	Enterotoxin Reduced absorption
Localisation	Colon (exclusively, or with small-intestinal involvement)	Predominantly small intestine
Diarrhoea	Often bloody and accompanied by tenesmus	Generally watery
Causative organisms	Salmonellae Shigellae Campylobacter jejuni Yersinia enterocolitica Escherichia coli 0157 (and other invasive types) Clostridium difficile Vibrio parahaemolyticus Entamoeba histolytica	Vibrio cholerae Salmonellae Escherichia coli (enterotoxigenic) Clostridium perfringens Clostridium difficile Bacillus cereus Staphylococcus aureus

in the stool and a prolonged fever. When, as frequently occurs, the infection is localised in the colon (but not when it is restricted to the small intestine), numerous granulocytes can be seen in a faecal smear stained with methylene blue.

The second form is *non-invasive, enterotoxic disease* (**cholera type**)**,** in which bacterial enterotoxin interferes with secretion and absorption in the small intestine, resulting in the loss of large quantities of fluid and electrolytes. The diarrhoea is watery and few granulocytes if any are passed in the stool. Fever is usually absent. As shown in Table 44, there are pathogens which cause a predominantly invasive infection and those which tend to be non-invasive. The same bacterial species (e. g. salmonella and Clostridium difficile) may contain strains which are more invasive and others which have a greater tendency to form enterotoxin. A few pathogenic species (e. g. salmonella, shigella, yersinia and campylobacter) possess both an antigen that causes invasive enteritis and an enterotoxin which causes watery diarrhoea. Which symptoms predominate then depends on the mode of transmission; faeco-oral infection gives rise to signs of invasive disease, whereas spread by means of a heavily contaminated item of food results in watery diarrhoea. As well as invasiveness and the ability to produce enterotoxin, there are other ways in which enteritis is produced.

The **adherence factor,** i. e. the ability of the causative organism to become attached to the cells of the mucous membrane of the intestinal wall and to colonise them, gives rise in the small intestine to a loss of absorptive villous surface. The resultant malabsorption leads to the chronic diarrhoea characteristic of Giardia lamblia and Cryptosporidium enteritis as well as of infection with enteropathogenic strains of Escherichia coli, which cause disease mainly through their adherence properties.

In addition to enterotoxin, some bacterial species such as Clostridium difficile are able to produce a **cytotoxin** which can give rise to extensive necrosis of the colonic mucosa. Some species of Escherichia coli produce a toxin which is cytotoxic *in vitro* to cultures of Vero cells and can give rise to severe ulceration *in vivo*. Such Vero cytotoxin-producing E. coli (VTEC), of which the commonest serotype is E. coli 0157, can cause haemolytic uraemic syndrome as well as haemorrhagic colitis and milder diarrhoeal illness (both bloody and non-bloody). The shigella group includes both Shigella dysenteriae type 1, which causes the life-threatening condition of dysentery with bloody diarrhoea, and other types of shigella which produce abundant enterotoxin but no cytotoxin and give rise to diarrhoeal disease with watery diarrhoea.

In bacterial food poisoning, the **incubation period** often gives a clue to the cause. The period between infection and the development of symptoms of nausea, vomiting and diarrhoea is generally 1–6 h for enterotoxin-forming staphylococci, 6–24 h for Clostridium perfringens and 6–48 h for salmonella enteritis. If a food has been contaminated with yersinia, campylobacter, shigellae or Vibrio parahaemolyticus, the interval is usually longer (17–72 h). Rota- and adenoviruses are usually spread by contact and have an incubation period of a few days. The diarrhoea of antibiotic-associated enterocolitis can begin during antibiotic therapy or at any time up to 6 weeks after its cessation.

Epidemiology: The time and place of the occurrence of the diarrhoea and the group of people affected will often suggest the cause (see Table 43). Thus the expected range of organisms in suspected food poisoning would be different from that expected in an outbreak of gastro-enteritis in a play group or in traveller's diarrhoea. In immunosuppressed patients, particularly those with AIDS, organisms should be sought which are of low virulence but can cause protracted diarrhoea (e.g. cryptosporidia).

Aetiological diagnosis: For mild and transient disease, investigation may not be necessary. Patients with fever, prolonged (one week or more) or bloody diarrhoea, or immunosuppression should always be investigated microbiologically, as should all hospital in-patients and food handlers.

The **macroscopic appearance** of the stool (presence of blood, water content etc.) and the presence or absence of *fever* give pointers to whether the enteritis is invasive or non-invasive, and hence to the range of expected causes. The presence of faecal granulocytes (for which a fresh specimen must be examined) is suggestive of a causative organism capable of invasion or cytotoxin formation.

The **microscopic investigation** of the stool (see Table 45) is also important in intestinal infections with protozoa and parasites (particularly in protracted diarrhoea). A wet mount of a liquid stool should be examined within 1 h of collection for living trophozoites of protozoa and for larvae of Strongyloides. Cysts and ova may be demonstrated in formed stools, if necessary after concentrating the sample by the merthiolate-iodine-formalin technique. The faecal specimen can be preserved with polyvinyl alcohol or 10% formalin for sending to another laboratory. Faecal smears can be examined microscopically after staining with trichrome or with iron-haemotoxylin. A duodenal mucosal biopsy (a spot preparation for giardia and a tissue snip for strongyloides and cryptosporidia) is preferable to faeces in the investigation of suspected protozoal or parasitic infection. A modified Ziehl-Neelsen (acid-fast) stain is necessary to demonstrate cryptosporidia, Isospora belli and Mycobacterium avium-intracellulare, and the identity of cryptosporidium-like bodies should be confirmed by specific immunofluorescence.

The stool should always be **cultured** for salmonellae, shigellae, campylobacter and yersinia. Additional investigations should be performed for E. coli 0157 when the diarrhoea contains blood, for vibrios when cholera is suspected, and for Clostridium difficile (by both culture and toxin detection) when an association with antibiotics is suspected. The possibility of infection with Mycobacterium avium-intracellulare (see p. 543) should be considered when investigating faeces from patients with AIDS. Rota- and adenoviruses can be demonstrated simply by a rapid commercial latex test. A blood culture should always be taken before starting treatment in patients with fever, since this may yield salmonellae, yersinia or campylobacter (bacteraemic form).

The demonstration of **serum antibodies** is of practical value only in cases of prolonged diarrhoea (e.g. in yersinia and amoebic infections). Serial antibody

Table 45. Diagnosis of enteritis.

Investigation	Causative organism	
Microscopy (stool, duodenal aspirate)	Giardia lamblia, Entamoeba histolytica, Strongyloides stercoralis	Wet preparation, stained smear
	Cryptosporidium, Isospora belli, Mycobacterium avium-intracellulare	Modified Ziehl-Neelsen (acid-fast) stain
Culture (stool)	Bacterial causes (which should be named on the request form when particularly suspected, e.g. E. coli 0157).	
Antigen detection in faeces (latex test or enzyme immunoassay)	Rotaviruses, adenoviruses, Clostridium difficile toxin, Giardia lamblia	
Sigmoidoscopy	Clostridium difficile (pseudomembranous enterocolitis), Entamoeba histolytica, cytomegalovirus (cytology)	
Demonstration of serum antibody	Limited use at present (in bacterial infections and amoebiasis)	
Examination of food residues when food poisoning suspected	Staphylococci, clostridia, aeromonas, Vibrio parahaemolyticus, Bacillus cereus	

determinations are necessary in such cases in order to establish whether the titres show current or recent infection.

Sigmoidoscopy and histological examination of a biopsy can be used to distinguish pseudomembranous enterocolitis (due to Clostridium difficile) from amoebic dysentery and colonic cytomegalovirus infection (in AIDS patients). In cases of chronic diarrhoea this can also help differentiate between ulcerative colitis and Crohn's disease, intestinal tuberculosis or Mycobacterium avium-intracellulare infection and amoebic dysentery.

In **food poisoning** (salmonella, Clostridium botulinum, Bacillus cereus, staphylococci etc.) the causative organism or its toxin may be detected in food residues or in vomit. Since these are often no longer available when symptoms develop, however, public health investigators now rely increasingly on sensitive epidemiological techniques which use questionnaires and case-control study, particularly in large outbreaks and where complex and variable menus at large catering functions are involved.

In the **differential diagnosis** of diarrhoea of unclear aetiology, many other conditions must be considered such as ulcerative colitis, Crohn's disease, food allergy, irritable colon, malabsorption, pancreatic insufficiency, lactose intolerance, fructose intolerance, Addison's disease, hyperthyroidism, phaeochromocytoma, laxative abuse and poisoning or intoxication.

Principles of treatment: Most enteric infections are self-limiting and heal spontaneously. Chemotherapy is not necessary in mild, non-invasive infections. Severe cases of enteric infection with fever, blood-stained or purulent diarrhoea (dysentery type) and enteric infections complicating primary diseases such as leukaemia, hepatic cirrhosis and occurring during immunosuppressive treatment should be treated with systemic antibiotics. Antibiotic treatment in such cases can shorten the period of symptoms and prevent or cure complications. It can also reduce the infectivity of shigellas and cholera. Co-trimoxazole and ampicillin are the drugs of choice for the blind therapy of bacterial enteritis. Tetracyclines are useful in cases of suspected yersinia infection and cholera. New quinolones (norfloxacin, ofloxacin, ciprofloxacin etc.) are active against all bacterial causes of enteritis except for Clostridium difficile and other species of clostridia. Non-absorbed antibiotics such as neomycin, polymyxin and poorly absorbable sulphonamides are often inactive or only weakly active, and so are best avoided. Parenteral antibiotics should only be given to patients with enteric infections in exceptional circumstances, such as vomiting or extra-intestinal complications. Fluid and electrolyte replacement can be more important in severe enteric infections than chemotherapy.

Shigella dysentery: Acute febrile diarrhoea (bacillary dysentery) with tenesmus and mucous, often blood-stained, stools. In addition to the invasive (dysenteric) form of the infection, there is a diarrhoeal form with watery stools which is caused by Shigella dysenteriae type I. The resistance of shigellae to sulphonamides, ampicillin, co-trimoxazole and tetracyclines is increasing, especially among strains of Shigella sonnei, so that treatment must be chosen on the basis of tested sensitivities, especially during an epidemic. Because of the high infectivity and destructive colitis, all patients should be treated for at least 5 days with oral antibiotics according to results of sensitivity testing. Co-trimoxazole (2 tablets twice daily for adults, 10–15 mg/kg twice a day for children), ampicillin (2 g daily for adults, 50 mg/kg for children) or tetracycline (1 g daily for adults, 50 mg/kg for children) are the antibiotics of choice. Ofloxacin (0.4 g twice daily) and ciprofloxacin (0.5 g twice daily) are effective, but are only licensed for use in adults. Poorly absorbed sulphonamides and local antibiotics that do not achieve tissue concentrations are unsuitable. Amoxycillin is also unreliable in bacillary dysentery.

Salmonella enteritis is an acute, sometimes febrile gastro-enteritis of variable intensity which usually occurs 8–24 hours after a meal contaminated with salmonellae. It often occurs in outbreaks. Typhoid and paratyphoid fevers, which are septicaemic illnesses, should not be confused with salmonella enteritis as they are treated quite differently (see p. 504). Depending on the properties of the causative strain, salmonella enteritis can lead to mucosal invasion with inflammation, to watery diarrhoea (through enterotoxin formation) and/or to ulceration and pseudomembranous enterocolitis (through cytotoxin formation) with a risk of metastatic foci of infection.

Mild, transient infections resolve spontaneously and are self-limiting, so antibiotics are unnecessary. More severe infections with fever and bloody diarrhoea with positive blood cultures or in the first year of life should be treated with systemic antibiotics because of the risk of metastatic infection of other organs (e.g. osteomyelitis, septic arthritis). Antibiotics should also be used in immunosuppressed patients and in the elderly (over 65 years of age). Until recently these have been ampicillin (3–5 g a day for adults, 100–150 mg/kg for children) or co-trimoxazole (960 mg twice a day). The new quinolones (ofloxacin, ciprofloxacin) are always effective. Despite its good clinical effect, chloramphenicol should not be used for the treatment of mild salmonella enteritis because of its haemotoxicity and because of the increasing resistance of salmonellae to chloramphenicol. Antibiotics used in the past have often not prevented the persistence of intestinal carriage. The new quinolones, however, can be used to treat chronic salmonella carriage.

Salmonella gastroenteritis in patients with severe underlying diseases (leukaemia, AIDS, organ transplantation, cirrhosis etc.) carries a considerable risk of septicaemia and metastatic infection. Treatment with ofloxacin, ciprofloxacin, mezlocillin or cefotaxime is then always indicated.

Yersiniosis: Intestinal infection with Yersinia pseudotuberculosis and Yersinia enterocolitica usually present as enteritis, sepsis or even suspected appendicitis, on account of the associated swelling of the mesenteric lymph nodes. The enteritis is usually acute, sometimes protracted, and may be localised in the ileum or the colon. Ulcers, which can bleed, often arise. Severe right lower abdominal pain is characteristic. Older children often also develop acute polyarthritis or erythema nodosum. The causative organisms can be recovered from mesenteric lymph nodes excised at appendectomy or from faeces. The diagnosis can also be made serologically by demonstration of a rising titre of specific antibodies. The disease generally follows a benign course with a tendency to spontaneous healing. Tetracyclines and co-trimoxazole are effective, as are the new quinolones (e.g. norfloxacin, ofloxacin or ciprofloxacin). β-Lactam antibiotics are unsuitable because most strains of yersinia produce β-lactamases.

Campylobacter enteritis: Painful, bloody diarrhoea with fever and sometimes vomiting. The causative organism (Campylobacter jejuni) is widely distributed in animals and man. Foods (meat products, particularly poultry, and milk) are common vehicles of infection. Epidemic outbreaks have been reported, particularly after failures of pasteurisation in dairies. Culture of campylobacters requires selective media and anaerobic incubation with CO_2 enrichment for several days. Characteristic curved ("seagull-like") bacilli are seen in a gram-stained smear, and motile, curved bacilli can be demonstrated in the stool by phase-contrast microscopy. Tetracyclines and erythromycin are effective, as are the new quinolones (ofloxacin or ciprofloxacin).

Cholera and cholera-like illnesses present as acute enteritis with persistent watery stools, fluid and electrolyte loss due to toxin, hypovolaemic shock, metabolic acidosis, muscle cramps, and aphonia. Severe cases show a characteristic clinical picture. The causative bacteria can be demonstrated by microscopy and culture. Cholera is not encountered in Northern, Central or Western Europe, but can still be acquired in the Mediterranean area and by travellers to the tropics. A cholera-like illness is sometimes found in other forms of gastroenteritis due, for example, to salmonella, cryptosporidia and enterotoxigenic strains of Escherichia coli.

Treatment is primarily by fluid and electrolyte replacement with infusions containing glucose, and correction of the metabolic acidosis. If the infusion is continued (maintenance therapy), the fluid loss must be carefully monitored by clinical and laboratory tests to prevent relapse into shock. If parenteral fluids are not available or cannot be given, oral replacement is recommended (20 g glucose, 4 g NaCl, 4 g $NaHCO_3$, 1 g KCl in 1 litre of water). In countries where cholera is endemic, sachets of the WHO Oral Rehydration Formula are widely available from retail pharmacists (or their equivalent). Opiates and inhibitors of peristalsis are contra-indicated, for they may be conducive to shock.

Antibiotic treatment with tetracycline (1 g daily by mouth for adults and older children) or co-trimoxazole for at least 5 days is effective in rapidly eliminating Vibrio cholerae. Co-trimoxazole is particularly useful when tetracycline-resistant cholera vibrios are found during an epidemic. *Prophylaxis:* Vaccination is not fully effective and careful hygiene in endemic areas is very important.

Escherichia coli gastro-enteritis: Escherichia coli can cause different forms of enteritis.

Enterotoxigenic strains cause severe intestinal infection in infants which is not accompanied by fever. Leukocytes cannot be demonstrated microscopically in the stool. Enterotoxin can be detected by colony hybridisation or PCR-based methods. The second form is caused by *entero-invasive* strains of Escherichia coli which can lead to a dysentery-like clinical picture, especially in older children and adults.

Bleeding gastric ulcers without fever have recently been reported with increasing frequency in intestinal infections with *Vero-cytotoxin-producing strains* of E. coli (VTEC), of which the commonest serotype, O157, can give rise to the complication of the haemolytic-uraemic syndrome. VTEC can be detected by a latex test performed on suspicions colonies from a selective medium. Hospital infections with *enteropathogenic E. coli* of serogroups such as 055 and 0111 used to be common in the past, but now occur so infrequently that routine investigation for these strains is no longer worthwhile.

Treatment: Severe infections with enterotoxigenic E. coli and dysentery-like E. coli infections may be treated with co-trimoxazole or ampicillin and in adults also with norfloxacin, ofloxacin or ciprofloxacin (see Table 46). Antimicrobial therapy is always advisable when E. coli 0157 is isolated.

Travellers' diarrhoea: Travellers to Southern Europe and other warm climates often suffer acute, usually afebrile diarrhoea. There is no clear single cause. Enterotoxigenic strains of Escherichia coli, to which the indigenous populations are mostly immune, are apparently the cause in many cases, although other agents such as salmonellae, shigellae, yersinias, campylobacter, entero-invasive Escherichia coli, aeromonas, Vibrio parahaemolyticus, Giardia lamblia and viruses can also be involved.

Treatment: In mild cases where fever and systemic symptoms are absent, the condition resolves rapidly and spontaneously. Severe cases should be treated with co-trimoxazole, 1.92 g a day orally, ampicillin, 2 g a day orally or tetracycline, 1 g a day orally (Table 46). Norfloxacin is active against all the currently recognised bacterial causes of this condition and may be given as a single dose of 0.4 g, but this antibacterial should only be used in adults. Other causes (amoebae, rotaviruses) should be sought in cases which fail to respond to norfloxacin; metronidazole may then be effective. Treatment and prophylaxis with quinoline derivatives (e. g. clioquinol) should be avoided because of neurotoxicity. Proprietary antidiarrhoeal drugs are usually ineffective and can have dangerous side-effects; of these drugs, only bismuth carbonate, which increases the consistency of the stool, is worth considering.

Oral rehydration (see Table 47) is important. Balanced sugar and electrolyte solutions as used in cholera are important here. Loperamide (Imodium), which inhibits peristalsis, can be taken if necessary by older children and adults for 1–2 days in cases of severe illness with watery diarrhoea caused by enterotoxigenic organisms. Loperamide is contra-indicated in younger children because of the danger of toxic megacolon through ileus. The dose for adults is 4 mg initially (capsules or drops) followed by 2 mg after every unformed stool up to a maximum of 8 mg a day; children from 8 years of age should be given an initial dose of 2 mg, then as for adults.

Prophylaxis through prolonged taking of a poorly absorbed sulphonamide, of neomycin, colistin, polymyxin B or paromomycin is ineffective. For shorter stays of 1–2 weeks, chemoprophylaxis with co-trimoxazole (0.96 g a day) or doxycycline (0.1 g a day) may be successful. There are, however, substantial arguments against

Table 46. Specific treatment of enteritis.

Cause	Recommended treatment	Alternatives	
Salmonella (not S. typhi)	Co-trimoxazole (0.96 g twice a day for 14 days)	Ciprofloxacin (0.5 g twice a day) Ampicillin (1 g 4 times a day)	for 14 days
Yersinia	Co-trimoxazole (0.96 g twice a day for 7 days)	Ciprofloxacin (0.5 g twice a day) Tetracycline (0.25 g 4 times a day)	for 7 days
Campylobacter jejuni	Erythromycin (0.25 g 4 times a day for 7 days)	Ciprofloxacin (0.5 g twice a day) Tetracycline (0.25 g 4 times a day)	for 7 days
Shigella	Co-trimoxazole (0.96 g twice a day for 5 days)	Ciprofloxacin (0.5 g twice a day) Ampicillin (0.5 g twice a day)	for 2–5 days for 5 days
Escherichia coli (invasive, enterotoxic, VTEC)	Co-trimoxazole (0.96 g twice a day for 5 days)	Norfloxacin (0.4 g twice a day) Ofloxacin (0.2 g twice a day) Ciprofloxacin (0.5 g twice a day) Ampicillin (0.5 g 4 times a day)	for 1–5 days for 5 days
Clostridium difficile	Vancomycin (0.125 g 4 times a day for 10 days)	Metronidazole (0.5 g 4 times a day)	for 10 days
Giardia lamblia	Metronidazole (0.25 g 3 times a day for 7 days)	Tinidazole (1 dose of 2 g)	for 1–2 days
Isospora belli	Co-trimoxazole (0.96 g 4 times a day for 10 days, then twice a day for 21 days)		
Entamoeba histolytica	Metronidazole (0.75 g 3 times a day for 5–10 days) plus diloxanide furoate (0.5 g for 10 days)	Chloroquine (0.6 g twice a day on the first day, then 0.3 g twice a day for 14 days)	

Table 47. Traveller's diarrhoea (severity, treatment).

Severity	Symptoms	Treatment
Mild	Up to 3 unformed stools a day	Fluids only by mouth (with glucose and salts)[1]
Moderate	4–5 unformed stools a day	Fluids only by mouth (with glucose and salts)[1] + bismuth subsalicylate[2]
Severe	>5 unformed stools a day, often accompanied by blood and fever	Fluids only by mouth (with glucose and salts)[1] or i. v. rehydration + co-trimoxazole[3] or (in adults) a single dose of norfloxacin 0.4 g

[1] WHO oral rehydration solution: 3.5 g NaCl, 2.5 g sodium bicarbonate, 1.5 g KCl are added to 1 litre of water and given in one cup of orange juice or with 2 bananas, + 20 g glucose. Sachets are widely available from pharmacies throughout the tropics (WHO Rehydration Formula).
[2] Give for no longer than one week, and not at the same time as drugs which reduce motility.
[3] 0.96 g by mouth every 12 h for 3–5 days.

this course (e. g. emergence of resistance, and photodermatosis, through doxycycline). Scrupulous food hygiene is more reliable and also protects against other infections (typhoid fever, cholera, amoebiasis, hepatitis A and poliomyelitis).

Tap water, ice cubes, dessert ices, salads, unpeeled fruit, raw vegetables, mayonnaise, cream desserts, unboiled milk, dairy products such as cheese, inadequately cooked meat, raw fish, shellfish, and cold buffets should all be avoided. Cooked foods are generally safe if still hot, as are fresh bread, boiled or chlorinated water, wine, beer, tea, coffee, and carbonated bottled drinks.

Necrotising enterocolitis is a life-threatening disease of the newborn with severe abdominal distention, sometimes with blood-stained stools and often accompanied by perforation of ulcers, peritonitis and ileus. The course is rapid and often fatal.

The cause is unknown, but ischaemia and damage to the intestinal mucosa by local toxin are assumed to facilitate the penetration of bacteria. The associated peritonitis is always a mixed infection.

Treatment in cases with peritonitis and septicaemia is with cefotaxime + piperacillin + clindamycin (i. v.) or cefotaxime + gentamicin + metronidazole. Intestinal perforation (free air in the abdomen) requires immediate operation. Other measures include fluid replacement, the treatment of shock and possibly mechanical ventilation, a nasogastric tube and peritoneal dialysis.

Viral gastroenteritis: Often occurs in younger children, usually as a mild intestinal illness due to rotaviruses, coronaviruses, enteroviruses (echo, coxsackie) and adenoviruses. Virus can be detected in the stool by the ELISA technique and by latex agglutination. There is no effective chemotherapy. Treatment is with diet and, if necessary, i. v. infusions or oral rehydration therapy.

Antibiotic-associated enterocolitis: Antibiotic treatment can interfere with the normal intestinal flora and can lead to an overgrowth of facultative pathogens in the gut. A connection with antibiotic therapy may be difficult to demonstrate. The risk of diarrhoea is particularly attributed to those antibiotics which are either poorly absorbed when given orally, or which are extensively excreted in the bile, and which have an effect on intestinal anaerobes. Milder forms of antibiotic-associated colitis arise as a result of the displacement of the normal intestinal flora and the multiplication of staphylococci, Bacteroides fragilis, Pseudomonas aeruginosa and other resistant bacteria. **Pseudomembranous enterocolitis,** which occurs as a result of the selection of Clostridium difficile and can be life-threatening, is particularly associated with treatment with clindamycin, ampicillins and tetracyclines. It is expressed by profuse diarrhoea, vomiting, collapse and circulatory failure (see p. 593). Other drugs that can cause pseudomembranous enterocolitis are other penicillins, cephalosporins, aztreonam, imipenem, co-trimoxazole, erythromycin, and cytotoxic agents.

Severe pseudomembranous enterocolitis may become chronic and can be fatal. The clinical picture is similar to that of ulcerative colitis and is due to the formation of cytotoxin and enterotoxin by Clostridium difficile. Watery diarrhoea without blood can occur, however. In both forms of this condition large numbers of leukocytes can be demonstrated microscopically in the faeces. Clostridium difficile can be grown profusely from faecal culture. The definitive test is the detection of toxin in either tissue culture or by a specific immunoassay. The diagnosis can also be confirmed by a careful colonoscopy.

Treatment must be started as soon as the condition is suspected. Severe cases of pseudomembranous enterocolitis with a sudden onset and systemic symptoms have a poor prognosis. The treatment of choice is oral vancomycin 0.125 g (5 mg/kg in children) every 4–6 h for 10 days. Oral metronidazole 0.25 g (7 mg/kg in children) 4 times a day or oral fusidic acid 0.5 g 3 times a day are also effective against Clostridium difficile. When oral administration is not possible, metronidazole by i.v. infusion is also effective. Relapse after treatment has stopped occurs in 10–20% of cases and usually responds to a further course of vancomycin or metronidazole. In severe forms of the disease with profuse diarrhoea and shock, intensive therapy with the replacement of water and electrolyte losses is important. The antibiotics responsible must be discontinued immediately.

Bacterial food poisoning: The most important bacterial causes are salmonellae (incubation period 8–24 h) and enterotoxin-producing staphylococci (incubation period 1–6 h). Other bacteria can also cause mild or severe diarrhoea when present in food in large amounts (e.g. Pseudomonas aeruginosa, Bacillus cereus, Aeromonas hydrophila, Plesiomonas shigelloides, Clostridium perfringens etc.). If Clostridium perfringens produces a cytotoxin in addition to enterotoxin, it can also cause pseudomembranous enterocolitis with blood-stained stools. The causative agents should always be sought first in the stool and may also be recoverable from food residues if they are still available. Staphylococci produce a heat-stable enterotoxin, and the absence of bacterial growth from a suspect item of cooked food does not exclude a staphylococcal aetiology.

In mild cases, *symptomatic treatment* is sufficient, e.g. with chalk or kaolin mixtures, active charcoal, electrolyte infusions or oral rehydration therapy, because the symptoms are often due purely to the toxins present in the food. Antibiotic treatment of salmonella food poisoning is sometimes necessary (see above).

Botulism: Diarrhoea and vomiting with symmetrical cranial nerve paralysis in a fully conscious patient. Risk of respiratory arrest. Toxin may be detected in the serum and in food remnants by animal inoculation. Intestinal botulism has occasionally been described in infants who develop the typical neurological features and disturbances of cardiac rhythm but no diarrhoea despite the presence of toxin-producing clostridia in the intestine. Wound botulism is very rare.

Treatment: Immediate administration of trivalent botulinum antitoxin (except in infantile intestinal botulism), corticosteroids, treatment of shock, intensive care, mechanical ventilation if necessary, and a cardiac pacemaker. Unabsorbed toxin is removed with magnesium sulphate, active charcoal tablets or an enema. Wound botulism should be treated with benzylpenicillin.

Enteritis caused by Vibrio parahaemolyticus: Halophilic vibrios have frequently caused food infections in Japan and the U.S.A., associated mainly with mussels, raw fish or contaminated meals. Vibrio parahaemolyticus has only occasionally been described in Europe. The disease follows a similar course to that of salmonella enteritis with diarrhoea (sometimes blood-stained), abdominal pain, nausea, vomiting, headache and moderate fever. Spontaneous resolution usually occurs within 2–5 days. Co-trimoxazole or tetracycline can be useful in severe cases.

Amoebic dysentery: An acute or chronic condition, although many patients are asymptomatic cyst passers, carrying the cysts in the lumen of the bowel only. The diagnosis is made by the microscopical demonstration of cysts and minuta forms of amoebae in the faeces, if necessary by sending a preserved stool to a reference laboratory (see p. 398). Intestinal mucosal involvement is confirmed by the presence of tissue (magna) forms which only occur in the fresh stool. The presence of an amoebic liver abscess can be confirmed by a CT scan or by ultrasound. Antibodies are detectable in the serum in tissue infections by latex agglutination, an indirect haemagglutination antibody test, by indirect immunofluorescence and by CFT.

In *treatment,* a distinction must be made between asymptomatic infestation of the lumen of the bowel and tissue infection. The severe consequences of unrecognised amoebic infection and the difficulty of making the diagnosis justify liberal treatment on reasonable suspicion of exposure (e.g. symptoms after travel to India). The drug of choice is metronidazole 0.75 g (10–15 mg/kg in children) by mouth 3 times a day for 3–5 days in mild infections and 10 days in severe infections. An alternative is tinidazole. The nitroimidazoles are effective in all forms of the disease, including liver abscess and, because of the risk of tissue invasion, should also be used to treat asymptomatic infections of the bowel lumen and cyst carriers.

Amoebic liver abscess, which is usually solitary, should additionally be managed by hospital admission, bed rest, restriction of solids or a liquid diet, and correction of fluid and electrolyte imbalance. The clinician should be alert for signs of rupture of the abscess into the pleura, pericardium or peritoneum. Chloroquine should be considered for cases in whom nitroimidazoles are not tolerated or fail. Large liver abscesses may need single or repeated closed needle aspiration under careful ultrasound or CT imaging. Other complications are secondary infection and hepatic vein thrombosis. Relapses can occur in the first 6 weeks after commencing treatment, and patients should be carefully watched during this period. Because of its rapid absorption, metronidazole is less effective than diloxanide in invasive infection from the intestinal lumen and, to avoid relapse, luminal cysts should be eradicated by a sequential course of diloxanide furoate 0.5 g three times a day by mouth for 10 days; in some European countries this drug is not licensed and so may have to be prescribed on a named-patient basis.

Giardiasis: Acute or chronic infestation with Giardia lamblia can be transmitted in drinking water, food, or direct contact (human or domestic animals). The infection is commoner in children, the immunosuppressed, and patients with hypogammaglobulinaemia, IgA deficiency, gastric ulcer, biliary disease and pancreatitis, and gives rise to acute or chronic (watery) diarrhoea, sometimes with malabsorption. The parasites can be detected microscopically more reliably in duodenal aspirate than in faeces because they are excreted intermittently. Direct antigen detection in the stool is now possible by means of a total genomic probe.

Treatment: Metronidazole, 0.75 g a day for adults (in three single oral doses), 0.25 g a day for children aged 4–8 years and 0.125 g a day for children under 4 years, all for 7 days. A single dose of tinidazole 2 g (adults) or 1 g (children aged 6–12 years) is a suitable alternative. Asymptomatic carriers should be treated at the same time.

Balantidial dysentery: Acute or protracted colitis with watery, mucous or blood-stained stools. A rare infection in which the large, motile trophozoites can easily be seen under the microscope. Pigs and other animals are the sources of infection.

Treatment: Oral metronidazole, 0.75–1.0 g for 5 days, or tetracycline, particularly oxytetracycline, 2 g per day by mouth.

Coccidial infections: Isospora belli and Cryptosporidium spp. are coccidial protozoa which can infect man at any age, as well as domestic and farm animals, and can cause severe, protracted illness in immunosuppressed patients, particularly those with AIDS. The diarrhoea can be cholera-like, sometimes with a low fever and abdominal colic. In the immunosuppressed the diarrhoea is often protracted with malabsorption syndrome (subtotal small intestinal villous atrophy), whereas in immunocompetent patients it is of shorter duration and self-limiting. The diarrhoea of Isospora belli infections is not usually so severe. The parasites can be demonstrated microscopically in a small intestinal biopsy (an alcohol-fixed spot preparation stained by the Giemsa method) or in the faeces by a modified acid-fast stain, if necessary after faecal concentration). The cryptosporidia adhere to the villous membrane of the small intestinal epithelium. Various developmental forms of this organism may be found in a small intestinal biopsy even when oocysts cannot be demonstrated in the faeces.

Treatment: In *cryptosporidium infections,* oral spiramycin (1 g 3 times a day for 2–4 weeks) sometimes leads to an improvement. Other agents are ineffective. Intravenous fluid therapy and parenteral nutrition are often necessary. The diarrhoea can sometimes be alleviated by prostaglandin inhibitors (indomethacin or naproxen).

In *Isospora* infections, oral co-trimoxazole (0.96 g 4 times a day for 10 days, then 0.96 g twice a day for 21 days) is usually effective. A longer period of suppressive therapy with 0.48 g of co-trimoxazole once a day by mouth is advisable in order to prevent relapse.

Whipworm infections: The large intestine is infested with Trichuris trichiura. A large worm load can give rise to mucous and sometimes blood-stained diarrhoea with colic and occasionally rectal prolapse. Commoner in tropical countries. The characteristic yellowish, lemon-shaped ova with bipolar button-like thickening may be demonstrated in the stool.

Treatment: Mebendazole (200 mg twice a day for 3 days) or thiabendazole (25 mg/kg twice a day for 3 days).

Strongyloides infections: This dwarf whipworm occurs in tropical and subtropical climates. Infection is brought about by the filariform larvae contained in the ground which penetrate the skin of the foot, pass through the circulation to the lungs and from there to the small intestine. The female worms, which are 2 mm long, attach themselves firmly to the mucosa, and about 4 weeks after infection is established start to lay eggs. Larvae capable of causing infection hatch while the eggs are still in the intestine, and pass out in the faeces. These larvae can also penetrate the intestinal well or the anal skin, thus leading to an increasing parasitic infestation.

In addition to skin and pulmonary symptoms, intestinal symptoms such as mucous diarrhoea, vomiting and abdominal pain can occur. Chronic strongyloides infection can lead to a malabsorption syndrome with protein loss through the intestine and loss of weight. In immunosuppressed patients with the so-called hyperinfection syndrome, the stool is usually bloody and the infection often disseminated, with larval invasion of most internal organs, and not uncommonly a fatal outcome. Eosinophilia may be absent in such cases.

Treatment: Thiabendazole is a relatively effective agent when given for 2 days (or two weeks in disseminated infection). A new alternative is ivermectin (proprietary name Mectizan, developed by MSD and now the drug of choice). Because of the danger of progressive autoinfection, treatment is also indicated in non-infected persons to avoid the possibility of a long course over many years.

Ulcerative colitis: Non-infectious, ulcerative inflammation of the large intestine of uncertain aetiology; bacterial infections play a secondary role. The antibacterial treatment does not therefore eliminate the cause.

The following drugs are recommended: sulphasalazine, 4–6 g initially, then 1.5–3 g/day as a maintenance dose for long-term treatment once improvement occurs. Its effect depends on the release and absorption of 5-aminosalicylic acid in the intestine, and not on antibacterial activity. Close monitoring is required because of frequent side effects (allergic rashes, fever). If sulphasalazine fails, treatment with metronidazole may be attempted.

Antibiotic combinations effective against anaerobes and enterobacteria are indicated in acute toxic colitis or severe exacerbation of a secondary bacterial infection (e. g. cefotaxime + metronidazole, or cefoxitin + azlocillin). The chances of success are not high, however. The disorder can also be treated with prednisone, sedatives, diet, blood transfusions (in emergencies), and psychotherapy. Surgical measures (colectomy) are required in 15–20%.

Crohn's disease: Non-infectious granulomatous inflammation of the distal small intestine and less often of the colon. Aetiology unknown. Bacterial infections may play a secondary role in the development of fistulae. As with ulcerative colitis, long-term treatment with sulphasalazine is recommended. Fever, fistula and local collection of pus often require additional antibiotic therapy. Metronidazole or combinations with activity against anaerobes and enterobacteria (e. g. gentamicin + clindamycin, cefoxitin + piperacillin, cefotaxime + metronidazole) can be used.

c) Appendicitis

Uncomplicated appendicitis should not be treated with antibiotics alone; prompt appendicectomy is the treatment of choice. Antibiotics should always be given in complicated cases (perforation, peritonitis, portal vein phlebitis, intra-abdominal abscess). Chemotherapy is also required if an operation cannot be performed immediately. This treatment (including metronidazole) is also necessary when appendicitis is suspected but an amoeboma cannot be excluded, as in patients who have stayed in the tropics. Severe systemic reactions such as a poor general condition and high fever are also indications for preoperative antibiotic treatment. The *chemotherapy of appendicitis* should cover the commonest agents found in mixed infections (Bacteroides fragilis, anaerobic streptococci and enterobacteria). Treat with combinations such as gentamicin + clindamycin or cefotaxime + metronidazole. Perioperative prophylaxis (as a single dose or a very short course) reduces the risk of secondary infection.

d) Peritonitis

Peritonitis may be primary or secondary. *Primary peritonitis*, to which patients with cirrhosis and ascites are predisposed, frequently arises haematogenously during the course of a systemic infection. Primary peritonitis can also occur in otherwise healthy people with a bacteraemia.

Secondary bacterial peritonitis is usually a perforation or penetration peritonitis and is frequently the consequence of a penetrating injury, a malignant tumour, appendicitis, diverticulitis, enteritis, cholecystitis or a duodenal ulcer. The result can be a circumscribed or diffuse peritonitis, an intra-abdominal abscess or a bacteraemia. A circumscribed or diffuse peritonitis can also arise in the presence of a pancreatic or splenic abscess. Pelvic peritonitis (see p. 447) and peritonitis in continuous ambulatory peritoneal dialysis (CAPD) are special forms of this condition.

Causative organisms: *Primary peritonitis* is usually an infection with a single organism, most commonly Escherichia coli (40–60%). Other causes are pneumococci (15%), enterococci (Enterococcus faecalis), group A streptococci (Streptococcus pyogenes), staphylococci, gonococci, other gram-negative bacilli, anaerobes and pseudomonas. A microscopic preparation of peritoneal exudate or pus usually shows a single bacterial type and more than 300 granulocytes per microlitre (µl). A culture for aerobic and anaerobic oranisms, including gonococci, should be set up in every case, as well as a blood culture.

Secondary peritonitis is always a mixed infection, usually of aerobic and anaerobic organisms from the gastro-intestinal tract. These will include Escherichia coli, other enterobacteria, enterococci, Bacteroides fragilis and other anaerobes.

Treatment: In *primary peritonitis* a laparotomy can often be avoided. When gram-negative bacilli are seen in a microscopic preparation, a good choice would be cefoxitin (8 g a day) + gentamicin (5 mg/kg/day). Metronidazole is indicated when anaerobes are cultured. In pseudomonas infection, azlocillin (or piperacillin) + tobramycin, or aztreonam or ciprofloxacin or imipenem are all effective. In pneumococcal and group A streptococcal peritonitis, benzylpenicillin i. v. (3–6 g daily) is sufficient. Gonococci are always susceptible to cefotaxime (6 g a day) and staphylococci to imipenem (although benzylpenicillin is preferable for specific treatment if the isolate is shown to be susceptible). Ampicillin or mezlocillin i. v. are the most effective agents against enterococci.

In *secondary peritonitis* an operation is almost invariably necessary to drain and remove the underlying cause. The peritoneal exudate should be sent for microbiological investigation, and antibiotic treatment should begin before the operation. Since infection complicating intestinal perforation is always mixed, an organism isolated in apparently pure culture should never be regarded as the sole cause; anaerobes readily die during transport to the laboratory. Antibiotic therapy should therefore cover the entire potential range of bacteria involved. Suitable combinations are cefotaxime + metronidazole, cefoxitin + piperacillin, ampicillin + gentamicin + metronidazole or imipenem + gentamicin. Alternatives are cefoxitin + amikacin or tobramycin + metronidazole. Treatment should be given for 14 days. The antibiotics should also reduce the chance of secondary septicaemia and abscess formation. Renal failure often accompanies peritonitis and must be taken into account when determining the antibiotic dosage.

Most antibiotics are well distributed in the inflamed peritoneum and achieve therapeutic concentrations there when given systemically. The intraperitoneal instillation of antibiotics is inadequate for treatment and can evoke a number of side-effects. Aminoglycosides and polymyxins can give rise to a dangerous neuromuscular blockade with respiratory arrest (antidote: prostigmine and calcium gluconate i. v.). The intraperitoneal use of tetracyclines can cause considerable peritoneal irritation. Chloramphenicol succinate, the injectable form, is inactive when instilled directly. Most antibiotics, and particularly the penicillins and cephalosporins, are absorbed so rapidly when given intraperitoneally that local treatment has no advantage. Peritoneal irrigation with povidone iodine is of questionable value on account of its low antibacterial activity and absorption of iodine and povidone.

Continuous ambulatory peritoneal dialysis (CAPD) is complicated not infrequently by peritonitis with or without bacteraemia. Infections of the catheter entry site ("tunnel infections") are commoner. The commonest bacterial causes are Staphylococcus epidermidis (40%), Staphylococcus aureus, enterococci and viridans streptococci; anaerobes and atypical mycobacteria are rare. Cultures are sterile in 30% of cases.

A single i. v. dose of vancomycin (1 g) and gentamicin (1.5 mg/kg) is the recommended treatment, followed by 25 mg of vancomycin and 4 mg of gentamicin into each litre of dialysate fluid for about 2 weeks. If bacteria can still be cultured after 7 days, the infected peritoneal catheter should be removed. In *candida infection,* amphotericin B (1–3 mg/l) should be added to the dialysate and oral flucytosine (30 mg/kg initially, then 15 mg/kg a day) given. The serum concentrations of flucytosine should be monitored and kept between 50 and 100 mg/l. A new alternative, less toxic antifungal therapy is fluconazole, which should be given in a reduced dose in renal failure of 200 mg initially, then 50 mg daily orally; an i.v. preparation is also available. When peritonitis becomes frequent and recurrent (> 3 episodes in 6 months), CAPD usually has to be discontinued.

e) Pancreatitis

Pancreatitis is usually due to autodigestion. Bacterial infection, which is usually mixed, plays a relatively minor role in the late stages of the disease. Ultrasound and CT imaging can demonstrate a pancreatic abscess or an infected pseudocyst. Treatment consists of the management of shock, analgesics, aspiration of the gastric contents, fasting, parenteral nutrition, atropine, calcium gluconate i.v. (in hypocalcaemia), and the treatment of any known cause, e.g. gallstones, by operation if necessary. If antibiotic treatment is required, mezlocillin i.v. (6–15 g a day for adults, 150 mg/kg for children in 3–4 divided doses) may be used. Cefotaxime, ceftriaxone, imipenem or piperacillin may also be considered.

f) Liver Abscess

Occurs as a complication of biliary sepsis after infected portal vein thrombosis and in amoebiasis.

Bacterial causes include Bacteroides species, anaerobic and microaerophilic streptococci, enterobacteria and staphylococci. In leukaemic patients multiple abscesses can be caused by candida or aspergillus. The diagnosis of liver abscess is difficult (liver tenderness on percussion, ultrasound or CT imaging, hepatic scintigraphy, and possibly the detection of amoebic antibodies in the serum and of amoebae in the stool). In multiple haematogenous abscesses the blood culture can be positive. Large abscesses may need aspiration under antibiotic cover. Trophozoites can be demonstrated microscopically in the aspirate from an amoebic abscess. An increased gallium uptake in the abscess wall, but reduced uptake in the centre is also typical of an amoebic abscess. 10% of amoebic abscesses are complicated by bacterial secondary infection.

The *treatment* must cover all the likely causes, including Entamoeba histolytica; antibiotic combinations are therefore necessary, such as mezlocillin + metronidazole, cefotaxime + metronidazole or ampicillin + gentamicin + metronidazole. A number of other combinations including another aminoglycoside, imipenem, flomoxef, piperacillin, aztreonam or tobramycin are also suitable.

Surgical intervention is required if the abscess ruptures, is very large, or is accompanied by cholangitis, diverticulitis or appendicitis. The treatment of amoebic abscess is described on p. 408.

g) Infections of the Biliary Tract

There is no clear correlation between particular agents and the clinical picture. Bile duct infections are nearly always secondary to a mechanical obstruction such as a stone, tumour, papillary stenosis etc. Primary bacterial cholangitis with no mechanical cause occurs only in Southeast Asia. Cholecystitis and empyema of the gall bladder are also nearly always due to obstruction.

The *causative organisms* include Escherichia coli, aerobic and anaerobic streptococci, Bacteroides species, and occasionally other enterobacteria, salmonellae, Clostridium perfringens etc., often in mixed infections. Culture of the causative agents is difficult, because not all patients have positive blood cultures. Culture of the duodenal contents is not helpful. Bile should always be sent for a cultural examination after operation or ERCP.

An *antibiotic* used for treating biliary infections should fulfil the following *criteria:*
1. Activity against organisms associated with biliary infection.
2. High blood and tissue levels.
3. Effective concentrations in the hepatic bile (not only as inactive metabolites).
4. Adequate biliary concentrations in cholestasis.
5. No antagonistic effect of bile on the activity of the antibiotic.

The antibiotic treatments of cholecystitis and cholangitis are broadly similar and also severe to prevent septic complications. Tetracyclines used to be the drugs of choice, and they are excreted in the bile in high concentrations. Their spectrum of activity includes most of the causes of bile duct infections. Treatment with tetracyclines has often been disappointing, however, and the high failure rate may be explained by an antagonism of the bile to the activity of the tetracyclines. Tetracyclines are not active at the normal slightly alkaline pH of the bile. The inactivation of tetracyclines in the bile is also reflected by the failure to eliminate bacteria. β-Lactam antibiotics, on the other hand, rapidly clear the bile of bacteria. Mezlocillin and cephalosporins which achieve satisfactory biliary concentrations (e. g. cefotaxime, ceftriaxone) are generally suitable for the treatment of biliary infections. β-Lactam antibiotics such as ampicillin, cefazolin, cefazedone, and cefoxitin are not concentrated in the bile and should only be used when there is no cholestasis. Aminoglycosides can also be used in combination therapy; the concentrations in bile are lower than in blood, but aminoglycosides are more active in the bile than in the serum.

In severe biliary infections, use a combination of a β-lactam antibiotic with an aminoglycoside. The importance of adequate biliary concentrations in the treatment of biliary infections should not be overestimated, for tissue concentrations also play an important role. Recommended treatment for uncomplicated biliary infections: cefotaxime, ceftriaxone or cefoperazone (4–6 g a day), imipenem (2 g a day) or mezlocillin (6–15 g a day), alone or with gentamicin (160–240 mg a day). If there is no cholestasis, amoxycillin (6–15 g a day), cefazolin (4–6 g a day), cefazedone (4–6 g a day) or cefoxitin (6 g a day) may also be used.

Mild biliary infections may be treated orally with amoxycillin (3 g a day) or ciprofloxacin (1 g a day) by mouth.

Further treatment: The most important measure for the effective treatment of cholangitis is the removal of the obstruction by operation or papillotomy. Without these measures, the biliary infection will recur.

When there is an *empyema of the gall bladder,* cholecystectomy under antibiotic cover is necessary either as an acute operation or at an interval after the acute infection has been brought under control by antibiotics. *Perforation* of the gall bladder with peritonitis is also an indication for immediate operation under antibiotic cover. The temporary improvement brought about by chemotherapy does not remove the necessity for a subsequent definitive operation. Antibiotic treatment of biliary infections is generally of limited value.

Because bacterial infections (fever, septicaemia, cholangitis, pancreatitis) often complicate *endoscopic surgery* of the bile ducts (e. g. ERCP), such procedures may be carried out under antibiotic prophylaxis. Mezlocillin, cefazedone or cefotaxime are suitable for this purpose, and should be started shortly before the procedure and only continued for a short period afterwards.

References

ABRAHAM, G., S. I. VAS: Treatment of fungal peritonitis in patients undergoing continuous ambulatory peritoneal dialysis (letter; comment). Am. J. Med. *88:* 825–827 (1990).

BARTLETT, J. G.: Clostridium difficile: Clinical considerations. Rev. Infect. Dis. *12* (Suppl. 2): S243 (1990).

BENNION, R. S., J. E. THOMPSON, E. J. BARON, S. M. FINEGOLD: Gangrenous and perforated appendicitis with peritonitis: treatment and bacteriology. Clin. Ther. *12* Suppl. C: 31–44 (1990).

BERBE, T. V. et al.: Antibiotic management of surgically treated gangrenous or perforated appendicitis. Am. J. Surg. *144:* 8 (1982).

BOGAERTS, J., P. LEPAGE, D. ROUVROY, J. VANDEPITTE: Cryptosporidium, a frequent cause of diarrhea in Central Africa. J. Clin. Microbiol. *20:* 874–876 (1984).

BRADLEY, E. L.: Antibiotics in acute pancreatitis. Current status and future directions. Am. J. Surg. *158:* 472–477 (1989).

BYRNE, J. J., T. L. TREADWELL: Treatment of pancreatitis. When do antibiotics have a role? Postgrad. Med. *85:* 333–334, 337–339 (1989).

CIMOLAI, N., J. D. ANDERSON, B. J. MORRISON: Antibiotics for Escherichia coli 0157: H7 enteritis?. J. Antimicrob. Chemother. *23:* 807–808 (1989).
DE ZOYSA, I., R. G. FEACHEM: Interventions for the control of diarrhoeal diseases among young children: chemoprophylaxis. Bull. WHO *63:* 295–315 (1985).
DIPERRI, G., M. STROSSELLI, E. G. RONDANELLI: Therapy of entamebiasis. J. Chemother. *1:* 113 (1989).
DUPONT, H. L., D. C. ERICSSON, P. C. JOHNSON: Chemotherapy and chemoprophylaxis of traveler's diarrhea. Ann. Intern. Med. *102:* 260 (1985).
ERICSSON, C. D. et al.: Treatment of traveler's diarrhea with sulfamethoxazole and trimethoprim and loperamide. J.A.M.A. *263:* 257 (1990).
FEKETY, R. et al.: Treatment of antibiotic-associated Clostridium difficile colitis with oral vancomycin: Comparison of two dosage regimens. Am. J. Med. *86:* 15 (1989).
GILAT, T., G. LEICHTMAN, G. DELPRE, J. ESHCHAR, P. BAR-MEIR, Z. FIREMAN: A comparison of metronidazole and sulfasalazine in the maintenance of remission in patients with ulcerative colitis. J. Clin. Gastroenterol. *11:* 392 (1989).
GLASS, R. I., B. J. STOLL, M. I. HUQ, M. J. STRUELENS, M. BLASER, A. K. M. G. KIBRIYA: Epidemiologic and clinical features of endemic Campylobacter jejuni infection in Bangladesh. J. Infect. Dis. *148:* 292–296 (1983).
HILL, D. R.: Giardia lamblia. In: G. L. MANDELL, R. G. DOUGLAS, JR., J. E. BENNETT (eds.): Principles and Practice of Infectious Diseases (3rd ed.). New York: Churchill Livingstone, 1990.
HORTON, M. W., R. G. DEETER, R. A. SHERMAN: Treatment of peritonitis in patients undergoing continuous ambulatory peritoneal dialysis. Clin. Pharm. *9:* 102–118 (1990).
HYAMS, J. S., W. A. DURBIN, R. J. GRAND, D. A. GOLDMANN: Salmonella bacteremia in the first year of life. J. Pediat. *96:* 57 (1980).
KIPPERMAN, H., M. EPHIROS, M. LAMBDIN, K. WHITE-ROGERS: Aeromonas hydrophila: a treatable cause of diarrhea. Pediatrics *73:* 253 (1984).
KOLMOS, H. J., K. E. H. ANDERSEN, L. HANSEN: The dialysis catheter and infectious peritonitis in intermittent peritoneal dialysis. Scand. J. Infect. Dis. *16:* 181 (1984).
KROTHAPALLI, R. K., H. O. SENEKJIAN, J. C. AYUS: Efficacy of intravenous vancomycin in the treatment of gram-positive peritonitis in long-term peritoneal dialysis. Am. J. Med. *75:* 345 (1983).
LUDLAM, H. A., I. BARTON, L. WHITE: Intraperitoneal ciprofloxacin for the treatment of peritonitis in patients receiving continuous ambulatory peritoneal dialysis (CAPD). J. Antimicrob. Chemother. *25:* 843–851 (1990).
MANDAL, B. K., M. E. ELLIS, E. M. DUNBAR, K. WHALE: Double-blind placebo-controlled trial of erythromycin in the treatment of clinical campylobacter infections. J. Antimicrob. Chemother. *13:* 619 (1984).
PAI, C. H., F. GILLIS, E. TOUMANEN et al.: Placebo-controlled double-blind evaluation of trimethoprim-sulfamethoxazole treatment of Yersinia enterocolitica gastroenteritis. J. Pediatr. *104:* 308 (1984).
PAPE, J. W. et al.: Treatment and prophylaxis of Isospora belli infection in patients with the acquired immunodeficiency syndrome. N. Engl. J. Med. *320:* 1044 (1989).
PEHRSON, P. E., E. BENGTSSON: A long-term follow up study of amoebiasis treated with metronidazole. Scand. J. Infect. Dis. *16:* 195 (1984).
PETERSON, P. K., W. F. KEANE: Infections in chronic peritoneal dialysis patients. In: REMINGTON, J. S., M. N. SWARTZ (eds.), Current Clinical Topics in Infectious Diseases. New York: McGraw-Hill, pp. 239–260 (1985).
PITARANGSI, C., P. ECHEVERRIA, R. WHITMIRE, C. TIRAPAT, S. FORMAL, G. J. DAMMIN, M. TINGTALAPONG: Enteropathogenicity of Aeromonas hydrophila and Plesiomonas

shigelloides: prevalence among individuals with and without diarrhea in Thailand. Infect. Immun. *35:* 666–673 (1982).
RAVDIN, J. I.: Amebiasis. Churchill Livingstone, London 1987.
ROMEU, J., B. CLOTED, C. TURAL et al.: Therapeutic challenge for Isospora belli enteritis in an AIDS patient who developed Lyell syndrome after co-trimoxazole therapy. Am. J. Gastroenterol. *84:* 207–209 (1989).
SAEZ-LLORENS, X.: Spiramycin for treatment of Cryptosporidium enteritis. J. Infect. Dis. *160:* 342 (1989).
SAKLAYEN, M. G.: CAPD peritonitis. Incidence, pathogens, diagnosis, and management. Med. Clin. North. Am. *74:* 997–1010 (1990).
SOAVE, R., W. D. JOHNSON: Cryptosporidium and Isospora belli infections. J. Infect. Dis. *157:* 225 (1988).
TEASLEY, D. G., D. N. GERDING, M. M. OLSON et al.: Prospective randomized trial of metronidazole versus vancomycin for Clostridium difficile-associated diarrhea and colitis. Lancet *2:* 1043 (1983).
THOMPSON JR., J. E., S. FORLENZA, R. VERMA: Amebic liver abscess: a therapeutic approach. Rev. Infect. Dis. *7:* 171 (1985).
TIEMENS, K. M., P. L. SHIPLEY, R. A. CORREIA et al.: Sulfamethoxazole-trimethoprim-resistant Shigella flexneri in Northeastern Brazil. Antimicrob. Ag. Chemother. *25:* 653 (1984).
WEINKE, T., W. SCHERER, U. NEUBER, M. TRAUTMANN: Clinical features and management of amebic liver abscess. Experience from 29 patients. Klin. Wochenschr. *67:* 415 (1989).
WISTROM, J., M. JERTBORN, S. A. HEDSTROM et al.: Short-term self-treatment of travellers' diarrhoea with norfloxacin: a placebo-controlled study. J. Antimicrob. Chemother. *23:* 905 (1989).

8. Infections of the Urogenital Tract

Introduction: The classification of infections of the urinary tract into pyelonephritis and cystitis, i.e. upper and lower urinary tract infections, gives rise to certain difficulties. There are a number of infections which cannot be clearly classified into one or other group and which should simply be called urinary infections. Cystitis can, of course, be the first stage of a pyelonephritis, but the likelihood of a lower urinary infection developing into chronic pyelonephritis has apparently been overrated in the past. This risk seems to be higher in children than in adults because replacement of damaged renal tissue by scar tissue is more likely to occur in the growing kidneys. Any cause of obstruction such as outflow obstruction, stones, ureteric valves, ureterocele or prostatic hypertrophy is an important factor in the development of urinary infection. Recurrent urinary infections should be thoroughly investigated by urinary flow studies, urography, micturating cystography and ultrasound.

Urinary infections may be *obstructive* or *non-obstructive*. Congenital malformations such as hydronephrosis, megaureter, urethral valves and other anomalies are the cause of 10–20% of recurrent urinary infections in children, particularly in boys.

Urinary infections are common in diabetes mellitus and pregnancy, in both of which regular urine tests are necessary. Repeated urinary infections are virtually inevitable in patients with a paraplegic bladder, and often lead to chronic renal failure. Infections of an obstructed urinary tract carry a considerable risk of septicaemia, the prognosis of which is often poor.

Microbiological examination of the urine: Reliable methods of examination and culture of urine, and the correct evaluation of the results, are essential for rational treatment. Unnecessary treatment is often given on the basis of results from urine culture which has been performed incorrectly (e. g. unsterile container, incorrect method of collection, delay in transit to the laboratory, misinterpretation of vaginal flora in dip-slide cultures). On the other hand, failure to examine the urine appropriately may lead to an acute infection being overlooked.

Collection of urine for microbiological examination: Mid-stream urine is normally used for urine microscopy and culture. It is important to clean the urethral meatus or vulva with physiological saline or a weak disinfectant such as 2% hydrogen peroxide solution first. In infants, use a special sterile urine collection bag which should be attached to the vulva or over the penis at the time of collection. The urine is collected from adults into a sterile container and should be cultured within 30 min or cooled at once to 4° C and sent as soon as possible to the laboratory. In small children and in emergencies, a catheter specimen may be necessary, particularly if the leucocyte count in a spontaneously voided urine is raised. Suprapubic aspiration of a full bladder is a safe and reliable method of urine collection even in infants and the newborn. If there is no local bacteriological laboratory, a dip-slide culture can be used (see below), and supplemented by a cell count and a methylene-blue stain of a voided sample. Alternatively, 1% boric acid may be used as a urine preservative.

Examination for cells: The fresh, uncentrifuged mid-stream urine is examined microscopically in a counting chamber for white cells (counts above $20/mm^3$ are abnormal) and red cells, and the sediment is examined for casts, particularly granular casts, as a wet preparation on a microscope slide. The white cell count in a urine deposit can be misleading, since large variations can occur due to mechanical causes.

Granulocytes can be detected in the urine by the use of test strips (e. g. Cytur, Chemstrip). The method estimates the chloroacetate esterase content of both intact and lysed granulocytes and has a 90–95% correlation with quantitative cell counts. False positive and false negative results can both occur. Provided the urine is collected correctly, this method can be readily used in the consulting room or patient's home, including self-monitoring by the patient.

Bacteria can also be detected microscopically in a fresh, uncentrifuged midstream urine, particularly if stained with methylene blue. Bacteria are not normally present and, if seen in large numbers in a fresh specimen, are suggestive of significant bacteriuria; in such cases, a direct disc sensitivity test (see below) can often give a readable result the next day.

Quantitative bacterial count: A bacterial count of more than 100000/ml of urine indicates significant bacteriuria. Contaminants or bacteria from the urethral flora occur in smaller numbers, usually less than 100000/ml, and a count between 10000 and 100000 bacteria/ml is borderline. In untreated pyelonephritis, the bacterial and cell counts rise in parallel. A high urinary bacterial count in the presence of a normal leucocyte count can be due to incorrect specimen collection, though it can also constitute an asymptomatic bacteriuria which may be an early phase of pyelonephritis. Equivocal findings without clinical symptoms are best checked before starting antibiotic treatment. Dip-slide cultures are easily performed in any general practice or clinical laboratory. The interpretation of a 12–18 h culture is quite straightforward and can even be done by trained ancillary staff. When acute pyelonephritis is of haematogenous origin, the blood culture is often positive. The absence of demonstrable bacteriuria usually rules out a urinary tract infection, except in occasional cases of infections due to anaerobes and other fastidious organisms which do not grow on the dip-slide culture media. A full antibiotic sensitivity test is not always necessary in uncomplicated urinary infections diagnosed by dip-slide in general practice. However, the identification of bacteria and performance of antibiotic sensitivity tests always require a well equipped bacteriological laboratory. In complicated urinary infections, therefore the incubated dip-slide and not the urine should be sent to the bacteriological laboratory if it is very remote from the patient. The nitrite test is unreliable.

Antibiotic sensitivity testing: Because of the high urine concentrations of antibiotics *in vivo,* bacteria disappear rapidly from the urine during treatment. This may seem to render *in vitro* testing superfluous, but the antibiotic sensitivity profile enables the drug with the highest activity in concentrations corresponding to blood and tissue levels to be selected. Because bacterial causes of urinary infection may respond in different ways to antibiotics, and because antibiotic resistance, particularly in hospital, is increasing, antibiotic sensitivity testing has become essential.

Frequency of different pathogens in acute, uncomplicated urinary infection: Escherichia coli 60–80%, enterococci, proteus (mainly Proteus mirabilis), klebsiella, enterobacter and Pseudomonas aeruginosa about 5% each. Staphylococcus epidermidis and S. saprophyticus, group B streptococci, anaerobes, providencia, alcaligenes, serratia and candida are less common in uncomplicated cases. Changes of infecting organism, mixed infections and infections with multi-resistant organisms occur more frequently in chronic pyelonephritis and after urological operations. The culture of diphtheroids, enterococci or staphylococci in scanty numbers is suggestive of contamination of the urine by genital flora. Urine obtained through a freshly inserted catheter or by suprapubic aspiration often contains the causative organisms in pure culture and is normally sterile.

Principles of treatment of urinary infections: Urinary infections used to be treated by antibiotics or chemotherapeutic agents for 10 to 14 days to produce effective tissue and urine levels. Urinary antiseptics or chemotherapeutic agents which act mainly by high urinary concentrations were thought to be inferior to chemotherapeutic agents which produce high blood and tissue levels. In recent years, however, it has become apparent that almost all uncomplicated infections of the lower urinary tract and some of the upper urinary tract in young women can successfully be treated with a single dose of the agent. The common urinary infections in older women with prolapse or other obstructive factors require a longer course of treatment (e. g. 3–5 days).

It has become practical to divide, urinary infections into those responsive to single dose treatment and those which do not respond. Single-dose therapy should not be given in the presence of obstruction (e. g. stenosis), recent urological operations or clinical evidence of pyelonephritis. The former recommendation of 10–14 days of treatment for chronic pyelonephritis is probably too short, and longer courses should be given, at least in males.

After treatment, all urinary infections should be followed up by repeated urine culture in order to detected any relapse (by the same organism) or reinfection (by a different organism). In either case, a further course of an appropriate antimicrobial agent should be given. Long-term treatment should be considered for urinary tract obstructions which cannot be removed (e. g. infected renal calculi), and also used for the prophylaxis of ascending infection in recurrent urinary infections of young females.

Intravesicular instillation of an antibiotic is not an adequate treatment of a urinary tract infection. If a bladder washout has to be performed, a disinfectant should be used in accordance with the recommended dosage (Table 48) to avoid irritation.

Table 48. Concentration of solutions for intravesicular instillation and irrigation.

Drug	Concentration
Chlorhexidine	0.02%
Ethacridine lactate	0.05%
Nitrofurantoin for instillation*	0.05–0.1%
Gentamicin	0.5–1.0%
Neomycin	0.5% and 1.0%
Noxythiolin	1.0–2.5%
Polymyxin B sulphate	0.1%
Polymyxin B sulphate (75000 units) + neomycin (20000 units) + bacitracin (1000 units)	Powder for reconstitution
Amphotericin B	100 mg/l
Miconazole	100 mg undiluted i. v. solution

* not available in Britain

Patients at particular risk can be given oral amoxycillin or trimethoprim or i. m. gentamicin for several days after a diagnostic procedure (e. g. catheterisation or cystoscopy). A closed drainage system is recommended for long-term indwelling catheters in order to prevent ascending bacterial infection. In catheters that are *in situ* for only a short time, chemoprophylaxis usually only postpones a urinary tract infection. If a catheter is required for a longer period, the possibility of intermittent catheterisation should be considered. Suprapubic drainage of the bladder gives rise to infection less frequently than an indwelling urethral catheter and is therefore preferable, particularly in men. The most important measure in a catheter-induced urinary infection is removal or replacement of the colonised catheter.

Criteria of effective treatment: Sterilisation of the urine after 48 hours, with the disappearance of urinary leucocytes, defervescence, resolution of dysuria and loin pain and the return of the peripheral white cell count, ESR and blood urea to normal. Regular microscopy and culture of the urine during and after treatment are advisable, and a persistent bacteriuria, irrespective of the bacterial count, suggests a failure of treatment or change of infecting agent. An acute pyelonephritis can only be regarded as cured if the culture is negative two weeks after the completion of treatment.

Change of infecting agent: The antibacterial treatment of mixed infections not infrequently selects strains of resistant bacteria. Treatment with ampicillin frequently selects ampicillin-resistant klebsiellae, in which case the antibiotic should be changed or another agent added, based on the sensitivities of the bacteria involved.

There are various *reasons for failure of antibiotic therapy*, including mixed infection, a change of infecting organism, secondary resistance, mechanical factors (obstruction, calculus, anatomical abnormalities), prostatitis, incorrect diagnosis (renal tuberculosis, chlamydial infection, trichomoniasis), or inadequate treatment (underdosage, too short a course, wrong choice of drug).

a) Treatment of Acute Urinary Infections (Tables 49 and 50)

Directed therapy: The most effective drug tested against the bacterial isolate (usually amoxycillin, trimethoprim, co-amoxiclav, an oral cephalosporin, norfloxacin or ciprofloxacin) should be given. 10–14 days used to be considered the necessary duration of treatment, but this has now largely been superceded in women by a single dose which is less expensive, associated with fewer side-effects, and carries no problems of patient compliance. Amoxycillin, the new quinolones (norfloxacin, ofloxacin and ciprofloxacin) and co-trimoxazole are effective orally in a single dose, as are injectable antibiotics such as cefotaxime, gentamicin and other aminoglycosides. Signs of acute pyelonephritis or obstruction are contra-indications to single-dose treatment. If relapse or reinfection are found at regular follow-up, treatment has to start again. In single-dose treatment, the urine should be checked at 48 hours, 5 and 10 days. Women with recurrent urinary infections may need subsequent prophylaxis of ascending infection with a urinary chemotherapeutic agent. Acute urinary infections in men and all complicated urinary tract infections (with outflow obstruction) should be treated appropriately for at least 20 days (or longer if the infection recurs).

Table 49. Antibiotic treatment of urinary infections, based on sensitivity testing.

Causative organism	Oral antibiotic	Parenteral antibiotic	Second-line antibiotic	Prophylaxis of ascending infection
Escherichia coli	Ampicillins, co-trimoxazole, quinolones[1]	Cefazolin, mezlocillin	Cefotaxime, gentamicin, cefixime	Cephalexin, co-trimoxazole, nitrofurantoin
Klebsiella	Quinolones[1], co-trimoxazole, co-amoxiclav	Gentamicin, cefotaxime	Mezlocillin, amikacin, cefixime	Cephalexin, co-trimoxazole, nitrofurantoin
Enterobacter spp.	Quinolones[1], co-trimoxazole	Cefotaxime, gentamicin	Aztreonam, imipenem, amikacin	Co-trimoxazole, nitrofurantoin
Serratia marcescens	Quinolones[1], co-trimoxazole	Ceftazidime, gentamicin	Imipenem, amikacin, mezlocillin, cefixime	Co-trimoxazole, nitrofurantoin
Proteus mirabilis	Ampicillins, co-trimoxazole, quinolones[1]	Cefazolin, gentamicin	Amikacin, mezlocillin, cefixime	Cephalexin, co-trimoxazole
Proteus vulgaris, Pr. rettgeri, Morganella morganii	Quinolones[1], co-trimoxazole	Cefotaxime, piperacillin, gentamicin	Imipenem, cefoxitin, amikacin, mezlocillin, cefixime	Co-trimoxazole
Pseudomonas aeruginosa	Quinolones[1]	Azlocillin, piperacillin, tobramycin, gentamicin	Ceftazidime, cefsulodin, amikacin, imipenem	Carfecillin
Enterococci	Ampicillin, quinolones[1]	Mezlocillin	Erythromycin, tetracycline, co-trimoxazole	Nitrofurantoin
Staphylococci	Phenoxypenicillins, flucloxacillin	Benzyl-penicillin, cefazolin	Quinolones[1], co-trimoxazole	Cephalexin, nitrofurantoin

[1] Norfloxacin, ofloxacin, ciprofloxacin

Table 50. Dosage for chemotherapy of urinary infections.

Drug	Mean daily dose on continuous therapy Children (mg/kg)	Mean daily dose on continuous therapy Adults (g)	Dose interval (h)	Safe to use in pregnancy	Dose for single-dose treatment (g)
Amoxycillin	50	1.5	8	Yes	2.0–3.0
Co-amoxiclav	45	1.875	8	No	1.875 (3 tabs)
Cephalexin, cephradine, cefaclor,	50–100	2.0–4.0	8	Yes	2.0
Cefuroxime axetil	10	0.25	12	Yes	?
Cefixime	8	0.4	12	?	?
Co-trimoxazole	40	1.92	12	No	unsuitable
Trimethoprim	6–9	0.4 or 0.3	12–24	No	unsuitable
Norfloxacin	contra-indicated	0.8	8	No	0.4
Ofloxacin	contra-indicated	0.4	12	No	0.2
Ciprofloxacin	contra-indicated	0.5	12	No	0.25
Nitrofurantoin	5	0.15–0.3	8	No	unsuitable
Cefuroxime	60	2.25–4.5	8	Yes	3
Cefotaxime	60	3.0–4.0	8–12	Yes	1.0
Azlocillin, mezlocillin piperacillin	100	6.0	8–12	Yes	2–5
Imipenem	30	1.5	8–12	?	1.5
Gentamicin, tobramycin	2–3	0.16–0.24	8–12	No	0.16
Amikacin	15	0.5–1.0	12	No	0.5

Blind therapy: Patients with severe symptoms of acute urinary infection may need to start treatment before bacteriological results are available. The history is important in such cases. Resistant bacteria (pseudomonas, enterobacter) rarely cause the first urinary infection in a patient unless there is preceding urological surgery. Treatment may be started with amoxycillin, trimethoprim or a new quinolone, and changed if necessary when antibiotic sensitivities become available. In women, a single dose of cefotaxime or an aminoglycoside or (in adults) a quinolone may also be effective. Follow-up cultures are particularly important after single-dose treatment. Multiresistant organisms are more common in urinary infections after urological surgery, bladder catheterisation or the relapse of pyelonephritis. An antibiotic such as gentamicin, a cephalosporin or (in adults) a new quinolone should then be used for initial treatment, continuing or changing when antibiotic sensitivities are known. Single-dose treatment is not suitable for complicated urinary infections or for urinary tract infections in the male. If a parenteral agent cannot be given initially, the quinolones are more effective in complicated urinary infections in adults than co-trimoxazole or ampicillin. The urine should be cultured before treatment begins and, where possible, 2–3 days after treatment has started to confirm the clearance of bacteria. A persistent significant bacteriuria is a sign of inadequate treatment due to a change of pathogen, resistance, incorrect intake of the drug etc.

b) Pyelonephritis

Acute pyelonephritis with fever, loin pain, peripheral leucocytosis and a high ESR puts the patient at risk of septicaemia and necrotising pyelonephritis with permanent renal damage, including possible renal calculi or stenosis.

The causes of acute pyelonephritis are often mechanical (stones, outflow obstruction, malformations) which can be relieved surgically. Like other urinary infections, mild disease can be treated with ampicillin derivatives or trimethoprim. Complicated forms and pyelonephritis after urological surgery require bactericidal antibiotics such as one of the newer cephalosporins or an acylaminopenicillin in high dosage and possibly combined with an aminoglycoside. The new quinolones (norfloxacin, ofloxacin and ciprofloxacin), which can be given orally, are effective, but their use in children is restricted on account of the risk of arthropathy and epiphyseal damage. After one or more relapses, a longer course of treatment is given (6–12 weeks or longer) than for a reinfection.

Chronic pyelonephritis has not been adequately defined as an entity in the past. The term includes recurrent pyelonephritis, chronic obstructive urinary tract infections (e.g. infected renal calculi, nephrocalcinosis) and secondarily infected interstitial nephritis of other causes (e.g. phenacetin kidney). Exacerbations of chronic pyelonephritis should be treated in the same way as the acute disease, once the urine has been investigated microbiologically. Regular urine cultures are particularly important in chronic pyelonephritis because of the high rate of relapse, reinfection, secondary resistance and change or persistence of the infecting agent. Every recurrence and reinfection should be treated with a further course of the appropriate antibiotic.

Since bacteria can persist for long periods in the renal medulla in chronic pyelonephritis, treatment for several months is justifiable. Long-term suppression with an agent such as co-trimoxazole may become necessary in chronic pyelonephritis when there are marked anatomical or functional changes. Cases of chronic pyelonephritis which are resistant to treatment may require intermittent high doses of a penicillin or cephalosporin, possibly in combination with an aminoglycoside.

Suppressive treatment of chronic pyelonephritis should not be confused with the **prophylaxis of ascending infection in the female.** The cause of recurrent urinary infections in women is much more likely to be due to a failure of the mechanisms which prevent the ascension of bacteria through the urethra. Poor genital hygiene, sexual activity and infrequent micturition may play a part. If such patients take a chemotherapeutic agent for long periods in small doses, the risk of recurrent urinary infections can be reduced. Agents frequently used for this purpose are co-trimoxazole (240–480 mg per day), cephalexin (250 mg daily) or nitrofurantoin (50 mg a day).

Pyelonephritis in pregnancy: Pyelonephritis is more likely to occur in pregnancy, which can precipitate an acute attack of a pre-existing but asymptomatic chronic pyelonephritis. Simple urinary infection in pregnancy is treated in the same way as acute pyelonephritis, except that many antibiotics (gentamicin, tobramycin, amikacin, netilmicin, tetracycline, co-trimoxazole, nitrofurantoin and quinolones such as nalidixic acid, pipemidic acid, norfloxacin, ofloxacin, ciprofloxacin, enoxacin and pefloxacin) are best avoided because of their potential toxicity. To this list should be added new antibiotics (e. g. imipenem) which are probably safe, but which should nevertheless be avoided on the grounds of insufficient evidence of their safety at present. Sulphonamides are contraindicated in the first four months of pregnancy because of their teratogenicity in animal experiments, and in the two weeks before the expected date of delivery because of the risk of neonatal jaundice and, in severe cases, kernicterus. Urinary infections in pregnancy are in practice treated with ampicillins or oral cephalosporins. Suitable alternatives are cefazolin, cefuroxime, cefotaxime, piperacillin, azlocillin and mezlocillin. Regular bacteriological monitoring after treatment for the remainder of pregnancy is very important, and definitive investigation of the urinary tract may be indicated after delivery.

Acute pyelonephritis of pregnancy is often preceded by asymptomatic bacteriuria, and can be prevented by screening all pregnant women at the end of the first trimester, and treating those who are positive. If a simple screening test such as microscopy for white cells or a dip-slide is positive, a full urine culture of a spontaneous mid-stream urine should be performed. Amoxycillin is generally suitable for asymptomatic bacteriuria. Single-dose therapy for uncomplicated lower urinary tract infections during pregnancy is less effective than in the nonpregnant women on account of the obstruction. If regular semiquantitative urine cultures show persistence of the bacteriuria, an appropriate antibiotic may be needed long-term, possibly throughout the pregnancy.

c) Cystitis

Clinical symptoms do not always distinguish clearly between simple cystitis and pyelonephritis. Dysuria and frequency are not solely caused by acute cystitis; they can also be due to urethritis (e. g. in gonorrhoea or trichomonas infection). Simple cystitis is not accompanied by fever, leucocytosis, a high ESR or loin pain. Cystitis can, however, be part of the picture of pyelonephritis. Recurrent cystitis resistant to standard antibiotic therapy can be the presenting symptom of chronic pyelonephritis, and is occasionally due to renal tuberculosis or a bladder tumour. Every case of cystitis must, therefore, be properly investigated by urinary microscopy and culture. Enterobacteria are the commonest causes of both cystitis and pyelonephritis. Acute haemorrhagic cystitis can also be caused by adenoviruses or, in oncological patients, by cyclophosphamide.

Treatment should be based on the common bacterial isolates. A single high dose (Fig. 61) of norfloxacin, co-trimoxazole or amoxycillin is usually adequate in women; an alternative is a single parenteral dose of a cephalosporin or an aminoglycoside. Failure of single-dose therapy when the causative organism remains sensitive is suggestive of occult renal involvement.

When cystitis is treated effectively, the symptoms resolve promptly. Persistence of symptoms is a sign of inadequate treatment, and gonorrhoea or an infection due to trichomonas or chlamydia should be ruled out.

d) Urethritis

Non-gonococcal urethritis can be caused by Chlamydia trachomatis (see below), Ureaplasma urealyticum, gardnerella, Escherichia coli, proteus, enterococci or staphylococci, which can be detected in men in the urethral secretions and in women by testing cervical secretions. The white cell count of the forestream urine is higher than in the remainder. Urethritis can be due to meatal stenosis, foreign bodies, a tumour, a periurethral abscess or a diverticulum. Juvenile urethritis can be due to threadworms or to vulvovaginitis which results from poor hygiene. Herpes simplex viral infection in the patient may be associated with herpes genitalis in the sexual partner.

As with acute pyelonephritis, bacterial urethritis should be *treated* with a long course of an effective antibiotic in order to prevent periurethral abscesses, urethral stricture, ascending infection or epididymitis. Systemic treatment with more effective agents has replaced the local instillation of antiseptics. Oral tetracycline is the only effective treatment for mycoplasma infections (Ureaplasma urealyticum). Systemic acyclovir (see p. 278) is useful in herpes simplex urethritis.

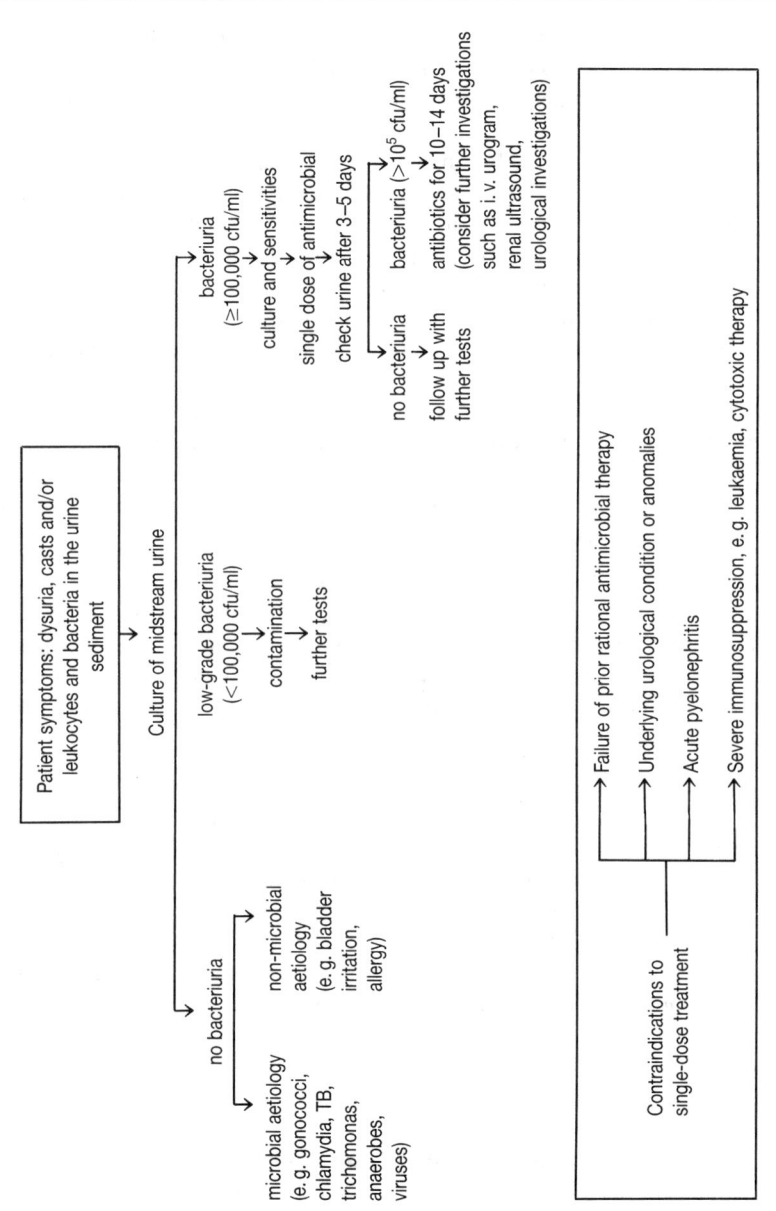

Fig. 61 Protocol for single-dose treatment of uncomplicated urinary tract infection in women.

Gonorrhoea is shown by the presence of gram-negative intracellular diplococci in the urethral secretion, confirmed where possible by culture. The treatment of choice is cefuroxime, cefotaxime, cefoxitin or a new quinolone such as ciprofloxacin (see p. 488).

Chlamydial urethritis caused by Chlamydia trachomatis has become one of the commonest sexually transmitted diseases and is a frequent cause of postgonococcal urethritis. Inclusion bodies appear in the affected urethral epithelial cells and are seen as red cytoplasmic granules in a Giemsa stain of a urethral smear; they are often crescent-shaped around the nucleolus. The agent can also be shown by direct immunofluorescence with a monoclonal antibody in a microscopic preparation using a Micro-Trak test kit. It can also be grown in cell culture in a special laboratory.

Treatment: Doxycycline, erythromycin, a new quinolone (ofloxacin, ciprofloxacin) or a sulphonamide for at least 2 weeks, with appropriate antibiotic treatment of any underlying secondary bacterial infection. Doxycycline is also effective against simultaneous infection with ureaplasmas. Where possible, the sexual partner should be treated at the same time.

Candida urethritis: Irrigation with nystatin is useful when Candida albicans is detected in the urethra by microscopy or culture. Cutaneous candidiasis on the external genitalia may be treated with a suitable cream (e.g. clotrimazole, miconazole). Endogenous reinfection may occur. Where candidiasis is confirmed, resistant cases can often be successfully treated with oral fluconazole, which has good renal elimination.

Trichomonas urethritis: Trichomonas vaginalis is a frequent cause of urethritis in women and men, in whom it may also be latent; the partner of a woman with trichomonal vaginitis should therefore also be treated. Milky, sometimes frothy, mucopurulent or even frankly purulent secretion is discharged from the urethra, sometimes with prostatic involvement also. Typical flagellates are seen in a wet preparation or in a gram- or Pappenheim-stained smear of the urinary deposit or in a urethral swab, which should be taken at least 2 h after the last micturition.

Like trichomonal vaginitis (see p. 446), *treatment* is with metronidazole or a single dose of tinidazole 2 g or ornidazole 1.5 g. The infected sexual partner should also be treated.

e) Prostatitis, Epididymitis, Orchitis

There are *various causes,* including gram-negative bacilli, gonococci, staphylococci, streptococci, anaerobes, Chlamydia trachomatis and tubercle bacilli. Prostatitis is often accompanied by cystitis and urethritis with dysuria and bacteriuria.

Directed treatment is often not possible because the bacterial cause is difficult to demonstrate. Where possible, prostatic secretion should be obtained for culture by massage. Co-trimoxazole diffuses better into the prostatic tissue than any other antibiotic and is thus the oral treatment of choice. Acute prostatis may also be treated blind with doxycycline, possibly in combination with gentamicin (240 mg per day). If parenteral administration is effective, change to the oral route after 1 week and continue for at least 4 weeks to reduce the risk of recurrence. Treatment with cefotaxime (6 g a day) is also often effective, especially if gonorrhoea is suspected. The best alternatives on the grounds of good tissue penetration and clinical efficacy are ofloxacin or ciprofloxacin. Surgical treatment may be unavoidable, particularly if abscesses form.

Antibiotics are less effective in *chronic infection*, particularly in chronic prostatitis. Pathogens are difficult to isolate, though comparative quantitative cultures of prostatic secretion, bladder urine, obtained by needle aspiration, and a forestream urine for urethral flora may be worthwhile. Possible bacterial causes include enterobacteria, Pseudomonas, enterococci and tubercle bacilli. Treatment can be attempted with co-trimoxazole, 2 tablets twice a day for 1–3 months, provided the peripheral blood count is regularly checked. Alternatively, one of the new quinolones may be used.

References

ANGEL, J. L., W. F. O'BRIEN, M. A. FINAN, W. J. MORALES: Acute pyelonephritis in pregnancy: a prospective study of oral versus intravenous antibiotic therapy. Obstet. Gynecol. *76:* 28–32 (1990).

CHILDS, S. J.: Ciprofloxacin in treatment of chronic bacterial prostatitis. Urology. *35* (1 Suppl). 15–18 (1990).

FINE, J. S., M. S. JACOBSON: Single-dose versus conventional therapy of urinary tract infections in female adolescents, Pediatrics *75:* 916 (1985).

HOOTON, T. M., K. RUNNING, W. E. STAMM: Single-dose therapy for cystitis in women. A comparison of trimethoprim-sulfamethoxazole, amoxicillin and ciclacillin. JAMA *253:* 387 (1985).

HUMPHREYS, H., D. C. SPELLER: Acute epididymo-orchitis caused by Pseudomonas aeruginosa and treated with ciprofloxacin. J. Infect. *19:* 257–261 (1989).

LIPSKY, B. A.: Urinary tract infections in men. Epidemiology, pathophysiology, diagnosis and treatment. Ann. Intern. Med. *110:* 138–150 (1989).

REIN, M. F.: Urethritis: In: G. L. MANDELL, R. G. DOUGLAS, JR., and J. E. BENNETT, (eds.), Principles and Practice of Infectious Diseases (3rd ed.). New York: Churchill Livingstone, 1990. Pp. 942–952.

SANDBERG, T., G. ENGLUND, K. LINCOLN, L. G. NILSSON: Randomised double-blind study of norfloxacin and cefadroxil of acute pyelonephritis. Eur. J. Clin. Microbiol. Infect. Dis. *9:* 317–323 (1990).

SCHAEFFER, A. J., F. S. DARRAS: The efficacy of norfloxacin in the treatment of chronic bacterial prostatitis refractory to trimethoprim-sulfamethoxazole and/or carbenicillin. J. Urol. *144:* 690–693 (1990).

SOBEL, J. D., D. KAYE: Urinary Tract Infections. In: G. L. MANDELL, R. G. DOUGLAS, JR., J. E. BENNETT (eds.): Principles and Practice of Infectious Diseases (3rd ed.). New York: Churchill Livingstone, 1990.
STAMM, W. E. et al.: Urinary tract infections: From pathogenesis to treatment. J. Infect. Dis. *159:* 400 (1989).
WATANAKUNAKORN, C., D. H. LEVY: Pharyngitis and urethritis due to Chlamydia trachomatis. J. Infect. Dis. *147:* 364 (1983).
WONG, E. S. et al.: Management of recurrent urinary tract infections with patients administered single dose therapy. Ann. Intern. Med. *102:* 302 (1985).

9. Surgical Infections

a) Wound Infections

Wound infections generally occur postoperatively (as hospital infection) and after trauma. Local antibiotics will reach the site of infection in concentrations adequate for treatment only if the wound is very superficial. Deep wounds require treatment with systemic antibiotics when there is clinical evidence of inflammation or the onset of more general spread (lymphangitis).

Wound infections, particularly abscesses, tend to heal spontaneously. The aim of chemotherapy as an adjunct to surgical measures is to accelerate the healing process and prevent complications such as lymphangitis and septicaemia.

Causative organisms: Predominantly staphylococci, although antibiotic-resistant gram-negative bacilli such as Pseudomonas aeruginosa, Proteus vulgaris and Enterobacter cloacae as well as anaerobes of the bacteroides group are increasing in frequency, whereas streptococci and clostridia are becoming less common, although they remain potentially life-threatening. Mixed infections are frequent.

Diagnosis: A provisional diagnosis may be made from a gram-stained smear of pus from the wound and confirmed by culture and sensitivity testing of significant bacterial isolates. In principle, all clinically infected wounds should be examined bacteriologically. Where the infection fails to resolve, further cultures should be taken during treatment to detect superinfection with resistant organisms.

The **initial therapy** of *postoperative wound infections* must cover staphylococcal infection, for which the best treatment is a penicillinase-stable penicillin such as oral flucloxacillin (2–3 g a day for adults in 3–4 divided doses) or cefazolin or cefazedone i.v. (3–6 g a day).

Less severe post-traumatic wound infections acquired outside hospital may be treated with flucloxacillin, co-amoxiclav or a basic (first-generation) cephalosporin such as cefazolin or cephradine. Trivial infections may even respond to phenoxymethyl-penicillin. *Severe post-traumatic wound infections,* which are frequently mixed, require a broad-spectrum combination such as cefoxitin + azlocillin, cefotaxime + piperacillin, cefotaxime + clindamycin, ampicillin + gentamicin + metronidazole, or imipenem. Any of these combinations may be expected to cover all the important pathogens. Cephalosporins of the cefotaxime group are less suitable as single agents for the treatment of severe wound infections because of their poor activity against bacteroides, staphylococci and pseudomonas. Tetracyclines are unsuitable for the blind treatment of wound infections because a large percentage of staphylococci and almost all strains of pseudomonas are resistant. Ampicillin and co-trimoxazole are now only effective against a minority of causes of wound infection. Aminoglycosides given alone have poor clinical efficacy, but may be combined with β-lactam antibiotics to good effect. The value of the quinolones in wound infections is still not established; ofloxacin and ciprofloxacin are effective in infections with gram-negative bacteria.

Directed therapy: according to the pathogen and antibiotic sensitivities (see Table 51).

Prophylaxis of wound infections: The routine use of antibiotics after aseptic operations is not advisable because it is unlikely to benefit the individual patient, and may select resistant strains which may then disseminate through the hospital environment. Strict asepsis at operation and postoperative wound toilet still afford

Table 51. Antibiotic treatment of wound infections.

Causative organism	Antibiotic(s) of choice	Second-line antibiotics
Staphylococci	Penicillinase-stable penicillin, cefazolin	Clindamycin, fusidic acid, vancomycin
Streptococci	Benzylpenicillin, phenoxymethylpenicillin	A cephalosporin, erythromycin
Enterococci	An ampicillin	Erythromycin, doxycycline, mezlocillin, a quinolone
Pseudomonas aeruginosa	Azlocillin + tobramycin, ciprofloxacin	Gentamicin, amikacin, ceftazidime, piperacillin, aztreonam, imipenem
Proteus vulgaris	Cefotaxime, gentamicin, ceftazidime, cefoxitin	Piperacillin, a quinolone, aztreonam, imipenem
Klebsiella	Cefotaxime, gentamicin, mezlocillin	A quinolone, piperacillin, aztreonam, imipenem
Escherichia coli	An ampicillin or cephalosporin or co-trimoxazole	Gentamicin, co-amoxiclav, a quinolone, imipenem
Pasteurella multocida	Benzylpenicillin	Doxycycline
Bacteroides fragilis	Metronidazole, clindamycin	Cefoxitin, imipenem, flomoxef, co-amoxiclav
Clostridium perfringens	Benzylpenicillin	Doxycycline, a cephalosporin, metronidazole

the best protection from wound infection; even in trivial lesions, antibiotic therapy is no substitute for good wound care. Antibiotic prophylaxis should only be given in exceptional cases where the risk of infection is particularly high (see Table 52). Many such indications may justifiably be regarded as the early treatment of infections which are already present.

To be effective, prophylaxis must be given as near to the start of the operation as possible, usually at the time of induction of anaesthesia. If antibiotic prophylaxis becomes necessary during the course of an operation as a conse-

Table 52. Indications for chemoprophylaxis in surgery.

Indication	Antibiotics	Reason
Heavily contaminated wounds and delay in initial wound care	Benzyl- or phenoxy-methyl-penicillin	Prevention of tetanus, gas gangrene and streptococcal infection
Compound fractures, traumatic penetration of joints or body cavities	Cefoxitin or cefuroxime, possibly + aminoglycoside and metronidazole	Mixed infections (including anaerobes) common; risk of gas gangrene
Gunshot and stab wounds	Benzylpenicillin; in chest and abdominal injuries, broad-spectrum combinations (see p. 581)	Infection inevitable; risk of gas gangrene or other mixed anaerobic infections
Severe burns	Benzylpenicillin 12–18 g daily for the first week	Prophylaxis of streptococcal infection
Human and animal bites	Benzyl- or phenoxy-methyl-penicillin	Streptococci (human) or Pasteurella multocida (animal)
Metal and plastic implants	Flucloxacillin, cefazolin, vancomycin	Foreign bodies predispose to wound infection (usually staphylococcal)
Cardiac surgery	Flucloxacillin, cefazolin, vancomycin	Prophylaxis of post-operative endocarditis (usually staphylococcal)
Transplant operations	Flucloxacillin, cefazolin, vancomycin	Prophylaxis of staphylococcal and streptococcal infection
Neurosurgical operations	Cefotaxime, latamoxef	Infections uncommon but dangerous
Operations in heavily contaminated areas (oesophagus, colon, rectum)	Cefotaxime + azlocillin + metronidazole, imipenem	Mixed infections with aerobic and anaerobic bacteria inevitable
Operations in the immunosuppressed patient	Cefotaxime + azlocillin, ceftazidime + gentamicin	Increased risk of infection
Lower limb amputation for gangrene	Benzylpenicillin	Prevention of gas gangrene

quence, for example, of the opening of a viscus, a suitable agent should be given immediately. The administration of antibiotic prophylaxis during an operation usually falls to the anaesthetist. Such prophylaxis should be brief, although opinions about the optimal length vary between one dose and a 3-day course. Ten to fourteen days of prophylaxis against surgical infection, which may still be practised in some units, is inappropriate. General restraint in the prophylactic use of antibiotics in surgery should never lead to the omission of prophylaxis for gas gangrene (see p. 498). The risk of short courses of prophylactic antibiotics is often overestimated, and bears no relationship to the risk of omitting prophylaxis when clearly indicated.

b) Infected Burns

Minor burns are treated as other skin injuries. The progress of extensive, third degree burns depends on the severity of any complicating infection. The indiscriminate prophylactic use of antibiotics is inappropriate because of the possible selection of resistant bacteria.

The main **causative organisms** are Pseudomonas aeruginosa and multi-resistant staphylococci (e.g. MRSA), though proteus, klebsiella, enterobacter, enterococci and fungi (aspergillus, mucor, candida) occur occasionally. Infections with group A streptococci are particularly dangerous, though infrequent, and can prevent the adherence of skin grafts and destroy residual epithelial tissue. Septicaemia is most commonly caused by Pseudomonas aeruginosa, Staphylococcus aureus, enterobacter and proteus, all of which carry a high mortality.

Diagnosis: Wound swabs before starting antibiotics, then once or twice a week during treatment, are helpful, since the wound flora can change. Since colonising bacteria are unlikely to be eradicated by antibiotics, the indications for treatment are the presence of clinical signs of infection. If septicaemia develops, blood cultures should be taken. Other infectious complications such as pneumonia and thrombophlebitis should be investigated if appropriate.

Suggested treatment protocol for extensive infected burns:
Week 1: Benzylpenicillin in high dosage (12–18 g daily for adults, or 0.3 g/kg/day for children, in 2–3 short infusions).
Week 2: A combination such as azlocillin (6 g daily i.v.) + flucloxacillin (3 g daily i.v.) + tobramycin (80–160 mg daily i.m.). For paediatric dosage, see p. 589).
The protocol may need to be modified in the light of bacteriological results. *Renal insufficiency,* which commonly complicates severe burns, must be taken into account when calculating the antibiotic dosage (see p. 598).

Local antibiotic treatment can be very useful in severe burns but is often impaired by tissue necrosis. During the first few days after injury, moist compresses with 0.5% silver nitrate solution have proved effective, not only because of their bactericidal effect on Pseudomonas aeruginosa but also because of their healing effect on the wound surface. Silver sulphadiazine (Flamazine) and povidone iodine may also be used locally on burns. When the burns are extensive, however, local agents may be absorbed percutaneously with possible systemic side-effects or direct toxicity; aminoglycosides, polymyxin B and bacitracin can be toxic in this situation. The risk of skin sensitisation makes penicillins, cephalosporins and neomycin unsuitable for local treatment. The quinolones would appear to be suitable for topical therapy of severe infections, although there is a risk of emergence of resistance when they are used alone; clinical experience of their use in burns is still lacking.

General measures, particularly the treatment of shock by intravenous infusion therapy, the replacement of fluid, electrolyte and protein losses, treatment of acidosis, analgesia, oxygen, tetanus immunisation, treatment of renal failure, and protection from hospital infection are all vital to the management of burns. When smoke has been inhaled, pneumonia may also develop, often through secondary bacterial infection with gram-negative bacilli. The burned area must be thoroughly cleaned, debrided and, if full thickness, grafted. Severe burns are best managed in a bacteriologically controlled environment with regular microbiological monitoring, conditions that are best provided in a specialised burns unit.

c) Hand Infections

The *causative organisms* are predominantly staphylococci, and occasionally streptococci, gram-negative bacilli (e.g. pseudomonas) or bacteroides (in mixed infections). Candida albicans can cause infections of the nails.

Cutaneous paronychia: Incision, drainage and immobilisation. Antibiotics are not essential to the treatment of staphylococcal infections, but should be used in streptococcal infections (risk of tenovaginitis). Where there is a risk of complications or the patient is immunodeficient (leukaemia, HIV infection etc.), even superficial paronychia should be treated with antibiotics.

Subcutaneous, osseous or articular paronychia, and purulent tenovaginitis: Surgical treatment is as important as antibiotics, which are effective only if given very early, to prevent the collection of pus. Antibiotics may protect against the development of complications such as lymphangitis, septicaemia, chronic osteomyelitis and palmar cellulitis. The choice of antibiotics is influenced by the direct microscopy of pus and the sensitivities of the pathogens cultured, which in rapidly progressive infections are almost always staphylococci. In chronic infections, anaerobes, enterobacteria and candida may also be isolated.

When *gram-positive cocci* in clusters (staphylococci) are seen in a stained smear, or when no organisms are seen (but staphylococcal infection is still probable), flucloxacillin, which is penicillinase-stable, should be given in an oral daily dose of 2–3 g to adults and children of school age and 100 mg/kg to infants. In patients allergic to penicillins, give clindamycin 0.9 g daily by mouth. Because of the risk of relapse, treatment should not be discontinued too soon.

When *gram-positive cocci* in chains (streptococci) are seen in a stained smear, phenoxymethylpenicillin 2–4 g daily should be given in four divided doses.

Gram-negative organisms are treated according to their antibiotic sensitivity pattern; if sensitivities are not available, a cephalosporin or co-amoxiclav are suitable for initial use.

Candida paronychia is best treated systemically with fluconazole, but not incision.

d) Postoperative Septicaemia

The general recommendations for the antibiotic treatment of septicaemia (see p. 327) also apply to postoperative septicaemia. Since these infections are almost always hospital-acquired, the causative organisms (staphylococci, Pseudomonas aeruginosa, Bacteroides fragilis, proteus, Escherichia coli, klebsiella, enterobacter) are likely to display *antibiotic resistance*. If perioperative prophylaxis is not given, streptococci, clostridia and sensitive anaerobes can also cause septicaemia. A bacteriological diagnosis is therefore essential. Successful treatment depends upon the detection and removal or treatment of the initial septic focus, such as an infected wound, venous catheter, foreign body, indwelling urethral catheter, or septic thrombophlebitis. Blood cultures and wound swabs (or free pus if present) should always be collected for microbiological examination before starting antibiotics.

Where the **pathogen is not known,** treatment is based on the likely range of pathogens ("blind" therapy). In severe infections broad-spectrum treatments indicated, such as with cefotaxime + azlocillin, or imipenem. Following operations that carry a risk of anaerobic infection, metronidazole or clindamycin should be added. The combination of ampicillin, gentamicin and metronidazole is still useful for less severe postoperative abdominal sepsis. The "blind" initial treatment may need modification in the light of bacteriological results and clinical progress.

Where the **pathogen is known,** treatment should be as described in the section on septicaemia (p. 335).

e) Postoperative Pneumonia

Factors which predispose to postoperative pneumonia include hypoventilation, atelectasis, inhalation anaesthesia, aspiration, lengthy and difficult operations, pre-existing lung disease, and chest or abdominal operations after which coughing is painful. The use of bacterially contaminated anaesthetic or ventilatory equipment can give rise to severe pneumonias in the immediate postoperative period. The *causes* include resistant staphylococci, klebsiella, enterobacter and pseudomonas. Endogenous infections with pneumococci, Haemophilus influenzae and anaerobes may also occur. Every effort should be made to isolate the causative organism, including chest physiotherapy to obtain deeply expectorated sputum, blood culture and transtracheal aspiration where available (see p. 377).

f) Infected Gangrene

Underlying cause: Impaired arterial perfusion of the leg, frequently complicated by secondary, usually mixed infection, with staphylococci, aerobic and anaerobic streptococci, clostridia and gram-negative bacteria (Pseudomonas aeruginosa, proteus, bacteroides etc.).

Treatment: Relief of the vascular obstruction is essential if amputation is to be avoided. Secondary infection (wet gangrene) may be treated with benzylpenicillin 6–24 g i.v. daily (to which anaerobic streptococci are only moderately sensitive), flucloxacillin 6–10 g i.v. daily (for penicillinase-producing staphylococci), gentamicin 0.24 g i.m. or i.v. and/or azlocillin 15–20 g i.v. daily (active against Pseudomonas aeruginosa and other gram-negative bacteria), with the possible addition of clindamycin or metronidazole i.v. Ofloxacin and ciprofloxacin penetrate well into the poorly perfused tissue. The local use (not yet licensed) of 0.1% ciprofloxacin in methylcellulose gel can reduce in the short term the likelihood of introducing infection of the necrotic area from the external surface, but carries the risk of emergence of bacterial resistance to quinolones. Because these infections can be life-threatening, combinations of two or three antibiotics should be used to reinforce the antibiotic effect by synergy and to broaden the spectrum. Severe infected gangrene can in some circumstances give rise to disseminated clostridial infection (see p. 498).

References

Gorbach, S. L., J. Bartlett, N. R. Blacklow: Infectious Diseases in Medicine and Surgery. Saunders, Philadelphia 1991.
Simmons, R. L., R. J. Howard (Eds): Surgical Infectious Diseases. Appleton-Century Hemel Hempstead 1988.

THOMSEN, P. D., T. E. TADDONIO, M. J. TAIT, J. K. PRASAD: Susceptibility of Pseudomonas and Staphylococcus wound isolates to topical antimicrobial agents: a 10-year review and clinical evaluation. Burns *15:* 190–192 (1989).
YOGEV, R.: Cerebrospinal fluid shunt infections: A personal view. Pediatr. Infect. Dis. *4:* 113 (1985).

10. Osteomyelitis and Septic Arthritis

a) Osteomyelitis

Osteomyelitis can occur in **four forms,** each of which should be treated differently. These are:
1. acute haematogenous osteomyelitis (mainly in children);
2. acute postoperative or post-traumatic osteomyelitis;
3. osteomyelitis with direct spread;
4. chronic osteomyelitis.

Aetiology: Acute haematogenous osteomyelitis is most frequently caused by staphylococci, and occasionally by group B streptococci, bacteroides, klebsiella, salmonella, brucella etc., and Haemophilus influenzae in infants and the elderly. Pseudomonas is an increasingly frequent cause of vertebral or pubic osteomyelitis in heroin addicts. Fungi such as candida and aspergillus are additional causes in the immunosuppressed and, not infrequently, atypical mycobacteria (e.g. Mycobacterium avium-intracellulare) in patients with AIDS. Post-traumatic osteomyelitis can be caused not only by staphylococci, but also (usually in mixed infection) by proteus, Pseudomonas aeruginosa, Escherichia coli and other bacteria. Osteomyelitis with direct spread is also usually a mixed aerobic and anaerobic infection; it can arise from dental foci, for example, or, in diabetics with peripheral vascular disease, from trophic foot ulcers. A special form of osteomyelitis is Brodie's abscess, which is usually staphylococcal in origin.

Diagnosis: Culture and antibiotic sensitivities are important if treatment is to be effective. Attempts should be made to isolate the causative organism before starting treatment, if possible from blood culture or an initial septic focus (frequently pyoderma). When a subperiosteal abscess has formed, pus may be aspirated by needle or drill biopsy. If blood cultures remain sterile or have not been obtained, a bone biopsy should be attempted for histological and cultural investigation for aerobic and anaerobic organisms, mycobacteria and fungi. Any material obtained at operation (in chronic osteomyelitis) must be very thoroughly investigated (subdivision of the specimen, a range of media and prolonged incubation).

In staphylococcal osteomyelitis the antistaphylolysin titre usually rises from its normal value (1–2 units/ml in adults) to 5–10 units/ml or more (except in infections due to Staphylococcus epidermidis). The diagnosis of osteomyelitis with group A streptococci, salmonellae or brucellae can also be made serologically. Haemophilus type b and group B streptococcal osteomyelitis can be detected by rapid direct latex agglutination of serum or urine. Radiological changes are not usually seen until the third week (or in infants the second week) of illness. The diagnosis may be confirmed earlier by skeletal scintigraphy or nuclear magnetic resonance studies.

Acute haematogenous osteomyelitis is treated according to the same principles as septicaemia. Bactericidal antibiotics should be used at maximal dosage. Because many antibiotics penetrate poorly into bone and to prevent relapse, treatment should continue for a considerable period.

Directed therapy: Infections with penicillin-sensitive staphylococci are best treated with *benzylpenicillin,* which is more active than other penicillins against sensitive strains, in doses of 6–18 g daily in 2–3 short i.v. infusions. Infections with penicillin-resistant staphylococci should be treated intravenously with a penicillinase-stable penicillin or with clindamycin as follows:

Flucloxacillin i.v.: Adults 6–10 g and children 0.2–0.3 g/kg daily.

Clindamycin: Adults 0.3–0.6 g i.v. or i.m. and children 15 mg/kg 3 times a day, followed by 0.9–1.2 g daily for adults and 20 mg/kg for children in 4 divided doses by mouth.

Fusidic acid (suitable pharmacokinetics but a risk of resistance emerging during treatment) has also been used successfully to treat osteomyelitis. The daily dose for adults is 2 g and for children 30 mg/kg in 3–4 divided doses after meals. Fusidic acid should always be given in combination with a second antistaphylococcal agent.

The *basic cephalosporins* are similar in their antistaphylococcal activity to the penicillinase-stable penicillins, and show extensive cross-resistance with flu- and dicloxacillin. The newer cephalosporins (e.g. ceftazidime) are less active against staphylococci, however. Cephalosporins should only be considered in patients with penicillin allergy.

When a *large subperiosteal abscess* has formed, pus should be aspirated and an antibiotic instilled if necessary (see septic arthritis, p. 440).

Vancomycin and teicoplanin (despite poor penetration into bone) or *fosfomycin* (which penetrates bone well) are useful in osteomyelitis caused by multi-resistant Staphylococcus epidermidis, which sometimes infects joint prostheses. Combination with fusidic acid or rifampicin is appropriate, however, in such cases.

Osteomyelitis caused by other agents is treated according to antibiotic sensitivity. When the causative organisms are penicillin-sensitive (e.g. streptococci), benzylpenicillin in high dosage is the treatment of choice; Haemophilus influenzae should be treated with ampicillin i.v. or, if resistant, cefotaxime. Pseudomonas infections should be treated with tobramycin in combination with azlocillin or ciprofloxacin. Ceftazidime, aztreonam and imipenem are alternatives. Salmonella osteomyelitis should be treated with cefotaxime in high dosage, ciprofloxacin or ofloxacin, according to sensitivity results.

Blind therapy of acute haematogenous osteomyelitis should be with high doses of antibiotics as soon as the clinical diagnosis has been made and blood cultures and a swab from any focus of initial infection taken. A combination of benzylpenicillin i.v. (18 g daily) and flucloxacillin i.v. (6–10 g daily for adults and 200 mg/kg for children) covers more than 90% of the likely bacterial causes (staphylococci, streptococci). In *children aged 1–6,* haemophilus can occur as well as staphylococci and cefotaxime + clindamycin is appropriate initial therapy. In the *newborn* or in patients with severe underlying illness or *immunodeficiency,* Pseudomonas and other gram-negative bacilli (e.g. salmonellae) should be considered, for which broad-spectrum combinations such as cefotaxime + piperacillin are suitable. Once the antibiotic sensitivity pattern is known, the most appropriate agent should be continued. Staphylococcal osteomyelitis is best treated with a combination of either benzylpenicillin or flucloxacillin and fusidic acid, or with clindamycin. If there is no clinical response, further bacteriological investigation may be necessary.

For sequential oral therapy, clindamycin, phenoxymethylpenicillin, fusidic acid and, in adults, ofloxacin or ciprofloxacin are suitable, according to the bacterial sensitivity.

Duration of therapy: Clinical improvement usually occurs rapidly after the initial high-dose intravenous therapy, and antibiotics may then be continued orally. After 4 weeks of intravenous benzylpenicillin or flucloxacillin, staphylococcal osteomyelitis may be treated with oral clindamycin (0.6 g daily for adults, 10 mg/kg for children), flucloxacillin (3 g daily for adults, 100 mg/kg for children) or phenoxymethylpenicillin (2 g daily for adults, 1 g daily for children) until the infection has completely resolved.

Osteomyelitis by direct spread: Osteomyelitis of the jaw, which can arise by direct spread from a dental root infection or maxillary sinusitis, may have various causes, but is usually staphylococcal or mixed, including anaerobes (streptococci, bacteroides, fusobacteria etc.), in origin.

High doses of antibiotics are indicated as an adjunct to operative drainage. If staphylococcal infection can be excluded, initial treatment with benzylpenicillin in high dosage is rational, and clindamycin i.v. as an alternative if penicillin fails.

Chronic osteomyelitis usually arises after operations or trauma, as well as after certain directly spreading infections and as a result of inadequately treated acute osteomyelitis. Surgical intervention is required (for removal of sequestra, osteoplasty etc.). When the cause is unclear, tuberculosis, actinomycosis and brucellosis should be ruled out. Local intra- or periosseous instillation of antibiotics or irrigation and drainage of the osteomyelitic cavity may be performed, supplemented if necessary by the insertion of gentamicin polymethylmethacrylate (PMMA) beads (see p. 139). Infected hip prostheses may have to be replaced under high-dose antibiotic cover. The success rate of new prosthetic implantation is increased by the use of a bone cement containing gentamicin.

Treatment should be guided wherever possible by the bacterial isolate and its sensitivities. High doses of systemic antibiotics have little chance of success unless used as adjuncts to surgical measures; they should be continued for a considerable period after clinical improvement is established. Chronic staphylococcal infections are usually treated with flucloxacillin, fusidic acid or clindamycin. Infections with enterobacteria should be treated with cefotaxime or ciprofloxacin, or possibly with a combination of piperacillin and gentamicin. Pseudomonas osteomyelitis is best treated with azlocillin + tobramycin, ciprofloxacin or aztreonam. Ofloxacin and ciprofloxacin penetrate well into bone and have proved their value in brucella osteomyelitis. The most effective agents in anaerobic infections, which are often mixed, are benzylpenicillin (except against Bacteroides fragilis), clindamycin, metronidazole and imipenem.

b) Acute purulent arthritis

Purulent arthritis arises haematogenously, after trauma or by direct spread from an infected focus of osteomyelitis or soft tissue infection. It is occasionally iatrogenic following the intra-articular injection of corticosteroids. The *commonest causes* are staphylococci, occasionally streptococci, pneumococci, gonococci, meningococci, salmonellae, enterobacteria, anaerobes (often mixed) and (in children) Haemophilus influenzae. Bacterial infection of a prosthetic joint is caused frequently by staphylococci (S. aureus, S. epidermidis) but also by gram-negative bacilli and anaerobes.

Treatment: After needle aspiration of the joint and collection of blood cultures, antibiotic treatment is based on the likely origin of the arthritis and the culture results. The dosage and duration of treatment are similar to that recommended for acute osteomyelitis and septicaemia. Irrigation of the joint with antibiotics is not usually necessary. Exceptionally, in resistant infections, systemic antibiotic therapy may be supplemented by intra-articular antibiotics given in the following concentrations:

gentamicin	0.5%	amikacin	0.25%
oxacillin	1.0%	amphotericin B	5 mg/ml

In prosthetic joint infection surgical drainage, antimicrobials for ≥6 weeks and retention of prosthesis are successful in 20–30%. In other cases removal of prosthesis, bactericidal antibiotics for 6 weeks and reimplantation succeed in nearly 30%.

References

DAN, M., Y. SIEGMAN-IGRA, S. PITLIK, R. RAZ: Oral ciprofloxacin treatment of Pseudomonas aeruginosa osteomyelitis. Antimicrob. Ag. Chemother. *34:* 849–850 (1990).
DELLAMONICA, P., E. BERNARD, H. ETESSE, R. GARRAFFO, H. B. DRUGEON: Evaluation of pefloxacin, ofloxacin and ciprofloxacin in the treatment of thirty-nine cases of chronic osteomyelitis. Europ. J. clin. Microbiol. Infect. Dis. *8:* 1024 (1989).
FASANO, F. J., D. R. GRAHAM, E. S. STAUFFER: Vertebral osteomyelitis secondary to Streptococcus agalactiae. Clin. Orthop. *256:* 101–104 (1990).
GENTRY, L. O.: Antibiotic therapy for osteomyelitis. Infect. Dis. Clin. North. Am. *4:* 485–499 (1990).
GENTRY, L. O., G. G. RODRIGUEZ: Oral ciprofloxacin compared with parenteral antibiotics in the treatment of osteomyelitis. Antimicrob. Ag. Chemother. *34:* 40–43 (1990).
MACGREGOR, R. R., A. L. GRAZIANI, J. L. ESTERHAI: Oral ciprofloxacin for osteomyelitis. Orthopedics. *13:* 55–60 (1990).
MADER, J. T. et al.: Oral ciprofloxacin compared with standard parenteral antibiotics therapy for chronic osteomyelitis in adults. J. Bone Joint Surg. [Am.] *73:* 104 (1990).
NORDEN, C. W. et al. Osteomyelitis. Infect. Dis. Clin. North Am. *4:* 361 (1990).
SCOTT, R. J., M. R. CHRISTOFERSEN, W. W. ROBERTSON: Acute osteomyelitis in children: a review of 116 cases. J. Pediatr. Orthop. *10:* 649–652 (1990).
WALDVOGEL, F. A.: Use of the quinolones for the treatment of osteomyelitis and septic arthritis. Rev. Infect. Dis. *11* (Suppl. 5): S1259 (1989).
WISPELWEY, B., W. M. SCHELD: Ciprofloxacin in the treatment of Staphylococcus aureus osteomyelitis. A review. Diagn. Microbiol. Infect. Dis. *13:* 169–171 (1990).

11. Gynaecological Infections

The general rules of antibacterial chemotherapy also apply to gynaecological and obstetric infections. During pregnancy, however, some antibiotics are potentially toxic to the fetus and others should be used only with caution (see p. 610). Deep infections of the female genital tract are potentially serious and are best treated with systemic antibiotics in high doses. Directed chemotherapy may be difficult to achieve because the causative organisms in pelvic infections may only be isolated in certain circumstances such as from curettings, pus or tissue obtained at operation, or blood culture. The more accessible superficial genital infections are often mixed, involving facultative pathogens, and material for culture fails to clarify which organism is the primary cause. Initial therapy may therefore have to be blind, and based on a knowledge of the frequency with which potential pathogens are found.

a) Bartholinitis

The commonest *causes* are Staphylococcus aureus and gonococci, with occasional mixed anaerobic infections.

Treatment should where possible be directed, and guided initially by a gram-stained film. When staphylococci are cultured or when no pathogen is found, a penicillinase-stable penicillin such as flucloxacillin, 2–3 g daily by mouth, should be given until the local symptoms resolve. Gonococcal infection should be treated with benzylpenicillin 2 g daily for at least 1 week. If the patient is allergic to penicillin or the strain produces β lactamase, alternatives are cefuroxime (which is also active against β-lactamase-producing strains, see p. 66) or ciprofloxacin. Incision and drainage may be necessary. Anaerobic infection (foul-smelling pus) should be treated with clindamycin or with ciprofloxacin + metronidazole.

b) Vulvitis

Treatment on the basis of culture results with local antibiotic preparations is usually sufficient. Systemic antibiotics are normally only necessary for deep infections such as abscesses, cellulitis or gangrene.

Infections with Candida albicans are relatively common and are treated with topical antifungals. Imidazoles such as clotrimazole, miconazole, econazole or isoconazole are suitable, as are nystatin, amphotericin B, pimaricin or ciclopiroxolamine. Underlying diseases such as diabetes mellitus, triggering factors such as ovulation inhibitors or broad-spectrum antibiotic therapy, skin diseases, senile vaginitis, allergies and venereal disease should also be considered.

c) Vulvovaginitis in Children

The *causative organisms* are occasionally gonococci but more frequently gardnerella, pneumococci, trichomonads and Candida albicans. Culture often yields intestinal bacteria, usually contaminants, and microscopic examination of a smear or wet preparation is more reliable. Herpetic vulvovaginitis is also not uncommon. Small blisters or ulcers are present on the labia minora, sometimes associated with bilateral painful inguinal lymphadenitis (for treatment see p. 446).

Treatment depends on the isolate. Culture-positive gonococcal infection should be treated with benzylpenicillin 0.5–1 g daily for 5 days, combined if necessary with an oestrogen (caution: risk of uterine bleeding) or, if penicillin-resistant, with cefuroxime (30 mg/kg daily). Ciprofloxacin, which is used for the treatment of gonococcal infection in adults, should not be used in children because of the risk of arthropathy. Infections with gardnerella, bacteroides or anaerobic cocci should be treated with oral metronidazole (7 mg/kg twice daily for 1 week), amoxycillin (25 mg/kg 3 times a day) or co-amoxiclav (25 mg/kg 3 times a day). Twice-daily baths using a mild soap are also helpful. Threadworm infestation should be treated with pyrantel or mebendazole (see 567) and hygienic measures (changing underwear, cutting fingernails short, treat all members of family). Infections with Trichomonas vaginalis are treated with oral metronidazole, tinidazole or ornidazole (see p. 428). The presence of a congenital or acquired rectovaginal fistula, or a foreign body in the vagina, should be excluded.

d) Vaginitis in Adults

Vaginitis is often combined with vulvitis, cervicitis or urethritis. Vaginal infections, whose principal symptom is a discharge, are often secondary to an underlying disease such as carcinoma, diabetes or hormonal imbalance. The investigation of an infection should therefore always include a search for the underlying cause. When the cause of the discharge is not apparent, syphilis, gonorrhoea and tuberculosis should be excluded. Some deodorant sprays and foreign bodies (tampons, pessaries) can cause contact vaginitis, and the postmenopausal physiological oestrogen deficiency predisposes to atrophic ("senile") vaginitis. Disruption of the normal vaginal flora (Lactobacillus acidophilus) allows potentially pathogenic bacteria to invade.

Vulvovaginitis, which is usually manifest as an increased discharge, burning or itching, dyspareunia and often dysuria as well, is of three principal types (Table 53), namely:

Table 53. Types and causes of vulvovaginitis in adults.

Type	Bacterial vaginosis (gardnerella, anaerobes)	Candida vaginitis (Candida species)	Trichomonas vaginitis (Trichomonas vaginalis)
Main symptoms	Pungent discharge ("amine vaginitis")	Severe itching (vulva), scanty, friable, odourless discharge	Profuse, thin or watery discharge (often foul-smelling)
Vulvitis	Uncommon	Frequent	Sometimes
Vaginal mucosa	Slight inflammation	Erythema with thick white coating	Erythema, sometimes with petechiae (cervix)
Vaginal pH	≥ 4.5	≤ 4.5	≥ 5.0
Amine odour (with 10% KOH)	Strong	Absent	Often present
Microscopy	Scanty granulocytes, scanty lactobacilli, numerous gram-negative cocci and bacilli	Moderate numbers of granulocytes and epithelial cells, and (in 80%) yeast buds and pseudomycelia	Moderate numbers of granulocytes, and motile trichomonads (in 80–90%)

1. Bacterial vaginosis;
2. Candida vaginitis;
3. Trichomonas vaginitis.

Since relapses are common with inappropriate treatment, the cause should always be established by clinical and microscopic investigations before treatment begins. Vaginal secretions are collected with a swab and spread on a slide. Two drops of 10% KOH solution are added and the wet preparation examined microscopically for cells, bacteria, fungi and trichomonads. A gram-stained smear will show to what extent the normal gram-positive lactobacilli have been replaced by gram-negative bacilli (gardnerella) and cocci. Bacterial vaginosis is not infrequently associated with trichomonas infection. Simultaneous treatment of the sexual partner is particularly important in trichomonas vaginitis.

Bacterial vaginosis (amine colpitis): This is also described as non-specific vaginitis or Gardnerella vaginitis. The vaginal secretions contain few or no lactobacilli and granulocytes, but numerous Gardnerella vaginalis (previously named Haemophilus vaginalis) in addition to non-sporing anaerobes (Bacteroides, anaerobic cocci) and curved motile rods (Mobiluncus). The desquamated epithelial cells are covered on their surface with bacteria and appear granulated ("clue cells"). When potassium hydroxide is added to the slide, a penetrating fishy odour develops which is due to amines and is particularly noticeable after coitus (because of the alkaline reaction of seminal fluid). The pH of the vaginal secretion, which can be readily tested with litmus paper, is higher than 4.5. The vaginal wall in bacterial vaginosis is uniformly covered with a greyish-white, non-viscous secretion and is only minimally inflamed. Vulvitis, with burning and pruritus, is usually absent.

Treatment (Table 54) with oral metronidazole (0.5 g twice daily for 7 days) eliminates Gardnerella vaginalis and the various anaerobes and promotes the recolonisation of the vagina with lactobacilli. During pregnancy the condition can be treated with amoxycillin or co-amoxiclav (0.5 g 3 times a day for 7 days), although these are less effective than metronidazole. Erythromycin and doxycycline are ineffective, as is local treatment with povidone iodine, sulphonamides or neomycin. Simultaneous treatment of the sexual partner is not necessary. Supportive treatment may be given with styli or pessaries containing lactic acid, or vaginal capsules containing freeze-dried viable lactobacilli. Relapse usually requires a further course of metronidazole if repeated investigations show no other cause for the discharge.

Candida vaginitis: A white, sometimes friable, odourless vaginal discharge, often accompanied by severe pruritus vulvae and dysuria. The vaginal pH is low (<4.5). A thick white coating covers the reddened vaginal mucosa. The yeasts can be shown microscopically in a methylene blue preparation as budding yeast cells and pseudomycelia, and can be cultured on Sabouraud's or malt agar or on a slide culture (Mycoslide).

Table 54. Treatment of gynaecological infections.

Disease	Treatment of choice	Treatment in pregnancy
Vulvovaginitis		
Bacterial vaginosis	Metronidazole (0.4 g orally twice daily for 7 days)	Amoxycillin (0.5 g orally 3 times a day for 7 days)
Candidosis	Clotrimazole (topically for 3–6 days)	Nystatin (topically)
Trichomoniasis	Metronidazole or tinidazole (2 g in a single oral dose)	Clotrimazole or natamycin (topically)
Cervicitis		
Chlamydial	Doxycycline (0.1 g orally twice a day for 14 days)	Erythromycin (0.5 g orally 4 times a day for 14 days)
Gonococcal (usually chlamydial also)	Cefoxitin or cefuroxime (2 g in a single i.v. or i.m. dose) + doxycycline (0.1 g orally twice a day for 14 days)	Cefoxitin or cefuroxime (2 g in a single i.v. or i.m. dose) + erythromycin (0.5 g orally 4 times a day for 14 days)
Herpes simplex primary	Acyclovir (0.2 g orally 5 times a day or 5 mg/kg i.v. 3 times a day for 5 days)	–
recurrent	Acyclovir (0.4 g orally twice daily, reduced to 0.2 g twice daily, interrupted every 6–12 months)	–
Salpingitis		
in hospital	Cefoxitin or cefuroxime (2 g i.v. 4 times a day for 14 days) + doxycycline (0.1 g orally twice a day for 14 days)	Cefoxitin or cefuroxime (2 g i.v. 4 times a day for 14 days) + erythromycin (0.5 g orally 4 times a day for 14 days)
out of hospital	Ceftriaxone (4 g every 24 h for 14 days) + doxycycline (0.1 g orally twice a day for 10–14 days)	Ceftriaxone (4 g every 24 h for 14 days) + erythromycin (0.5 g orally 4 times a day for 14 days)

Treatment: Locally with clotrimazole as vaginal tablets or cream, either as a single application or for 3–6 days, with simultaneous treatment of the vulva with an antimycotic skin cream. Alternatives are miconazole vaginal cream, econazole, ciclopiroxolamine and povidone iodine. When nystatin is used locally, applications are usually necessary twice daily for 2 weeks. Fluconazole may be used systemically for candida vaginitis, particularly in immunosuppressed patients. Single to short term therapy is possible but relapses are frequent. The sexual partner, who may have candida balanitis or urethritis, should be treated simultaneously. Factors which can predispose to candida infection (diabetes, pregnancy, oral contraceptives, AIDS and antibiotic therapy) should be considered.

Trichomonas vaginitis may be acute or chronic, symptomatic or asymptomatic. A profuse watery, often foul-smelling discharge is typical, sometimes accompanied by dysuria. The KOH test is positive (amine odour). The vaginal mucosa is red and inflamed, often with petechiae on the cervix, and the discharge may be frothy. The vigorously motile trichomonads can be best demonstrated microscopically in a wet preparation of fresh material on a pre-warmed slide, or in a smear stained with methylene blue. The organisms may be cultured in a special nutrient medium. Mixed infections with Gardnerella are not uncommon.

Treatment: Metronidazole 200 mg (adults), 100 mg (girls aged 6–12) or 50 mg (girls aged 2–5), all twice a day orally for 7 days, with no repeat course for 4–6 weeks. Single-dose therapy with tinidazole (2 g) or ornidazole (1.5 g) is also effective. The sexual partner should always be treated simultaneously; trichomonas urethritis in the male can be asymptomatic. Some infections are relatively resistant to metronidazole, in which case a repeat course with 2 g daily for 2 weeks is usually effective.

During the first few months of pregnancy oral nitroimidazoles should be avoided; alternatives are local treatment with clotrimazole or pimaricin pessaries (twice daily for 10 days).

Herpes simplex vulvovaginitis may be acute or chronically recurrent and in adults is usually due to herpes virus type 2. An extensive vesicular eruption which may ulcerate is found in the vagina and vulva and on the cervix and perineum. It is very painful, especially during micturition, and can cause urinary retention. During pregnancy there is a risk of miscarriage, premature delivery and neonatal death as a result of generalised herpes. When primary infection occurs within 14 days of term, elective caesarian section is advisable. A vaginal smear stained by the Papanicolaou method shows intranuclear inclusion bodies in multinucleate giant cells. Secondary infection can occur with bacteria or fungi.

Local *treatment* with povidone iodine (vulval toilet, vaginal gel and pessaries) is unreliable. Baths, compresses and a trial of acyclovir cream (0.5%) 1–2 times daily for 2–3 weeks are better. In severe cases (primary herpes simplex infection and immunological impairment), acyclovir can be given systemically in a dose of 0.2 g orally 5 times a day or 5 mg/kg i.v. 3 times a day for 5 days. Recurrences are usually less severe and of shorter duration.

e) Pelvic Inflammatory Disease

Infections of the cervix with chlamydia, gonococci and herpes simplex virus can give rise to severe complications. Progression to endometritis and salpingitis can result in ectopic pregnancy, infertility, premature rupture of the membranes, chorioamnionitis and puerperal sepsis. An aetiological diagnosis in cervicitis is therefore very important for successful treatment. Endocervical secretion containing numerous granulocytes is found almost exclusively in chlamydial infection. In gonorrhoea a gram-stained smear of cervical secretion will contain gram-negative diplococci. In herpes simplex cervicitis a smear stained by the Papanicolaou method contains multinucleate giant cells and epithelial cells with intranuclear inclusion bodies. Culture can be positive for gonococci or herpes simplex virus even when microscopy is negative. Double infections (chlamydia and gonococci) and mixed infections (of aerobic and anaerobic bacteria) are frequent. The demonstration of staphylococci, enterococci or intestinal bacteria in a cervical smear is usually of no pathogenic significance.

In *adnexitis, endometritis, parametritis and pelvo-peritonitis,* Chlamydia trachomatis, gonococci and anaerobic bacteria (streptococci, bacteroides, clostridia) are most commonly found. An aetiological diagnosis is often difficult and requires investigation of pus, material obtained at operation or laparoscopy, and blood culture.

Chlamydiae can be grown in cell culture from material obtained at operation or biopsy if sent in special transport medium. Culture is unreliable, however, and alternative, rapid tests include a commercial immunoassay and the microscopic detection of antigen by direct immunofluorescence of a smear (MikroTrak®).

Gonococci can be demonstrated by immunofluorescence, in a methylene blue or gram smear of cervical secretions or a urethral or rectal swab, or by prompt inoculation and culture on selective media (e.g. Thayer-Martin), if necessary after sending to the laboratory in Stuart's or Amies' transport medium.

Successful culture of anaerobic bacteria requires a suitable transport medium (e.g. Amies') or the prompt inoculation of material into an evacuated container (anaerobic culture bottle).

If tuberculosis is suspected, menstrual blood should be inoculated on to special media. Carcinoma should always be ruled out when the cause of a cervical discharge is not obvious.

Treatment of acute pelvic infections: The initial treatment of cervicitis, endometritis and/or salpingitis, when the cause is still not known, should be with an antibiotic combination with reliable activity against the commonest causes (chlamydiae, gonococci and anaerobes). A combination recommended by the Centers for Disease Control (CDC) in the USA is cefoxitin (or cefuroxime) + doxycycline; for dosage, see Table 54. Erythromycin may be used instead of doxycycline during pregnancy. Treatment for at least 14 days is generally necessary, preferably supervised in hospital. Clinical progress can also be monitored by ultrasound. If treatment has to be given on an outpatient basis, a cephalosporin active against gonococci and anaerobes should be given parenterally in high dosage. If sensitive gonococci are isolated, benzylpenicillin (6 g twice daily as a short i.v. infusion) may be used. An alternative (e.g. in penicillin or cephalosporin allergy) is imipenem (1 g twice daily i.v.) which is highly active against gonococci and anaerobes, in combination with doxycycline (against chlamydia). If pathogens other than chlamydiae, gonococci or anaerobes are found, the initial therapy may need to be corrected. In tubal or ovarian abscess, i.v. antibiotics for at least 2 weeks should be followed by oral treatment for 6–8 weeks because of the danger of relapse. Treatment with ofloxacin or ciprofloxacin covers both gonococci and chlamydiae.

In *post-abortal adnexitis,* infection with penicillin-resistant staphylococci should be considered; i.v. clindamycin is often effective here as well as against Bacteroides, but not against gonococci.

When local suppuration has occurred (pyosalpinx, ovarian or pelvic abscess), the chances of success with antibiotics alone are slight and operative drainage is necessary.

Chronic adnexitis may be due to tuberculosis, which should be treated with standard triple antituberculous therapy for 6–12 months.

f) Febrile Abortion

This infection is usually with mixed aerobic and anaerobic bacteria including Bacteroides fragilis, various enterobacteria, streptococci and enterococci. Clostridia, staphylococci and other bacteria are less common. Culture of blood, a cervical swab and placental tissue is important, but the results must be interpreted carefully. Even when only a single pathogen is isolated, the infection is often mixed. When spontaneous febrile abortion occurs in the middle trimester of pregnancy, infection with Listeria monocytogenes should be strongly suspected, and early confirmation may be given by direct examination of a gram-stained smear of aborted material.

High dose *antibiotic treatment* should be started as soon as possible. Mild cases may be treated initially with i.v. benzylpenicillin (6–18 g daily) which is effective against the particularly dangerous streptococci and clostridia. In more severe cases, particularly where the uterus has perforated or there are signs of peritonitis, treatment should also cover non-sporing anaerobes of the Bacteroides group and enterobacteria. Suitable combinations are imipenem + gentamicin or cefotaxime + gentamicin + metronidazole. If chlamydiae are present or suspected on account of antecedent sexually transmitted disease, doxycycline should be given for 2 weeks in addition. Ampicillin + gentamicin is the treatment of choice for maternal and neonatal listeriosis.

Antibiotics should be continued for at least 6–8 days after the patient has become afebrile and until all signs of local infection have resolved. Surgical measures such as curettage are often necessary. The control of shock and the prevention or treatment of anuria or coagulopathies are also vital. Tetanus hyperimmune globulin (250 I.U. i.m.) + active tetanus immunisation should be given after an artificially induced "back-street" abortion. In gas gangrene, for which the treatment of choice is benzylpenicillin, hyperbaric oxygen treatment in a high pressure chamber may be given, and heparin if diffuse intravascular coagulation develops (see p. 497).

Septic thrombophlebitis of the pelvic veins can occur with infected abortion and *post partum,* and is usually the result of a mixed infection with Bacteroides fragilis and anaerobic cocci. The treatment of choice is a combination of a cephalosporin + metronidazole, together with anticoagulant therapy.

Before performing a *termination of pregnancy,* gonorrhoea and chlamydial infection should be ruled out if at all possible; otherwise, the procedure must be carried out under appropriate antibiotic cover (see pp. 488 and 491).

In women with congenital or acquired heart defects all invasive procedures involving the internal genital tract must be carried out under the recommended prophylactic regime with ampicillin and gentamicin, or, if penicillin-allergic, vancomycin.

g) Puerperal Fever

The *causative organisms* are generally the same as for febrile abortion. Infections with β-haemolytic streptococci and clostridia (gas gangrene) are particularly dangerous. The portals of entry of these organisms are either the puerperal uterus, perineal wounds or the opened uterus after caesarian section. Mixed infections are the rule.

Antibiotic treatment is largely as for septic abortion, but antibiotics should always be given in high dosage because of the risk of fatal puerperal sepsis.

Any fever in the puerperium should give rise to suspicion of a puerperal infection; a swab of the lochia and of any purulent discharge, as well as blood cultures, should be taken, after which antibiotics should be commenced in high dosage (e.g. benzylpenicillin 6–12 g a day i.v. in 2–3 divided doses). Obstetric intravaginal manipulations can give rise to an infection with anaerobes and resistant staphylococci, for which broader spectrum treatment is necessary, e.g. with imipenem or with gentamicin + clindamycin.

When *puerperal sepsis* is suspected, very broad-spectrum treatment such as cefotaxime + gentamicin + metronidazole, or imipenem, is indicated. The maintenance of blood pressure and diuresis are important, as are surgical measures such as the drainage of abscesses, curettage and, in emergency, hysterectomy.

The *prophylactic use of antibiotics* after an uncomplicated delivery is not generally recommended, since it can encourage postpartum uterine infection with multi-resistant bacteria. Patients with heart valve abnormalities should, however, receive prophylaxis against endocarditis.

h) Mastitis

The *causative organisms* of puerperal mastitis are almost always staphylococci, and only exceptionally streptococci or other pyogenic bacteria. The bacteria are demonstrable first in the breast milk and later in pus from the abscess also. The usual portals of entry are fissures and cracks on the nipple.

Treatment should be started promptly with an antistaphylococcal antibiotic, such as oral flucloxacillin 3–4 g daily. Should the organism be sensitive to penicillin, however, benzylpenicillin is then still the treatment of choice. Patients allergic to penicillin or whose staphylococci are methicillin-resistant (MRSA) may be treated with clindamycin 1.2 g daily, fusidic acid 4 g daily (in combination with another antistaphylococcal agent), or erythromycin 2 g daily.

Antibiotic treatment alone will be effective only if started promptly and continued at full dosage for an adequate period of time. The initial treatment should therefore be parenteral at high dosage, and continued orally once the local signs of infection regress. If an abscess has already formed, antibiotics serve to prevent further extension and metastatic spread to distant septic foci. Other symptomatic measures which support antibiotic treatment include the suppression of lactation, binding of the breast in an elevated position and cold compresses, as well as incision or aspiration of an established abscess. A mother with mastitis should not allow her baby to feed from the inflamed breast because of the risk of transmission of infection to the child through pus and bacteria in the milk.

Opinions vary as to the prophylactic value of the local application of antibacterial skin preparations to the nipple. Strict hygienic measures in the delivery suite and maternity wards are, however, important preventive measures.

Mastitis of a non-lactating breast is less common and is usually caused by mixed anaerobic bacteria (bacteroides, peptostreptococci), for which clindamycin, cefoxitin or metronidazole are the best choices. An underlying tumour of the lactiferous ducts is occasionally the cause.

i) Pyrexia During Labour

If signs of chorioamnionitis occur after premature rupture of the membranes or if any fever of uncertain origin develops during labour, antibiotic treatment is indicated.

The *range of causative organisms* is largely as found in febrile abortion, with the addition of group B streptococci and listeria.

Treatment should be with antibiotics that readily cross the placenta, enter the fetal circulation and pass through the fetal urinary tract to achieve adequate concentrations in the amniotic fluid. Penicillins and cephalosporins have this property, and they may be present in much higher concentrations in amniotic fluid than in the fetal blood. An active, well tolerated combination with a broad spectrum of activity is azlocillin or piperacillin + cefotaxime, all of which can be given in high dosage to the mother. Because of the possibility of bacterial resistance, blood cultures should be taken from the newborn baby immediately after delivery and the blood count monitored, so that if necessary the baby can be treated without delay with a combination of azlocillin or piperacillin + cefotaxime (or gentamicin). If the mother develops septicaemia, which may be accompanied by shock and a consumption coagulopathy, treatment should be with the same agents as given to the baby and according to the sensitivities of the bacteria isolated.

j) Pyelonephritis During Pregnancy

Urinary infections are common in pregnancy, and the *causative organisms* are similar to those of uncomplicated urinary infections in the non-pregnant woman. Escherichia coli is still the commonest bacterial cause. A mid-stream urine should always be investigated by bacterial culture and sensitivity testing. Because of the risk of relapse, treatment should be given for at least one week. The choice of antibiotic (see p. 423) must take into account the possibility of toxicity to the fetus (see p. 425).

The *treatment* of choice is a penicillin or cephalosporin. Co-trimoxazole, quinolones, aminoglycosides and tetracyclines should be avoided. If significant bacteriuria is repeatedly found in pregnancy, the patient should be treated even if asymptomatic, since acute pyelonephritis may otherwise develop.

k) Toxic Shock Syndrome

The staphylococcal toxic shock syndrome is based on the formation of a *special toxin by Staphylococcus aureus* (TSST-1). The disease occurs in people who have a deficiency of specific antitoxin in their serum, and is commonest at the end of menstruation in teenage girls and young women who use tampons. The condition occurs less fequently in non-menstruating women, in younger children and in men with a TSST-1-producing staphylococcal infection on their skin or mucous membranes (e.g. postoperatively). Women with vaginitis, *post partum*, or who are using pessaries are also at risk.

The *diagnosis* is first made clinically. The disease is characterised by the sudden onset of a high fever, abdominal pain, vomiting, diarrhoea, a generalised rash resembling that of scarlet fever, hypotension and hypovolaemic shock (as a result of severe intravascular and extravascular fluid loss) and functional disturbance of several organs, with an increase in serum creatinine, bilirubin and transaminases, impaired consciousness, thrombocytopenia, muscle weakness and increase in creatine kinase. Hypocalcaemia, hypophosphataemia, hypokalaemia and disseminated intravascular coagulation are also usually present. The typical coarse, flaky desquamation of the skin, particularly on the hands and feet, first appears 1–2 weeks after the onset of the illness. Toxin-producing strains of staphylococci can be isolated from the vagina and sometimes also from lesions on other areas of the skin and mucous membranes; their identification usually requires the facilities of a reference laboratory. Bacteraemia is very unusual in this condition. The *differential diagnosis* includes septic shock, scarlet fever, Kawasaki syndrome, exfoliative dermatitis (Lyell's syndrome), drug rashes, measles, endometritis, salpingitis, and septic abortion.

Treatment: Fluid and electrolyte replacement and the treatment of shock lung, acute renal failure, cardiac failure and consumption coagulopathy are all urgent. Antibiotic treatment with flucloxacillin 4 g daily i.v. or cefazolin 4 g daily i.v., followed by oral cephradine, cephalexin or another oral antistaphylococcal agent for a further week, all have no effect on the course of the disease, but reduce the relapse rate from 60% to less than 1%. Women who have recovered from the toxic shock syndrome should no longer use tampons. Frequent changing of tampons is not in itself sufficient to protect susceptible women from this condition.

References

Austin, T. W., E. A. Smith, R. Darwish et al.: Metronidazole in a single dose for the treatment of trichomoniasis. Failure of a 1 g single dose. Brit. J. Vener. Dis. *58:* 121 (1982).

Balsdon, M. J.: Gardnerella vaginalis and its clinical syndrome. Eur. J. Clin. Microbiol. *1:* 288–293 (1982).

Bardi, M., G. Manenti, D. Mattioni, L. Lasala: Metronidazole for non-specific vaginitis. Lancet *1:* 1029–1030 (1980).

Blackwell, A. L., I. Phillips, A. R. Fox, D. Barlow: Anaerobic vaginosis (non-specific vaginitis): Clinical, microbiological, and therapeutical findings. Lancet *17:* 1379 (1983).

Brammer, K. W.: A comparison of single-dose oral fluconazole with 3-day intravaginal clotrimazole in the treatment of vaginal candidiasis. Br. J. Obstet. Gynaecol. *96:* 226–232 (1989).

BRIGGS, G. G., P. AMBROSE, M. P. NAGEDOTTE: Gentamicin dosing in postpartum women with endometritis. Am. J. Obstet. Gynecol. *160:* 309–313 (1989).
GALL, A. A., L. CONSTANTINE: Comparative evaluation of clindamycin versus clindamycin plus tobramycin in the treatment of acute pelvic inflammatory disease. Obstet. Gynecol. *75:* 282–286 (1990).
HUNTER, J. M., R. G. SOMMERVILLE: Erythromycin stearate in treating chlamydial infections of the cervix. Brit. J. Vener. Dis. *60:* 387–389 (1984).
LEDGER, W. J.: Selection of antimicrobial agents for treatment of infections of the female genital tract. Rev. Infec. Dis. *5:* 98 (1983).
LIVENGOOD, C. H., J. L. THOMASON, G. B. HILL: Bacterial vaginosis: diagnostic and pathogenetic findings during topical clindamycin therapy. Am. J. Obstet. Gynecol. *163:* 515–520 (1990).
LOSSICK, J. G.: Treatment of sexually transmitted vaginosis/vaginitis. Rev. Infect. Dis. *12,* Suppl. 6: S665–S681 (1990).
MARDH, P. A.: Treatment of pelvic inflammatory disease and related matters. J. Antimicrob. Chemother. *25:* 729–731 (1990).
MARTENS, M. G., S. FARO, H. A. HAMMILL et al.: Sulbactam/ampicillin versus metronidazole/gentamicin in the treatment of postcesarean sectio endometritis. Diagn. Microbiol. Infect. Dis. *12* (4 Suppl.): 189S–194S (1989).
MONIF, G. R.: Infectious Diseases in Obstetrics and Gynecology. 3rd. edition. Raven Press, New York 1992.
SIMON, C., D. SCHRÖDER, D. WEISNER, M. BRÜCK, U. KRIEG: Bacteriological Findings After Premature Rupture of the Membranes. Arch. Gynecol. Obstet. *244:* 69–74 (1989).

12. Eye Infections

The antibiotic treatment of eye infections requires a detailed knowledge of ophthalmology. Acute conjunctivitis is not the only cause of red eye, and a full ophthalmological examination together with identification of the causative organism (bacterial, viral, fungal or protozoal) are essential if the infection is to be rapidly cured.

Diagnosis of eye infections: Cases of neonatal, pseudomembranous and chronic conjunctivitis, corneal inflammation, orbital cellulitis and endophthalmitis should always be investigated by microscopy and culture. A conjunctival smear is best made from a sterile calcium alginate or dacron swab moistened with physiological saline. In order to avoid contamination from the lid margins and eyelashes, the swab is wiped once along the length of the lower conjunctival sac and if possible plated immediately on to special media, or else put in suitable transport medium (e.g. Stuart's or Amies') for prompt dispatch to the bacteriological laboratory. A smear should be made at the time for gram and giemsa staining. Special transport media should be used for chlamydial culture (e.g. saccharose phosphate broth) and viral culture, or special slides prepared for rapid chlamydial immunofluorescence (MikroTrak®), fixed or air-dried, and sent as rapidly as possible to the laboratory.

The cellular picture seen in the giemsa preparation gives a pointer as to the cause. Neutrophil granulocytes are predominant in bacterial and fungal infections, lymphocytes in viral infections, and a mixture of lymphocytes and granulocytes in chlamydial infections. Eosinophils predominate in allergic conjunctivitis. In corneal ulcers that are infected with bacteria or fungi, the ophthalmologist should collect ulcer material with a special scraper and inoculate immediately on to culture media and microscope slides.

Systemic treatment with antibiotics is indicated in all severe bacterial infections of the outer eye (e.g. gonococcal conjunctivitis, corneal ulceration etc.) and in intraocular or orbital infections which are inaccessible to local treatment. Antibiotics diffuse at different rates from the blood into the various parts of the eye, with the poorest concentrations in the bradytrophic tissues of the cornea, lens and vitreous body. Treatment of intraocular infections must overcome the barriers between blood and the aqueous humor and between blood and the vitreous body.

Chloramphenicol is a particularly suitable agent for the treatment of many eye infections and achieves an intra-ocular concentration that is 50% of its serum concentration. Sulphonamides vary according to the preparation, but achieve some 40–80% of serum concentrations intra-ocularly, oxytetracycline and tetracycline about 15–20%, benzylpenicillin, ampicillin, gentamicin and tetracycline about 10%. Thus exceptionally high doses of antibiotic are necessary to achieve an adequate intraocular concentration; examples are benzylpenicillin 6–12 g, ampicillin 10 g, chloramphenicol 3 g. Cefotaxime and metronidazole penetrate the eye relatively well. The barrier between blood and the aqueous humor may be more permeable in the infected eye, enabling even higher concentrations to be achieved.

Local treatment may be given by external application, subconjunctival and retrobulbar injection, and by direct injection into the anterior chamber or vitreous body.

External application is usually adequate for the treatment of bacterial infections of the conjunctiva and cornea. The ability of an antibiotic to penetrate the anterior parts of the eye depends on its solubility not only in water but also in lipids, since the corneal epithelium is rich in lipids and presents a barrier to lipid-insoluble drugs. Most sulphonamides and antibiotics diffuse through the intact cornea in minimal quantities, if at all, though corticosteroids and isoniazid penetrate more readily. Epithelial lesions and changes in the lipid barrier, e.g. through iontophoresis, allow some drugs to penetrate more deeply, but they never pass the ciliary body by this route.

When giving antibiotics externally, an isotonic solution or ointment in a suitable base is applied to the conjunctival sac. *Ointments* remain in the eye longer than solutions (eye drops) and they are more stable; however, they may impair vision, cause contact dermatitis more frequently than solutions, and may inhibit corneal epithelial mitosis, which is not usually affected by eye drops. It is sometimes practical to use eye drops by day and eye ointment at night. The addition of hemicellulose to eye drops increases their viscosity and prolongs their retention time. Since treatment will only be effective if the antibiotic is present in adequate concentrations for long periods, the drug must be given regularly at short intervals. Eye drops should be given every 15 min initially, then every 2 h, whereas an eye ointment should first be used every 1–2 h, then every 4 h. It may be practical to give eye drops by day and ointment overnight; this will also soften crusts which cause the lids and eye lashes to adhere together when the patient is asleep. Eye baths can be used several time a day for 10–30 min. When the cornea is inflamed or oedematous, the antibiotic may penetrate into the aqueous humor.

Subconjunctival injection may be given by the ophthalmologist for certain corneal and anterior chamber infections, and permits antibiotics to diffuse through the sclera into the anterior chamber of the eye. Thus a high antibiotic concentration can be achieved in the aqueous humor for several hours. This is especially useful in intra-ocular infections, keratitis, serpiginous keratitis and blennorrhoea. Once or twice a day, 0.3–0.5 ml of an antibiotic solution containing e.g. benzylpenicillin 180–300 mg or gentamicin 20 mg is injected, in general for not longer than 3 days.

The subconjunctival injection of benzylpenicillin once a day is relatively well-tolerated but painful, and often gives rise to an inflammatory reaction which limits the number of injections that can be given. Pain associated with subconjunctival injection can be minimised by the injection 5 min beforehand of 0.1 to 0.2 ml of 2% lignocaine or a longer-acting anaesthetic (e.g. bupivacaine) into the subconjunctival space. For certain infections, other antibiotics may be injected subconjunctivally, such as ampicillin (50 mg), piperacillin (50 mg), methicillin (50 mg), cefazolin (50 mg), amikacin (25 mg), gentamicin and tobramycin (10–20 mg), amphotericin B (0.05–0.1 mg), miconazole (5 mg) or isoniazid (10–20 mg). The subconjunctival injection of amphotericin B can cause persistent yellow discoloration of the conjunctiva; at higher doses (>5 mg), red nodules can develop, which gradually regress after treatment has been stopped.

The **retrobulbar injection** of an antibiotic in severe intraorbital infections is used to attain an adequate antibiotic concentration in the retrobulbar space and around the optic nerve. Higher intraocular concentrations are attained than after subconjunctival injection. This form of treatment should always be complemented with high i.v. doses of the same antibiotic.

Direct **injection into the anterior chamber** of the eye not infrequently damages the lens or cornea, and should only be used in exceptional circumstances.

Injection into the vitreous body may be indicated in endophthalmitis.

Choice of antibiotic for local treatment: For eye infections which tend to resolve spontaneously, such as most cases of conjunctivitis, bacterial culture and sensitivities are not essential. When a trial of treatment of conjunctivitis fails, however, cultures and sensitivity tests should be performed. In severe eye infections such as corneal ulceration and endophthalmitis, an attempt should always be made to establish a bacteriological diagnosis; if this fails, the clinical picture may give some clues. Central corneal ulcers, for example, are often due to pneumococci, other streptococci or pseudomonas. If the initial treatment does not produce an improvement in 2–3 days, a different antibiotic should be tried.

There is a range of empirically formulated local preparations which do not always fulfil the criteria of true chemotherapy. In principle, only single substances in precisely formulated vehicles with well-tolerated, fully declared preservatives should be used. Preparations should always be sterile when used, and presentation in single-use containers is also important.

Aminoglycosides such as gentamicin, tobramycin, neomycin, kanamycin and framycetin, which are active against staphylococci, Proteus and other enterobacteria, are suitable for local treatment. Gentamicin and tobramycin are well-tolerated as drops or ointment and have a broad spectrum of action, but little activity against pneumococci and none against chlamydiae. Neomycin gives rise not infrequently to allergic reactions. Local preparations containing chloramphenicol or tetracycline are only bacteriostatic, but rarely cause sensitisation and have proved effective in practice. Eye drops and ointment containing rifampicin are active against staphylococci and chlamydia, but can give rise to secondary resistance and are not currently available in Britain. Tetracycline hydrochloride 1% eye drops or ointment should be used to treat chlamydial conjunctivitis; regular use for long periods (6 weeks to 6 months) is necessary for the treatment of trachoma. Eye drops containing fusidic acid 1% in a gel which liquefies on contact with the eye have recently been introduced. Ophthalmic preparations containing quinolones, which have a broad spectrum and good diffusion properties, are available in several countries.

Polymyxin B is active only against Pseudomonas aeruginosa and other gram-negative bacilli, and occasionally causes allergy. Some eye ointments and drops contain combinations such as gramicidin + neomycin + polymyxin B, gramicidin + neomycin, polymyxin B + bacitracin, and polymyxin B + trimethoprim. Tyrothricin, which is only active against gram-positive bacteria, is available as an eye ointment in some countries but not Britain. Erythromycin eye ointment (0.5%) is used in the USA, particularly for the prophylaxis and treatment of chlamydial ophthalmitis in the newborn.

Topical natamycin (pimaricin) can be used to treat candida infections. Ocular preparations of miconazole and amphotericin B (Table 55) are only available in specialist centres, to which all patients with fungal infections of the eye should be referred. There are various high-concentration sulphonamide-containing eye

Table 55. Concentration of antimicrobials for topical use in the eye.

Drug	Eye drops or ointment	Subconjunctival injection
Amikacin	0.5%	25 mg
Ampicillin	–	50–100 mg
Bacitracin	300 units/g (or ml)	–
Benzylpenicillin	–	300 mg
Chloramphenicol	0.4–1%	100 mg
Cefazolin	–	50–100 mg
Clindamycin	–	15 mg
Erythromycin	0.5%	–
Fusidic acid	1%	–
Gentamicin	0.3%	10–20 mg
Gramicidin	0.025%	–
Kanamycin	0.5%	30 mg
Neomycin	0.5%	–
Oxacillin	–	100 mg
Piperacillin	–	50–100 mg
Polymyxin B	0.1–0.2%	5 mg
Sulphacetamide	10%	–
Tetracycline	0.5–1%	–
Tobramycin	0.3%	10–20 mg
Tyrothricin	0.06%	–
Amphotericin B	0.5%	0.05–0.1 mg
Miconazole	1%	5 mg
Natamycin (pimaricin)	1%	–
Nystatin	100000 units/g (or ml)	–
Acyclovir	3% (ointment)	–
Idoxuridine	0.1%	–
Trifluridine	2% (ointment) 1% (drops)	–
Tromantadine	1% (ointment)	–
Vidarabine	3% (ointment)	–

drops which are still sometimes used to treat trachoma in the tropics, although tetracycline is preferred. Sulphacetamide should no longer be used topically to treat eye infections, since it is rarely of any value. Because of the risk of sensitisation, penicillin eye drops and ointment have been withdrawn. Preparations containing silver have a disinfectant action, but should only be given for short periods because of the risk of silver deposition.

Preparations for topical use which are active against herpes simplex virus include idoxuridine (see p. 295), trifluridine (see p. 296), tromantadine and vidarabine (see p. 292). Interferon α (see p. 298) protects against recurrence of herpes simplex and may be used topically in the eye at the same time as a virustatic agent.

Possible side-effects of topical antimicrobial treatment:
1. Irritation of the eye may occur when the concentration in the solution is too high, when large crystals are present in the ointment, when there is a shift in pH or when the drops or ointment have become contaminated with pseudomonas, proteus, other bacteria, fungi or viruses.
2. Allergic reactions, particularly to penicillin, streptomycin and sulphonamides, may develop as eczema or oedema of the eyelid, conjunctivitis or, in the case of systemic treatment, a systemic response. The sensitising factor is frequently the preservative.
3. Post-antibiotic keratoconjunctivitis after topical therapy may be caused by Pseudomonas aeruginosa, staphylococci or fungi (e.g. Candida albicans). Glucocorticoids in some antibiotic eye drops or ointments can also predispose to fungal infection (e.g. mycotic keratitis) or activate a latent herpes simplex infection, which is recognisable in its early stages only with the aid of a slit lamp. Since corticosteroids are contraindicated in superficial keratitis caused by herpes simplex and in corneal epithelial defects, antibiotic-containing eye drops or ointments which contain corticosteroids should only be prescribed by an ophthalmologist after a full examination.

a) Lid Infections

Blepharitis: Ulcerating blepharitis is usually caused by staphylococci or streptococci. Angular blepharitis is often associated with infection by Moraxella. Secondary bacterial infections often occur in eczematous dermatitis of the lids and in chronic seborrhoeic blepharitis. Mites and lice should be ruled out as causes. Viral infections of the lids (herpes simplex, herpes zoster, molluscum contagiosum, papovaviruses) require special treatment.

Locally: First remove crusts with warm compresses moistened with physiological saline or olive oil. If ulceration has occurred, give gentamicin or neomycin + bacitracin eye ointment.

Systemically: For severe infections use flucloxacillin, or benzylpenicillin if causative organisms sensitive. Moraxella infection responds best to doxycycline.

External hordeolum (stye involving sebaceous glands in the lid margin) and **internal hordeolum** (stye of the Meibomian glands in the tarsal plate) are usually caused by Staphylococcus aureus. Orbital cellulitis may occur, and there is a risk of thrombosis of the angular vein.

Locally: Warm compresses or dry heat. If the abscess does not perforate spontaneously, incision may be necessary. Local preparations are usually ineffective.

Systemically (for internal styes): flucloxacillin or erythromycin.

Chalazion is a chronic granulomatous inflammation of the meibomian glands and is sometimes due to secondary infection.
Locally: operative removal when the infection has subsided.

Abscess and **cellulitis of the lid** are usually caused by staphylococci, and less frequently by streptococci, haemophilus or anaerobes. They occur after trauma, by direct spread from pyogenic infection of the paranasal sinuses or local osteomyelitis, or very occasionally as a septic metastasis. There is a risk of orbital cellulitis or of septic thrombosis of the orbital veins.
Locally: Incision (by an ophthalmologist) if necessary.
Systemically: Flucloxacillin or cefazolin (according to the causative organism and its sensitivities). In cases of septicaemia a broad-spectrum agent such as imipenem (see p. 103) should be used.

Furuncle of the lid is caused by staphylococci and carries a risk of thrombophlebitis of the orbital veins and of meningitis.
Systemic treatment is as for a furuncle of the nose or lip (see p. 479), e.g. with flucloxacillin or cefazolin.

Erysipelas of the lid is caused by Streptococcus pyogenes.
Systemically: Benzylpenicillin (see erysipelas, p. 479).

Mycosis of the skin of the lid should be treated according to the fungal cause with local preparations which are tolerated by the eye (see Table 55). Candida infection sometimes leaves an ulcer on the lid margin, which has small granulomas on the edge of the ulcer.

Herpes simplex virus infections of the lid give rise to small blisters with an umbilicated centre, which often occurs on the lips as well. All cases should be examined by an ophthalmologist in order to localise the infection precisely and check whether there is corneal involvement.
Topical treatment to protect the conjunctiva and cornea: acyclovir eye ointment every 4 h. Secondary bacterial infection should be treated with e.g. polymyxin + bacitracin eye ointment. Steroids are *contraindicated*.
Systemically: Treat severe cases with acyclovir 5 mg/kg 3 times daily in short i.v. infusions for 5 days.

Dacryoadenitis: Acute infection associated with infectious diseases such as mumps, or spreading from nearby infections caused by staphylococci, streptococci, Klebsiella pneumoniae etc. Chronic infection can occur in leukaemia, lymphogranulomatosis, tuberculosis, syphilis and trachoma.
Treatment: Moist or dry warm compresses and, in the case of bacterial infection, systemic treatment with flucloxacillin for staphylococci and guided by sensitivity results for other bacteria. Chronic infections should be treated according to their cause. When insufficient tears are formed, artificial tears may be used.

Dacryocystitis (inflammation of the lacrimal sac) may be acute or chronic. *Cause:* obstruction to the outflow of tears, with secondary infection due to pneumococci, streptococci, staphylococci, Candida albicans etc. In the newborn, stenosis of the nasolacrimal duct is a frequent underlying cause of dacryocystitis, and carries a risk of abscess formation or cellulitis of the lacrimal gland which may discharge to the exterior and form a fistula. In chronic dacryocystitis, rule out tuberculosis, syphilis and trachoma. Infection of the nasolacrimal duct (canaliculitis) is sometimes caused by Actinomyces israeli or nocardia; in actinomycosis, typical "sulphur" granules can be seen in the pus which can be expressed from the characteristically hyperaemic, pouting punctum on the inner margin of the lower lid.

Topically: Once the acute infection has subsided, the obstruction to flow should be removed by an ophthalmologist, irrigating if necessary with an antibiotic solution according to the causative organism. When an abscess has formed, incision may be necessary, but carries the risk of fistula formation. Chronic dacryocystitis may be treated by dacryocystorhinostomy.

Systemically: For the acute infection, benzylpenicillin, cefazolin or cefotaxime according to the causative organism.

Orbital cellulitis: Spreading infection of the orbital or periorbital tissue from a suppurative blepharitis, dacryocystitis, sinusitis, osteomyelitis of the jaw or dental root abscess. Haematogenous spread secondary to septicaemia also occurs. Typical symptoms of orbital cellulitis are protrusion of the eye, restricted eye movement, reduced corneal sensitivity and blurred vision. A wide range of organisms may be involved, including anaerobes of dental origin, and zygomycetes (= Mucor) in diabetics and immunosuppressed patients. Haemophilus type b and pneumococci are frequently found in blood culture, and the serum and urine latex agglutination tests for these organisms may then be positive.

Treatment: Operative drainage and removal of the cause. Treatment guided by the isolate or "blind" with cefotaxime + clindamycin or with imipenem.

b) Conjunctival Infections

There are many infectious and non-infectious causes of conjunctivitis. Every case should be examined by slit-lamp for corneal changes (foreign body, injury or ulcer). A red eye may also be due to iridocyclitis or acute glaucoma. Antibiotic drops or ointment containing steroids should never be used before herpes simplex infection has been excluded by examination with a slit-lamp.

The *commonest infective causes* of conjunctivitis are pneumococci, staphylococci, haemophilus and adenoviruses. Isolates of Staphylococcus epidermidis, Sarcina sp., saprophytic corynebacteria ("diphtheroids"), viridans streptococci, Branhamella etc. are all commensal flora and normally of no pathogenic significance.

Acute bacterial conjunctivitis is usually associated with an exudate (serous, mucopurulent or frankly purulent) and often resolves spontaneously.

Causative organisms include pneumococci, staphylococci, Streptococcus pyogenes, haemophilus, proteus, Escherichia coli, Pseudomonas aeruginosa, gonococci, meningococci and moraxella. Effective antibiotics will shorten the course of the infection. An acute, non-purulent, *follicular* conjunctivitis is caused either by chlamydiae (see inclusion conjunctivitis and trachoma) or by adenoviruses (or other viruses). Follicular conjunctivitis can also occur in infections of the lid margin with herpes simplex virus (for treatment, see p. 459).

Topically: Eye drops or ointment containing chloramphenicol, gentamicin, neomycin + bacitracin, gramicidin + neomycin + polymyxin B, and, for chlamydial follicular conjunctivitis, tetracycline.

Systemically: Systemic antibiotics should always be given in severe purulent conjunctivitis to reduce the risk of complications. For pneumococci, streptococci, gonococci and meningococci, use benzylpenicillin; for staphylococci, use flucloxacillin; for haemophilus, use amoxycillin, co-amoxiclav, cefaclor or cefuroxime; for pseudomonas, use azlocillin or tobramycin; for enterobacteria or resistant gonococci, use cefotaxime, ceftazidime, aztreonam, or a quinolone (except in children).

Conjunctival diphtheria: Give diphtheria antitoxin and benzylpenicillin, as for other forms of diphtheria (see p. 370). A pseudomembranous conjunctivitis is also found in infections with certain adenoviruses and with Streptococcus pyogenes.

Topically: Gentamicin eye drops or ointment.

Neonatal conjunctivitis (ophthalmia neonatorum) may be catarrhal or purulent. Infection can occur before, during or after birth, and is associated *(ante partum)* with premature rupture of the membranes. *Causative organisms* include staphylococci, streptococci, pneumococci, gonococci, Escherichia coli, Pseudomonas aeruginosa and Chlamydia trachomatis (inclusion conjunctivitis). A bacteriological examination will make the distinction from chemical conjunctivitis due to silver nitrate drops ("silver catarrh"), in which the pus is sterile. Infections with herpes simplex virus can also occur in the neonate, and are difficult to distinguish from other forms of conjunctivitis.

Topically: Bacterial infections (excluding chlamydial) should be treated with chloramphenicol, gentamicin, neomycin + bacitracin, or gramicidin + neomycin + polymyxin B eye drops or ointment.

Systemic treatment guided by sensitivity tests is necessary in severe bacterial infections. For "blind" therapy, give i.v. cefotaxime (which includes activity against gonococci), possibly with azlocillin (active against pseudomonas).

Prophylaxis: The recommendations of the American Academy of Pediatrics for the prophylaxis of gonococcal ophthalmia of the newborn in the USA include, in addition to 1% silver nitrate solution, 1% tetracycline or 0.5% erythromycin eye ointment which, when used from the first day of life, can also prevent chlamydial conjunctivitis (inclusion blennorrhoea). For this purpose a single piece of ointment 0.5–1 cm long is applied once into each conjunctival sac. Only single-dose containers are permissible, using a fresh one for each child. If the mother has gonorrhoea, the newborn baby should be given as prophylaxis cefuroxime or cefotaxime (single dose of 100 mg i. v. or i. m.).

Gonococcal ophthalmia in the newborn or adult carries the risk of corneal involvement and blindness. Gonococci may be demonstrated in a methylene blue- or gram-stained smear of pus and on culture. Credé's 1% silver nitrate prophylaxis (1 drop in each conjunctival sac) gives more effective prophylaxis than penicillin drops, but still fails in 0.1–0.2% of cases. Treatment should be started as soon as the condition is suspected clinically, to give the best chance of full recovery without residual corneal scarring.

Topically: Irrigation, compresses, chloramphenicol or gentamicin eye drops or ointment. Protect the healthy eye.

Systemic treatment should be started without delay, with cefuroxime or cefotaxime 60 mg/kg (neonates) or 2–6 g (adults) i. v. daily for 7 days. If the isolate is known to be sensitive, benzyl penicillin 240 mg (neonates) or 6 g (adults) i. v. daily for 7 days may be used.

Inclusion conjunctivitis (blennorrhoea) in the newborn, children and adults is caused by transfer of Chlamydia trachomatis from the genitalia or birth canal and gives rise to a mucopurulent exudate. The onset in the newborn is usually 5–7 days after birth but can be later, up to 4 weeks. Typical basophilic cytoplasmic inclusion bodies are seen in the epithelial cells in a giemsa-stained smear, fluoresce brightly with immunofluorescence, and grow in cell culture in 2–3 days. Spontaneous healing usually occurs in a few weeks or months, and this period is shortened by chemotherapy, although late changes or development of chronic keratoconjunctivitis can occur. Chlamydial pneumonitis can develop in children aged 1–6 months who have not been treated with systemic erythromycin at the same time.

Topically: Tetracycline eye ointment 6 times a day for at least 2 weeks.

Systemically: Supplementary doxycycline in adults and older children, and erythromycin 50 mg/kg/d in the newborn for at least 3 weeks.

Trachoma: Infection with Chlamydia trachomatis of a serotype different from that found in temperate countries. The various stages are acute catarrhal discharge, granular follicles on the conjunctiva, corneal lesions, pannus formation, blindness, deformation of the eyelids and frequently secondary infection with staphylococci and other bacteria. Inclusion bodies in the epithelial cells can be shown by giemsa staining. The traditional *drugs of choice* for both treatment and prophylaxis have been sulphonamides, which are initially given both topically and systemically. Tetracyclines (e. g. doxycycline), erythromycin, rifampicin and chloramphenicol are also effective. In older children and adults systemic treatment should be given for at least 3 weeks, because topical treatment alone is not sufficient. Because of the danger of relapse, topical therapy should be given over a longer period, e.g. twice daily for 2 months or, in difficult circumstances, twice daily for 5 days in each month for 6 months. The complications of trachoma, such as entropion, trichiasis and corneal leukoma, also require appropriate treatment.

Adenovirus conjunctivitis (epidemic keratoconjunctivitis), occurring alone or in association with pharyngoconjunctival fever, is a follicular conjunctivitis with preauricular lymphadenopathy. Adenoviruses types 8 and 19 can also give rise to pseudomembrane formation and subepithelial infiltration of the cornea. A stained smear contains small intranuclear inclusion bodies and numerous mononuclear cells. Most cases heal spontaneously after 3–4 weeks.

Topical and systemic treatment: Antibiotics have no effect. Treatment is symptomatic with cold compresses and anti-inflammatory eye drops. Topical steroids may be used at the discretion of an ophthalmologist to reduce corneal infiltration.

Chronic bacterial conjunctivitis is frequently caused by staphylococci or Moraxella and is often manifest as blepharoconjunctivitis. It can also arise as a result of the use of infected eye drops or cosmetics, or be secondary to rosacea or stenosis of the nasolacrimal duct. Treat topically with neomycin + bacitracin eye ointment, and in rosacea give supplementary doxycycline 0.1 g daily. Tetracycline eye ointment is effective against moraxella. Chronic mucopurulent conjunctivitis can be due to chlamydiae.

c) Corneal Infections

Corneal ulcers and hypopyon: *Causative organisms* are pneumococci, pseudomonas, staphylococci, streptococci and enterobacteria. Mixed infections are common. Fungi (e.g. Candida albicans, aspergillus, fusarium) can cause a central corneal ulcer. Bacterial keratitis (e.g. with Pseudomonas aeruginosa) develops not infrequently as a result of contaminated contact lenses. Culture of exudate from the ulcer will usually yield the causative organism, and antibiotic sensitivities are important for treatment. Severe complications (e.g. secondary glaucoma) can occur, and the condition should always be managed by an ophthalmologist, who can determine what other measures are necessary. Systemic antibiotics are always needed, should be started promptly without awaiting bacteriological results, and should include all the common causative organisms.

Topically: Gramicidin + neomycin + polymyxin B, neomycin + bacitracin, or gentamicin (except in streptococcal or pneumococcal infection). Deep ulcers with hypopyon may require the subconjunctival injection of benzylpenicillin or another antibiotic by an ophthalmologist (see p. 455). Topical amphotericin B, miconazole or pimaricin (natamycin) may be used for fungal infection (see Table 55); if a subconjunctival antifungal is required, miconazole (5 mg) is tolerated best.

Systemically: Initial treatment with cefotaxime or imipenem. If pneumococci, streptococci or sensitive staphylococci are isolated, high-dose benzylpenicillin may be used. Flucloxacillin, cefazolin or clindamycin are usually effective against penicillinase-producing staphylococci. A combination (e.g. ceftazidime or azlocillin + tobramycin, ciprofloxacin + gentamicin) is always necessary for Pseudomonas infection. In fungal infection, the topical therapy, which is particularly important, may be supplemented by oral fluconazole or itraconazole.

Infections of the corneal margin usually spread from conjunctivitis but are occasionally primary corneal infections (staphylococci, Haemophilus, Moraxella) and may also be allergic, pharmacotoxic, traumatic or trophic in origin. Antibiotic treatment is as for conjunctivitis (according to cause).

Circumorbital abscesses frequently follow injury or operation or can be metastatic from septicaemia. The prognosis is poor because of the risk of panophthalmitis. The usual causes are pneumococci or pseudomonas.

Topically: depending on the causative organism, benzylpenicillin or gentamicin by subconjunctival injection, or gramicidin + neomycin + polymyxin B eye ointment.

Systemic treatment with benzylpenicillin (in pneumococcal infection), azlocillin + tobramycin (in Pseudomonas infection), or other antimicrobials according to sensitivity results, should be started as soon as possible.

Herpetic keratitis: *Cause:* Herpes simplex virus. Occurs at all ages, including the newborn, who can be infected during birth from genital herpes in the mother. The epithelial cells contain microscopic eosinophilic intranuclear inclusion bodies demonstrated in a giemsa or, better, an immunofluorescent preparation. The diagnosis and treatment should be carried out by an ophthalmologist.

Topically: Superficial forms only *(dendritic keratitis)* may be treated with acyclovir eye ointment (3%) or trifluridine eye drops (1%) or ointment (2%). The drops should be used every 1–2 h and the ointment 4–5 times a day (where drops are prescribed, use ointment at night). Gentamicin eye drops may be given for secondary bacterial infection. Corticosteroids are strongly contraindicated because of the risk of corneal ulceration.

The deeper *disciform keratitis* is clearly due to hypersensitivity to viral antigens, since viable virus is absent. It usually heals with symptomatic treatment only.

In severe disease with involvement of the stroma combined topical treatment with a corticosteroid and an antiviral agent can be effective. Idoxuridine eye drops and ointment are not very well tolerated. Acyclovir orally is indicated in severe herpetic keratouveitis.

Ophthalmic zoster: Keratitis, iridocyclitis, hyperaemic conjunctivae, often with blisters on the lid. There is a risk of scleritis, secondary glaucoma, optic neuritis and ocular palsy. Topical treatment should only be given by an ophthalmologist.

Acyclovir 10 mg/kg 3 times a day by short i.v. infusion for 5 days eliminates the virus rapidly. The use of topical or systemic steroids (not in patients with malignancies) is controversial. An antibiotic should be given for secondary bacterial infection, guided by the isolate and its sensitivities. Severe disease may benefit from the addition of high doses of i.v. immunoglobulin.

Parenchymatous keratitis: *Topically* with steroids under the guidance of an ophthalmologist, with simultaneous treatment of the underlying disease (see syphilis, p. 484 and tuberculosis, p. 513). There are a number of other causes of interstitial keratitis, e.g. Chlamydia trachomatis, Herpes simplex and Varicella zoster viruses, which should be treated appropriately.

Allergic keratoconjunctivitis (e.g. phlyctenular keratoconjunctivitis): Treat secondary bacterial infection in addition to other therapy.

Topically: Tetracycline eye ointment, a preparation containing polymyxin B, or gentamicin eye drops or ointment.

Keratomycosis: *Cause:* Candida albicans, Aspergillus, Fusarium, or other fungi. Keratomycosis is often recognised too late, after being initially mistaken for herpetic keratitis. Usually follows an injury or a primary bacterial or viral infection of the cornea, often after local steroid therapy. Corneal ulceration and involvement of the lid and conjunctiva may occur. The causative organism can be demonstrated by microscopy and culture.

Topically: Pimaricin + chloramphenicol eye ointment, econazole 1%, and possibly also amphotericin B or nystatin (see Table 55, p. 457).

Systemically: Amphotericin B in severe cases (for dosage, see p. 193), which is active against Candida, Aspergillus and other fungi, and may be combined with flucytosine. Alternatives are fluconazole or intraconazole (systemically). Antibiotics with no antifungal activity and corticosteroids should not be used.

Bacterial endophthalmitis: Usually postoperative or following a perforating injury, and occasionally complicating a corneal ulcer or as a metastatic focus in septicaemia in a patient with immunosuppression, endocarditis or an intravenous drug abuser.

Causative organisms are mainly staphylococci, streptococci, anaerobes, enterobacteria, Haemophilus, Pseudomonas and occasionally fungi (Candida, Aspergillus etc.). Mixed infections occur. The causative organism may be isolated from an aspirate or a blood culture; it is important to make a bacteriological diagnosis if possible because of the range of possible infecting organisms and the need to differentiate non-bacterial forms of endophthalmitis and tumours. The prognosis depends on the promptness with which treatment is begun, and the infecting organism. Infections with staphylococci have a considerably better prognosis than those with enterobacteria. Poor results of treatment (blindness) are generally due to poor penetration of antibiotics into the vitreous, so that the most important local treatment is the intravitreal injection of an appropriate antibiotic, for which the following single doses are used: ampicillin 0.2 mg, oxacillin 0.5 mg, cefazolin 1–2 mg, gentamicin or tobramycin 0.2 mg, amikacin 0.4 mg, benzylpenicillin 0.36 mg, vancomycin and clindamycin 1 mg.

Topical treatment (topical, subconjunctival, intravitreal) should always be supplemented by *systemic treatment* at high dosage. Initial treatment should be with a combination which covers not only staphylococci, but also Pseudomonas and anaerobes, and which penetrates into the eye as well as possible. These criteria are fulfilled only by certain combinations, such as vancomycin + amikacin + metronidazole or imipenem or ciprofloxacin + rifampicin. Metronidazole, which diffuses very well, is the best agent against anaerobes. In severe infections, particularly those due to anaerobes and fungi, early vitrectomy can improve the outcome. A fungal infection can, if sensitive, be treated with systemic amphotericin B + flucytosine. Miconazole i.v. or fluconazole are the only effective agents against certain fungi. Miconazole 0.01 mg and amphotericin B 0.005 mg are suitable for intravitreal injection.

Perioperative prophylaxis: In vitreal and retinal operations, in all eye surgery on patients at special risk and in those on steroid therapy, a brief course of systemic antibiotics, e.g. cefazolin + tobramycin in high dosage for 1–2 days beginning 2 h before the operation, is recommended. This may be supplemented by topical antibiotics.

References

BAUM, J., et al.: Bilateral keratitis as a manifestation of Lyme disease. Am. J. Ophthalmol. *105:* 75 (1988).

BORRMANN, L. R., I. H. LEOPOLD: The potential use of quinolones in future ocular antimicrobial therapy. Am. J. Ophthalmol. *106:* 227 (1988).

CHEESBROUGH, J. S., C. L. WILLIAMS, R. RUSTOM, R. C. BUCKNALL, R. B. TRIMBLE: Metastatic pneumococcal endophthalmitis: report of two cases and review of literature. J. Infect. *20:* 231–236 (1990).

FARBER, B. B., D. L. WEINBAUM, J. S. DUMMER: Metastatic bacterial endophthalmitis. Arch. Intern. Med. *145:* 1 (1985).

HAMMERSCHLAG, M. R.: Neonatal ocular prophylaxis. Pediatr. Infect. Dis. J. *7:* 81 (1988).

HAMMERSCHLAG, M. R. et al: Efficacy of neonatal ocular prophylaxis for the prevention of chlamydial and gonococcal conjunctivits. N. Engl. J. Med. *320:* 769 (1989).

HEGGIE, A. D., A. C. JAFFE, L. A. STUART et al.: Topical sulfacetamide vs oral erythromycin for neonatal chlamydial conjunctivitis. Am. J. Dis. Child. *139:* 564 (1985).

LAGA, M. et al.: Prophylaxis of gonococcal and chlamydial ophthalmia neonatorum. N. Engl. J. Med. *318:* 653 (1988).

MCCLOSKEY, R. V.: Topical antimicrobial agents and antibiotics for the eye. Med. Clin. North Am. *72:* 717 (1988).

ORIEL, J. D.: Ophthalmia neonatorum: relative efficacy of current prophylactic practices and treatment. J. Antimicrob. Chemother. *14:* 209 (1984).
RAPOZA, P. A. et al.: Assessment of neonatal conjunctivitis with a direct immunofluorescent monoclonal antibody stain for chlamydia. J.A.M.A. *255:* 3369 (1986).
TABBARA, K. F., and R. A. HYNDIUK, eds.: Infections of the Eye. Boston: Little, Brown, 1986.
WEBER, D. J., et al.: Endophthalmitis following intraocular lens implantation. Report of 30 cases and review of the literature. Rev. Infect. Dis. *8:* 12 (1986).
WOLFSON, J., and D. C. HOOPER: Quinolone Antimicrobial Agents and Ophthalmologic Infections. In: J. S. WOLFSON and D. C. HOOPER (eds.), Quinolone Antimicrobial Agents. Washington, D. C.: American Society for Microbiology, 1988.

13. Infections of the Ear, Nose and Throat

In general practice a bacteriological diagnosis of ENT infections is often difficult to obtain. If conditions such as sinusitis, laryngitis and otitis media are inadequately treated, however, every effort should then be made to obtain bacterial isolates and sensitivities in order that antibiotics can be used effectively to reduce the risk of more dangerous complications such as otogenic meningitis, mastoiditis and jugular vein thrombosis.

The evaluation of *bacteriological results* from these sites requires a detailed understanding of the normal bacterial flora of the mucous membranes of the nose, mouth and outer ear. Whereas viridans and nonhaemolytic streptococci, nonpathogenic neisseriae and corynebacteria, Staphylococcus epidermidis, sarcina and occasionally even Staphylococcus aureus are normal isolates from the nose and mouth, gonococci and haemolytic streptococci of groups A, C or G are usually pathological. Pseudomonas aeruginosa will colonise the oropharynx after tracheostomy or tracheal intubation and Candida albicans will do so in the immunosuppressed, particularly if the patient is receiving broad-spectrum antibiotics.

The assessment of bacteriological findings is made more difficult by the fact that a number of pyogenic bacteria (aerobic and anaerobic streptococci, bacteroides and fusobacteria) are commensal flora in the nose, mouth and throat. Antibiotic therapy often selects coliforms such as klebsiella and Escherichia coli in the mouth, particularly after abdominal operations. The healthy external auditory canal normally contains only harmless skin organisms such as staphylococci, sarcina and diphtheroids. Pneumococci, haemolytic streptococci, branhamella, Escherichia coli, klebsiella and Mycoplasma pneumoniae should not be isolated from the outer ear, and Staphylococcus aureus does not occur in large numbers. Pseudomonas aeruginosa and proteus may colonise the external auditory canal when there is a chronic discharge from the middle ear (e. g. in sero-mucinous otitis media, or "glue ear"). Though abnormal, these organisms are not necessarily of pathogenic significance when isolated from this site.

Mixed infections with bacteria and viruses are not uncommon in ENT practice. Pus with a foetid odour is a sign of mixed infection with aerobic and anaerobic bacteria. Viruses can predispose to more serious secondary bacterial infection. When bacteriological findings are normal despite obvious clinical signs, a viral infection which would not respond to antibiotics should be considered. Failure to recognize anatomical abnormalities such as septal deviation or congenital malformations hinders effective antibiotic treatment, since surgical correction may be necessary before the infection can be eradicated. The insufflation, instillation or irrigation with antimicrobials should be carried out only by a specialist, who is best able to assess the chances of success of topical treatment. Systemic antibiotics are most effective in acute infections; chronic processes, especially in closed cavities, are less likely to respond to antibiotics alone.

Maxillary, ethmoidal, frontal or **sphenoidal sinusitis** usually originates in the nose. Maxillary sinusitis can also be of dental origin, e.g. periostitis of a dental root, which may be chronic with foetid pus. Haematogenous spread is possible. Catarrhal forms sometimes occur after acute rhinitis. Purulent infections are frequently unilateral and seldom bilateral or part of a pansinusitis. Necrotising infections can occur in scarlet fever and influenza. A collection of fluid in a sinus may be demonstrated by ultrasound and sometimes also radiologically as a fluid level in the erect posture, or by CT scan.

Whereas acute sinusitis generally causes severe symptoms, in chronic disease the fever, headache and purulent nasal discharge are often absent. Chronic purulent sinusitis is usually recognized by its consequences (laryngitis, pharyngitis, bronchitis, otitis media or anosmia), and the diagnosis may be confirmed by endoscopy, aspiration or irrigation, and by imaging. Any unilateral cold which lasts for more than 3 weeks is suggestive of sinusitis. Careful distinction between allergic and chronic polypoid sinusitis is important. Nasal pus, preferably obtained by direct aspiration or sinus washout, should be examined bacteriologically in every case. A discharge can be produced by releasing a compressed politzer bag. The usual bacterial pathogens are staphylococci, Streptococcus pyogenes (group A), pneumococci, Haemophilus influenzae, Branhamella catarrhalis, Klebsiella pneumoniae and anaerobes.

Acute sinusitis is best treated with high doses of antibiotics in order to prevent serious complications as well as to treat the primary infection. The choice of antibiotic is based mainly on the severity of the infection and on the bacteriological results. Parenteral treatment is necessary in acute frontal, ethmoidal and sphenoidal sinusitis and when complications arise (see below). Suppurative infections may be treated with cefuroxime or cefotaxime (effective against pneumococci, other streptococci, haemophilus and staphylococci) or, in adults, with ciprofloxacin i.v. (although streptococci, particularly pneumococci, are usually resistant to quinolones). When sinusitis is of dental origin, the focus of infection (the tooth) should be removed and benzylpenicillin 3–6 g given daily; this is effective against peptostreptococci and Bacteroides melaninogenicus, as is metronidazole (in most cases). Severe cases with fever may also be treated with imipenem (active also against anaerobes) or doxycycline i.v. + clindamycin i.v. These antibiotics should be continued i.v. and later orally for at least 3 weeks. Less severe cases may be treated with a new oral cephalosporin or co-amoxiclav. *Ethmoidal sinusitis* may be complicated by orbital cellulitis and *frontal sinusitis* by osteomyelitis, each requiring appropriate treatment. Meningitis, epi- or subdural empyema, cerebral abscess and cavernous sinus thrombosis can all be complications of ethmoidal, sphenoidal or frontal sinusitis and are usually detectable by CT scan.

In **subacute and chronic maxillary sinusitis,** systemic antibiotic therapy is not very successful. An operation may be necessary to improve sinus drainage. Neomycin, neomycin + bacitracin, gentamicin or polymyxin B may all be instilled locally every fifth day for 2–3 weeks. *Chronic fungal sinusitis,* caused by aspergillus or mucor, is a rare form of this condition. It should be treated by instillation of an antifungal (e.g. miconazole) and, in life-threatening infections in the immunosuppressed patient, with i.v. amphotericin B + flucytosine followed, if necessary, by oral itraconazole.

Furuncles of the nose and lip are caused by staphylococci. Thrombophlebitis of the angular and ophthalmic veins can give rise to a life-threatening orbital cellulitis, cavernous sinus thrombosis, and meningitis. Nasal furuncles should therefore always be treated promptly with flucloxacillin or an oral cephalosporin in a daily dose of 3–4 g (adults) or 100 mg/kg (children). Sensitive infections may be treated with benzylpenicillin or phenoxymethylpenicillin in a daily dose of 2–3 g, or oral erythromycin or clindamycin if the patient is allergic to penicillin. Extensive incision should if possible be avoided, since it may encourage the infection to spread into veins or lymphatics. Bed rest, a fluid diet and speech prohibition are recommended for patients with large nasal or labial furuncles with perifocal oedema.

Osteomyelitis of the upper and lower jaws is caused by staphylococci, streptococci or anaerobes and is often a mixed infection. Any initial focus of infection such as a tooth or sinus should first be treated. Benzylpenicillin may be used if the causative organism is known to be sensitive; alternatives for staphylococcal infection are flucloxacillin or a cephalosporin. Cefoxitin (6 g daily), clindamycin (1.2 g daily for adults, and 30 mg/kg for children) or metronidazole (500 mg i.v. three times a day) should be used for anaerobic infection. A quinolone (ofloxacin, ciprofloxacin) may also be considered in adults. Operative drainage is usually necessary.

Suppurative parotitis is usually caused by staphylococci, occasionally by streptococci. It occurs either in the presence of severe primary disease or after operation, mainly as an ascending infection, but also secondary to salivary calculi or blockage of secretions. Suppurative parotitis should be distinguished from mumps, chronic or recurrent parotitis (in which dilatation of the duct can be demonstrated by sialography), tumours, tuberculosis, syphilis, sarcoidosis and Sjögren's syndrome. By applying pressure to the parotid gland, pus can be expressed from the orifice of the parotid duct and then examined bacteriologically. Suppurative parotitis should be treated with flucloxacillin, an oral cephalosporin or erythromycin by mouth and, in severe cases, with a cephalosporin i.v. (6 g daily). When there is liquefaction of pus, several stab incisions should be made by an ENT surgeon parallel to the course of the facial nerve.

Stomatitis can take several forms and have various causes:

Ulcerating or *gangrenous stomatitis* occurs with underlying diseases and impaired resistance (e.g. leukaemia, AIDS). *Causative organisms:* anaerobes, occasionally staphylococci or streptococci. *Treatment* is with benzylpenicillin in high doses combined if necessary with metronidazole; if treatment fails or the disease is severe, cefoxitin i.v. may be used, possibly in combination with gentamicin.

Candida stomatitis (thrush): White plaques which can be wiped away. Yeasts can be shown microscopically in methylene blue or gram preparations and in culture. Thrush generally occurs during broad-spectrum antibiotic therapy and in the seriously ill patient, particularly if immunosuppressed. *Treatment:* Nystatin or amphotericin B suspension by mouth, 1–2 ml 3–4 times a day, or natamycin (pimaricin) or amphotericin B lozenges or miconazole oral gel.

Aphthous stomatitis: Causative organisms are herpes or coxsackie viruses. Antibiotics should not be used. Herpes stomatitis may improve with acyclovir. For local treatment, zinc sulphate mouthwash, hydrocortisone lozenges and, for major aphthae, ointment or lozenges containing a local anaesthetic may be useful. Solitary aphthae of uncertain aetiology will usually respond neither to antibiotic therapy nor to acyclovir.

Angular stomatitis (perlèche): Usually due to secondary infection with Candida albicans, staphylococci or streptococci. *Topical treatment* with nystatin cream (for candida) or neomycin or gentamicin cream (for bacterial infection).

Auricular perichondritis is an infection (usually with Pseudomonas aeruginosa or staphylococci) which arises secondary to injury. *Systemic* and *topical* antibiotic treatment should be guided by sensitivity testing, and any associated abscess incised and drained, with debridement of the necrotic cartilage. A life-threatening necrotising otitis externa caused by Pseudomonas aeruginosa is described in diabetics and can progress to severe osteomyelitis (malignant otitis externa, see below), so auricular perichondritis in these patients must be treated promptly and adequately with antibiotics.

Erysipelas of the auricle spreads from lesions at the external auditory meatus or the skin of the head and is a group A streptococcal infection. Treat *systemically* with benzylpenicillin or phenoxymethylpenicillin (see p. 479).

Otitis externa, infected eczema of the auditory canal and **furuncle of the ear:** Look for an underlying disease, e.g. diabetes. Bacterial, viral (herpes) and fungal (candida, aspergillus) infections can all occur. Infected eczema of the auditory canal can result from a chronic purulent cholesteatoma. Vesicles are found on the posterior wall of the auditory canal in otitic herpes zoster.

Treatment should be directed towards the organism concerned (Pseudomonas aeruginosa, staphylococci, Escherichia coli, proteus etc.) and based on sensitivity testing. Treat topically with antibiotic-containing ear drops or ointment, but for not longer than one week because excessive use may result in fungal infections. Topical anti-infectives which are not used systemically, containing framycetin, polymyxin B, neomycin, chlorhexidine or clioquinol, are suitable; if such preparations are used in patients who have a perforation of the tympanic membrane, however, there is an increased risk of drug-induced deafness. Compound preparations, some with the addition of a corticosteroid, are also available. Chloramphenicol ear drops, which contain propylene glycol, cause hypersensitivity in about 10% of users; this may be avoided by the use of chloramphenicol eye ointment. Aspergillus otitis may be treated with topical 2% alcoholic salicyclic acid or natamycin (pimaricin); other fungal infections may be treated with clotrimazole 1% in polyethylene glycol. Herpes simplex otitis may respond to 3% vidarabine ointment or to systemic acyclovir. Furuncle of the ear with marked perifocal swelling and lymphadenitis should be treated with systemic antibiotics, e.g. flucloxacillin or an oral cephalosporin; incision is seldom necessary.

Malignant otitis externa: In severe diabetes mellitus and certain other underlying illnesses, a malignant otitis externa can develop. The causative organism is almost always Pseudomonas aeruginosa. Inflammation arises in the cartilage of the auditory canal and spreads to cause osteomyelitis of the base of the skull.

Treatment of choice: Initially azlocillin 20 g daily + tobramycin 0.24 g daily, then, after 4 weeks, oral ciprofloxacin for several months.

Otitis media: The *commonest causes* are pneumococci (>40%), Streptococcus pyogenes (group A), Haemophilus influenzae (especially in young children), Branhamella catarrhalis, anaerobes and (in infants) Escherichia coli.

Acute, serous otitis media associated with a viral infection seldom requires antibiotics unless the patient is immunosuppressed. Secondary bacterial infection arises relatively frequently.

Acute suppurative otitis media and *necrotising otitis media* should always be treated with antibiotics because of the risk of mastoid involvement. Local treatment with ear drops (e. g. chloramphenicol) is ineffective unless the ear-drum has already perforated, and then it carries the risk of inner ear damage if drops containing an aminoglycoside (neomycin, gentamicin) are instilled. A pulsating reflex on the discharge or a teat-like protuberance on the mucous membrane are signs of spontaneous perforation of the drum. If perforation has not yet occurred, regular re-examination of the ear-drum is important so as not to miss the optimal time for tympanocentesis by a specialist. Where the course of the otitis media is prolonged, the possibility of mastoiditis should not be overlooked.

For *blind therapy,* amoxycillin is generally effective against pneumococci, streptococci and Haemophilus influenzae. Cefixime and co-amoxiclav are additionally effective against penicillinase-producing strains of haemophilus and branhamella. Cefaclor and cefuroxime axetil also have good activity against haemophilus, including ampicillin-resistant strains. Antibiotics should generally be given for 7–10 days. In children over the age of 5, in whom haemophilus infections are less common, phenoxymethylpenicillin is usually adequate. Erythromycin is effective against most strains of pneumococci, Branhamella catarrhalis and Mycoplasma pneumoniae but unreliable in Haemophilus infections. Where complications arise, antibiotics should be given parenterally in high dosage.

Directed treatment: Where blind therapy fails or mastoiditis develops, an ENT specialist should obtain pus or exudate from the middle ear by tympanocentesis using a fine cannula and send the material for microbiological examination. Otitis media caused by mucoid strains of pneumococci is often prolonged, associated with pallor of the ear-drum, and can progress insidiously to mastoiditis; this condition should be treated with benzylpenicillin in high doses (6–10 g daily). The serum latex agglutination test for pneumococcal antigen is usually positive in these cases. Such mucoid pneumococcal infections can occur at any age but are commoner in infants, the elderly and in males, and can give rise to a conductive deafness of sudden origin.

Special forms include the otitis media which may accompany *scarlet fever* and which should also be treated with benzylpenicillin. This complication usually occurs late in the disease as a simple otitis media, although a severe necrotizing otitis externa can sometimes develop in the first few days of this infection, progress rapidly and lead to perforation of the ear-drum, mastoiditis or labyrinthitis. Bilateral otitis media often develops 1–2 weeks after the onset of the rash of *measles,* and results in prolonged suppuration and frequently in secondary bacterial infection.

Blood blisters are seen on the ear-drum in the otitis or myringitis which accompanies infection with Mycoplasma pneumoniae; they are also seen in *influenzal otitis,* in which a serosanguinous or purulent haemorrhagic discharge can then develop. Influenzal otitis does not require antibiotics, whereas mycoplasma otitis is best treated with erythromycin or doxycycline. In *diphtheria*, otitis media with pseudomembranous inflammation can spread from foci of nasal or pharyngeal infection (for treatment see p. 370).

If acute otitis media is *recurrent*, a predisposing cause should be sought. Some cases may be relieved by myringotomy with the insertion of ventilatory grommets, a procedure also used for chronic sero-mucinous otitis media ("glue ear").

In *chronic otitis media* there is persistent purulence of the mucous membrane, accompanied sometimes by destruction of bone (secondary cholesteatoma formation), which can progress in severe cases to intracranial complications (e.g. cavernous sinus thrombosis, meningitis, cerebral abscess) or to purulent labyrinthitis. The ear-drum tends to perforate centrally in mucosal suppuration and peripherally where bone is involved, with the discharge of (usually) foul-smelling pus, from which gram-negative bacteria (commonly Pseudomonas aeruginosa, proteus, klebsiella, Escherichia coli or serratia) and staphylococci can be isolated. The infection is frequently mixed, with aerobic and anaerobic bacteria (bacteroides, peptococci or peptostreptococci).

Because of the difficulties in treatment of this condition, the pus should always be examined microbiologically. There is also a risk of increasing hearing loss, so chronic otitis media should always be managed by an ENT specialist. Once *bone* becomes involved, a drainage operation or tympanoplasty is usually inevitable, together with supportive topical measures such as irrigation with antiseptics as appropriate, or antibiotics (e.g. polymyxin B) as guided by antibiotic susceptibility results. The prolonged topical use of framycetin, gentamicin, kanamycin or neomycin may damage the inner ear. Systemic antibiotic therapy is almost always ineffective. *Chronic sero-mucinous otitis media* ("glue ear") requires investigation by an ENT specialist to establish the underlying cause (e.g. adenoids) and is often successfully treated by myringotomy and the insertion of grommets.

Mastoiditis can develop in weeks 2–4 of acute suppurative otitis media and is accompanied by marked hearing loss, pain on pressure on the mastoid, swelling of the posterior wall of the external ear, and sometimes a purulent discharge to the exterior or into the auditory canal. A peripheral facial palsy may also occur. Since antibiotics cannot penetrate the avascular foci of suppuration, chemotherapy alone is unlikely to be curative.

The main value of antibiotics in this condition is to treat or suppress intracranial complications such as cerebral abscess, epidural or subdural empyema, and cavernous sinus thrombosis, all of which may be recognized and localized by a CT scan. The prompt use of appropriate antibiotics (e.g. cefuroxime or cefotaxime, 6 g or 100 mg/kg daily) at the onset of acute mastoiditis can lead to rapid improvement and avoid the need for operation. Many cases will require an operation (mastoidectomy or antrotomy), however, and this should always be performed under antibiotic cover (e.g. a cephalosporin), continued for 3–6 weeks postoperatively.

Infections with mucoid strains of pneumococci should be treated with benzylpenicillin in high dosage. Chronic mastoiditis that arises as a complication of chronic otitis media is often associated with gram-negative bacilli (particularly pseudomonas) and non-sporing anaerobes (bacteroides, peptococci etc.) as well as with staphylococci. Treatment should then be started with imipenem i.v. or a combination of cefotaxime + gentamicin + clindamycin or metronidazole. An operation in such cases is inevitable.

Cervical lymphadenitis: When acute, the lymph nodes involved are painful and may form abscesses. When chronic, they are coarse and indolent. Their site depends on the initial focus; the submental and submandibular lymph nodes drain the lower jaw and teeth, whereas the superior cervical nodes drain the tonsils, nasopharynx and larynx. The cervical lymph nodes can also be involved haematogenously in generalised infections. Non-specific cervical lymphadenitis usually results from staphylococcal or streptococcal infection, whereas specific infections may be due to tuberculosis, nontuberculous ("atypical") mycobacteria, actinomycosis, syphilis, toxoplasmosis, AIDS, cat-scratch disease or infectious mononucleosis. Non-infectious causes such as leukaemia, lymphogranulomatosis or tumours should also be considered.

Treatment of non-specific cervical lymphadenitis: If streptococcal, phenoxymethylpenicillin; if staphylococcal, flucloxacillin or an oral cephalosporin (which would also be effective against streptococci), together with treatment of the primary focus (e.g. tonsils, adenoids, teeth, gums). If this fails, rule out other causes of infection, if necessary by aspiration or biopsy. Infections with nontuberculous ("atypical") mycobacteria (e.g. M. scrofulaceum or M. avium-intracellulare) are less likely to respond to chemotherapy and should be removed urgently by operation.

References

BLUESTONE, C. D.: Management of otitis media in infants and children: Current role of old and new microbial agents. Pediat. Infect. Dis. J. *7:* S129 (1988).
HICKEY, S. A., G. R. FORD, A. F. O'CONNOR, S. J. EYKYN, P. H. SONKSEN: Treating malignant otitis with oral ciprofloxacin. Brit. med. J. *299:* 550 (1989).
JOHNSON, M. P., R. RAMPHAL: Malignant external otitis: Report on therapy with ceftazidime and review of therapy and prognosis. Rev. Infect. Dis. *13:* 173 (1990).
JONES, R. A. K.: Ototoxicity of gentamicin ear-drops. Lancet *1:* 1161 (1978).
LANG, R. et al.: Successful treatment of malignant external otitis with oral ciprofloxacin: Report of experience with 23 patients. J. Infect. Dis. *161:* 537 (1990).
NADAL, D., P. HERRMANN, A. BAUMANN et al.: Acute mastoiditis: clinical, microbiological, and therapeutic aspects. Eur. J. Pediatr. *149:* 560–564 (1990).
RUBIN, J., V. L. YU: Malignant external otitis: Insights into pathogenesis, clinical manifestations, diagnosis, and therapy. Am. J. Med. *85:* 391 (1988).

14. Skin Infections

When treating skin infections, the first decision is whether a **systemic antibiotic** is necessary. Although topical antimicrobials may suffice for mild conditions, systemic treatment is always advisable for more extensive infections, whether superficial or deep.

Topical antimicrobial treatment, which is only justifiable when the infection is very superficial, allows the antibiotic to have an immediate effect on the causative organism at the site of application. Antibiotics do not diffuse through intact skin, so agents applied topically will not be effective in skin infections that are more deeply situated. Moreover, not all skin conditions that are oozing, crusted or pustular are actually infected. Skin infections for which topical treatment may be appropriate include superficial pyoderma, impetigo, some purulent wounds, second- and third-degree burns, and secondarily infected leg ulcers or eczema. Antibacterials should not be used topically for cutaneous and subcutaneous infections such as erysipelas, cellulitis, furunculosis, erysipeloid, cutaneous anthrax or tuberculosis.

To minimise the risk of selection of resistant organisms, it is advisable to limit the choice of antimicrobials applied topically to those which are not used systemically. Resistant organisms are more common in hospitals and, where possible, samples for microbiological examination should be taken before beginning treatment. Some drugs, e.g. neomycin, may cause sensitization; if large areas are being treated, aminoglycosides such as neomycin and gentamicin can also cause ototoxicity, particularly in children and in the elderly.

As a general rule, narrow-spectrum antimicrobials are preferable for infections whose cause is known, and broad-spectrum agents for mixed infections. Tables 56 and 57 summarize the available topical antimicrobials, of which neomycin, framycetin, gentamicin, chloramphenicol and tetracycline are broad-spectrum agents. Polymyxin B is effective only against gram-negative bacteria. Bacitracin, erythromycin, fusidic acid, mupirocin and tyrothricin are effective against gram-positive bacteria. Ciclopiroxolamine, clotrimazole, miconazole, nystatin and pimaricin (natamycin) are effective against certain fungi (see Table 58).

The *antiviral agents* acyclovir, idoxuridine, tromantadine and vidarabine may all be used topically for herpes simplex. Acyclovir cream is the most effective for primary and recurrent labial and genital infections with herpes simplex, and treatment should begin as early as possible. Systemic treatment (see p. 278) is necessary for buccal or vaginal infections and for herpes zoster (shingles). Idoxuridine (IDU) solution (5% in dimethyl sulphoxide) is used less frequently for herpes simplex because acyclovir is more effective; IDU has the best chance of success if started early, is applied frequently and is continued for 3–4 days.

Since superficial skin infections are frequently mixed or changing, proprietary preparations for topical use often contain combinations of antimicrobials in order to broaden their spectrum. Mild antiseptics containing benzalkonium, cetrimide, chlorhexidine, dibromopropamidine isethionate, hexachlorophane, polynoxylin, povidone iodine, proflavine or triclosan may be used as disinfectant cleansers in minor wounds, burns or abrasions, and for the topical treatment of superficial skin infections. Their therapeutic efficacy should not be overestimated, however, and they are not free from toxicological effects. In particular, topical preparations containing hexachlorophane should be used with caution in neonates and should not be used on extensive raw surfaces.

Topical agents have advantages over systemic therapy in the treatment of minor skin infections because they can often produce higher, usually bactericidal, antibiotic concentrations at the site of infection. Antibiotic sensitivity testing is therefore only of limited value in topical therapy.

Table 56. Topical skin antibacterials which are not used systemically.

Drug	Combination with	Application form
Amphomycin*	neomycin	ointment
Colistin	–	powder
Framycetin	– gramicidin	cream cream, ointment, tulle
Nitrofurazone*	–	ointment, powder
Mupirocin	–	ointment, nasal ointment
Neomycin	– bacitracin gramicidin bacitracin polymyxin B	cream, ointment cream, powder ointment spray, powder spray
Polymyxin B	bacitracin neomycin	ointment spray, powder spray
Tyrothricin*	–	ointment, powder

* Not available for this use in Britain.

Table 57. Topical skin antibacterials that are also available for systemic use.

Drug	Combination with	Application
Chloramphenicol	–	ointment (primarily for eyes)
Clindamycin	–	solution (for acne)
Erythromycin	–	solution (for acne)
Fusidic acid	–	cream, gel, ointment, tulle
Gentamicin	–	cream, ointment
Tetracycline	–	ointment, solution (for acne)

14. Skin Infections

Table 58. Topical skin antifungals.

Drug	Combination with	Application
Amphotericin**	–	ointment
Benzoic acid	salicyclic acid	ointment (Whitfield's)
Benzoyl peroxide	–	cream
Bifonazole*	–	cream, gel, powder, solution
Ciclopiroxolamine*	–	cream, powder, solution
Clotrimazole	–	cream, dusting-powder, spray-solution, solution
Econazole*	–	cream, dusting-powder, lotion, spray-powder, spray-solution
Ketoconazole**	–	cream, shampoo
Miconazole**	–	cream, dusting-powder, spray-powder
Naftifin*	–	cream, gel, solution
Natamycin (Pimaricin)	– neomycin	cream lotion, ointment*
Nystatin	–	cream, dusting-powder, gel, ointment
Salicyclic acid	– benzoic acid	cream, paint ointment (Whitfield's)
Sulconazole nitrate	–	cream
Povidone iodine	–	cream, solution
Tioconazole	–	nail solution
Tolnaftate	–	cream
Undecanoates	–	cream, dusting powder, paint, spray-solution

* Not available for this use in Britain
** Preparations for systemic use are also available

When treating skin infections topically, it is important to choose the most suitable **preparation** (cream, lotion, ointment, paint, powder, spray-powder, spray-solution or solution). Sprays and solutions are usually more efficient vehicles of the active drug than creams or ointments, and a cream (as an emulsion of oil in water) is generally better in this respect than an ointment, which is water-free. An ointment is preferable for dry skin, however, especially for longer courses of treatment. The removal of exudate, crusts and areas of epidermal thickening with a keratolytic ointment will improve the conditions for the use of topical antibiotics.

Topical preparations containing penicillins, cephalosporins and sulphonamides should not be used because of the risk of **sensitisation.** Tetracycline and chloramphenicol ointments, on the other hand, are widely used and seldom give rise to allergy. Neomycin occasionally causes hypersensitivity reactions such as contact dermatitis, but these are seldom reported with the other antibiotics that are available for topical use only. Many instances of sensitisation are attributable not to the active constituent but to additives such as hydroxybenzoates (parabens). Other side-effects of topical antimicrobial therapy include disruption of the normal commensal bacterial flora, overgrowth with fungi such as candida, and systemic toxicity as a result of cutaneous absorption, particularly when extensive lesions are treated, as in burns (see p. 434).

Frequent causes of skin infections include staphylococci, streptococci, Pseudomonas aeruginosa, Escherichia coli, proteus, klebsiella and Candida albicans. Staphylococcus epidermidis, other micrococci, sarcinas, propionibacteria, non-pathogenic corynebacteria, aerobic sporing bacilli and Candida albicans (in small numbers) are normally found on the skin, as are other facultative pathogens on occasion (see above). The demonstration of the primary cause of a skin infection is often made more difficult by the secondary infection which develops subsequently.

a) Acute Bacterial Infections

Pyoderma (impetigo, follicular impetigo, bullous impetigo, sycosis barbae, pemphigus neonatorum, ecthyma simplex etc.). The *causative organisms* are usually staphylococci (often with Streptococcus pyogenes in impetigo); other bacteria rarely cause pyoderma.

Local treatment: Neomycin + bacitracin, gentamicin, mupirocin.

Systemic treatment: In severe infections and in immunodeficient patients (including the newborn), systemic spread is relatively common, so a penicillinase-stable penicillin (flucloxacillin), or benzylpenicillin where penicillinase-sensitive staphylococci or streptococci have been isolated, should be used. Patients allergic to penicillin may be treated with erythromycin. Systemic treatment with benzylpenicillin or phenoxymethylpenicillin is preferable to topical antibiotics in streptococcal pyoderma because it accelerates healing and reduces the rate of relapse and of complications.

Exfoliative dermatitis (caused by exfoliatin-forming staphylococci) should be distinguished from the drug-induced Lyell syndrome. Fever, redness of the skin and blister formation are all typical of this condition. Staphylococci cannot be isolated from the blisters, but only from the initial focus.

Treatment: Flucloxacillin initially i.v., then orally. Erythromycin and oral cephalosporins are also effective.

Ecthyma gangrenosum is caused by Pseudomonas aeruginosa.
Local treatment: Polymyxin B, gentamicin or povidone iodine.
Systemic treatment: When extensive, give azlocillin + tobramycin i.v. in high doses. Alternatives, particularly in the elderly and in patients with poor renal function, are ceftazidime, aztreonam, ciprofloxacin or imipenem. Lesions which arise through haematogenous spread in leukaemia may require long courses of treatment.

Abscesses, cellulitis, sweat gland abscess, whitlow, gangrene: The *causative organisms* are staphylococci, streptococci and other microorganisms (see also surgical infections, pp. 430 and 436).
Local treatment: Incision if necessary.
Systemic treatment (according to isolate): Flucloxacillin orally or i.v. (staphylococci), benzylpenicillin (streptococci), erythromycin or an oral cephalosporin. In young children, Haemophilus influenzae can also cause cellulitis, which should be treated with cefotaxime (100 mg/kg daily i.v.).

Erysipelas: The *causative organisms* are streptococci of group A (Streptococcus pyogenes), and occasionally of groups B or C.
Systemic treatment: Benzylpenicillin 1.2–2.4 g daily for 1–2 weeks, or phenoxymethylpenicillin; erythromycin is an alternative for patients who are allergic. Chronic or recurrent erysipelas should be treated with benzylpenicillin 6 g i.v. or i.m. daily for 10 days, followed if necessary with benzathine penicillin 1 g i.m. once a month for several months.

Furuncles (boils) are caused by staphylococci and can take several forms.
Small, solitary boils: Antibiotics are unnecessary, except for boils of the lips, nose or eyelid.
Large furuncles or *carbuncles:* Incision if necessary, together with oral flucloxacillin for 7–10 days to prevent further spread. Erythromycin is an alternative in patients with penicillin allergy, and either may be combined with fusidic acid.
Furunculosis (multiple, recurrent) often accompanies underlying diseases such as diabetes which lower general resistance. Treat with oral flucloxacillin or erythromycin for 1–2 weeks. The application of neomycin/bacitracin ointment around the boil may protect the surrounding skin from further infection.

Erysipeloid is caused by Erysipelothrix rhusiopathiae.
Systemic treatment: Phenoxymethylpenicillin 1–2 g daily for 10 days, or doxycycline in patients with penicillin allergy (see p. 499).

Cutaneous anthrax (malignant pustule) is caused by Bacillus anthracis (see p. 499).

Tularaemia (cutaneo-glandular type) is caused by Francisella tularensis.
Systemic treatment: Gentamicin i.m. for 1 week, usually in combination with doxycycline (see p. 508).

Cutaneous diphtheria is caused by toxigenic strains of Corynebacterium diphtheriae.
Systemic treatment is with a single i.m. dose of diphtheria antitoxin 10,000 units, together with benzylpenicillin 1.2–2.4 g daily or, in patients with penicillin allergy, erythromycin 1–1.5 g (50 mg/kg in children) daily for one week.

Erythrasma: The *causative organism* is Corynebacterium minutissimum. Gram-positive rods may be seen in a gram-stained smear, and the skin lesions fluoresce red under Wood's light. The organism may be cultured on special media.
Topical treatment: Tetracycline ointment twice daily for 3 weeks; tolnaftate is also effective.
Systemic treatment: Oral fusidic acid or erythromycin 1 g daily for 2 weeks. Doxycycline is an alternative.

Borreliosis (Lyme disease) occurs acutely as erythema migrans and chronically as Acrodermatitis atrophicans.
Causative organism: Borrelia burgdorferi. The risk of serious chronic forms of this infection (see also p. 361) is justification for the treatment of every case of erythema migrans and every inflamed tick bite with phenoxymethylpenicillin 2 g daily, doxycycline 0.2 g daily or erythromycin 1 g daily, for 10 days. Ceftriaxone 2 g daily may also be used.

b) Chronic Bacterial Infections

Cutaneous tuberculosis (Lupus vulgaris, tuberculosis cutis verrucosa, scrophuloderma) is nowadays very rare; it responds well to chemotherapy, especially isoniazid (adults 300 mg, children 8–10 mg/kg daily by mouth). Combination with other antituberculous drugs such as ethambutol, rifampicin or pyrazinamide is essential in order to prevent the development of bacterial resistance (see p. 516).

Swimming pool granuloma: Ulcerating nodes on the chin, elbows, lower leg or feet, due to Mycobacterium marinum or M. balnei.
Treatment: Local excision of subcutaneous nodes, and systemic rifampicin + ethambutol. Tetracyclines (e.g. minocycline) are also effective.

Buruli ulcer: A chronic ulcerating condition which particularly affects the extremities. The *causative organism* is Mycobacterium ulcerans, which grows slowly and prefers 33° C. Relatively common in tropical Africa, this condition also occurs in other tropical countries. The ulcer is nearly always solitary, almost painless, and difficult to treat; surgical excision with skin grafting if necessary is the most effective treatment. Although a few strains of M. ulcerans are sensitive to ethambutol, streptomycin is the only antibiotic to which the organism is always susceptible *in vitro*. Chemotherapy alone is seldom effective, however; local heat is sometimes beneficial.

Actinomycosis (cervicofacial form) is *caused* by Actinomyces israeli (p. 512).
Topical treatment: Incision and drainage where necessary.
Systemic treatment: Initially benzylpenicillin 6 g as a short i.v. infusion twice daily for 4–6 weeks, followed by phenoxymethylpenicillin 1–3 g daily by mouth for 2–6 months or longer if necessary.

In mixed infections which involve staphylococci, anaerobes etc., i.v. flucloxacillin, clindamycin or metronidazole may be added. Doxycycline may be used as an alternative to penicillin in patients who are penicillin-allergic. Sulphonamides are inferior to penicillin and are no longer used to treat this condition, even in combination with other agents.

c) Bacterial Infections Secondary to Viral Infections

Secondary bacterial infections, which are frequently mixed, occur in herpes simplex and zoster, chickenpox and eczema herpeticum. Severe cases should be treated systemically with an antistaphylococcal, penicillinase-stable penicillin (flucloxacillin) or with a broader-spectrum agent such as a cephalosporin. Topical treatment with mupirocin may be beneficial.

d) Viral Infections of the Skin

Severe herpes, zoster and chickenpox may be treated with acyclovir (see p. 278).

e) Secondary Infections in Dermatoses

Eczema, exudative neurodermatitis, dermatoses with blister formation, contact dermatitis, leg ulcers and acne can all become secondarily infected with staphylococci or streptococci, and sometimes also with proteus, Escherichia coli, Pseudomonas aeruginosa or Candida albicans. Chronic ulcers of the lower leg are almost always heavily colonised with bacteria and should be treated with antimicrobials only when there is clear clinical evidence of inflammation.

Treatment: Topical gentamicin, polymyxin B (for gram-negative bacteria), mupirocin or amphomycin (for gram-positive cocci), and nystatin, miconazole or clotrimazole (for Candida albicans). Systemic antimicrobials are only necessary in severe cases or in the presence of potentially dangerous pathogens (e.g. Streptococcus pyogenes).

f) Acne and Rosacea

Acne: Systemic treatment with a tetracycline such as oral minocycline (which is particularly lipophilic) 50 mg daily, or with oral doxycycline 100 mg daily, promotes healing of the skin lesions by reducing the production and release of locally irritant free fatty acids by Propionibacterium acnes into the comedones. A low dose of tetracycline (250 mg) taken daily over a long period is sometimes also effective, as is oral erythromycin used in the same way. Systemic treatment is only justifiable in severe disease, and milder cases will usually respond to topical clindamycin, tetracycline or erythromycin. Supportive treatment with ultraviolet light, expression of the comedones, benzoyl peroxide, and possibly vitamin A acid may also be beneficial.

In **rosacea,** doxycycline 100 mg orally once daily for 4–6 months may be beneficial even though the lesions are non-infective. Topical metronidazole gel (applied twice daily) has been approved for this indication, particularly in the pustular forms of the disease.

g) Fungal Infections of the Skin

If fungal infection is suspected, the **diagnosis** should be confirmed by microscopy (squash preparation with 10% KOH) and culture, since there are dermatoses which resemble fungal infection, and since some antifungal agents are only effective against certain fungal species. Bacterial infections and allergic reactions can occur secondarily. Fungal infections are frequently associated with a defect in host resistance which should, if possible, be corrected. Other predisposing factors include diabetes mellitus and treatment with topical steroids or broad-spectrum antibiotics. The treatment of dermatophyte infections may be unsuccessful until the animal source has been removed or controlled.

The **imidazole derivatives** clotrimazole, econazole, ketoconazole, miconazole, sulconazole and tioconazole have greatly improved the topical therapy of fungal infections of the skin (see Table 58, p. 477). They have a broad spectrum of antifungal activity. Indications for topical use of these agents include clinically suspected or confirmed infections with dermatophytes or yeasts, erythrasma and pityriasis versicolor. Ketoconazole cream is effective in seborrheic dermatitis if caused by the yeast Pityrosporum orbiculare.

Nystatin, natamycin (pimaricin) and **povidone iodine** are alternative topical treatments for superficial skin infections with Candida albicans, such as perlèche, interdigital infections, intertrigo and paronychia. For anal intertrigo due to candida, nystatin should be used orally as well as topically in order to reduce the colonic reservoir.

Ciclopiroxolamine* is very effective when used topically, and penetrates particularly well into affected nails. **Tolnaftate** is beneficial in skin infections with dermatophytes, particularly tinea pedis. **Naftifin*** is unrelated to other antifungal agents and is well tolerated. It is used as a cream, gel or solution (for nails) for infections with dermatophytes, yeasts and moulds.

Systemic treatment with **griseofulvin** is indicated in tinea (epidermophytosis and trichophytosis but not tinea versicolor), microsporum infections and favus. Resistance to griseofulvin has been found in some infections with Trichophyton rubrum, Microsporum canis and Epidermophyton floccosum. Failure of griseofulvin treatment is sometimes attributable to inadequate absorption and hence low serum concentrations. Since griseofulvin is more soluble in lipids than in water, it is better taken after a fatty meal.

Infections of the toes do not usually respond well to griseofulvin. Since treatment is based on the incorporation of the antibiotic in the deeper layers of the skin, from which it passes gradually to the surface, superficial lesions and hairs should be treated from the outset with a suitable topical antifungal such as tolnaftate. Removal of affected hairs or nails and keratolytic treatment with 1–2% salicylic acid ointment improve the effectiveness of local measures.

Once improvement is seen, the initial daily dose of 0.5–1 g may be halved, or given in full on alternate days. Treatment may be required for 1–6 months, depending on the site and extent of the lesion. Improvement is seen at the earliest after 3–4 weeks in skin lesions, after 4–6 weeks in the hair, after 6–8 weeks in the palms and soles, after 3–6 months in the fingernails and often only after 1–2 years in the toenails. Because of its possible side-effects, griseofulvin should only be used in severe infections which are unlike to respond to alternative forms of treatment.

An alternative to griseofulvin in severe fungal infections is the systemic use of an imidazole such as fluconazole or itraconazole. These agents have now largely replaced the i.v. use of miconazole. All these drugs have side-effects and should therefore only be used where topical therapy is unlikely to succeed.

Fluconazole is a triazole antifungal indicated for local and systemic candidiasis and cryptococcal infections. It is given in a single oral dose of 150 mg for acute or recurrent candidosis, and at a dose of 50 mg daily by mouth for 7 days in oropharyngeal candidosis and 14 days in other mucosal infections such as

---

* not available in Britain

oesophagitis and candiduria. It may also be used i.v. for systemic fungal infections, including cryptococcal meningitis, which occur as a complication in immunosuppressed patients, and particularly those with AIDS.

Itraconazole is given in an oral dose of 200 mg twice daily for one day in vulvovaginal candidosis, 200 mg once daily for 7 days in pityriasis versicolor, 100 mg daily for 15 days in tinea corporis and tinea cruris, and 100 mg daily for 30 days in tinea pedis and tinea manuum. This drug should not be given for longer than 30 days.

Ketoconazole is given in an oral dose of 200 mg (3 mg/kg in children) once daily with food for 14 days or until at least 1 week after symptoms have resolved or cultures cleared. Because of the risk of severe, potentially fatal hepatotoxicity, this drug should be used only in exceptional cases and regular liver function tests during treatment are mandatory.

Amphotericin B i.v. is indicated in generalised candidosis and in granulomatous candida and cryptococcal infections localised in the deeper layers of the skin. Prolonged therapy is almost always necessary and should be combined with flucytosine when the isolate is sensitive. The synergistic effect of this combination allows a lower dose of amphotericin B to be used than would otherwise be necessary. For the use and dosage of amphotericin B, see p. 193. Amphotericin B is *contraindicated* in pregnancy and in severe hepatic and renal disease.

References

DONTA, S. T., P. W. SMITH, R. E. LEVITZ, R. QUINTILIANI: Therapy of Mycobacterium marinum infections. Use of tetracyclines vs. rifampin. Arch. Intern. Med. *146:* 902 (1986).
EADY, E. A., K. T. HOLLAND, W. J. CUNLIFFE et al.: The use of antibiotics in acne therapy: oral or topical administration. J. Antimicrob. Chemother. *10:* 89 (1982).
KLOTZ, S. A.: Malassezia furfur. Infect. Dis. Clin. North Am. *3:* 53 (1989).
KOHLHEPP, W., P. OSCHMANN, H. G. MERTENS: Treatment of Lyme borreliosis. Randomized comparison of doxycycline and penicillin G. J. Neurol. *236:* 464 (1989).
Medical Letter. Topical metronidazole for rosacea. Med. Lett. Drugs Ther. *31:* 75 (1989).
SCHMADEL, L. K., G. K. MCEVOY: Topical metronidazole: a new therapy for rosacea. Clin. Pharm. *9:* 94–101 (1990).

15. Sexually Transmitted Diseases

a) Syphilis

Penicillin remains the drug of choice for the treatment of all stages of syphilis (lues). Tetracycline and erythromycin, both of which are only bacteriostatic against treponemes, or a cephalosporin, are alternatives in penicillin-allergic patients. Penicillin is best given as a depot preparation by deep i.m. injection; procaine penicillin should be given daily, and a compound preparation of procaine, benethamine and benzylpenicillins (Triplopen) every 2–3 days in this way. Benzathine penicillin for parenteral use is available as a depot preparation in some countries, but not in Britain.

Because of the consequences of inadequate treatment, oral penicillins should not be used to treat syphilis. When treating primary and secondary syphilis, the serum concentration of penicillin should not be allowed to fall below 18 mg/l for 10–14 days, because treponemes replicate slowly in the body, and penicillin only kills actively dividing bacteria. Tertiary and neurosyphilis should be treated for at least 3 weeks. Higher dosage does not improve results except in cases of AIDS, tertiary syphilis and neurosyphilis; starting treatment as early as possible gives the best chance of success. Supplementary topical steroids may be needed to treat parenchymatous keratitis.

Diagnosis: Diagnostic tests should be completed before the first dose of penicillin is given. These include dark-ground microscopy of secretions from the primary lesion or from condylomata lata. Blood and, where indicated, CSF should be obtained for serological tests for syphilis. Whatever the serological method used, results may be falsely positive in pregnancy and rheumatic conditions, and falsely negative in the early phase of the disease. The Treponema pallidum haemagglutination (TPHA) test is suitable for screening. The non-specific cardiolipin reaction, as the VDRL slide test or the cardiolipin CFT, first becomes positive later in the primary phase of syphilis, when regional lymphadenitis has developed. This test can revert to negative in tertiary disease. If positive, confirmatory serological tests should be carried out. The indirect immunofluorescence technique (FTA-ABS test) will detect specific anti-treponemal IgG and IgM; the latter is an index of active infection.

Although penicillin treatment is rapidly effective, the patient does not become seronegative for several months. The cardiolipin titre usually falls to about one-third of its maximal level after adequate treatment. Treponema-specific 19S (IgM) antibodies are no longer detectable 3–24 months after the end of treatment, whereas specific 7S (IgG) antibodies usually persist for life ("serological scars"). The total serum IgM and IgG remain within normal limits. Since syphilis responds less readily to treatment in patients who are HIV-positive, patients with positive syphilitic serology should also be tested for HIV.

In the **newborn babies** of syphilitic mothers, it used to be difficult to distinguish between maternal antibody acquired by placental transfer and antibody formed as a result of infection in the baby. If the mother has been treated adequately with penicillin, IgG antibodies transferred passively to the infant will fall steadily during the first year of life. On the other hand, a rise in titre and the detection in the infant's blood of IgM antibody specific to Treponema pallidum, which does not cross the placenta, is always evidence of infection in the child. When the child does not become infected until the end of pregnancy, its syphilitic serological titres at and immediately after birth can still be negative. Screening tests for syphilis should therefore be performed at the beginning of pregnancy and, if omitted then or if clinical suspicion of infection arises, also in the third trimester and at delivery.

Guidelines for treatment: There are a number of views about the size of the *penicillin dosage* and the duration of treatment required. In the USA and certain other countries, 3 injections of 1.44 g benzathine penicillin (at weekly intervals) are considered sufficient for primary and secondary syphilis, whereas in Britain and Germany a daily injection of procaine penicillin 0.72 g for 15 days is preferred. In tertiary syphilis and in latent syphilis of longer standing, which can progress to neurosyphilis, there is general agreement that a higher dosage is needed.

Serological tests should be repeated 3, 6 and 12 months after treatment in order to detect relapse or reinfection, and a fourth test after a further year is necessary in patients whose disease was present for longer than 1 year at diagnosis. Patients with neurosyphilis should be followed up with serological tests of blood and CSF for at least 3 years. Declining titres can be demonstrated up to 1–2 years after penicillin therapy. A further course of penicillin is indicated if serological titres rise, if there is clinical deterioration, or if there are CSF changes and positive serological titres in the CSF. Reinfections can occur after successful initial treatment. The sexual partner should also be treated at the same time. Before any further courses of treatment are given, serological titres in the CSF should be measured in order to exclude asymptomatic neurosyphilis, which is also accompanied by an increase in CSF cells and protein. Patients with HIV infection are likely to show an atypical serological response and a lower rate of response to treatment.

Treatment: **Acquired syphilis,** either primary or secondary, of less than one year's duration is treated with a depot penicillin such as procaine penicillin 0.72–1.44 g (according to body weight) daily for 15 days. HIV-positive patients should be given higher doses of penicillin for longer (6 g twice daily for 3 weeks); despite this, relapses and more rapid progression to neurosyphilis are reported.

Patients with tertiary and neurosyphilis should be treated with i.v. benzylpenicillin 7.2–14.4 g daily for 15 days.

A Herxheimer reaction (fever, chills, increase in syphilitic lesions), due to the release of treponemal endotoxins, may occur on the first day of treatment. This should not be mistaken for penicillin allergy but should be treated with bedrest and antipyretics and, if severe, with prednisone. Treatment should not be interrupted.

Patients allergic to penicillin should be given either tetracycline 2 g twice daily for 20 days, or minocycline 100 mg twice daily for 2 weeks (30 days in neurosyphilis or latent syphilis of more than one year duration). These alternative regimes require long-term follow-up to detect possible relapse. If cross-allergy with penicillins can be ruled out, cefuroxime 1 g i. m. twice daily for 2 weeks or ceftriaxone 1 g i. v. once daily for 2 weeks are more reliable than tetracycline and minocycline and are particularly useful in pregnancy. The quinolones are ineffective in syphilis.

Congenital syphilis in *neonates* and *infants* should be treated with procaine penicillin i. m. or aqueous benzylpenicillin i. v. in a dose of 30 mg/kg daily for 14 days (total dose 420 mg/kg). Because of the increased danger of a Herxheimer reaction at this age, a simultaneous dose of prednisone (2 mg/kg) is recommended on the first day of treatment. Benzathine penicillin is not sufficiently reliable for use in congenital syphilis with CNS involvement because it does not achieve adequate CSF concentrations. The skin and mucosal lesions rapidly improve with treatment, but the regression of the hepatosplenomegaly and bone changes is more gradual. Serological titres usually become negative after 3–6 months. The patient should be followed up serologically, clinically and, where necessary, with CSF examination every 3 months at first, then 6-monthly and finally annually. Oral treatment with phenoxymethylpenicillin 120 mg daily for 14 days (total dose 1.68 g) should only be undertaken in hospital, where regular dosage can be ensured.

Pre-school children should be treated with i. m. procaine penicillin 300 mg daily, and *children of school age* 600 mg daily, each for two weeks.

Syphilis in pregnancy is treated with procaine penicillin 720 mg daily for 15 days. For safety, this course may be repeated at the same dosage 1–2 months before the expected date of delivery, and should be repeated if titres rise. Patients allergic to penicillin may be treated with ceftriaxone or cefotaxime 2 g daily.

Postnatal prophylaxis in the newborn is necessary when the seropositive mother was not treated for her syphilis at all, or only inadequately, or not treated with benzylpenicillin until the end of her pregnancy, or treated with erythromycin on account of her penicillin allergy. Since the newborn baby may initially be symptom-free and, when infected in the final stage of pregnancy, may not seroconvert until after a latent period, the safe course is to treat the child as soon as possible after birth in the same way as for manifest congenital syphilis, particularly if regular follow-up of the child cannot be guaranteed. Serological titres should be regularly checked thereafter.

References

Centers for Disease Control. Guidelines for the prevention and control of congenital syphilis. M.M.W.R. *37* (Suppl. 1): 1–13 (1988).
Centers for Disease Control. 1989 Sexually transmitted disease treatment guidelines. M.M.W.R. *38* (Suppl. 8): 1–43 (1989).
Csonka, G. W. and J. K. Oates: Sexually Transmitted Diseases. Ballière Tindall, London 1990.
Handsfield, H. H.: Old enemies. Combating syphilis and gonorrhea in the 1990s (editorial comment). J.A.M.A. *264*: 1451–1452 (1990).
Holmes, K. K.: Sexually Transmitted Diseases. 2nd Edition. McGraw-Hill, New York 1990.
Lowhagen, G. B.: Syphilis: test procedures and therapeutic strategies. Semin. Dermatol. *9:* 152–159 (1990).
1989 sexually transmitted diseases treatment guidelines: extracted from the Centers for Disease Control guidelines. Pediatr. Infect. Dis. J. *9:* 379–382; discussion 382–384 (1990).
Tramont, E. C.: Treponema pallidum (Syphilis). In: G. L. Mandell, R. G. Douglas, Jr., J. E. Bennett (eds.), Principles and Practice of Infectious Diseases (3rd ed.). New York: Churchill Livingstone, 1990. Pp. 1794–1808.
Treatment of sexually transmitted diseases. Med. Lett. Drugs Ther. *32:* 5–10 (1990).
Zenker, P. N., R. T. Rolfs: Treatment of syphilis. Rev. Infect. Dis. *12*, Suppl. 6: S590–609 (1990).

b) Gonorrhoea

This common sexually transmitted disease often goes unrecognised, particularly in the female. The diagnosis should always be confirmed bacteriologically by microscopy (gram, methylene blue, immunofluorescence) and culture on selective media, e.g. Thayer-Martin, with full identification of suspect colonies to species. In women, gonococci are best demonstrated in samples of cervical discharge; they may also be found in anal swabs (in women and homosexuals), urethral discharge and sometimes also from the oropharyngeal mucosa and pharyngeal swabs (in gonococcal pharyngitis). Swabs should be placed immediately in special transport medium (Amies' or Stuart's) for transmission to the laboratory where cultures on selective media should be incubated in a CO_2-enriched atmosphere (candle jar or CO_2 incubator).

Asymptomatic carriers of gonococci are common. The microscopic demonstration of intra- or extracellular gram-negative diplococci is not in itself sufficient to make a diagnosis of gonorrhoea, since other neisseriae may also be isolated from the vagina, and other microorganisms can be mistaken for neisseriae in gram smears. *Double infection* with gonococci and Treponema pallidum can occur, with syphilis not becoming apparent until after the gonorrhoea has resolved. A rise in temperature at the beginning of a course of penicillin for gonorrhoea may be due to a Herxheimer reaction from undetected syphilis. Gonorrhoea is frequently accompanied by a chlamydial cervicitis or urethritis, and not infrequently by mycoplasma infection (Ureaplasma urealyticum).

Follow-up should include culture after 2 weeks of a urethral swab in men, and of a cervical and rectal swab in women, because of the possibility of relapse.

Treatment: Until recently, benzylpenicillin was the antibiotic of choice. In the past 10 years, however, an increase in penicillin-resistant strains has occurred everywhere, most of which are also resistant to tetracycline and erythromycin. Single-dose therapy should nowadays therefore be with a β-lactamase-stable cephalosporin from the outset, or with another agent whose activity can be relied upon. There is now considerable experience with cefoxitin, cefuroxime (parenteral), ceftriaxone and cefotaxime. Failure of cephalosporin treatment is attributable either to diagnostic error or to reinfection, particularly if both partners were not treated simultaneously. Postgonococcal urethritis with other bacteria can sometimes occur. Apparent failures of treatment in patients from whom gonococci have not been cultured are frequently due to primary infections with resistant microorganisms such as chlamydiae, gardnerella, ureaplasma, candida, trichomonas etc. An unrecognised herpes simplex cervicitis or urethritis should also be considered.

Recently acquired gonorrhoea: Whereas benzylpenicillin in a single i. m. dose of 2.88–3.6 g used always to be sufficient, it is now considered better to give i. m. cefuroxime 1.5–2 g, injected into 2 sites, before sensitivities are available. An alternative is a single injection of cefotaxime (0.5 g i. v. or i. m.) or cefoxitin (2 g i. v.). There are recommendations that the possible simultaneous presence of chlamydial infection should always be treated with supplementary oral doxycycline 0.1 g twice a day for 2 weeks at the outset, without awaiting the results of microbiological investigations. If possible, the sexual partner should be treated in the same way.

Spectinomycin may also be used in a single dose of 2 g in uncomplicated gonorrhoea, but has a failure rate of up to 10%.

Oral tetracycline 2 g daily or erythromycin 3 g daily for one week used to be recommended as an alternative in patients allergic to penicillin, but has a failure rate of up to 20%. A course of co-trimoxazole 1.92 g (2 tablets) twice daily for 8 days is also unlikely to be effective against penicillin-resistant strains. The quinolones have so far proved reliable against all strains of gonococci, and are now the treatment of choice in gonorrhoea. The recommended single oral dose of ciprofloxacin is 0.25–0.5 g, of ofloxacin 0.2 g, of norfloxacin 0.8 g and of pefloxacin 0.4 g. With the exception of norfloxacin, these agents will also eliminate chlamydial infection, but co-existent syphilis will be unaffected.

Long-standing gonorrhoea, gonococcal proctitis or gonorrhoea with other complications such as salpingitis, endometritis, prostatitis or epididymitis, where sensitive, should be treated with benzylpenicillin i. v. in a daily dose of 2.4–7.2 g daily for 10 days, or cefuroxime i. v. 6 g daily for 10 days. Deep foci such as pyosalpinx and ovarian abscess may need surgical treatment under antibiotic cover, which is usually undertaken after the acute infection has subsided.

Septicaemia, arthritis and meningitis should be treated where sensitive with aqueous benzylpenicillin (not a depot preparation) in a daily dose of 6–12 g for 2–3 weeks (4 weeks for endocarditis), or with cefuroxime, cefoxitin or cefotaxime 6 g i. v. daily for 10 days. Generalised infection in the newborn as a result of amnionitis from premature rupture of the membranes should be treated with cefuroxime i. v. in a daily dose of 100 mg/kg.

Gonococcal ophthalmia: Cefuroxime and cefotaxime are now more reliable as initial treatment than benzylpenicillin. The daily dose of cefuroxime i. v. is 60 mg/kg in the newborn and 4–6 g in adults, both given for 7 days. Sensitive infections may be treated with i. m. procaine penicillin 240 mg daily in the newborn and 2.4 g in adults for 7 days, together with topical chloramphenicol or gentamicin eye drops. When a diagnosis of gonorrhoea is made in the mother before delivery, the newborn baby should be treated as soon as possible after birth not only with erythromycin (0.5%) or tetracycline (1%) eye ointment, but also with a single i. v. or i. m. injection of cefuroxime or cefotaxime 100 mg/kg.

Vulvovaginitis in children: When sensitive, give i. m. procaine penicillin 600 mg daily, or cefuroxime 60 mg/kg daily, each for 5 days. A single dose of cefuroxime 100 mg/kg is an alternative.

Gonococcal pharyngitis: Single-dose treatment is less effective and should always be monitored bacteriologically. Treatment failures should be given a longer course (5–10 days) of either procaine penicillin 600 mg daily, cefuroxime i. v. 2 g daily or ciprofloxacin i. v. 1 g daily. Spectinomycin and ampicillin are ineffective in this situation.

References

BRYAN, J. P., S. K. HIRA, W. BRADY et al.: Oral ciprofloxacin versus ceftriaxone for the treatment of urethritis from resistant Neisseria gonorrhoeae in Zambia. Antimicrob. Agents. Chemother. *34:* 819–822 (1990).

Centers for Disease Control: Sexually transmitted diseases treatment guidelines. Pediatr. Infect. Dis. J. *9:* 379–382 (1990).

COVINO, J. M., M. CUMMINGS, B. SMITH et al.: Comparison of ofloxacin and ceftriaxone in the treatment of uncomplicated gonorrhea caused by penicillinase-producing and non-penicillinase-producing strains. Antimicrob. Agents. Chemother. *34:* 148–149 (1990).

JUDSON, F. N.: Management of antibiotic-resistant Neisseria gonorrhoeae. Ann. intern. Med. *110:* 5 (1989).

MORAN, J. S., J. M. ZENILMAN: Therapy for gonococcal infections: options in 1989. Rev. Infect. Dis. *12*, Suppl. 6: S633–644 (1990).

c) Lymphogranuloma venereum

Causative organism: Chlamydia trachomatis of serotypes 1, 2 or 3. The primary stage is an isolated papule on the genitalia, which progresses to a superficial, indolent ulcer with a sharp edge. Swelling and suppuration develop in the inguinal lymph nodes, and late sequelae are proctitis and genital elephantiasis. Primary infections of the vagina or rectum lead to marked swelling of the pelvic and perirectal lymph nodes, and oropharyngeal infections involve the cervical lymph nodes. The serum CFT is positive in >80% of patients, and sometimes in chlamydial urethritis as well. Cross-reactions can occur in psittacosis/ornithosis and trachoma.

Treatment: Tetracycline, e. g. doxycycline 0.2 g daily by mouth for 3 weeks, or longer in chronic infections. Relapse can occur. The buboes may, if necessary, be drained by aspiration. Rectal strictures may require dilatation and in severe cases anoplasty. Sulphonamides (4 g a day) and co-trimoxazole (0.96 g a day) for 3 weeks are also effective (failure rate 7–10%).

References

BECKER, L. E.: Lymphogranuloma venereum. Int. J. Dermatol. *15:* 26 (1976).
BURGOYNE, R. A.: Lymphogranuloma venereum. Prim. Care *17:* 153–157 (1990).
LAL, S., B. G. GARY: Further evidence of the efficacy of co-trimoxazole in granuloma venereum. Br. J. Vener. Dis. *56:* 412–413 (1980).
MCLELLAND, B. A., P. C. ANDERSON: Lymphogranuloma venereum. JAMA *235:* 56 (1976).

d) Chancroid

Causative organism: Haemophilus (Streptobacillus) ducreyi. Usually gives rise to multiple painful genital ulcers with a narrow margin of erythema, lymphangitis and inguinal lymphadenitis (bubo). The organism can be seen microscopically and cultured from secretions at the margin of the ulcer or from pus; dark-ground microscopy for treponemes should also be performed. Double infections (chancroid + syphilis, chancroid + lymphogranuloma inguinale) may occur, and the condition may be confused with ulcerating vesicular herpes simplex.

Treatment: The treatment of choice is now oral erythromycin 2 g daily for 7 days. An alternative if the response is unsatisfactory is oral co-trimoxazole 1.92 g daily for 7 days. A single dose of i. m. ceftriaxone 0.5 g, ciprofloxacin 1 g or oral co-trimoxazole 3.84 g may also be used. Aspiration and drainage of the buboes may be necessary. Even if asymptomatic, the sexual partner should be treated wherever possible at the same time. Other antibiotics (tetracyclines, streptomycin, cephalothin, cefoxitin, ampicillin, benzylpenicillin and chloramphenicol) are no longer effective because of the frequency with which resistant strains are found.

References

DANGOR, Y., R. C. BALLARD, S. D. MILLER et al.: Treatment of chancroid. Antimicrob. Agents. Chemother. *34:* 1308–1311 (1990).
DUNCAN, M. O., Y. R. BILGERI, H. G. FEHLER, R. C. BALLARD: Treatment of chancroid with erythromycin. A clinical and microbiological appraisal. Brit. J. Vener. Dis. *59:* 265 (1983).
DYLEWSKI, J., H. NSANZE, L. D'COSTA et al.: Trimethoprim sulphamoxole in the treatment of chancroid: comparison of two single dose treatment regimens with a five day regimen. J. Antimicrob. Chemother. *16:* 103 (1985).
MACDONALD, K. S., D. W. CAMERON, L. D'COSTA, J. O. NDINYA-ACHOLA, F. A. PLUMMER, R. A. RONALD: Evaluation of fleroxacin (RO 23-6240) as single-oral-dose therapy of culture-proven chancroid in Nairobi, Kenya. Antimicrob. Agents Chemother. *33:* 612 (1989).
PLUMMER, F. A., H. NSANZE, L. J. D'COSTA, P. KARASIRA, I. W. MACLEAN, R. H. ELLISON, A. R. RONALD: Single-dose therapy of chancroid with trimethoprim-sulfametrole. N. Engl. J. Med. *309:* 67–71 (1983).
SCHMID, G. P.: Treatment of chancroid. Rev. Infect. Dis. 12, Suppl. *6:* S580–589 (1990).
TAYLOR, D. N., C. PITARANGSI, P. ECHEVERRIA, K. PANIKABUTRA, C. SUVONGSE: Comparative study of ceftriaxone and trimethoprim-sulfamethoxazole for the treatment of chancroid in Thailand. J. Infect. Dis. *152:* 1002–1006 (1985).

e) Granuloma inguinale (Donovanosis)

Causative organism: Calymmatobacterium (Donovania) granulomatosis; gram-negative rods with bipolar staining which will not multiply on non-living culture media. Both intra- and extracellular organisms may be seen in ulcer exudate and biopsy material. Clumps of bacteria in the intracytoplasmic vacuoles of large mononuclear cells or neutrophil granulocytes in the ulcer exudate are typical. The disease is sexually transmitted. One or more indurated papules, which develop into irregular, painless ulcers, arise at the site of entry (external genitalia). The granulation tissue at the base of the ulcer has a reddened, cobblestone appearance. The ulcer margins are thickened and shiny. There is no inguinal lymphadenopathy, though subcutaneous granulomata sometimes form in the inguinal region. The lesions tend to extend locally and can severely distort the external genitalia and rectum.

Diagnosis: Clinical and cytological or histological (malignant degeneration possible). Simultaneous infection with gonorrhoea or syphilis must be ruled out.

Treatment: Oral tetracycline 0.5 g 4 times daily or doxycycline 0.1 g twice a day for 3 weeks, or oral erythromycin 0.5 g 4 times a day for 3 weeks during pregnancy. I. m. gentamicin 1 mg/kg twice daily or oral co-trimoxazole 0.96 g twice daily for 2–3 weeks are also effective. Newer antibiotics (cefotaxime, ciprofloxacin) may be suitable, but experience of their use is at present lacking.

References

HART, G. Donovanosis: In: K. K. HOLMES et al. (eds.), Sexually Transmitted Diseases (2nd ed.). New York: McGraw-Hill, 1990. Pp. 273–277.
RAMANAN, C., P. S. SARMA et al.: Treatment of donovanosis with norfloxacin. Int. J. Dermatol. *29:* 298–299 (1990).
SEHGAL, V. N., SHYAM-PRASAD, A. L. Donovanosis: Current concepts. Int. J. Dermatol. *25:* 8 (1986).

16. Rheumatic Fever

Rheumatic fever is a disease predominantly of children and young adults in which fever, arthralgia, carditis, subcutaneous nodules and erythema develop some 2–3 weeks after a group A streptococcal infection. The symptoms are variable and may be confused with those of other conditions, such as lupus erythematosus and polyarteritis nodosa.

The importance of rheumatic fever to the patient is its legacy of damage to the heart valves, which can not only cause disorders of cardiac blood flow in later life, but can also act as foci for bacterial endocarditis. A suspected diagnosis of rheumatic fever must, therefore, be fully investigated and confirmed because of its implication to the patient of many years of penicillin prophylaxis against further attacks of rheumatic fever and hence worsening of the sequelae.

Treatment: Residual foci of streptococcal infection can be eradicated by treatment for two weeks with oral phenoxymethylpenicillin 250 mg 3 times a day, i. m. procaine penicillin 360 mg daily, or oral erythromycin 1 g daily if the patient is allergic to penicillin. Sulphonamides, co-trimoxazole and tetracyclines are unreliable in streptococcal infection and should not be used. The patient may also be given an antipyretic analgesic such as aspirin and, where necessary, prednisone in an initial dose of 50–100 mg (adults) or 2 mg/kg (children). The latter treatment is preferably managed in hospital with gradual reduction of the dose until the patient is free of symptoms and the ESR has returned to normal.

The purpose of **long-term penicillin prophylaxis** after rheumatic fever is to protect the patient from further infection with group A streptococci (Streptococcus pyogenes), which would cause the rheumatic fever to recur in 30–50% of cases if penicillin were not given. Streptococcal reinfection can be suppressed with a relatively low dose of penicillin given once a day. This prophylaxis should be continued for 5 years after every episode of rheumatic fever. After rheumatic carditis, particularly when valvular damage or several relapses have occurred, penicillin may need to be given life-long, or until at least the age of 25 when the first attack has occurred during childhood.

The long-term prophylaxis after rheumatic fever to prevent further infection with Streptococcus pyogenes should not be confused with the prophylaxis of bacterial endocarditis in patients with congenital or post-rheumatic heart valve abnormalities. For the latter, short perioperative courses of phenoxymethylpenicillin, amoxicillin, erythromycin, vancomycin or a cephalosporin are used to prevent the development of endocarditis on damaged heart valves secondary to the transient bacteraemia with viridans streptococci, enterococci or coagulase-negative staphylococci which can arise during dental, gynaecological, urological, orthopaedic and some colonic procedures (see p. 347).

Four regimens are acceptable for the prevention of recurrent rheumatic fever. These are:

1. Benzathine penicillin injected i. m. once a month. This regimen gives adequate serum penicillin concentrations for 4 weeks and has the lowest failure rate (0.4%), but sometimes causes local induration at the injection site and is strongly contraindicated in patients with penicillin allergy. Dosage: 0.72 g for adults and children of school age, and 0.48 g for pre-school children once a month (Fig. 62).
2. Oral phenoxymethylpenicillin 150 mg twice a day. Because the patient sometimes forgets to take the drug the failure rate is 3–5%.
3. In penicillin allergy, sulphonamides can be as effective as phenoxymethylpenicillin, e. g. sulphadiazine 1 g for adults, 0.5 g for children, once a day. Oral erythromycin 0.25 g twice daily is an alternative in patients who cannot tolerate sulphonamides.
4. When continuous long-term prophylaxis of rheumatic fever is not taken, the patient should be given a generous course of penicillin whenever symptoms arise which could even remotely be attributed to group A streptococci, i. e. for every sore throat or acute respiratory or wound infection.

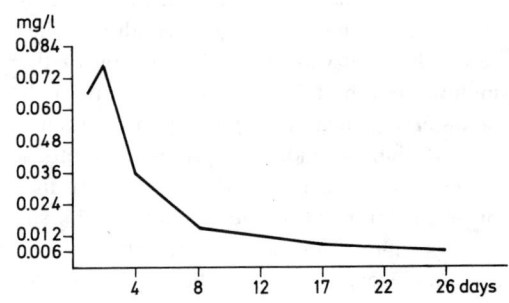

Fig. 62. Blood concentrations after a single i. m. injection of 0.72 g of benzathine penicillin.

Acute glomerulonephritis seldom recurs and so does not require long-term penicillin prophylaxis.

References

DAJANI, A. S. et al.: Prevention of rheumatic fever: A statement for health professionals by the Committee on Rheumatic Fever, Endocarditis and Kawasaki Disease of the Council on Cardiovascular Disease in the Young, the American Heart Association. Pediatr. Infect. Dis. J. *8:* 263 (1989).
ESPINOZA, L.: Infections in the Rheumatic Diseases. Grune and Stratton, New York 1988.
Leading Article: Prevention of rheumatic heart disease. Lancet *1:* 143 (1982).
WHITELAW, D. A.: Acute rheumatic fever in adults. S. Afr. Med. J. *78:* 305–308 (1990).

17. Scarlet Fever

Scarlet fever is an infection (usually a sore throat) caused by a toxigenic strain of *group A streptococci* (Streptococcus pyogenes), accompanied by a rash due to the erythrogenic toxin and in which the complication of nephritis or myocarditis can arise. The antibody response after convalescence gives no protection from future group A streptococcal infections, but will prevent any accompanying rash of scarlet fever. Prompt penicillin therapy shortens the course of the infection and reduces the risk of complications. Scarlet fever should always, therefore, be treated with antibiotics, generally penicillin for 10 days. In the third or fourth weeks after onset the urine should be examined to exclude post-streptococcal glomerulonephritis and an ECG performed if myocarditis is suspected. The differential diagnosis from toxic shock syndrome (see p. 451), Kawasaki syndrome, Lyell's syndrome and drug rashes is sometimes difficult.

Treatment: Although group A streptococci are susceptible to many antibiotics, penicillin is the most active and is the treatment of choice. Oral phenoxymethylpenicillin should be given for 10 days in a daily dose of 250 mg (preschool children), 375–500 mg (children of school age) and 750 mg (adults). Alternatives are an oral cephalosporin, i. m. benzathine penicillin* in a single dose of 360 mg (children) or 720 mg (adults), which ensures an adequate serum concentration for at least 10 days. Patients from whose throats group A streptococci can still be isolated after such treatment do not require further penicillin if they remain free of symptoms, and may be assumed to be non-infectious. Insistence on negative throat swabs before return to play group or school is no longer justifiable.

Patients who are *allergic to penicillin* should be given erythromycin in a daily dose of 1 g (adults) or 40 mg/kg (children). The relapse rate after erythromycin is

---

* Injectable form no longer available in Britain

higher than after penicillin. Sulphonamides, co-trimoxazole and tetracycline are unsuitable.

Contacts of streptococcal pharyngitis or scarlet fever can avoid infection by taking oral phenoxymethylpenicillin at therapeutic dosage for 10 days.

18. Tetanus

Causative organism: Clostridium tetani. The clinical picture, with tonic muscle spasm in a fully conscious patient, is caused by tetanus toxin. In the newborn the disease begins 3–10 days after birth and is expressed as difficulties in feeding and swallowing, as prolonged screaming and as tonic spasms and muscular rigidity.

Antibiotic treatment can limit further toxin production by eliminating bacteria from the site of primary infection. Benzylpenicillin is the most suitable antibiotic, or i.v. tetracycline if the patient is allergic to penicillin. In deeply penetrating wounds the clostridia may be associated with foreign bodies and therefore only susceptible to antibiotics at high dosage. The antibiotic treatment of tetanus should also cover the possibilities of aspiration pneumonia and of mixed wound infection involving other bacteria. The treatment of choice is benzylpenicillin 6–12 g a day (0.6 g/kg in tetanus neonatorum) given in 2–3 short i.v. infusions; penicillin-allergic patients may be given either cefazolin or cefotaxime 6 g daily i.v. (after exclusion of cross-allergy) or i.v. tetracycline 1–2 g daily. The antibiotics should be given for at least 10 days.

Intensive care and the control of symptoms determine the outcome of the disease. This supportive treatment includes adequate sedation with diazepam, muscle relaxants, betablockers if required, early tracheotomy and mechanical ventilation, aspiration of respiratory secretions, maintenance of fluid and electrolyte balance, parenteral nutrition, control of hyperpyrexia by drugs and physical means, surgical measures where necessary, and supplementary pyridoxine in the newborn.

A single i.m. dose (never i.v.) of 6000 units of *human tetanus immunoglobulin* should always be given, even though the quantities of circulating toxin available for neutralisation may be small. Because of the risk of later relapse, the patient should be actively immunised at the same time with the first injection of tetanus toxoid (tetanus vaccine or adsorbed tetanus vaccine) 0.5 ml i.m. into the contralateral site.

Tetanus prophylaxis after injury:

Fully immunised persons whose last immunisation was more than 1 year previously should be given a booster dose of tetanus toxoid 0.5 ml i.m. If the wound is contaminated, oral phenoxymethylpenicillin, or tetracycline if the patient is penicillin-allergic, should be given for 10 days. Human tetanus

immunoglobulin 250 units should be given to patients not known to have received active immunisation if the wound:
- was sustained more than 6 hours before treatment was received;
- is a puncture wound;
- is potentially heavily contaminated with tetanus spores;
- is septic, or
- contains much devitalised tissue.

500 units should be given if more than 24 hours have elapsed or there is particularly heavy contamination.

Nonimmunised or incompletely immunised persons should always be given simultaneous active and passive protection with human tetanus immunoglobulin 250 or 500 units i.m. (see above) and tetanus toxoid 0.5 ml i.m. into the contralateral site.

A second dose of toxoid is given after 4 weeks and a third after a further 4 weeks.

Human tetanus immunoglobulin alone cannot be relied upon to protect fully against tetanus.

Neonatal tetanus when the mother is non-immune can be prevented by 2 doses of tetanus toxoid during pregnancy.

References

CATE, T. C.: Clostridium tetani (Tetanus). In: G. L. MANDELL, R. G. DOUGLAS, JR., J. E. BENNETT (eds.), Principles and Practice of Infectious Disease (3rd ed.). New York: Churchill Livingstone, 1990.

STANFIELD, J. P., A. GALAZKA: Neonatal tetanus in the world today. Bull. WHO 62: 647–669 (1984).

19. Gas Gangrene

The most important *cause* of gas gangrene is Clostridium perfringens (welchii), although other anaerobic clostridia such as C. novyi, C. septicum, C. histolyticum, C. bifermentans and C. fallax can also give rise to this condition. The infections are commonly mixed with other anaerobes (peptostreptococci, bacteroides) and enterobacteria. These bacteria are almost ubiquitous and enter deep wounds through dirt or soil following road traffic accidents, particularly those involving motorcycles, agricultural accidents and gunshot wounds. They produce toxins under anaerobic conditions.

There are several clinical forms. **Clostridial cellulitis** of skin and subcutaneous adipose tissue develops slowly, with marked crepitation. It does not involve muscle, unlike acute, fulminating **clostridial myositis,** which develops suddenly and progresses rapidly to severe systemic intoxication, intravascular haemolysis, metastatic septic foci and acute renal failure. Gas formation is slight or absent.

Postoperative gas gangrene can follow lower limb amputation for arteriosclerosis; the organisms enter the stump wound through local lymphangitis. Other clinical forms include the severe uterine gas gangrene which can follow illegal abortion, and postoperative gas gangrene in the abdominal wall after gall bladder operations. **Clostridial septicaemia** can arise from the gut in conditions such as leukaemia and neoplasms of the large bowel.

The **diagnosis** of gas gangrene is primarily clinical, but can rapidly be confirmed by the microscopic demonstration of typical gram-positive rods in material from the wound. Culture is not difficult, but requires special media. Other forms of cellulitis associated with extensive subcutaneous gas formation and myonecrosis are caused by gram-negative bacilli, streptococci and/or bacteroides; they have a generally more favourable prognosis.

Treatment: When gas gangrene is suspected, benzylpenicillin in high doses (12–24 g daily in 3–4 short i. v. infusions) should be started at once in an attempt to prevent further spread of the infection. The clostridia of gas gangrene are always susceptible to penicillin. High doses are needed to reach organisms in necrotic tissue. Metronidazole, a parenteral cephalosporin or tetracycline are alternatives in patients allergic to penicillin. Gangrenous myositis requires a surgeon radically to excise all necrotic tissue, drain pus and lay open the wound. Septic abortion requires thorough curettage and possibly hysterectomy. The value of *hyperbaric oxygen* is controversial; to be effective, this treatment has to be started early, and the patient needs to be transported with care to a hyperbaric chamber in the vicinity. Clostridia are quite commonly seen in material from wounds, the uterus, bile obtained at operation and abdominal surgical wounds. Such findings are always an indication for treatment with benzylpenicillin. Mixed infections with Bacteroides fragilis should be treated with additional i. v. metronidazole, and mixed infections with gram-negative aerobes with additional cefotaxime and gentamicin.

Intensive supportive treatment including transfusion of blood or plasma, maintenance of fluid and electrolyte balance, and haemodialysis in renal failure is extremely important. The administration of clostridial antiserum (horse) is unnecessary and dangerous; corticosteroids and immunoglobulins also have no place in the treatment of gas gangrene.

Prophylaxis: Benzylpenicillin in high dosage (3–12 g daily) can prevent the development of gas gangrene in patients with contaminated wounds or severe tissue damage. Prophylaxis with moderate doses of penicillin should be given to any patient with a severely contaminated wound or who is about to undergo lower limb amputation for ischaemia; failure to do so may be regarded as medical negligence. Prophylactic antitoxin is no longer recommended.

20. Anthrax

The **causative organism** is Bacillus anthracis. Anthrax has become a rare infection, found usually in persons who work with animals or hides, or who handle bone-meal fertiliser. The characteristic malignant pustule of anthrax is the commonest and least severe form and may heal spontaneously. Pulmonary, intestinal, septicaemic and haemorrhagic meningitic anthrax have a poor prognosis and are often fatal despite treatment. The large gram-positive bacilli may be demonstrated by microscopy and culture of pus, sputum or blood. Penicillin susceptibility is variable, and high doses of benzylpenicillin should always be given.

Treatment: Benzylpenicillin i. v. (or i. m.). Cutaneous anthrax should be treated with at least 3 g (adults) or 60 mg/kg (children) daily, and other forms with 12 g (adults) or 300 mg/kg (children) daily.

Patients allergic to penicillin should be treated with tetracycline 0.5–1 g i. v. 12-hourly or doxycycline 0.2 g daily by mouth. Cutaneous anthrax should be treated for 2 weeks and other forms for at least 4 weeks according to the severity of the disease. In cutaneous anthrax even a single dose of doxycycline 0.3–0.5 g can lead to cure. Cephalosporins are also very effective. The organisms are susceptible to virtually every antibiotic.

References

DAVIES, J. C. A.: A major epidemic of anthrax in Zimbabwe. Cent. Afr. J. Med. *28:* 291–298 (1982).
NALIN, D. R., B. SULTANA, R. SAHUNJA: Survival of a patient with intestinal anthrax. Amer. J. Med. *62:* 130 (1977).
SAGGAR, S. N., M. M. JOSEPH, W. J. BELL: Treatment of cutaneous anthrax with a single oral dose. East Afr. Med. J. *51:* 889 (1974).

21. Erysipeloid

Causative organism: Erysipelothrix rhusiopathiae. Characteristic skin lesions on the hands have a good prognosis; arthritis or septicaemia with endocarditis are rare complications. The organism can be cultured micro-aerophilically from skin biopsy material. This infection is particularly associated with meat handlers.

Treatment of choice: Phenoxymethylpenicillin 750 mg daily for 10 days; for septicaemia, benzylpenicillin 3–12 g daily i. v. for 4–6 weeks. Doxycycline or erythromycin are alternatives in penicillin-allergic patients.

References

BAIRD, P. T., R. BENN: Erysipelothrix endocarditis. Med. J. Aust. 2: 743 (1975).
MUIRHEAD, N., T. M. S. REID: Erysipelothrix rhusiopathiae endocarditis. J. Infect. 2: 83 (1980).
VENDITTI, M., V. GELFUSA, F. CASTELLI et al.: Erysipelothrix rhusiopathiae endocarditis. Eur. J. Clin. Microbiol. Infect. Dis. 9: 50–52 (1990).

22. Listeriosis

Premature and neonatal listeriosis follows placental transfer of the organisms and frequently causes mid-trimester abortion, stillbirth, premature labour and inflammatory changes in the placenta. The following symptoms are suggestive of neonatal listeriosis: meconium-stained amniotic fluid, septic neonatal jaundice, posterior pharyngeal granulomas, purulent conjunctivitis, bronchopneumonia, meningitis or encephalitis. Infection of the newborn during birth from contact with vaginal fluid containing listeria can cause meningitis or isolated intestinal infection (late onset disease).

Early diagnosis is essential for successful treatment and can be made by demonstrating gram-positive rods in a gram-stained smear and on culture of the meconium, nasal or eye swabs, urine, CSF, blood, tracheal aspirate, placental tissue and lochia. The presence of gram-positive bacilli in the meconium, which is normally sterile, is an indication for blood culture from the baby, followed immediately by antibiotic treatment. Meconium from all babies whose mothers had spontaneous premature labour should be cultured for listeria, regardless of whether the babies have signs of sepsis, since premature labour is often the first sign of congenital listeriosis. Where possible, placental tissue (and products of conception in any unexpected mid-trimester abortion) should also be sent for culture. Blood cultures from a pregnant woman with unexplained fever, particularly if it is followed by premature labour or spontaneous abortion, may yield listeria. Serological tests on maternal and cord blood are not suitable for screening for listeriosis, but may be used to confirm infection with a particular serotype. Prompt treatment increases the chance of recovery to 50–80%. Despite good *in-vitro* activity, the effect of antibiotics against organisms sequestered in deep granulomatous tissue is unreliable, so prolonged treatment at high dosage is usually necessary.

Treatment of neonatal listeriosis: Ampicillin, mezlocillin and piperacillin have proved better than tetracyclines or chloramphenicol, which used to be recommended. Ampicillin or amoxycillin 200–400 mg/kg in 4 divided i. v. or i. m. doses are given daily for at least 3 weeks, and longer in meningitis; combination with gentamicin for the first 14 days is advisable. After 2–3 weeks a further 14-day course of ampicillin may be necessary to prevent relapse. Simultaneous treatment of the mother is not usually necessary unless she has symptoms. Cephalosporins are unreliable in listeriosis.

Meningoencephalitis (acquired form): Infection with listeria is usually sporadic but certain foods have been implicated in outbreaks, including coleslaw, meat pâté, milk and dairy products and some soft cheeses. Listeria is unusual in causing a predominantly granulomatous meningoencephalitis, affecting mainly the elderly and patients with impaired immunity or resistance to infection (e. g. diabetes, liver disease, leukaemias and lymphoma). Most cases only show a moderate CSF pleocytosis (300–1000 cells/µl, many of which are mononuclear). Lower cell counts (<300/µl) are sometimes found, as is purulent CSF as in acute pyogenic meningitis.

The *diagnosis* is made by CSF culture (which may need prolonged incubation); the organisms are sometimes missed by direct microscopy because of their small numbers. Serological methods are unreliable. Since listeria meningoencephalitis is always haematogenous in origin, there is no need to search for an initial nasal or otogenic focus.

Treatment: As with neonatal listeriosis, listeria meningitis is best treated with i. v. ampicillin (or amoxycillin) 6–12 g (adults) or 200–400 mg/kg (children) daily in 3–4 divided doses. Benzylpenicillin in high dosage (12 g daily) is also effective. Combination with gentamicin 6 mg/kg/day is synergistic. In penicillin-allergic patients, a tetracycline such as minocycline (which penetrates CSF relatively well) in combination with gentamicin may be considered. Because of the poor penetration of antibiotics into the granulomatous tissue, treatment must be continued for at least 4 weeks.

Septicaemia (acquired, a not uncommon complication of cirrhosis, lymphomas and renal transplantation): Since meningitis frequently follows listeria septicaemia, treatment should be as for meningitis with ampicillin or amoxycillin plus gentamicin. Cephalosporins have no useful activity.

Listeriosis in pregnancy is usually asymptomatic and may lead to premature labour. Fever, pyelonephritis and endometritis sometimes occur, and meningitis very rarely. The diagnosis is confirmed by blood culture.

Treatment: Ampicillin or amoxycillin 3–6 g daily i. v. or orally for at least 2–3 weeks.

Oculoglandular or **cutaneous forms:** *Treatment* with ampicillin or amoxycillin 3–6 g or 100 mg/kg daily until clinical resolution; tetracycline in patients allergic to penicillin.

References

BOUVET, E., F. SUTER, C. GIBERT et al.: Severe meningitis due to Listeria monocytogenes. A review of 40 cases in adults. Scand. J. Infect. Dis. *14:* 267 (1982).
GELLIN, B. G., and C. F. BROOME: Listeriosis. J.A.M.A. *261:* 1313 (1989).
HEARMON, C. J., S. K. GHOSH: Listeria monocytogenes meningitis in previously healthy adults. Postgrad. Med. J. *65:* 74–78 (1989).
MANCINI, J., M. CHOUX, N. PINSARD: A cerebral abscess due to Listeria monocytogenes in a 15-month-old infant. Ann. Pediatr. Paris. *37:* 299–302 (1990).
ORTEL, S.: Listeria-meningitis and -septicaemia in immunocompromised patients. Acta. Microbiol. Hung. *36:* 153–157 (1989).
PEETERMANS, W. E., H. P. ENDTZ, A. R. JANSSENS, P. J. VAN DEN BROEK: Recurrent Listeria monocytogenes bacteraemia in a liver transplant patient. Infection *18:* 107–108 (1990).
STAMM, A. M., W. E. DISMUKES, B. P. SIMMONS et al.: Listeriosis in renal transplant recipients: report of an outbreak and review of 102 cases. Rev. Infect. Dis. *4:* 665 (1982).
TRAUTMANN, M., J. WAGNER, M. CHAHIN, T. WEINKE: Listeria meningitis: report of ten recent cases and review of current therapeutic recommendations. J. Infect. *10:* 107 (1985).

23. Salmonella Infections

Typhoid and paratyphoid fever (*causative organisms:* Salmonella typhi, S. paratyphi A or B), collectively known as enteric fever, are septicaemic illnesses which differ in their pathogenesis, diagnosis and treatment from the less severe gastrointestinal salmonellosis (*causative organisms:* S. typhimurium, S. enteritidis and a range of other serotypes) which generally cause a gastroenteritis that is limited to the intestinal tract. This distinction is important in the epidemiological management of asymptomatic salmonella carriage, since excretors of S. typhi and S. paratyphi pose a greater risk to the public health than excretors of non-enteric-fever strains, whose faecal carriage almost always ceases spontaneously within a few weeks or months.

a) Typhoid and Paratyphoid Fevers

Causative organisms: Salmonella typhi, Salmonella paratyphi A, B and C.

Clinical features: A septicaemic illness in which bacteria can be isolated from blood culture. Not to be confused with salmonella gastroenteritis.

Laboratory diagnosis: Salmonellae can be isolated from the blood during the first week of illness and from faeces and urine from the second week onwards. The Widal test for specific serum agglutinins shows a rise in titre to serum O antibody. Antibiotic susceptibility testing is important because multiresistant strains of S. typhi, which include resistance to chloramphenicol, co-trimoxazole and ampicillin, are regularly isolated in some parts of the world. Quinolones such as ofloxacin, ciprofloxacin and pefloxacin have so far remained effective.

Treatment: Chloramphenicol, for many years the standard treatment of typhoid fever, was largely superceded in the 1970's by co-trimoxazole. The risk of side-effects was smaller and therapeutic results were similar, although treatment occasionally failed. Like chloramphenicol, co-trimoxazole produces a slow lysis of fever after an interval of 1–3 days, but complete defervescence does not occur before 5–6 days. Although they reliably improve the course of the disease, neither co-trimoxazole nor chloramphenicol can completely prevent complications such as intestinal haemorrhage, perforation, relapse (after completion of treatment) or chronic excretion. Because of bacteriolytic (Herxheimer) reactions, it was usual with chloramphenicol to start with a low dose and increase gradually over 3 days. Such reactions do not occur with co-trimoxazole.

Co-trimoxazole should be given in a high dosage of 2.88 g (3 tablets) to adults and 30 mg/kg to children, twice a day. The blood count should be regularly monitored. Since co-trimoxazole is generally well tolerated, treatment should be continued for at least 10 days after defervescence. Trimethoprim has also been used to treat typhoid fever in this way to good effect.

The introduction of the broad-spectrum cephalosporins and quinolones has made the treatment of typhoid safer and more reliable. *Cefotaxime* and *ceftriaxone* at normal dosage (Table 78, p. 591) are almost always curative. Despite a rapid clinical response, treatment should still be continued for at least 8–10 days.

Ofloxacin, ciprofloxacin and *pefloxacin* are also effective treatment of typhoid fever (see Table 78, p. 591 for dosage) and should be given for at least 10 days as well. Ciprofloxacin has proved very effective in the treatment of chronic excretion of S. typhi and paratyphi, as well as of other salmonellae.

Because of its toxicity and the increase in resistance, *chloramphenicol* is now seldom considered in westernised countries for the treatment of enteric fever; it still has an important role in tropical countries, however.

A *suitable regimen* for oral or parenteral chloramphenicol in 3 divided doses is as follows:
Day 1: 1 g (adults), 15 mg/kg (children);
Day 2: 2 g (adults), 30 mg/kg (children);
Day 3: 3 g (adults), 50 mg/kg (children).

The daily dose of chloramphenicol 3 g (adults) or 50 mg/kg (children) is given until defervescence, after which 1.5–2 g (adults) or 30 mg/kg (children) daily for a further 10–14 days is sufficient. When a critical total chloramphenicol dose of 25–30 g (adults) or 700 mg/kg (children) has been given, treatment may be changed to co-trimoxazole, ciprofloxacin or amoxycillin to avoid haematotoxicity.

Prednisone 20–60 mg daily for 2–3 days may be given for shock (usually at the start of treatment) or for particularly severe disease. Because of the risk of intestinal perforation, prednisone is contraindicated from the 3rd week of illness onwards, or in the presence of complications such as intestinal haemorrhage or perforation. Intestinal perforation is likely to give rise to peritonitis with mixed aerobic and anaerobic bowel organisms, for which a combination of antibiotics such as ampicillin + gentamicin + metronidazole, cefotaxime + metronidazole, ciprofloxacin + metronidazole, or imipenem + metronidazole should be given (see p. 411). Salicylates and other antipyretics should not be used because of enhanced sensitivity in typhoid fever which could result in hypothermia.

Ampicillin, which only achieves a slow defervescence and delayed improvement in symptoms, has been superceded by other antibiotics and should no longer be used to treat typhoid or paratyphoid fevers.

Tetracyclines are clinically ineffective in typhoid and paratyphoid fevers despite good *in vitro* activity and high biliary concentrations.

Relapses should be treated with an antibiotic which has not previously been used, e. g. cefotaxime if the initial treatment was with ciprofloxacin. If *metastatic foci* become established in other organs (osteomyelitis, septic arthritis, spondylitis, cholecystitis, empyema of the gall bladder, meningitis, orchitis), they should be treated with a broad-spectrum cephalosporin (e. g. cefotaxime) or ciprofloxacin.

b) Gastrointestinal Salmonellosis

The **causative organisms** are salmonellae other than S. typhi or S. paratyphi, many serotypes of which can give rise to gastrointestinal salmonellosis. These strains are seldom isolated from blood or urine, but are generally found in culture of faeces from the onset of the illness. The infection is usually acquired from contaminated food (see p. 400) and gives rise to a febrile gastroenteritis with diarrhoea and vomiting that is generally self-limiting, but can be severe or even life-threatening in patients with impaired resistance or severe dehydration.

Treatment: Mild infections may not be recognised as salmonellosis until the clinical picture has improved, and need symptomatic treatment only. In more severe infections for which an antibiotic is required, co-trimoxazole, trimethoprim or a quinolone may be considered. The principal aims of antibiotic treatment are to shorten the duration of symptoms, prevent the development of metastatic foci of infection, and reduce the likelihood of intestinal carriage after recovery. Gastrointestinal salmonellosis in patients with impaired immunity due, for example, to lymphoma, AIDS, bone marrow or solid organ transplantation, should always be treated with antibiotics; despite a response to therapy, such cases often relapse.

When bacteraemia develops, with a high fever and features of septicaemia, co-trimoxazole 1.92 g daily (adults) is usually effective. Alternative regimes are gentamicin in combination with high doses of parenteral ampicillin (if the salmonella is susceptible), cefotaxime, or ciprofloxacin. Salmonella meningitis is treated with cefotaxime or chloramphenicol.

c) Salmonella Excretors

Two categories of salmonella excretor should be carefully distinguished, namely:
1. *Excretors of S. typhi and S. paratyphi,* who have a reservoir of organisms, usually in the gallbladder but occasionally in the intestinal or urinary tracts, that is unlikely to clear spontaneously, and
2. *Excretors of other salmonella serotypes,* who pass the organisms temporarily in the faeces after gastroenteritis for a few weeks or months, after which there is almost always spontaneous clearance.

α) Persistent Excretors of Salmonella typhi and S. paratyphi

Patients who continue to pass Salmonella typhi or S. paratyphi A or B asymptomatically in their urine or faeces months after clinical treatment and resolution of the acute illness are persistent carriers. They often have chronic cholecystitis or gallstones. Attempts to clear a persistent typhoid or paratyphoid excretor with antibiotics should be preceded by bacteriological culture of aspirated duodenal fluid and ultrasound examination of the gallbladder. If gallstones are present, clearance of the carrier state will only be achieved by cholecystectomy under antibiotic cover (see below). The risk of operation has to be assessed for each case in the light of the benefit of eradication of persistent carriage. If the gallbladder is normal and free of stones, cholecystectomy is not usually necessary and high-dose antibiotic treatment should be tried first.

Conventional treatment regimes for persistent excretors: Ampicillin or amoxycillin 5–10 g a day in several short i. v. infusions for at least 14 days (if the strain has been shown *in vitro* to be susceptible), followed by oral treatment with amoxycillin 2–3 g or ampicillin 4 g daily for 2 months, or an ester such as pivampicillin 2 g or pivmecillinam 1.2–2.4 g daily for 14–28 days. Regular renal and liver function tests should be performed when pro-drugs are used for extended periods.

Good results have also been achieved with oral co-trimoxazole 1.92 g daily for 2–4 months. Chloramphenicol should not be used in chronic typhoid and paratyphoid carriage because of its toxicity and lack of effect.

Antibiotics that achieve high biliary concentrations such as cefoperazone, ceftriaxone, mezlocillin and the new quinolones have been extensively studied; ciprofloxacin in a dose of 500 mg twice a day for 4 weeks to 750 mg twice a day for 3 weeks (adults only) appears to be effective. These agents will undoubtedly replace earlier forms of treatment in due course.

β) Excretors of Other Salmonellae

The reservoir of organisms in chronic carriers of the salmonellae of gastrointestinal salmonellosis is usually the intestine and very rarely the gallbladder. Faecal carriage is usually self-limiting and seldom lasts more than a few weeks. Treatment with ampicillin or co-trimoxazole may temporarily suppress and even prolong the excretion of salmonellae. If treatment is attempted nevertheless because the patient is, for example, a food-handler, oral ciprofloxacin 0.5 g twice daily for 10 days should be used. Person-to-person spread is uncommon, but has been described in hospitals, pre-school play groups and institutions for the mentally handicapped.

References

BRYAN, J. P., H. ROCHA, W. M. SCHELD: Problems in salmonellosis: rationale for clinical trials with newer beta-lactam agents and quinolones. Rev. Infect. Dis. *8:* 189–207 (1986).
DATTA, N., H. RICHARDS, C. DATTA: Salmonella typhi in vivo acquires resistance to both chloramphenicol and co-trimoxazole. Lancet *I:* 1181 (1981).
EDELMAN, R. E., M. M. LEVINE: Summary of an international workshop on typhoid fever. Rev. Infect. Dis. *8:* 329–350 (1986).
LIMSON, B. M., R. T. LITTAUA: Comparative study of ciprofloxacin versus co-trimoxazole in the treatment of Salmonella enteric fever (letter). Infection *17:* 105 (1989).
RODRIGUEZ-NORIEGA, E. et al.: Quinolones in the treatment of Salmonella carriers. Rev. Infect. Dis. *11* (Suppl. 5): S1179 (1989).
SABBOUR, M. S., L. M. OSMAN: Experience with ofloxacin in enteric fever: J. Chemother. *2:* 113–115 (1990).
ST. GEME, J. W., et al.: Consensus: Management of Salmonella infection in the first year of life. Pediatr. Infect. Dis. J. *7:* 615 (1988).
THRELFALL, E. J., J. A. FROST, H. C. KING, B. ROWE: Plasmid-encoded trimethoprim resistance in salmonellas isolated in Britain between 1970 and 1981. J. Hyg. Camb. *90:* 55 (1983).
WITTLER, R. R., J. W. BASS: Nontyphoidal Salmonella enteric infections and bacteremia. Pediatr. Infect. Dis. J. *8:* 364–367 (1989).
YOUSAF, M., A. SADICK: Ofloxacin in the treatment of typhoid fever unresponsive to chloramphenicol. Clin. Ther. *12:* 44–47 (1990).

24. Brucellosis

Causative organisms: Six species of brucella have so far been associated with human brucellosis; they are B. abortus (cattle), B. melitensis (sheep and goats), B. suis (pigs), B. canis (dogs), B. ovis (sheep and hares) and B. neotomae (rats). The infection is usually acquired by direct contact with animals or their infected aborted material, or from the consumption of unpasteurised milk and its products. Brucellosis in man is a septicaemic illness with an acute, subacute or chronic course.

The **complications** of brucellosis include osteomyelitis, spondylitis, endocarditis, meningoencephalitis, granulomatous hepatitis, pneumonia and abortion. Epithelioid cells can be demonstrated histologically in the granulation tissue. The peripheral white cell count is normal or low. The organisms may be isolated from blood culture in special media incubated in a normal and a CO_2-enriched atmosphere. Agglutinating and complement-fixing antibodies may be demonstrated in the patient's serum (positive titre 1:100 or higher). The presence of blocking antibodies may make antibody detection difficult.

Treatment is difficult, particularly in subacute and chronic infection. Relapses are frequent despite effective chemotherapy. Infected patients become debilitated and easily fatigued, so general supportive measures are important. The antibiotics of choice are tetracyclines, e.g. oral doxycycline 0.2 g (adults) or 4 mg/kg (children) daily for 3–4 weeks. In severe infections, concomitant i.m. streptomycin 0.5–0.75 g (adults) or 25 mg/kg (children) daily for 2 weeks has been recommended (beware of toxicity to the inner ear). In *brucella osteomyelitis*, gentamicin is preferable to streptomycin for the 6 weeks of treatment because of its better tolerance. In *brucella endocarditis* and *meningoencephalitis* treatment with a tetracycline plus streptomycin (or gentamicin) should be supplemented with rifampicin, and doxycycline plus rifampicin for 6 weeks is emerging as the treatment of choice for all forms of acute brucellosis. Co-trimoxazole 1.44 g twice daily for 6–8 weeks has also been used but is associated with a high relapse rate. The new quinolones (e.g. ciprofloxacin) show promise but need further evaluation.

Relapses should be treated with a further course of a tetracycline such as doxycycline plus rifampicin; resistance to these agents has not been observed.

Chronic brucellosis causing endocarditis or osteomyelitis should be treated with maximal doses of a tetracycline for 6 weeks in combination with i.m. gentamicin + oral rifampicin for 3–4 weeks.

References

AL AWADHI, N. Z., F. ASHKENANI, E. S. KHALAF: Acute pancreatitis associated with brucellosis. Am. J. Gastroenterol. *84:* 1570–1574 (1989).
AL EISSA, Y. A., A. M. KAMBAL, M. N. AL NASSER et al.: Childhood brucellosis: A study of 102 cases. Pediatr. Infect. Dis. J. *9:* 74–79 (1990).
AL-IDRISSI, H. Y., A. K. UWAYDAH, K. T. DANSO, H. QUTUB, M. S. AL-MOUSA: Ceftriaxone in the treatment of acute and subacute human brucellosis. J. int. Med. Res. *17:* 363 (1989).
ARIZA, J., F. GUDIOL, R. PALLARÉS et al.: Comparative trial of co-trimoxazole versus tetracycline-streptomycin in treating human brucellosis. J. Infect. Dis. *152:* 1358 (1985).
ARIZA, J., F. GUDIOL, R. PALLARÉS et al.: Comparative trial of rifampin-doxycycline versus tetracycline-streptomycin in the therapy of human brucellosis. Antimicrob. Ag. Chemother. *28:* 548 (1985).
BOSCH, J., J. LIÑARES, M. J. LOPEZ DE GOICOECHEA et al.: In vitro activity of ciprofloxacin, ceftriaxone and five other antimicrobial agents against 95 strains of Brucella melitensis. J. Antimicrob. Chemother. *17:* 459 (1986).
CISNEROS, J. M., P. VICIANA, J. COLMENERO, J. PACHON, C. MARTINEZ, A. ALARCON: Multicenter prospective study of treatment of Brucella melitensis brucellosis with doxycycline. Antimicrob. Ag. Chemother. *34:* 881–883 (1990).

COLMENERO, J. D., J. M. REGUERA, F. P. CABRERA et al.: Serology, clinical manifestations and treatment of brucellosis in different age groups. Infection *18:* 152–156 (1990).
FARID, Z.: Brucella endocarditis cured by medical treatment (letter). J. Infect. Dis. *162:* 281 (1990).
FOUNTAIN, M. W., S. J. WEISS, A. G. FOUNTAIN et al.: Treatment of Brucella canis and Brucella abortus in vitro and in vivo by stable plurilamellar vesicle-encapsulated aminoglycosides. J. Infect. Dis. *152:* 529 (1985).
KIIAN, M. Y., M. DIZON, F. W. KIEL: Comparative in vitro activities of ofloxacin, difloxacin, ciprofloxacin, and other selected antimicrobial agents against Brucella melitensis. Antimicrob. Agents. Chemother. *33:* 1409–1410 (1989).
SHEHABI, A., K. SHAKIR, M. EL-KHATEEB, H. QUBAIN, N. FARARJEH, A. SHAMAT: Diagnosis and treatment of 106 cases of human brucellosis. J. Infect. *20:* 5–10 (1990).
VIEIRA, J. D. E. M.: Treatment of brucellosis with doxycycline and rifampicin: a study of 50 cases. Curr. Ther. Res. *35:* 944 (1984).

25. Tularaemia

Causative organism: Francisella tularensis. Transmitted by rodents, infected meat, droplets, animal bites and insect vectors. The primary focus is a sharply defined skin ulcer with marked swelling and occasionally suppuration of the regional lymph nodes. Pneumonia, conjunctivitis and septicaemia can also occur. Agglutinins may be demonstrated in the serum, a titre of 1:160 or more being considered positive. Animal inoculation is also used, and the organism may be cultured on special media.

Treatment: Because of its good bactericidal activity, streptomycin was considered the most suitable agent, though resistance rapidly develops. Gentamicin also appears to be effective. Good results have also been reported with tetracyclines when given early, so a combination of streptomycin (or gentamicin) and doxycycline would be reasonable. Oral doxycycline is used to prevent relapse. There is little reported experience with newer antibiotics.

Dosage: Streptomycin 1 g i. m. daily (increased to 2 g daily in cases of pneumonia or septicaemia), in combination with oral doxycycline 0.2 g daily for 10–14 days (until at least 5 days after defervescence). The daily dose of gentamicin is 0.24 g i. m. or i. v. (instead of streptomycin).

References

ALFORD, R. H., J. T. JOHN, R. E. BRYANT: Tularemia treated successfully with gentamicin. Amer. Rev. resp. Dis. *106:* 265 (1972).
BLOOM, M. E., W. T. SHEARER, L. L. BARTON: Oculoglandular tularemia. Pediatrics *61:* 660 (1978).
BUTLER, T.: Plague and tularemia. Pediat. Clin. North Amer. *26:* 355 (1979).
HALSTED, C. C., H. P. KULASINGHE: Tularemia pneumonia in urban children. Pediatrics *61:* 660 (1978).
MASON, W. L., T. EIGELSBACH, F. LITTLE, J. H. BATES: Treatment of tularemia, including pulmonary tularemia with gentamicin. Amer. Rev. Respir. Dis. *121:* 39 (1980).

26. Pertussis

Pertussis can occur from the first year of life onwards and is commonest in young children, though a milder form is occasionally found in adults also. In the catarrhal stage the cough is not characteristic of pertussis, but typical paroxysms of whooping cough and a peripheral lymphocytosis occur later. Before beginning antibiotic treatment, a pernasal swab should be inoculated promptly on to special media (e. g. Bordet-Gengou); this is valuable when the diagnosis is uncertain, to give early confirmation of the diagnosis and to differentiate B. pertussis from other pathogens. The best results are obtained when the patient attends the laboratory for specimens to be collected. Specific IgM antibodies are frequently detectable by immunoassay from the fourth week of illness onwards.

Pertussis-like symptoms may be caused in children by infection with Haemophilus influenzae, Bordetella parapertussis, Branhamella catarrhalis, Mycoplasma pneumoniae, Chlamydia trachomatis (in the first six months of life) and adenoviruses; foreign body aspiration should also be considered.

Antibiotics are used in whooping cough in an attempt to eliminate the causative organism and to prevent or treat complications. Early treatment in the catarrhal stage and at the start of the convulsive stage is generally only indicated in infants and young children, who are at the greatest risk of pneumonia and encephalopathy. Antibiotic treatment is unnecessary in children of school age except in those who have pre-existent brain damage or impaired immunity (e. g. leukaemia).

Because antibiotics are notoriously ineffective in controlling the distressing cough of pertussis, the best means of prevention is by active immunisation during the first year of life. The first dose of combined diphtheria, tetanus and pertussis vaccine may be given from the second month onwards. A single-antigen pertussis vaccine is also available. Concern which peaked in the 1970's about neurological damage from pertussis vaccine led to a fall in uptake in Britain which has only recently been reversed as public confidence in newer forms of the vaccine has been restored. The decade of low vaccine uptake was marked by several epidemics of whooping cough.

Treatment: Oral erythromycin 50 mg/kg daily, or parenteral cefotaxime 60 mg/kg daily in patients who are vomiting frequently, eliminates the bacteria rapidly but does not shorten the paroxysmal stage. A patient who has been treated with erythromycin for 2 weeks may be assumed to be no longer infectious.

Doxycycline syrup 2 mg/kg daily stains teeth, so should only be used in children aged 8 or over. Pertussis hyperimmune globulin is of no value, and active immunisation should not be given once symptoms have developed.

Supplementary treatment: Fresh air, bronchiolytics, frequent small meals, hospital care, careful aspiration of mucus or vomit, humidification of inspired air, and increased oxygen if necessary. Codeine should be avoided because of the increased risk of atelectasis and secondary pneumonia. Prednisone may be given for encephalopathy, and bronchoscopy with deep suction may be necessary for persistent major pulmonary atelectasis.

Pertussis pneumonia is often accompanied by secondary infection with organisms such as Haemophilus influenzae or pneumococci, in which case treatment with i. v. cefotaxime 60 mg/kg daily or oral cefixime is advisable.

Chemoprophylaxis after exposure is recommended in infants and non-immunised children at increased risk because of underlying conditions such as heart defects or cystic fibrosis. Erythromycin 30 mg/kg daily should be given for 10 days, or longer if contact is prolonged.

References

BANNATYNE, R. M., R. CHEUNG: Susceptibility of Bordetella pertussis to cephalosporin derivatives and imipenem. Antimicrob. Ag. Chemother. 26: 604 (1984).
BASS, J. W.: Pertussis: current status of prevention and treatment. Ped. Infect. Dis. 4: 614 (1985).
HOPPE, J. E., U. HALM, H. J. HAGEDORN, A. KRAMINER-HAGEDORN: Comparison of erythromycin ethylsuccinate and co-trimoxazole for treatment of pertussis. Infection 17: 227 (1989).

27. Leptospirosis

Causative organisms: Various pathogenic serovars (serotypes) of Leptospira interrogans can infect man. In Europe the commonest are Leptospira icterohaemorrhagiae (Weil's disease), L. grippotyphosa (swamp fever), L. sejroe *serovars* hardjo and saxkoebing (lymphocytic meningitis), L. canicola and L. pomona. Though traditionally leptospirosis was associated with sewer workers, miners and fish workers, agricultural workers are now the main occupational group at risk and account for more than half the cases reported in Britain, where infections with L. sejroe following contact with cattle have become the commonest form of leptospirosis in recent years.

Diagnosis: Leptospirosis is confirmed either by isolating the organism from blood, CSF or alkaline urine, or by detecting specific serum antibodies from the second week of illness onwards, by agglutination, complement fixation or ELISA. Serological testing for leptospirosis is appropriate only for the confirmation of an initial clinical suspicion and should not be used to decide whether or not to start treatment.

Treatment: The prognosis is dependent on the virulence of the infecting organisms and on the age of the patient, being less favourable in the elderly.

Antibiotic treatment is controversial and usually only effective if started within the first four days of illness, before the diagnosis can be confirmed, when it may reduce the likelihood of meningitis and shorten the course of the disease. Antibiotics are unlikely to be of value if started on or after the fourth day of illness, and many people recover without treatment. Thus benzylpenicillin 2.4–6.0 g or ampicillin i.v. 1 g should be given every 6 hours from when leptospirosis is first suspected (exposure, muscle pains etc.). In patients allergic to penicillin, doxycycline 0.2 g once daily can be used, also in patients with renal failure.

References

McClain, J. B. L., W. R. Ballou, S. M. Harrison, D. L. Steinweg: Doxycycline therapy for leptospirosis. Ann. Intern. Med. *100:* 696 (1984).

Takafuji, E. T., J. W. Kirkpatrick, R. N. Miller, J. J. Karwacki, P. W. Kelley, M. R. Gray, K. M. McNeill, H. L. Timboe, R. E. Kane, J. L. Sanchez: An efficacy trial of doxycycline chemoprophylaxis against leptospirosis. N. Engl. J. Med. *310:* 497–500 (1984).

28. Rickettsial and Coxiella Infections

Typhus fever (caused by Rickettsia prowazekii) and other rickettsial infections have become rare in north-western Europe in the past decade. Q-fever, which is caused by Coxiella burnetii and often gives rise to an interstitial pneumonia, is also uncommon. Exotic and classical forms of typhus are still occasionally imported, however; tick-borne typhus ("fièvre boutonneuse", caused by Rickettsia conorii) is quite frequently seen in travellers from parts of the Mediterranean and Africa. Sporadic infections with R. conorii occur in Central Europe. In the United States the common rickettsial diseases are Rocky Mountain spotted fever, endemic typhus, Rickettsial pox and Q-fever. The clinical diagnosis of typhus fever can be confirmed by the microscopic demonstration of rickettsiae in a skin biopsy from a typical petechial lesion by direct immunofluorescent antigen detection, and from the tenth day of illness onwards by the demonstration of specific antibodies in the patient's blood by latex agglutination, ELISA or indirect immunofluorescence, in high single or in rising titre. Isolation of the causative organisms in tissue culture or animals is possible, but for reasons of safety requires a high degree of laboratory containment.

Treatment of rickettsial infection is with doxycycline, initially i.v., then orally in a dose of 0.2 g twice daily until 6 days after defervescence. Single-dose treatment of louse-borne typhus (caused by R. prowazekii) with doxycycline 0.2 g has proved effective in Africa. Chloramphenicol has also been used in the past in an initial daily dose of 3 g orally, then 2 g a day after defervescence. Prednisone 50 mg daily for a few days may be added in severe cases. Chemoprophylaxis for scrub typhus (Tsutsugamushi fever) with a single weekly dose of doxycycline 0.2 g orally for 6 weeks after an infecting insect bite is effective in almost 90% of cases.

Treatment of Q-fever is with oral doxycycline 0.2 g (in children 4 mg/kg) daily for 10–12 days of until 3 days after defervescence. For the treatment of Q-fever endocarditis, see p. 346.

References

BELLA, F., B. FONT, S. URIZ et al.: Randomized trial of doxycycline versus josamycin for Mediterranean spotted fever. Antimicrob. Agents Chemother. *34:* 937 (1990).
BUTLER, T., P. K. JONES, C. K. WALLACE: Borrelia recurrentis infection: single-dose antibiotic regimens and management of the Jarisch-Herxheimer reaction. J. Infect. Dis. *137:* 573–577 (1978).
MUÑOZ-ESPIN, T., P. LÓPEZ-PARÉS, E. ESPEJO-ARENAS, B. FONT-CREUS, I. MARTINEZ-VILA, J. TRAVERIA-CASANOVA, F. SEGURA-PORTA, F. BELLA-CUETO: Erythromycin versus tetracycline for treatment of Mediterranean spotted fever. Arch. Dis. Child. *61:* 1027–1029 (1986).
PERINE, P. L., S. AWOKE, D. W. KRAUSE, J. E. MCDADE: Single-dose doxycycline treatment of louse-borne relapsing fever and epidemic typhus. Lancet *II:* 742–744 (1974).
RAOULT, D., H. GALLAIS, P. DEMICCO, P. CASANOVA: Ciprofloxacin therapy for Mediterranean spotted fever. Antimicrob. Ag. Chemother. *30:* 606–607 (1986).
TEKLU, B., A. HABTE-MICHAEL, D. A. WARRELL, N. J. WHITE, D. J. M. WRIGHT: Meptazinol diminishes the Jarisch-Herxheimer reaction of relapsing fever. Lancet *I:* 835–839 (1983).
WISSEMAN JR., C. L., S. V. ORDONEZ: Action of antibiotics on Rickettsia rickettsii. J. Infect. Dis. *153:* 626 (1986).

29. Actinomycosis

Causative organism: Actinomyces israeli, which is not a true fungus, but an anaerobic, branching, filamentous bacterium. Clinically, actinomycosis gives rise to a chronic, indurated inflammation with a tendency to abscess and fistula formation. Cervicofacial actinomycosis is the commonest form, and thoracic (sometimes with pleural empyema) and abdominal actinomycosis only account for about 20% of cases. Metastatic spread to the skin, bones, liver, testes, heart valves or brain (causing cerebral abscess) is rare. The organisms can be seen microscopically in microcolonies ("sulphur granules") in pus as branching, filamentous, gram-positive bacilli. For this reason, pus should always be sent to the laboratory in preference to a swab. Culture is on special media incubated anaerobically for up to 10 days. The diagnosis may also be made histologically.

Treatment: A. israeli is very sensitive to benzylpenicillin. As with other chronic infections, penicillin must be given at high dosage over long periods because of the poor antibiotic penetration into the granulation tissue.

Dosage: Thoracic and abdominal actinomycosis should be treated with benzylpenicillin 6 g twice daily as a short i. v. infusion for 4–6 weeks, followed by a depot penicillin or oral phenoxymethylpenicillin 1.2–3 g daily for 2–6 (or even 12) months. Patients with penicillin allergy or in whom penicillin has failed may be given tetracycline 2 g daily, or other antibiotics. Clindamycin i. v. is also effective. Lower doses of penicillin (1.8 g daily for 6 weeks) may suffice in cervical actinomycosis.

Mixed infections with other anaerobes (Actinobacillus actinomycetem comitans, Haemophilus aphrophilus, bacteroides, streptococci) are usual and may be treated with the addition of doxycycline or metronidazole. Combinations of sulphonamides with the penicillin, as formerly recommended, do not improve results. Cure may be accelerated in some cases by surgical intervention such as incision, drainage or resection. If antibiotic treatment fails, the rare but clinically and microscopically similar condition of nocardiosis should be considered; this infection usually responds to large doses of sulphonamides, co-trimoxazole or imipenem.

References

BERKEY, P., G. P. BODEY: Nocardial infection in patients with neoplastic disease. Rev. Infect. Dis. *11:* 407 (1989).
FORBES, G. M., F. A. HARVEY, J. N. PHILPOTT-HOWARD et al.: Nocardiosis in liver transplantation: variation in presentation, diagnosis and therapy. J. Infect. 20: 11 (1990).
LESTER, F. T., E. JUHASZ: Actinomycosis of the ear. Ethiop. Med. J. *28:* 41–44 (1990).
ROSE, H. D., M. W. RYTEL: Actinomycosis treated with clindamycin. J. Amer. med. Ass. *22:* 1052 (1972).

30. Tuberculosis

Since the introduction of antituberculous drugs the prognosis and mortality of tuberculosis have greatly improved. In north-west Europe, new infections continue to occur in the elderly, young adults, members of ethnic minorities and patients with AIDS and other underlying disease; since the start of the AIDS epidemic, the progressive downward trend in the incidence of new cases of tuberculosis has levelled out in the USA and now also in Britain. Tuberculosis can be the presenting feature of AIDS, particularly in populations in which widespread immunisation with BCG has not been carried out.

Since antituberculous chemotherapy is not without risk and has to be given systemically over a long period of time, every effort must be made to confirm the diagnosis of tuberculosis by bacteriological and other means. The following **diagnostic procedures** should therefore always be performed before starting treatment:

1. The *microscopic demonstration* of acid-alcohol-fast bacilli (AAFB) in specimens such as sputum and gastric aspirate is suggestive but not diagnostic of tuberculosis, since the AAFB may be saprophytic or "atypical" mycobacteria.

Saprophytic species such as M. chelonae are particularly likely to occur in sputum samples obtained by fibreoptic bronchoscopy and, if not recognised as such, can give rise to "pseudo-outbreaks" of tuberculosis.

2. A *positive culture* to confirm the diagnosis and allow antibiotic sensitivities to be determined is essential. Where appropriate, sputum, a laryngeal swab, fasting gastric washings in children, pus, urine, CSF, needle biopsy material and bronchial secretions obtained at bronchoscopy should sent for bacteriological investigation before starting chemotherapy. Excised tissue should always be examined by culture as well as histologically.

3. *Animal inoculation* is no longer necessary for the primary isolation of M. tuberculosis because *in-vitro* culture methods have greatly improved.

4. The *tuberculin test* is still of great practical value in both children and adults, since in some "western" countries, particularly where young teenagers are not routinely immunised with BCG, 60–80% or more of young adults are tuberculin-negative. Patients with active tuberculosis generally react on intracutaneous testing to low concentrations of tuberculin ($\frac{1}{100}$, $\frac{1}{10}$, or 1 unit). Reactions which are negative at 1, 10 or 100 tuberculin units are usually evidence for the absence of active tuberculosis, although false negative reactions can occur in <1% of infected patients (pre-allergic phase, negative anergy, corticosteroid or cytotoxic therapy, measles, AIDS). A positive skin reaction to tuberculin is not in itself proof that the patient has human or bovine tuberculosis, but is merely evidence of past or present infection with acid-fast bacteria, which can include other species such as Mycobacterium kansasii, M. avium-intracellulare and M. fortuitum (cross-allergy). A positive tuberculin skin reaction persists for at least 5–10 years after immunisation with BCG.

5. *Sensitivities* against a full range of antituberculous agents should be determined for all mycobacteria isolated, both initially and from follow-up specimens, in case drug resistance has emerged during therapy. *In-vitro* testing is technically complex and best performed by a reference laboratory with special expertise. Isotopic methods (e.g. BACTEC) have reduced the time needed for sensitivity results from 3–6 weeks to 7–15 days. Complete or partial resistance to a range of drugs early in the disease raises suspicions of atypical or saprophytic mycobacteria, which should always be identified to species. Cross-resistance may be found between ethionamide and prothionamide and also between some members of the streptomycin group (streptomycin, kanamycin, capreomycin).

6. *Histopathology:* Tissue granulomas with epithelioid and giant cells in biopsied material or excised organs are not pathognomonic of tuberculosis but can be found in other mycobacterial infections, fungal infections, brucellosis and other chronic infections. The differentiation between non-caseous tuberculosis and sarcoidosis can also be difficult.

7. All patients with tuberculosis should have HIV serology.

a) Principles of Antituberculous Chemotherapy

The classification of tuberculosis into uncomplicated and complicated cases (Fig. 63) is of practical importance because of differences in the principles of treatment of these two groups of patients (see below). The combination of several antituberculous agents in full dosage for a long period is common to both groups. Triple therapy with isoniazid, streptomycin and para-aminosalicylic acid (PAS) was standard for many years. PAS, which is poorly tolerated, was then replaced with ethambutol. The introduction of rifampicin, which is bactericidal, enabled the period of treatment to be shortened from 2 years to 6–9 months. Quinolones (ofloxacin, ciprofloxacin, pefloxacin) are active *in vitro* against mycobacteria, including M. tuberculosis, but the results of clinical trials are awaited before their clinical value can be assessed.

The **treatment of the uncomplicated case** is based on 5 standard drugs (rifampicin, isoniazid, ethambutol, pyrazinamide, and streptomycin). Of these, only ethambutol is not bactericidal. Streptomycin is less active than isoniazid and rifampicin but more active than ethambutol. Isoniazid and rifampicin are the most effective antituberculous agents.

Uncomplicated case	Early, localised, non-cavitating	X-ray findings	Disseminated with cavitation	Complicated case
	No previous treatment	Treatment history	Previous treatment, reactivation	
	Sputum negative, no underlying disease	Bacteriology, underlying disease	Sputum positive, underlying disease present	

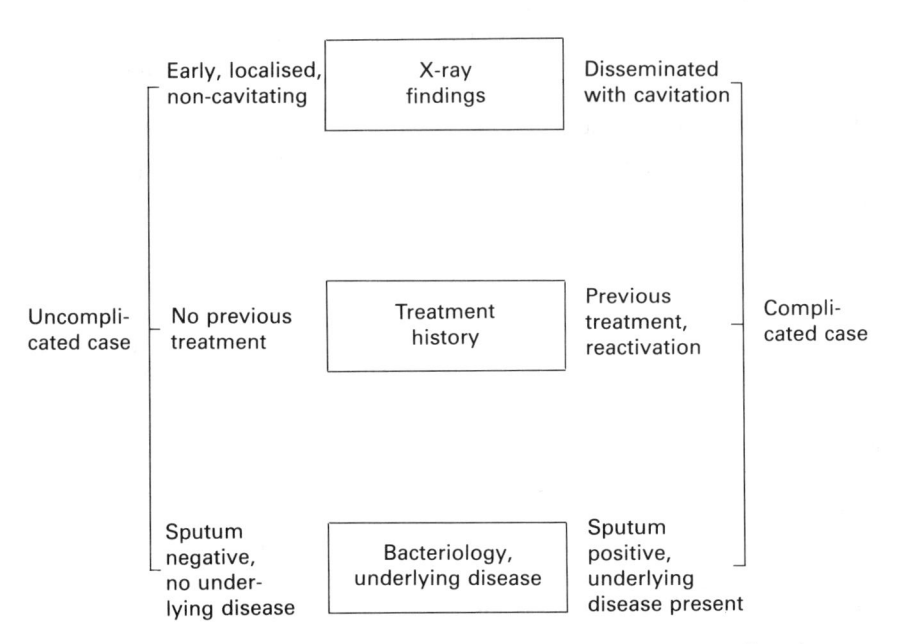

Fig. 63. Differentiation of pulmonary tuberculosis in uncomplicated and complicated cases.

The treatment of tuberculosis has two phases, namely an *initial phase* for 8 weeks and a *consolidation phase* for 4–7 months. At least 3 drugs are used during the **initial phase** in order to reduce the numbers of viable bacteria as rapidly as possible and to minimise the risk of ineffective treatment in those patients infected with antibiotic-resistant mycobacteria. The treatment of choice in the *initial phase* is a daily regimen of isoniazid, rifampicin and pyrazinamide; either ethambutol or streptomycin should be added if drug resistance is thought likely.

In the **consolidations phase,** treatment is continued with isoniazid and rifampicin if there are no contra-indications. Pyrazinamide is bactericidal against actively dividing forms of M. tuberculosis and therefore only effective in the first 2–3 months of treatment, after which it should be stopped. In the consolidation phase, ethambutol may be used with either isoniazid or rifampicin, but it requires a longer course and particular care to avoid ophthalmic toxicity. Streptomycin should only be used in the consolidation phase if there is no alternative, because of its cumulative oto- and nephrotoxicity.

During the consolidation phase, *intermittent treatment* under full supervision with high-dose isoniazid (15 mg/kg) and rifampicin (10 mg/kg up to a maximal dose of 0.9 g) twice a week (Table 59) has proved as effective as unsupervised therapy, particularly when patient compliance at home is unreliable. This regimen, which needs to be continued for only 6 months, has proved reliable and effective with a recurrence rate of less than 1%.

Antituberculous agents are always used in combination to increase antibacterial activity and prevent the emergence of bacterial resistance. Monotherapy of tuberculosis constitutes malpractice because any drug used singly will rapidly lose its effectiveness as resistance develops.

The **chemotherapy of the complicated case** is less easily standardised. Non-pulmonary tuberculosis always comes into this category because of the increased

Table 59. Dosage of antituberculous agents when given daily or intermittently.

Drug	Daily dose (mg/kg)	Usual total dose (g/day)	Intermittent dose
Rifampicin	10	0.45–0.6 (maximum 0.75)	10 mg/kg (maximum 0.75 g)
Isoniazid	5	0.3	15 mg/kg
Ethambutol	15	1	40 mg/kg
Pyrazinamide	25–30	1.5–2.0	60 mg/kg (3–4 g)
Streptomycin	15	0.75–1.0	0.75–1 g
Prothionamide	8–10	0.5–1.0	0.5–1 g

likelihood of relapse, of the emergence of resistant strains during treatment, and of the increased association with underlying diseases such as diabetes, alcoholism, neoplasia, or with factors which impair host resistance such as corticosteroid therapy. If the disease progresses or is reactivated despite treatment, the antituberculous drugs should if possible only be changed on the basis of the sensitivities of the patient's isolate. Complicated cases should always be given a full, standard, not a shortened course of treatment.

The **duration of treatment** depends on the combination of drugs used in the initial phase. Where isoniazid and rifampicin are given daily throughout treatment, a 9-month course is sufficient for patients with *pulmonary tuberculosis*, regardless of its extent. If in the initial phase pyrazinamide is included with isoniazid and rifampicin, and the latter 2 drugs are then used in the continuation phase, a total of 6 months of treatment gives equally good results.

Triple therapy of *open pulmonary tuberculosis* should be continued at least until sputum conversion (the disappearance of acid-fast bacilli from the sputum), which usually occurs within 2–3 months. Treatment should then be continued for a further 6–9 months with a combination of two active drugs, one of which should if possible be rifampicin.

Closed cases (primary tuberculous pleurisy or culture-negative pulmonary tuberculosis with minimal changes) may be treated with a double combination of rifampicin and isoniazid 6–9 months from the outset. The long-term treatment of tuberculosis requires much patience and understanding on the part of the patient, and psychological support by the doctor and his team. It is important to avoid both excessive and inadequate dosage. The major causes of treatment failure are incorrect prescribing by the physician and inadequate compliance by the patient. The initial treatment should be parenteral in unreliable patients (e.g. alcoholics) who may not take tablets regularly; isoniazid, rifampicin, ethambutol and streptomycin may all be given parenterally.

In **pregnancy,** active tuberculosis may be treated without serious risk to the fetus with isoniazid and ethambutol, and with rifampicin in the second half of pregnancy. Streptomycin, capreomycin and kanamycin can cause fetal damage and should be avoided, as should ethionamide and prothionamide (no longer marketed in Britain), and rifampicin in the first half of pregnancy.

In patients with **pre-existent liver damage,** streptomycin and ethambutol carry the lowest risk of side-effects. Isoniazid may be continued if the liver function does not deteriorate during the course of treatment. The combination of isoniazid and rifampicin should be avoided in patients with acute hepatitis. The risk of liver damage by isoniazid is greater in patients over 50 years of age than in younger adults and children.

In **renal impairment,** isoniazid and rifampicin may be given in normal dosage, since they are predominantly metabolised by the liver. The dose of ethambutol (see p. 266), pyrazinamide, streptomycin and capreomycin should be reduced and the two aminoglycosides avoided if renal failure is severe. Ethionamide, prothionamide and kanamycin should be avoided if at all possible.

Children should be treated according to the same principles as adults. Congenital tuberculosis is very rare; if treatment is required during the first month of life, potentially ototoxic antibiotics such as streptomycin and capreomycin should be avoided if possible, or only used in reduced dosage, because of the risk of accumulation as a result of immature renal function.

Bacterial resistance to isoniazid is rare (1–5%) in new cases of tuberculosis in Europe, but is commoner in second infections, which carries implications for treatment. Primary resistance to pyrazinamide and rifampicin is even less frequent. When a patient relapses or when the first course of treatment fails or causes unacceptable side-effects, a further course is given with another triple combination which should contain at least two drugs that have not previously been used and may include second-line drugs such as capreomycin, cycloserine or prothionamide. Subsequent treatment is based on the results of sensitivity testing which, with new and rapid methods, should become available within 1–2 weeks. If resistance to one of the drugs in this second-line combination is demonstrated initially or during treatment, further alternatives should be considered, of which ethionamide has proved effective in combination. If the isolate is resistant to streptomycin, cross-resistance and cumulative ototoxicity have been reported with capreomycin, which should not, therefore, be used until its sensitivity *in vitro* is known and inner ear damage has been ruled out.

Corticosteroids may be considered as an adjunct to antituberculous therapy in tuberculous empyema, meningitis or pericarditis, and miliary tuberculosis; they are of little value in other forms of the disease. The general contra-indications to steroid therapy should always be observed, and particular care taken when using steroids in patients with underlying diseases such as leukaemia, which can render antituberculous therapy less effective and lead to rapid dissemination of the tuberculosis. Corticosteroids should not, therefore, be started until several antituberculous drugs of known efficacy have been given in full dosage.

Dosage and side-effects. The risk of irreversible drug toxicity is small provided the patient is carefully monitored for side-effects and the relevant drug stopped at the first sign of intolerance (Table 60).

Isoniazid is cheap and highly effective; for pulmonary tuberculosis it is given in a dose of 300 mg (adults) or 6 mg/kg (children) daily, or up to 1 g (15 mg/kg) twice weekly. For tuberculous meningitis, a daily dose of 10 mg/kg is used. Its only common side-effect is *peripheral neuropathy,* which is more likely to occur at high

Table 60. Possible side-effects of the main antituberculous agents at normal dosage.

Side-effects	Isoniazid	Rifampicin	Ethambutol	Streptomycin	Prothionamide	Pyrazinamide
Normal daily dose for adults	0.3–0.5 g (6 mg/kg)	0.45–0.75 g (10 mg/kg)	1 g (15 mg/kg)	0.75–1 g (15 mg/kg)	0.5–1 g (8–15 mg/kg)	1.5–2.5 g (25–30 mg/kg)
Stomach and intestine		(+)			+	(+)
Liver	+	+			+	+
Kidneys		(+)		(+)		
Central nervous system	(+)		+	++	(+)	
Peripheral nervous system	+		(Optic nerve)	(Vestibular nerve)		
Bone marrow	(+)	(+)			(+)	
Skin	(+) (Pellagroid)			Allergy	(+) (Pellagroid)	(+) (Photo-dermatosis)
Joints						+ (gout)
Precautions and contra-indications	Consumption of alcohol, epilepsy, psychiatric illness	Liver damage, early pregnancy	Eye damage, consumption of alcohol	Renal failure, hearing loss, pregnancy	Liver damage, psychosis, epilepsy, alcohol abuse, early pregnancy, diabetes	Renal failure, liver damage, gout

dosage (as in meningitis) or where there are pre-existing risk factors. In these circumstances, pyridoxine 10 mg daily should be given prophylactically from the start of treatment. Other side-effects, such as hepatitis and psychosis, are rare.

Streptomycin is given intramuscularly in a standard dose of 1 g (15 mg/kg in children) daily, reduced to 0.5–0.75 g in small patients or those over the age of 40 years. Plasma concentrations of this drug should be monitored regularly, as should auditory and vestibular function, and an alternative drug (but not capreomycin) substituted at the first sign of inner ear damage. Aminoglycosides (streptomycin, capreomycin, kanamycin, gentamicin, tobramycin, netilmicin, amikacin) should never be combined with one another. If an aminoglycoside is used over a long period and plasma concentrations show no evidence of accumulation, treatment should only be continued with a different aminoglycoside when the patient's audiogram has remained normal and regular monitoring of cochlear and vestibular function can be continued. Side-effects increase after a cumulative dose of 100 g, which should only be exceeded in exceptional circumstances.

Rifampicin should be given in a single daily dose of 450 mg in adults of less than 50 kg, 600 mg in those above that weight, and up to 20 mg/kg (maximum 600 mg) in children. During the first two months of rifampicin administration, transient disturbance of liver function with elevated serum transaminases is common but generally does not require interruption of treatment. Occasionally, more serious liver toxicity requires a change of treatment, particularly in patients with pre-existing liver disease. On intermittent treatment, 6 toxicity syndromes have been recognised, namely influenzal, abdominal and respiratory symptoms, shock, renal failure and thrombocytopenic purpura; they can occur in 20–30% of patients. Rifampicin induces hepatic enzymes which accelerate the metabolism of several drugs including oestrogens, corticosteroids, phenytoin, sulphonylureas and anticoagulants. The effectiveness of oral contraceptives is reduced and alternative family planning advice should be offered.

Pyrazinamide is bactericidal against intracellular, dividing forms of M. tuberculosis, and is therefore only effective in the first 2–3 months of treatment. It is particularly useful in tuberculous meningitis because of its good meningeal penetration, and is not active against M. bovis. Pyrazinamide 20–35 mg/kg daily is given as 3–4 divided doses orally up to a maximum of 3 g a day. Side-effects include hepatotoxicity (fever, anorexia, hepatomegaly, jaundice, liver failure, nausea, vomiting, arthralgia, sideroblastic anaemia and urticaria) and hyperuricaemia (sometimes precipitating attacks of gout). Metabolic interactions with other drugs may be suspected but have not yet been described.

Ethambutol is used in conjunction with isoniazid or rifampicin in a daily dose of 15 mg/kg (adults and children over 6 years of age). Its principal side-effect is optic neuritis as shown by loss of visual acuity, red/green colour blindness and restriction of visual fields. These toxic effects are more common when excessive dosage is used or the patient's renal function is impaired. The earliest features of ocular toxicity are subjective, and patients should be advised to discontinue therapy immediately and seek further advice if their vision deteriorates. Early discontinuation of the drug is almost always followed by recovery of eyesight. Ethambutol should therefore be *avoided* in patients with renal impairment or who cannot understand warnings about visual side-effects (including children under 6 years of age).

If *symptoms of allergy* develop during combined therapy, the most likely cause (streptomycin) should be stopped and an alternative antituberculous agent substituted. *Women of child-bearing age* should take adequate contraceptive precautions because of the risk of teratogenicity if they become pregnant (note: rifampicin interferes with oral contraceptives).

The **criteria for successful treatment** are sputum conversion (disappearance of acid-fast bacilli), resolution and disappearance of a cavity or infiltrate, reduction in ESR and defervescence.

Failures of chemotherapy may be due to:
1. Too short or irregular a course of treatment.
2. Monotherapy.
3. Primary or secondary bacterial resistance.
4. Underlying disease (e.g. silicosis, leukaemia, lymphoma, AIDS).
5. Inadequate initial treatment (underdosage, omission of an active drug of first choice).
6. Infection with atypical mycobacteria.

Clinical improvement in pulmonary tuberculosis usually begins after 2–4 weeks and is followed by progressive improvement in the radiological changes. The sputum usually converts after 4–8 weeks. If acid-fast bacilli are still present after 6 months of combined chemotherapy, they will almost always be resistant to one or more of the drugs used.

Chemoprophylaxis with isoniazid 6–10 mg/kg/day for 3 months may be given after the exposure of a child or older family member even if symptoms are absent and the tuberculin test is negative. If the family contact remains tuberculin-negative (up to 100 units intracutaneously) after this period, BCG immunisation is recommended. The contact should then be kept away from any possible source of infection for at least 6 weeks. Immediate contacts of the patient should be tuberculin tested and have serial chest x-rays where necessary.

The newborn baby of a mother who was adequately treated during pregnancy or earlier and no longer has active tuberculosis does not need to be separated from the mother after delivery; the baby does not require isoniazid and may be given BCG. If the mother has signs of active, open tuberculosis and is infectious, the safest course is to separate mother and baby immediately after birth, give the baby chemoprophylaxis with isoniazid for 3 months, then give the baby BCG, and maintain the separation until the baby becomes tuberculin-positive (usually 6–12 weeks after BCG). Congenital tuberculosis should always be ruled out and, if present, should be treated with isoniazid and rifampicin. If the temporary separation of mother and child is impractical, the baby should be given prophylactic isoniazid under close medical supervision for 1 year and then be given BCG if still tuberculin-negative.

Preventive chemotherapy with isoniazid should be considered:
- when tuberculin conversion occurs during childhood. Dosage: isoniazid 6–10 mg/kg/day (maximum 300 mg) for 6–12 months. If the contact is infected with isoniazid-resistant bacteria, preventive therapy with rifampicin 600 mg + ethambutol 15 mg/kg daily is advisable. Indicated also in recent seroconverters (adults) with PPD ⩾10 mm increase within 2 year period for persons <35 years and ⩾15 mm increase for persons over 35 years.
- when there is a risk of reactivation of old tuberculosis by HIV infection, measles, leukaemia, or corticosteroid or immunosuppressive therapy. The dosage of isoniazid for adults is 300 mg daily and for children 10 mg/kg/day, for the period of exposure. Isoniazid is hepatotoxic and should be used with caution in the elderly and in patients with liver disease. If nevertheless radiological changes are detected by regular chest x-rays, combined chemotherapy should be given as in the acute case.

b) Treatment of Tuberculosis and their Chemotherapy

Pulmonary tuberculosis: *Initial treatment* is with a bactericidal combination, preferably isoniazid, rifampicin and ethambutol (or streptomycin). The addition of pyrazinamide leads to more rapid bacterial elimination. The following alternative regimens are acceptable treatments of uncomplicated pulmonary tuberculosis:

Initial treatment			Consolidation phase	
I. Rifampicin Isoniazid Ethambutol	10 mg/kg 5 mg/kg 15 mg/kg	2 months	Rifampicin Isoniazid	further 6 (–9) months
II. Rifampicin Isoniazid Streptomycin	10 mg/kg 5 mg/kg 15 mg/kg	2 months	Rifampicin Isoniazid	further 6 (–9) months
III. Rifampicin Isoniazid Streptomycin Pyrazinamide	10 mg/kg 5 mg/kg 15 mg/kg 25–30 mg/kg	2 months	Rifampicin Isoniazid	further 4 (–7) months

The *consolidation phase of treatment* is generally self-administered by outpatients. The drugs must be taken regularly and in unreliable patients may need monitoring. Regular medical follow-up including x-rays, blood counts, ESR and bacteriological examination of the sputum is important. Serum transaminases should be monitored in patients treated with rifampicin, isoniazid, pyrazinamide and ethionamide*. Regular tests of vision, visual fields, colour vision and fundoscopy are essential during ethambutol therapy. Frequent blood counts are particularly important in patients treated with isoniazid and rifampicin. Mycobacteria other than M. tuberculosis, which are often resistant to the usual antituberculous agents, may cause pulmonary tuberculosis in immunosuppressed patients; M. avium-intracellulare is particularly associated with AIDS. Culture from a lung biopsy is needed to confirm this diagnosis, because sputum culture is only suggestive. Possible treatments are discussed on p. 543, and may in future include the new quinolones.

In *absorption atelectasis* secondary to bronchial obstruction, bronchoscopy may be necessary to remove caseous material and avoid persistent pulmonary

---
* not marketed in Britain.

induration. *Segmental resection* or *lobectomy* are nowadays only needed in very few situations, such as large and persistent unilateral cavitation.

Exudative pleurisy: Treat as pulmonary tuberculosis with isoniazid + rifampicin for several months, but initially with the addition of a corticosteroid to accelerate absorption of the effusion and to minimise the formation of adhesions. *Dosage:* Prednisone 30–50 mg initially, reducing to 10–20 mg for about 4 weeks. The intrapleural instillation of isoniazid or streptomycin is not generally necessary.

Empyema: Systemic treatment as for pulmonary tuberculosis. Drugs may also be instilled into the pleural cavity, taking the possibility of absorption of agents also given systemically into account. Surgical intervention may also be necessary. Secondary infection with staphylococci or other organisms occurs not infrequently, and should be treated with appropriate antibiotics.

Tuberculosis of the cervical lymph nodes with human or bovine strains should be treated for several months with isoniazid and rifampicin, particularly when complete operative removal is not possible and there is a danger of recurrence. Surgical excision of the affected nodes shortens the course of the disease and reduces the likelihood of complications.

Infections of cervical lymph nodes due to atypical mycobacteria should be treated according to the species isolated and the results of sensitivity testing.

If the primary focus is in the tonsils or adenoids, tonsillectomy or adenoidectomy may be useful.

Tuberculosis of the mesenteric lymph nodes, intestine and peritoneum used to arise from a primary intestinal infection, but is now more usually the result of haematogenous spread or open pulmonary tuberculosis, and is increasingly reported in patients with AIDS. Combined chemotherapy should be given as for pulmonary tuberculosis, and isoniazid should never be given alone.

Miliary tuberculosis: Triple therapy with isoniazid, rifampicin and ethambutol or streptomycin, with the addition of a corticosteroid for a short time in patients with severe dyspnoea or toxicity. A lumbar puncture should be performed to rule out meningitis. A long course of treatment must be given even after early rapid improvement.

Tuberculous meningitis: Once a specimen of CSF has been examined, treatment should be started immediately with the following *four drugs in maximal dosage:*

- Isoniazid 10 mg/kg initially, then 5–7 mg/kg after 3–4 weeks (adults), or 15 mg/kg initially, then 10 mg/kg after 3–4 weeks (children). The maximum daily dose for adults is 1 g and for children 0.5 g.
- Rifampicin 10 mg/kg daily up to a maximal daily dosage of 0.75 g.

- Streptomycin 30 mg/kg i.m., with as maximal dose of 1 g daily (up to 1.5 g in adults) for the first month, reduced to twice weekly from the second month onwards.
- Ethambutol 15 mg/g daily.

If the strain of M. tuberculosis isolated proves resistant to any of these agents, pyrazinamide or prothionamide* may be substituted (for dosage, see Table 59, p. 516), both of which achieve good concentrations in the CSF. Pyrazinamide 30 mg/kg a day (daily maximum 2 g) may be used initially in place of ethambutol.

In severe cases with raised intracranial pressure, *prednisone* 50–100 mg (adults) or 1–2 mg/kg (children) may be given, reducing to a maintenance dose when clinical improvement is established.

Isoniazid achieves good CSF concentrations when given i.v. and need not therefore be given intrathecally. The intrathecal administration of streptomycin sulphate is unnecessary and dangerous.

Urogenital tuberculosis: As with other severe forms of nonpulmonary tuberculosis, treat with a combination of drugs, preferably isoniazid, rifampicin and ethambutol. Of these three agents, dosage reduction because of impaired renal function is only necessary for ethambutol. A prolonged course is necessary because of the increased risk of recurrence. Surgical intervention is now seldom necessary and should only occur when strongly indicated. Secondary infections worsen the prognosis, so unnecessary endourethral procedures such as catheterisation and cystoscopy should be avoided.

Bone and joint tuberculosis: A long course of combined chemotherapy as for other forms of non-pulmonary tuberculosis, with surgical clearance of foci if necessary, and orthopaedic measures.

Cutaneous tuberculosis: Isoniazid + rifampicin. Surgical intervention is nowadays rarely necessary.

Tuberculosis in AIDS: see p. 543.

References

ACOCELLA, G., A. NONIS, G. GIALDRONI-GRASSI, C. GRASSI: Comparative bioavailability of isoniazid, rifampin and pyrazinamide administered in free combination and in a fixed triple formulation designed for daily use in antituberculosis chemotherapy. Amer. Rev. resp. Dis. *138:* 882–885 (1988).

AHN, C. H., J. R. LOWELL, S. S. AHN et al.: Short-course chemotherapy for pulmonary disease caused by Mycobacterium kansasii. Amer. Rev. Respir. Dis. *128:* 1048 (1983).

Centers for Disease Control. The use of preventive therapy for tuberculosis infection in the United States. M.M.W.R. *39* (RR-6): 9–12 (1990).

---

* not marketed in Britain.

COHN, D. L., B. J. CATLIN, K. L. PETERSON, F. N. JUDSON, J. A. SBARBARO: A 62-dose, 6-month therapy for pulmonary and extrapulmonary tuberculosis. A twice-weekly, directly observed, and cost-effective regimen. Ann. intern. Med. *112:* 407 (1990).
COMBS, D. L., R. J. O'BRIEN, L. J. GEITER: USPHS Tuberculosis Short-Course Chemotherapy Trial 21: effectiveness, toxicity, and acceptability. The report of final results. Ann. intern. Med. *112:* 397 (1990).
DUTT, A. K., D. MOERS, W. W. STEAD: Smear- and culture-negative pulmonary tuberculosis: Four-month short-course chemotherapy. Am. rev. Respir. Dis. *139:* 867 (1989).
East and Central African/British Medical Research Council Fifth Collaborative Study: Controlled clinical trial of 4 short-course regimens of chemotherapy (three 6-month and one 8-month) for pulmonary tuberculosis: final report. Tubercle *67:* 5 (1986).
Hong Kong Chest Service/British Medical Research Council: Acceptability, compliance, and adverse reactions when isoniazid, rifampin, and pyrazinamide are given as a combined formulation or separately during three-times-weekly antituberculosis chemotherapy. Amer. Rev. resp. Dis. *140:* 1618 (1989).
HOWELL, F., R. O'LAOIDE, P. KELLY, J. POWER, L. CLANCY: Short-course chemotherapy for pulmonary tuberculosis. A randomised controlled trial of a six-month versus nine-month oral regimen. Ir. med. J. *82:* 11 (1989).
JANSSENS, J. P., R. DE HALLER: Spinal tuberculosis in a developed country. A review of 26 cases with special emphasis on abscesses and neurologic complications. Clin. Orthop. *257:* 67–76 (1990).
JAWAHAR, M. S., S. SIVASUBRAMANIAN, V. K. VIJAYAN et al.: Short-course chemotherapy for tuberculous lymphadenitis in children. Brit. med. J. *301:* 359 (1990).
KILPATRICK, M. E., N. I. GIRGIS, M. W. YASSIN, A. A. ABU EL ELLA: Tuberculous meningitis – clinical and laboratory review of 100 patients. J. Hyg. *96:* 231–238 (1986).
NYE, K., D. K. CHADHA, P. HODGKIN et al.: Mycobacterium chelonei isolation from broncho-alveolar lavage fluid and its practical implications. J. Hosp. Infect. *16:* 257 (1990).
PUN, W. K., S. P. CHOW, K. D. LUK et al.: Tuberculosis of the lumbosacral junction. Long-term follow-up of 26 cases. J. Bone. Joint. Surg. Br. *72:* 675–678 (1990).
REES, R. J. W. (ED.): Tuberculosis and Leprosy, Churchill Livingstone, London 1988.
SNIDER, D. E., J. GRACZYK, E. BECK et al.: Supervised six months treatment of newly diagnosed pulmonary tuberculosis using isoniazid, rifampin and pyrazinamide with and without streptomycin. Am. Rev. Respir. Dis. *103:* 1091 (1984).
WALLACE JR., R. J., J. M. SWENSON, V. A. SILCOX, M. G. BULLEN: Treatment of nonpulmonary infections due to Mycobacterium fortuitum and Mycobacterium chelonae on the basis of in vitro susceptibilities. J. Infect. Dis. *152:* 500 (1985).
ZIMMER, B. L., D. R. DEYOUNG, G. D. ROBERTS: In vitro synergistic activity of ethambutol, isoniazid, kanamycin, rifampin, and streptomycin against Mycobacterium avium-intracellulare complex. Antimicrob. Ag. Chemother. *22:* 148 (1982).

31. Leprosy

Causative organism: Mycobacterium leprae. A chronic infectious disease which is still widespread in developing countries and can affect the skin, mucous membranes, peripheral nerves and internal organs. The **various forms of the disease,** which are dependent on immune status, are:

1. Tuberculoid leprosy with maculo-anaesthetic foci. The lepromin skin test is strongly positive. Bacteria in affected tissues are scanty. Peripheral nerve involvement with secondary paralysis is common.
2. Lepromatous leprosy (anergic response to M. leprae antigen). The lepromin skin test is always negative. Numerous bacteria are found in the skin lesions; nerve involvement is absent until a very late stage of the disease.
3. Borderline leprosy (dimorphic or intermediate form) in which features of both tuberculoid and lepromatous forms are present at the same time. The lepromin skin test is weakly positive or negative. Moderate numbers of bacteria in affected tissues. Peripheral nerve involvement frequent. There are also transitional forms of borderline leprosy which are closer either to tuberculoid (borderline tuberculoid) or to lepromatous (borderline lepromatous) leprosy.
4. Indeterminate form at the onset of the disease, which can develop into either the tuberculoid or the lepromatous form. Bacteria in tissue sections are absent or very scanty. The lepromin skin test is weakly positive or negative, and nerves are not involved.

Clinically, tuberculoid leprosy is characterised by depigmented or erythematous areas of skin which are insensitive to touch or heat; later, palpable nerve cords, nerve pains and trophic changes in the hands and feet often develop, leading to ulcers and mutilation. In lepromatous leprosy there are nodular changes in the skin (particularly on the extensor surfaces of the arms and legs, forehead, cheek and outer ear), and later, through mucous membrane involvement, constant nasal discharge, dysphagia, hoarseness and dyspnoea. In lepromatous leprosy, a condition attributable to the formation of immune complexes and known as *erythema nodosum leprosum* develops in many patients a few months after starting treatment and may be accompanied by fever, synovitis or iridocyclitis.

The **diagnosis** is initially made clinically. In the lepromatous form, acid-fast bacilli may be demonstrated microscopically in smears stained by the Ziehl-Neelsen method of secretions from a shallow skin biopsy from the edge of the skin lesion, or from nasal discharge. Histological investigation of a biopsy permits a classification of the diseases and some prediction of the prognosis as well as an assessment of the efficacy of treatment. Injection of tissue material taken during dapsone therapy into the foot-pad of a mouse will establish whether the lepra bacilli are still living and hence whether the strain is resistant.

Treatment: For over 20 years the mainstay of treatment was dapsone monotherapy, but resistance to dapsone then became an increasing concern. A World Health Organisation Study Group has made recommendations to overcome the problem of dapsone resistance and to prevent the emergence of resistance to other antileprotic drugs. These recommendations are based on the same principles as those used in the treatment of tuberculosis and advocate combinations of drugs given over a long period. The drugs used are dapsone, clofazimine and rifampicin.

Primary resistance to clofazimine and rifampicin is rare; when resistance is proven, ethionamide* or prothionamide* may be considered (see p. 270) and perhaps in the future a new quinolone (ofloxacin, ciprofloxacin, pefloxacin). Antituberculous drugs such as isoniazid, ethambutol and streptomycin are ineffective.

For treatment purposes, the *WHO recommendation* of 1984 divides leprosy patients into those suffering from paucibacillary leprosy (tuberculoid, borderline tuberculoid and lepromatous forms) and multibacillary leprosy (lepromatous, borderline lepromatous and borderline forms). Their treatment is as follows:

1. In **paucibacillary leprosy,** 2 drugs should be used for at least 6 months, namely:
   - rifampicin 0.6 g once a month, supervised (0.45 g for patients weighing less than 35 kg), and
   - dapsone 0.1 g daily, self-administered.
2. In **multibacillary leprosy,** 3 drugs should be given for at least 2 years and continued where possible until smear negativity; these are:
   - rifampicin 0.6 g once a month, supervised (0.45 g for patients weighing less than 35 kg),
   - dapsone 0.1 g daily, self-administered, and
   - clofazimine 0.05 g daily, self-administered, and 0.3 g once a month, supervised.

Since persistence of the organisms can lead to relapse, follow-up investigations are necessary, including microscopic investigations if relapse is suspected. In some patients treatment must be continued for years and even for life. The patient must be carefully monitored for side-effects of dapsone (see p. 275), rifampicin (see p. 262) and clofazimine (see p. 276).

If type I **(reversal)** or type II **(erythema nodosum leprosum)** reactions develop, the antileprotic treatment should continue unchanged with the addition, if the reactions are severe, of a corticosteroid or clofazimine. The action of clofazimine is not only antibacterial, but also anti-inflammatory, although the latter effect is delayed and is not seen until after 4–6 weeks; in mild erythema nodosum, acetylsalicylic acid or paracetamol may be sufficient. Iridocyclitis should be treated topically with a corticosteroid and a mydriatic.

Neither the multibacillary nor the paucibacillary antileprosy regimens are sufficient to treat active pulmonary tuberculosis, so patients who also have the latter should be given an appropriate course of antituberculous chemotherapy in addition to the antileprosy regimen.

References

GUELPA-LAURAS, C. C., J. H. GROSSET, M. CONSTANT-DESPORTES, G. BRUCKER: Nine cases of rifampin-resistant leprosy. Int. J. Leprosy 52: 101 (1984).
HASTINGS, R. C.: Leprosy. Churchill Livingstone, New York, Edinburgh, London, Melbourne, 1986.

* not marketed in Britain

JI, B. H., J. K. CHEN, C. M. WANG, G. A. XIA: Hepatotoxicity of combined therapy with rifampicin and daily prothionamide for leprosy. Lepr. Rev. 55: 283–289 (1984).

KAR, P. K., A. S. SOHI: Study of multidrug therapy in paucibacillary leprosy. J. Indian med. Ass. 87: 34 (1989).

LANGUILLON, J.: Précis de Léprologie. Masson et Cie, Paris, 1986.

LEIKER, D. L.: Preliminary results of treatment of leprosy patients in The Netherlands with daily rifampicin, dapsone and clofazimine. Lepr. Rev. 57 (Supplement 3): 272–273 (1986).

PATTYN, S. R., L. JANSSENS, J. BOURLAND et al.: Hepatotoxicity of the combination of rifampin-ethionamide in the treatment of multibacillary leprosy. Int. J. Leprosy 52: 1 (1984).

PATTYN, S. R., J. BOURLAND, S. GRILLONE, G. GROENEN, P. GHYS: Combined regimens of one-year duration in the treatment of multibacillary leprosy. I. Combined regimens with rifampicin administered during one year. Lepr. Rev. 60: 109 (1989).

PATTYN, S. R., G. GROENEN, L. JANSSEN, J. DEVERCHIN, P. GHYS: Combined regimens of one-year duration in the treatment of multibacillary leprosy. II. Combined regimens administered during six months. Lepr. Rev. 60: 118 (1989).

PATTYN, S. R., J. A. HUSSER, G. BAQUILLON: Evaluation of five treatment regimens, using either dapsone monotherapy or several doses of rifampicin in the treatment of paucibacillary leprosy. Lepr. Rev. 61: 151–156 (1990).

REES, R. J.: Tuberculosis and Leprosy. Churchill Livingstone, London 1988.

32. Influenza

True influenza caused by influenza viruses A or B should not be confused with other influenza-like upper respiratory infections or with bronchitis due to Haemophilus influenzae. Uncomplicated cases of influenza require no antibacterial chemotherapy, but should be treated symptomatically with codeine, paracetamol or salicylates.

Since influenza virus often paves the way for secondary bacterial pneumonia, appropriate *antibiotics* should be given early to patients at particular risk such as the elderly, diabetics, pregnant women in the last trimester, and patients with cardiac failure, mitral valve defects, cirrhosis and bone marrow insufficiency. Suitable oral broad-spectrum agents that are active against Haemophilus influenzae, pneumococci and staphylococci are co-amoxiclav 375–750 mg every 8 hours, co-fluampicil (ampicillin plus flucloxacillin) 0.5–1 g every 6 hours, cefuroxime axetil 250–500 mg every 12 hours and cefixime 200 mg every 12 hours or 400 mg once daily. Co-trimoxazole and erythromycin are alternatives in patients allergic to penicillin but resistant strain occur.

Treatment of early influenza A with amantadine is less reliable, and controversial. *Prophylaxis* with daily doses of amantadine is effective but usually not practicable. The best prophylaxis, which is important for the chronically ill and elderly, is early, active immunisation with a vaccine that protects against the epidemic strain.

Influenzal pneumonia can occur in two forms. A *primary, haemorrhagic viral pneumonia* occasionally develops early in the infection and is caused by the influenza virus itself. It should be distinguished from the much commoner *secondary bacterial bronchopneumonia* that can complicate influenza (especially in elderly and debilitated patients). Since superinfection with staphylococci and other bacteria can also occur after primary viral pneumonia, a *trial of therapy* with imipenem or an intermediate cephalosporin such as cefuroxime is always advisable.

Many strains of staphylococci are now resistant to tetracycline.

Other *complications of influenza* include otitis media and sinusitis (which may also be bacterial), laryngo-tracheitis (influenzal croup) and myocarditis.

References

Capparelli, E. V. et al.: Rimantadine pharmacokinetics in healthy subjects and patients with end-stage renal failure. Clin. Pharmacol. Ther. *43:* 536 (1988).
Douglas, R. G., Jr.: Drug therapy: Prophylaxis and treatment of influenza. N. Engl. J. Med. *322:* 443 (1990).
Hall, C. B. et al.: Treatment of children with influenza A infection with rimantadine. Pediatrics *80:* 275 (1987).
Hayden, F. G. et al.: Emergence and apparent transmission of rimantadine-resistant influenza A virus in families. N. Engl. J. Med. *321:* 1696 (1989).
Prevention and control of influenza. Recommendations of the Immunization Practices Advisory Commitee (ACIP). MMWR *39* RR 7: 1–15 (1990).
Vale, J. A., K. S. Maclean: Amantadine-induced heart-failure. Lancet *1:* 548 (1977).

33. AIDS

AIDS (acquired immune deficiency syndrome) is caused by the retrovirus HIV (= human immunodeficiency virus) which can be isolated from the blood and body fluids of infected persons. Almost all cases in Europe and the USA at present are caused by HIV-1; in Western Africa, however, HIV-2 also accounts for a substantial proportion of infections. The virus is spread from person to person through unprotected sexual contact, the sharing of contaminated injection equipment (syringes, needles) by drug abusers (and occasionally when injection equipment and transfusion apparatus are re-used medically in countries with reduced economic resources), transfusion of contaminated blood and blood products, and transplacental or intrapartum infection of a child by its mother. Other routes of spread (droplets, splashes) appear to be less important epidemiologically.

This epidemic disease has now spread worldwide. Groups particularly affected are male homosexuals, intravenous drug abusers, the sexual partners of infected persons and the newborn babies of infected mothers. The number of cases of heterosexual transmission is increasing. In addition to recipients of blood transfusions, patients with haemophilia and the recipients of certain plasma products were initially infected, but new infections do not now occur in these groups, if control of donors and sterilization of plasma products is carried out correctly. There is a certain risk to all persons who received blood or certain blood products (e.g. factor VIII) between 1978 and 1985. The infection can be transferred from infected persons who are in the latent period but have not yet developed symptoms. In contrast to most other viral infections, persons with HIV antibodies generally also have infectious virus in their blood, regardless of their state of health, and are potentially infectious to others at this time. Infectivity clearly increases with the onset of symptoms. The period between infection and the formation of detectable serum antibodies is generally 6–9 weeks but may be longer.

Pathogenesis: The time between infection and the appearance of antibodies should be designated as the *incubation period*. There is then a variable *latent period* lasting from a few months to many years during which the patient feels quite well and is free of symptoms; however, investigations in this period often show immunological abnormalities to be present already. The virus targets cells of the immune system, principally the T4 (helper-inducer) subset of the T lymphocytes, which express the CD4 molecule on their surface. The CD4 molecule acts as a high-affinity receptor for the gp120 portion of HIV. Other monocytes and macrophages can also be infected. The depletion of infected CD4+ cells (both T4 lymphocytes and macrophages) permits the development of life-threatening opportunistic infections and certain malignant conditions (Kaposi's sarcoma, lymphoma).

Oncogenic viruses (e.g. Epstein-Barr virus) possibly play an important part as co-factors in the occurrence of malignant tumours. **Malignancies** that frequently occur in adults with AIDS are Kaposi's sarcoma (usually in an atypical form on the skin, and sometimes also with visceral involvement), Burkitt-like lymphoma, non-Hodgkin lymphoma, CNS lymphoma, Hodgkin's disease and also antral or genital carcinoma.

HIV infection progresses typically through **several stages,** for which various classifications have been produced as summarised in Table 61. HIV infection is a clinical entity. The separation into AIDS and pre-AIDS is artificial. A new WHO classification is based mainly on the number of T4 (helper) lymphocytes.

The virus itself can give rise several weeks after infection to a disease that resembles acute mononucleosis or an aseptic meningitis and resolves without treatment. After an asymptomatic stage, most patients develop the lymphadenopathy syndrome (LAS) which, when severe, is designated the AIDS-related complex (ARC). In this stage the patients have fever, lymph-node swelling, lassitude and may already show signs of opportunistic infections (oral thrush, seborrhoeic dermatitis, zoster and pneumonias caused by the usual agents).

Table 61. Classification of AIDS (based on published reports). The stage WR0 or FF1a can only be confirmed retrospectively. Suspicion may arise from the patient's circumstances, e.g. in the wife of an infected haemophiliac. The Frankfurt (FF) classification can be expanded by abbreviations of the principal manifestations (e.g. 3; neuro, KS).

Centers for Disease Control (CDC)	Trivial designation	Walter Reed (WR) stage	Frankfurt (FF) stage
No term	Incubation period	WR0	1a
Group I Acute infection	Acute HIV infection	–	1a–b
Group II (seropositive) A. Asymptomatic B. + pathological laboratory results	Asymptomatic Minor AIDS (with thrombocytopenia)	WR1 WR1T	1b
Group III (seropositive) A. Generalised lymphadenopathy B. + pathological laboratory results	LAS (lymphadenopathy syndrome)	WR2 WR3	2a 2b
Group IV (seropositive) A. General symptoms	ARC (= AIDS-related complex)	WR3B to WR6B	2b
B. Neurological symptoms		WR3CNS to WR6CNS	3
C.1 Opportunistic infections	AIDS	WR6	3
C.2 Other infections		WR6	3
● Oral hairy leukoplakia	OLP		
● Herpes zoster	Minor AIDS		
● Tuberculosis	Minor AIDS		
● Candida stomatitis	Minor AIDS		
D. Malignancies	AIDS		3
● Kaposi		WR2K to WR6K	
● CNS lymphoma		WR3CNS to WR6CNS	
E. Other			

HIV is markedly neurotropic. Even in early stages of the disease mild brain involvement is possible, which can progress to severe dementia (AIDS encephalopathy). It is often difficult to distinguish symptoms of AIDS encephalopy from those of secondary forms of encephalitis.

In full-blown AIDS numerous **opportunistic infections** can occur; the most important are listed in Table 62. Interestingly, the common facultative pathogens (e.g. staphylococci, Escherichia coli, pseudomonas) are relatively rare causes of infection in AIDS patients.

Presenting **symptoms** of AIDS and their rates of incidence are given in Table 63. However, it should be kept in mind that an AIDS patient will experience many different complications in the course of the disease.

Laboratory findings: Patients with ARC and AIDS have typical, though variable, laboratory results. The best correlation of the clinical state is with the absolute count of T4 lymphocytes; low T4 cell counts ($<200/mm^3$) in HIV-seropositive patients show the risk of imminent clinical AIDS. Other laboratory findings are lymphocytopenia, leucocytopenia, eosinophilia, a polyclonal hypergammopathy and a reduced response of lymphocytes to mitogens. Previously positive tuberculin skin tests become negative. In fully developed AIDS, serum antibodies that were previously present, including HIV antibodies, may become undetectable. Free p 24 antigen (a core protein) may appear. In the end-stage of

Table 62. Important opportunistic organisms and typical features of disease which mark the development of AIDS in persons with HIV infection.

Causative organism	Typical features of disease
Cryptosporidia	Intractable diarrhoea, resistant to therapy
Pneumocystis carinii	Bilateral interstitial pneumonia
Toxoplasma gondii	Toxoplasma encephalitis
Aspergillus species	Pneumonia, involvement of CNS and of internal organs
Candida albicans	Candida stomatitis and oesophagitis
Cryptococcus neoformans	Abscesses of internal organs, meningitis
Actinomycetes, nocardia	Pneumonia, suppuration, cerebral abscess
M. avium-intracellulare and other mycobacteria	Septicaemia, extrapulmonary involvement of several organs, generalised lymph-node involvement
Mycobacterium tuberculosis	Extrapulmonary tuberculosis, involvement of several organs, generalised lymph-node involvement
Salmonellae (other than S. typhi and S. paratyphi)	Septicaemia (recurrent), empyema, soft tissue and organ abscesses
Cytomegalovirus	Retinitis, pneumonia, widespread involvement of internal organs
Herpes simplex (Types I and II)	Cutaneous and mucocutaneous ulcers, encephalitis, proctitis
Molluscum contagiosum virus	Molluscum contagiosum (extensive and multiple)
Papovaviruses	Multifocal leucoencephalopathy, papillomas
Varicella zoster virus	Progressive varicella, varicella pneumonia, generalised zoster

Table 63. Presenting features of AIDS in the first 267 patients in Frankfurt am Main, Germany.

Presenting feature	Total
Pneumocystis carinii pneumonia (PCP)	101
Kaposi's sarcoma (KS)	73
PCP and KS	5
Toxoplasma encephalitis	17
Malignant lymphomas*	17
Candida oesophagitis	11
Necrotising anal herpes	10
HIV encephalopathy	9
Hodgkin's disease**	5
CNS cryptococcosis	4
Cryptosporidiosis	4
Generalised CMV infection or CMV retinitis	3
Atypical mycobacteriosis or disseminated tuberculosis	3
Generalised herpes zoster or zoster pneumonia	2
Other bacterial pneumonias***	2
Listeria meningitis	1

  * One primary CNS lymphoma
 ** At same time as severe oral candidosis
*** Nocardia pneumonia

AIDS, patients often have anaemia and sometimes thrombocytopenia as well, even when they have not been treated.

Principles of treatment: A distinction must be made between the treatment of the HIV infection itself, of secondary opportunistic infections, of secondary malignancies, and other symptomatic treatment in the seriously ill patient.

The treatment of the HIV infection itself is still in its infancy. The particular biological properties of a retrovirus theoretically require lifelong treatment with potentially cytotoxic antiviral agents, which have to attack the metabolic processes of the infected cells. The only established drug for the treatment of AIDS or ARC are the antimetabolites azidothymidine (AZT, zidovudine, see p. 288) and DDI. In the present state of knowledge, the use of azidothymidine should be considered when the absolute T4 lymphocyte count continues to fall in patients with ARC, at the first presentation of opportunistic infections (Pneumocystis carinii pneumonia, cerebral toxoplasmosis) or when neurological symptoms arise. Early treatment with AZT is still controversial.

Present experience suggests that azidothymidine can give the majority of patients a prolonged remission. Its use usually leads to an increase in body weight, an increase in the T4 lymphocyte count and an improvement in the state of bodily and intellectual well-being. Some mild infections, such as oral candidosis, regress, but severe infectious complications such as Pneumocystis carinii pneumonia can still arise. Controlled studies now suggest that the mortality in AIDS patients can be substantially reduced by azidothymidine. The side-effects are, however, considerable. Patients with neurological involvement can deteriorate, and fatal epileptic fits have been reported. About 20% of patients treated with high dosage develop severe anaemia which may require blood transfusion. The improvement in laboratory results is usually sustained for 6–12 months. Azidothymidine has no effect on secondary malignancies (e. g. Kaposi's sarcoma). Lower doses cause fewer side-effects. The contraindications, dosage and mode of administration of azidothymidine are given on p. 290. Early treatment, intermittent therapy and dose reduction, and the preventive efficacy after accidental inoculation with a contaminated needle have all been the subject of recent studies.

Azidothymidine is undoubtedly an important pioneering substance in the treatment of AIDS. The chemotherapy of HIV infection is at present the only effective, albeit expensive, treatment of the cause of AIDS. DDI (Didesoxy-

Table 64. Intervention therapy for infections in AIDS and ARC (AIDS-related complex). LAS = lymphadenopathy syndrome.

Symptoms	Possible causes	Treatment		
		First line	Second line	Third line
Fever of unknown origin (no localisation)	Salmonellae, mycobacteria, staphylococci, fungi	Ciprofloxacin (1 g daily)	Ciprofloxacin + rifampicin	Imipenem + fluconazole + rifampicin
Pneumonia (segmental or lobar) in LAS or ARC	Pneumococci, staphylococci, legionella, pneumocystis	Cefazolin	Rifampicin + ciprofloxacin	Co-trimoxazole (7.62 g daily)
Pneumonia (interstitial or atypical) in AIDS or ARC	Pneumocystis, mycobacteria	Co-trimoxazole (7.62 g daily)	Co-trimoxazole + rifampicin	Ciprofloxacin (1 g daily)
Enteritis in AIDS or ARC	Salmonellae, clostridia	Ciprofloxacin (1 g daily)	Ciprofloxacin + vancomycin	Metronidazole (1.5 g daily)
Abdominal pain of obscure origin, fever	Salmonellae, yersinia, anaerobes, mycobacteria	Ciprofloxacin (1 g daily)	Rifampicin + ciprofloxacin	Metronidazole (1.5 g daily)
Necrotising gingivitis	Staphylococci, anaerobes	Penicillin	Metronidazole + penicillin	Clindamycin
Vesicular rash	Herpes, varicella, zoster	Acyclovir	Fos carnet	Immuno-globulin (high doses)

inosine) is indicated if AZT has failed or if AZT is not tolerated. Substances which modulate the immune response, although often mentioned, do not influence the course of HIV infection significantly.

The appropriate and prompt **treatment of opportunistic infections** can substantially prolong the patient's life. This requires a detailed knowledge of the course of the illness and its complications and of the means by which an early diagnosis can be made. It is rare for the causative organism to be apparent at the time when a secondary infection presents, although some causes may be suspected on the basis of the organs involved, the history and the clinical picture. Since intracellular infections often occur, drugs with intracellular activity, which are often poorly tolerated, may need to be used. The incidence of side-effects of anti-infective treatment of patients with AIDS is generally high.

For the various clinical presentations of AIDS, which generally start with fever, there is now a well-established intervention therapy, the rules of which are summarised in Table 64.

If at all possible before starting intervention therapy, appropriate material (blood, sputum, urine, swabs) should be taken in order to make a microbiological diagnosis. Bronchoscopy is necessary to confirm the diagnosis of pneumocystis carinii pneumonia or a mycobacterial infection. Successful treatment always requires a team effort involving microbiologists, other pathologists, infectious disease physicians and other specialists.

a) Pneumocystis carinii Pneumonia (PCP)

PCP is the commonest life-threatening infection in patients with AIDS. When promptly recognised and treated, some 90% of patients can survive the first episode and then have a subsequent life-expectancy of up to 3 years. Unlike bacterial pneumonia, the onset is insidious, so that the initial symptoms, such as fever and unproductive cough, may be misinterpreted and the danger of the infection not immediately recognised. Since signs of consolidation are usually absent on auscultation, the patient may be thought only to have a simple viral infection. A chest X-ray is essential, therefore, in all patients with HIV infection who show the triad of fever, unproductive cough and increasing dyspnoea for more than 3 days. Even if relatively minor changes are seen on the X-ray, there may be a reduced arterial pO_2 and a considerable reduction in the vital capacity. A gallium scan of the lungs will show a diffuse uptake of the isotope in the tissues. The diagnosis of PCP may be made by induced sputum production using 3–5% saline via an ultrasonic nebuliser (large particle size) with postural drainage, but is best made by fibreoptic bronchoscopy with broncho-alveolar lavage with buffered isotonic saline, and microbiological demonstration of the pneumocystis by silver staining. Specimens obtained in this way can also be examined for mycobacteria and other opportunistic pathogens. If these techniques fail, transbronchial biopsy or open lung biopsy may be necessary to obtain material for histological examination.

The **treatment of choice** in pneumocystis pneumonia is co-trimoxazole at 4 times the normal dosage (7.68 g i. v.) for 20 days (Table 65). These high doses of co-trimoxazole are often poorly tolerated. Many patients with pneumocystis pneumonia react to co-trimoxazole with skin rashes, neutropenia, nausea and other symptoms for which treatment may have to be stopped. Trimethoprim alone is not satisfactory, but may be combined with dapsone (contraindicated in glucose-6-phosphate dehydrogenase deficiency).

Pentamidine dimethane sulphonate i. m. or i. v., until recently an alternative treatment of PCP but with unacceptably severe side-effects, has now been replaced by the better tolerated preparation pentamidine isethionate. Pentamidine should be given as a slow intravenous infusion in a dose of 4 mg/kg/day i. v. in 250 ml glucose. Almost all patients develop side-effects such as hypo- or hyperglycaemia, hypotension, renal or hepatic toxicity and leukopenia. The nephrotoxicity precedes the blood sugar changes that are obviously caused by pancreatic damage. Systemic treatment with pentamidine should therefore be

Table 65. Clinical symptoms, diagnostic measures and results, and treatment of Pneumocystis carinii pneumonia.

Symptoms	Diagnostic measures and results	Treatment
Insidious onset	*Auscultation:* usually unremarkable, occasional increased breath sounds and discrete crepitations	**Co-trimoxazole** i. v. (sulphamethoxazole 100 mg/kg + trimethoprim 20 mg/kg daily for 21 days)
Feeling of exhaustion		
Fever		
Unproductive cough	*Chest X-ray:* increased interstitial markings	If allergic reaction, reduce dose, possibly interrupt treatment, consider steroids
Increasing dyspnoea		
	Vital capacity: reduced	Possibly add **pentamidine by inhalation**
	Blood gas analysis: pO_2 reduced	If co-trimoxazole fails, try difluoromethyl ornithine (DFMO)
	Bronchoscopy with lavage and possible biopsy: Pneumocystis carinii in lavage or biopsy material, shown by silver staining	In advanced disease (white lungs), add **prednisone** 0.5 g, reducing dose rapidly in 10 days

avoided to the greatest possible extent. This does not, however, apply to inhalation therapy with pentamidine isethionate 600 mg or 8 mg/kg through a special inhaler, which is suitable not only as conventional treatment of PCP but also to prevent relapse.

There is an urgent need for better ways of treating PCP. One possibility is trimetrexate, a lipid-soluble analogue of methotrexate, which is a much stronger inhibitor of the hydrofolate reductase of Pneumocystis carinii than trimethoprim or pyrimethamine. When used in a dose of 30–60 mg/m^2 i.v. and combined with folinic acid, its toxicity is relatively low, and it may rationally be combined with either a sulphonamide or a sulphone.

Difluoromethyl ornithine (DFMO), an inhibitor of polyamine synthesis which can be used to treat trypanosomal infections, is also effective in PCP. The combination of pyrimethamine with clindamycin is active *in vitro* and in animal models, though there is as yet little clinical experience. Primaquine 15 mg daily by mouth plus clindamycin 600 mg four times a day i.v. is another alternative.

The prognosis in advanced Pneumocystis pneumonia is very poor. A "whiteout" of the lung fields on X-ray is an indication for the addition of high doses of corticosteroids (prednisone 0.5–1 g a day), although this treatment may cause a flare-up of zoster infection.

Pneumocystis carinii pneumonia recurs in about 25% of cases. Opinions about the value of prophylaxis with co-trimoxazole in a reduced dose (2 tablets once daily), sulfadoxine and pyrimethamine (Fansidar) 1 tablet weekly, or dapsone 25 mg four times a day, are divided. Pentamidine by inhalation (every 2–4 weeks) is effective as prophylaxis of PCP. The protective effect depends on high quality nebulisers (very small droplets).

b) Toxoplasmosis

Cerebral toxoplasmosis in AIDS is usually shown as a large, space-occupying process in the brain that can be demonstrated by CT imaging with contrast medium. The principal symptoms are the rapid onset of convulsions, focal neurological symptoms, changes in consciousness level, altered personality and paralysis (Table 66).

The distinction from AIDS encephalopathy and a cerebral lymphoma is difficult. Serological tests for toxoplasmosis in AIDS patients are unreliable. The diagnosis can best be confirmed by a brain biopsy, but in practice is inferred from the rapid response to treatment with pyrimethamine 0.1 g daily and sulphonamide for 3 weeks (see p. 558). Because of the thrombocytopenia expected with pyrimethamine, supplementary treatment with folinic acid 10–15 mg daily is recommended. In cases of sulphonamide intolerance or in extreme thrombocytopenia, treatment with high-dose clindamycin can be carried out. Cerebral toxoplasmosis has a strong tendency to recur, and long-term prophylaxis with

Table 66. Clinical symptoms, diagnostic measures and results, and treatment of toxoplasma encephalitis.

Symptoms	Diagnostic measures and results	Treatment
Fever	*Neurological examination:* Local failures, e. g. hemiparesis, hemianopia, aphasia	**Pyrimethamine** 50–100 mg daily + **sulphadiazine** 4 g initially, then 2–4 g daily from day 2 + folinic acid 15 mg daily
Headache		
Changes in personality	*EEG:* Focal abnormalities + generalised changes	
Disturbances of balance		Monitoring of treatment: a fall in platelet count may occur; clinical improvement within 1 week
Convulsions	*CT:* Translucent areas	
	CT with contrast medium: Ring-like foci	Regression of the foci seen on CT scan within 4 weeks
	CSF: Mild inflammatory changes, antibodies as in serum	Discontinue sulphonamide after 3–4 weeks
	Serology: Titres unreliable	For increased intracranial pressure, give **dexamethasone** 16 mg daily.
		For intolerance give **clindamycin** 2.4 g daily
		Danger of **relapse,** so lifelong **prophylaxis** with pyrimethamine 50 mg daily or Fansidar or clindamycin

pyrimethamine 50 mg/day or Fansidar 2 tablets weekly, or possibly with clindamycin 1.8 g daily is essential.

c) Cryptosporidial Infections

The important role of the coccidian parasite Cryptosporidium as a cause of enteritis in AIDS is well known. In patients with severe immunodeficiency, this protozoon may lead to intractable, non-bloody, very watery diarrhoea which cannot be influenced by dietary measures.

The demonstration of numerous cryptosporidia in the stool by means of a special stain is straightforward in principle but requires laboratory facilities.

There is at present no reliable treatment for cryptosporidial infection; spiramycin, recommended by some authors, almost always fails. Treatment has to be confined to symptomatic measures such as beef colostrum or antiperistaltic agents.

d) Candida Infections

Candida albicans is the commonest cause of secondary infection in AIDS. Almost all patients have severe oral thrush, not only in terminal disease but also in the early stages of LAS or ARC. The local appearance can be very typical, but the infection may also develop as a plaque on the oropharyngeal mucosa, with disturbances of taste and a burning sensation on the tongue. Dysphagia, a persistent sensation of a lump in the throat and retrosternal pain are all suggestive of candida oesophagitis (Table 67). The dysphagia may be so severe that eating becomes difficult or impossible. Because the symptoms can be so variable, semiquantitative demonstration of the organisms from serial dilutions of oral rinses is often necessary to confirm the diagnosis. The oesophageal involvement can be shown by careful endoscopy or X-rays (Table 67).

The oral candidiasis of AIDS is not usually cleared by topical antifungal agents; the lesions regress briefly in response to amphotericin B or nystatin suspension, only to recur soon after these agents are stopped. When the clinical diagnosis is obvious, a systemic antifungal agent should be started as soon as samples have

Table 67. Clinical symptoms, diagnostic measures and results, and treatment of candida oesophagitis.

Symptoms	Diagnostic measures and results	Treatment
Whitish plaques in mouth, sometimes only redness and burning	*Swab for microscopy and culture:* Candida albicans	Fluconazole 0.1 g twice daily; when fluconazole not tolerated, long-term treatment with 0.1 g once a day; simultaneous treatment with rifampicin may also be given
Taste disorders	*Oral rinses for organism counts:* $>10^3$ colonies/ml	
Sensation of a lump in the throat		or:
Pressure over the sternum	*Oesophagoscopy:* whitish plaques	Ketoconazole 0.2 g twice daily initially, then 0.2 g 3 times a day from day 2. Long-term therapy with 0.2 g once a day
Dysphagia	*Barium swallow and X-ray of oesophagus:* filling defects with appearance of a string of beads	

been taken for culture. The treatment of choice at present is fluconazole 0.1 g twice daily by mouth. After regression of the plaques within 3 days, recurrence may be prevented by continuing the fluconazole at the lower dose of 0.1 g daily. Gaps in treatment depend on the individual tendency to relapses. Treatment with ketoconazole can have a number of side-effects, and a range of interactions may occur, for example with rifampicin, which should not be given with ketoconazole. Because of the hepatotoxicity of ketoconazole, serum transaminases should be regularly monitored during treatment.

In severe systemic infections, including candida and cryptococcal meningitis, up to 0.4 g fluconazole daily may be given i.v. for 6–8 weeks or longer if necessary. Fluconazole may be continued for longer periods at a daily dose of 0.2 g to prevent recurrence in cryptococcal meningitis. In very severe systemic candida infections, treatment with amphotericin B + flucytosine may be necessary.

e) Cryptococcal Meningitis

Cryptococcal meningitis, which is otherwise very uncommon, occurs relatively frequently in patients with AIDS. The infection behaves as a subacute meningitis and is often preceded by headaches or symptoms resembling sinusitis (Table 68). On microscopy of the CSF, both stained and unstained cryptococci can be mistaken for lymphocytes. The mucoid capsules of the cryptococci are readily demonstrated in an India ink preparation. The diagnosis is confirmed by growth in culture and by the demonstration of cryptococcal antigen in the CSF, serum and urine. Rounded foci in the lung fields can often be seen on chest X-ray.

For many years, the recommended treatment of cryptococcal meningitis has been the combination of amphotericin B and flucytosine. Fluconazole has good activity against cryptococci, too; initial treatment with amphotericin B + flucytosine + fluconazole can be recommended. Clinical improvement is seen in a few weeks; long-term treatment should be continued with fluconazole 0.2 g once daily for several months or even lifelong. Itraconazole (see p. 202) is now an alternative in cryptococcal meningitis.

Table 68. Clinical symptoms, diagnostic measures and results, and treatment of cryptococcal meningitis and other severe cryptococcal infections.

Symptoms	Diagnostic measures and results	Treatment
Insidious onset	*Lumbar puncture:* CSF pleocytosis, low sugar, increased protein	**Amphotericin B** 0.3–0.6 mg/kg daily
Headaches		**+ flucytosine** 200 mg/kg daily
Fever	*India ink preparation:* Round yeast cells with a pale halo and mucoid capsule	in 4 divided doses **+ fluconazole** 0.4 g daily
Meningism		
Cranial nerve involvement	*Culture:* Typical colonies on special media	then
Increasing clouding of consciousness		Fluconazole 0.2 g daily
	Cryptococcal antigen in blood, CSF and urine: positive	for several months or even lifelong to prevent recurrence
	CT (skull): basal granulomatous changes, space-occupying lesion(s), interruption of CSF circulation	or: **Itraconazole** 0.2 g daily for no more than 30 days
	Chest X-ray: Rounded foci	

f) Aspergillus Infections

Whereas candida infections in patients with AIDS are very frequent and lead to typical disease, infections with aspergillus are less common and almost impossible to diagnose clinically. Nevertheless, aspergillus was demonstrated in the lungs of 6 percent of patients who died of AIDS in Frankfurt, in contrast to only one postmortem diagnosis of candida pneumonia. None of these patients had signs of aspergillus infection during life. Proven aspergillus infections should be treated with the combination of amphotericin B and flucytosine. The position of itraconazole is unknown – despite in vitro activity. Liposomal amphotericin B may be promising.

g) Mycobacterial Infections

AIDS patients frequently suffer from tuberculosis and from infections with other, non-tuberculous mycobacteria of environmental origin. Mycobacterial infections in patients with AIDS behave differently from mycobacterial infections in the immunocompetent person; for example, infections with M. tuberculosis and with non-tuberculous mycobacteria are clinically almost indistinguishable in patients with AIDS. The commonest presenting feature of mycobacterial infection is usually fever (Table 69), followed by weight-loss and lymph-node swelling. The cough in pulmonary tuberculosis may be productive, in contrast to the dry, unproductive cough of Pneumocystis carinii pneumonia. Tuberculosis in AIDS may mimic acute lobar pneumonia. Intractable diarrhoea and abdominal pain may be signs of abdominal tuberculosis. Attempts to demonstrate the organism by culture of body fluids and faeces are essential, as are imaging techniques such as ultrasound, X-rays and CT scans.

Non-tuberculous mycobacteria can frequently be isolated from blood culture by the use of special techniques. Since the typical radiological changes may be absent in AIDS patients with pulmonary tuberculosis, bronchoscopy with lavage should be undertaken whenever a causative pathogen cannot be demonstrated by microscopy and culture in an AIDS patient with fever and a productive cough. Cases of bronchial mucosal tuberculosis have occasionally been reported. In lymph-node tuberculosis, the tissue biopsy is the most important investigation; if typical granulation tissue is absent, the diagnosis may have to be confirmed by microscopy or culture. The tuberculin skin test is not helpful because it is usually negative in patients with AIDS, even in the presence of proven tuberculosis.

When the diagnosis of tuberculosis is made early, the prognosis is relatively good even in patients with severe immunodeficiency. Even when extensive, the lesions regress more rapidly than in immunocompetent patients, which may be explained by the absence of granulation tissue. As a rule of thumb, tuberculosis progresses and then disappears rapidly when treatment is started promptly, although this rapid clinical improvement does not permit the standard duration of treatment to be shortened.

The situation in infections with non-tuberculous mycobacteria is less favourable. Although the disease produced by these organisms is less severe and subacute, their elimination may be difficult because of partial resistance, and a cure may not be achieved. When acid-fast bacilli are demonstrated by microscopy, the usual triple combination of rifampicin, ethambutol and isoniazid should initially be started, in order to treat adequately any possible infection with Mycobacterium tuberculosis, which is much more fulminant. Infections with Mycobacterium avium-intracellulare are less responsive to treatment; clofazimine, the experimental derivative ansamycin, amikacin, clarithromycin and possibly also the quinolones (ofloxacin or ciprofloxacin) may be tried.

Table 69. Clinical symptoms, diagnostic measures and results, and treatment of mycobacterial infections (with both M. tuberculosis and non-tuberculous mycobacteria).

Symptoms	Diagnostic measures and results	Treatment
Fever Increasing weakness Night sweats Cough (usually productive) Local or general lymphadenopathy Persistent diarrhoea	*Chest X-ray, tomography of suspicious foci, CT scan:* Shadowing or rapidly enlarging cavitation (often unilateral), effusion, hilar enlargement, or no abnormality (tuberculosis of bronchial mucosa) *Investigation of sputum (bronchoscopy + lavage if negative), blood, needle aspirate, biopsy material, faeces, urine:* Acid-fast bacilli on microscopy, M. tuberculosis or other mycobacteria on culture of blood, biopsy, sputum *Biopsy of lymph nodes and skin:* Acid-fast bacilli on microscopy, often no typical granulation tissue *Ultrasound (abdomen, neck):* Lymph node enlargement	If clinical suspicion and microscopic demonstration of **acid-fast bacilli,** start treatment with isoniazid, rifampicin, ethambutol and possibly pyrazinamide Treatment may need modification of other mycobacteria **M. avium:** ethambutol + rifabutin + ethionamide, possibly clofazimine or a quinolone (ofloxacin) or clarithromycin or amikacin **M. xenopi:** streptomycin, isoniazid, ethionamide

h) Salmonella Septicaemia

The gastroenteritis-producing strains of salmonella (e.g. Salmonella typhimurium) typically give rise to a septicaemic picture in patients with AIDS. Thus blood cultures from patients with salmonellosis and ARC who have even relatively mild symptoms are likely to be positive. The treatment of choice is one of the new quinolones (ofloxacin or ciprofloxacin); cefotaxime or ceftriaxone may also be considered. Co-trimoxazole should be avoided because of the frequency of allergies in AIDS patients.

i) Herpes

Herpes simplex viral infections occur frequently in AIDS and have a particularly long and severe course with a tendency to deep necrosis. Painful ulceration occurs in the pharynx, on the lips, perianally, on the genitalia and in the rectum.

The drug of choice for prophylaxis and treatment is acyclovir 15 mg/kg i.v. daily, which is relatively well tolerated. In chronic recurrent herpes, acyclovir may also be given by mouth. For herpes encephalitis, which is uncommon in AIDS, the dose of acyclovir needs to be 2–3 times higher than normal. For mild disease, treatment with acyclovir tablets or even ointment may be considered.

j) Varicella and Zoster

A primary infection with zoster is typically an early feature of HIV infection, and may be accompanied by severe necrosis and pain if the immunodeficiency is masked.

Zoster infections in HIV-infected patients must always be treated systemically with an adequate course of acyclovir because serious complications (paralysis, myelitis) are frequent. Zoster-immune globulin (ZIG) may be considered. Varicella in patients with HIV is a life-threatening infection and should be treated with acyclovir 30 mg/kg/day i.v.

k) Cytomegalovirus

Cytomegalovirus (CMV) infection only shows a typical clinical picture in the presence of retinitis. The other symptoms of CMV-induced illnesses are uncharacteristic, and the diagnosis may only be confirmed histologically. Serological tests are of little value because the majority of the population have antibodies to CMV, and rises in titre do not occur in immunodeficient patients. More than half of all patients who have died of AIDS have evidence of widespread CMV infection, particularly involving the lungs, kidneys and gastro-intestinal tract. Cerebral symptoms can also be caused by CMV. The treatment of choice is the nucleoside analogue ganciclovir in a dose of 10 mg/kg/day i.v. (see p. 286). CMV retinitis often responds quite well to ganciclovir but relapses after cessation of therapy with further deterioration of vision. Long-term treatment with ganciclovir 5 mg/kg/day i.v. is an option at present. An alternative is the treatment with foscarnet. Foscarnet, a broad spectrum antiviral agent, is effective in CMV caused by ganciclovir-resistant strains. The dose is 180 mg/kg daily for 2 weeks and then 90–120 mg/kg daily thereafter. Foscarnet causes no myelosuppression, but a rise in serum creatinine may occur and require dose adjustment.

l) Papovaviruses

Another opportunistic viral infection in AIDS is multifocal leucoencephalopathy, which is caused by certain papovaviruses. The clinical symptoms are variable. The diagnosis of this infection in life is very difficult and there is at present no effective treatment, although interferon has been tried. Papovaviruses are the cause of the severe condylomata that affect HIV-positive patients, and possibly also play a part in the pathogenesis of AIDS-associated genital carcinoma.

References

Centers for Disease Control. Guidelines for prophylaxis against Pneumocystis carinii pneumonia for persons infected with human immunodeficiency virus. M.M.W.R. *38* (S-5): 1 (1989).

Centers for Disease Control. Public Health Service statement on management of occupational exposure to human immunodeficiency virus, including considerations regarding zidovudine postexposure use. M.M.W.R. *39:* 1–14 (1990).

CHIN, J., et al.: Treatment of disseminated Mycobacterium avium complex infection in AIDS with amikacin, ethambutol, rifampin, and ciprofloxacin. Ann. Intern. Med. *113:* 358 (1990).

CHUCK, S. L., M. A. SANDE: Infections with Cryptococcus neoformans in the acquired immunodeficiency syndrome. N. Engl. J. Med. *321:* 794 (1989).

Collaborative DHPG Treatment Study Group: Treatment of serious cytomegalovirus infections with 9-(1,3-dihydroxy-2-propoxymethyl) guanine in patients with AIDS and other immunodeficiencies. New Engl. J. Med. *314:* 801 (1986).

CONTE, J. E., Jr., D. CHERNOFF, D. W. FEIGEL Jr., P. JOSEPH, C. McDONALD, J. A. GOLDEN: Intravenous or inhaled pentamidine for treating Pneumocystis carinii pneumonia in AIDS. A randomized trial. Ann. intern. Med. *113:* 203 (1990).

COTTON, P.: Controversy continues as experts ponder zidovudine's role in early HIV infection. J.A.M.A. *263:* 1605 (1990).

CREAGH-KIRK, T., et al.: Survival experience among patients with acquired immunodeficiency syndrome receiving zidovudine: Follow-up of patients in a compassionate plea program. J.A.M.A. *260:* 3009 (1988).

DE WIT, S., D. WEERTS, H. GOOSSENS, N. CLUMECK: Comparison of fluconazole and ketoconazole for treatment of oropharyngeal candidiasis in AIDS patients. Lancet *1:* 746–748 (1989).

DISMUKES, W. E.: Cryptococcal meningitis in patients with AIDS. J. Infect. Dis. *157:* 624 (1988).

DOBLE, N., P. HYKIN, R. SHAW, E. E. KEAL: Pulmonary Mycobacterium tuberculosis in acquired immune deficiency syndrome. Brit. Med. J. *291:* 849 (1985).

FALLOON, J., et al.: Human immunodeficiency virus infection in children. J. Pediatr. *114:* 1 (1989).

FISCHL, M. A., et al.: Prolonged zidovudine therapy in patients with AIDS and advanced AIDS-related complex. J.A.M.A. *262:* 2405 (1989).

GALASSO, G. J., R. J. WHITLEY, T. C. MERIGAN: Antiviral agents and viral diseases of man. Raven Press, New York 1990.

GELMON, K.: AIDS, San Francisco. Lancet *335:* 1581 (1990).

GOTTLIEB, M. S., S. KNIGHT, R. MITSUYASU et al.: Prophylaxis of Pneumocystis carinii infection in AIDS with pyrimethamine-sulfadoxine. Lancet *ii:* 398 (1984).
HORSBURGH Jr., C. R., U. G. MASON III, D. C. FARHI, M. D. ISEMAN: Disseminated infection with Mycobacterium avium-intracellulare. A report of 13 cases and a review of the literature. Medicine *64:* 36 (1985).
HOY, J., A. MIJCH, M. SANDLAND: Quadruple-drug therapy for Mycobacterium avium-intracellulare bacteremia in AIDS patients. J. Infect. Dis. *161:* 801–805 (1990).
ISRAELSKI, D. M., REMINGTON, J. S.: Toxoplasmic encephalitis in patients with AIDS. Infect. Dis. Clin. North Am. *2:* 429 (1988).
JACOBSON, M. A., et al.: Effect of foscarnet therapy on infection with human immunodeficiency virus in patients with AIDS. J. Infect. Dis. *158:* 862 (1988).
LEVY, J. A. (ed.): AIDS Pathogenesis and Treatment. New York: Marcel Dekker, 1989.
MCKINSEY, D. S., et al.: Long-term amphotericin B therapy for disseminated histoplasmosis in patients with the acquired immunodeficiency syndrome (AIDS). Ann. Intern. Med. *111:* 655 (1989).
MERIGAN, T. C., et al.: Circulating p24 antigen levels and responses to dideoxycytidine in human immunodeficiency virus (HIV) infections: A phase I and II study. Ann. Intern. Med. *110:* 189 (1989).
MONTAGNIER, L., W. ROZENBAUM, J. C. GLUCKMAN: Aids and HIV Disease. Mosby, St. Louis 1990.
MONTGOMERY, A. B., J. M. LUCE, J. TURNER: Aerosolised pentamidine as sole therapy for pneumocystis carinii pneumonia in patients with acquired immunodeficiency syndrome. Lancet *2:* 480–483 (1987).
MONTGOMERY, A. B., et al.: Aerosolized pentamidine as second line therapy in patients with AIDS and Pneumocystis carinii pneumonia. Chest *95:* 747 (1989).
REED, E. C., et al.: Treatment of cytomegalovirus pneumonia with ganciclovir and intravenous cytomegalovirus immunoglobulin in patients with bone marrow transplants. Ann. Intern. Med. *109:* 783 (1988).
SANDE, M. A., P. A. VOLBERDING: The medical management of AIDS. Saunders, Philadelphia 1990.
SCHMITT, F. A., et al.: Neuropsychological outcome of zidovudine (AZT) treatment of patients with AIDS and AIDS-related complex. N. Engl. J. Med. *319:* 1573 (1988).
SHERR, L.: HIV and AIDS in mothers and babies. Blackwell Scientific Publications, Oxford (1991).
SUGAR, A. M., C. SAUNDERS: Oral fluconazole as suppressive therapy of disseminated cryptococcosis in patients with acquired immunodeficiency syndrome. Am. J. Med. *85:* 481 (1988).
VOLBERDING, P. A., et al.: Zidovudine in asymptomatic human immunodeficiency virus infection. N. Engl. J. Med. *322:* 941 (1990).
WHARTON, J. M., D. L. COLEMAN, C. B. WOFSY et al.: Trimethoprim-sulfamethoxazole or pentamidine for Pneumocystis carinii pneumonia in the acquired immunodeficiency syndrome. A prospective randomized trial. Ann. Intern. Med. *105:* 37 (1986).
YARCHOAN, R., et al.: Phase I studies of 2'3'-dideoxycytidine in severe human immunodeficiency virus infection as a single agent and alternating with zidovudine (AZT). Lancet *1:* 76 (1988).
YARCHOAN, R., et al.: Initial clinical studies of 2'3'-dideoxyadenosine (ddA) and 2'3'-dideoxyinosine (ddI) in patients with AIDS or AIDS-related complex (ARC) (abstr.). J. Cell. Biochem. *138:* 313 (1989).

34. Fungal Infections

For practical purposes, fungi that are facultative pathogens in man may be classified as follows:
1. Dermatophytes (Trichophyton, Microsporum, Epidermophyton).
2. Facultatively pathogenic yeasts (e.g. Candida, Torulopsis).
3. Facultatively pathogenic moulds (e.g. Aspergillus, Mucor).
4. Dimorphous fungi that cause systemic mycoses (e.g. Histoplasma, Coccidioides).

Filamentous bacteria such as actinomyces and nocardia were at one time classified with the fungi; the resemblance is morphological only, however, since these organisms are, like bacteria, inhibited by antibacterial agents.

Laboratory diagnosis: The facultative fungal pathogens are readily identified morphologically and in culture. Since they can be part of the normal body flora or be present in the inanimate environment, however, the interpretation of the pathogenic significance of fungal isolates is sometimes difficult. The presence of a fungal skin infection is best shown by a squash preparation in 10% potassium hydroxide on a microscope slide; fungal elements are most likely to be seen in skin scrapings from the edge of the lesion or, if a vesicle, from the wall (not the base or the fluid). Hair should be removed intact with forceps. Nail clippings should be full thickness and taken as close as possible to the base of the nail. Budding cells and pseudomycelia are characteristic of infections with candida. Where possible, the yeast or mould causing the infection should be identified, because Candida albicans and Aspergillus fumigatus have greater clinical significance than other species. Correlation with the clinical picture is important and an isolate in the absence of supportive clinical features does not normally justify antifungal therapy.

The diagnostic procedures for fungal septicaemia and organ mycoses are described elsewhere. The failure of blind, broad-spectrum antibacterial therapy is often attributed to a systemic fungal infection, and this is sometimes the case in patients with neutropenia, AIDS, or who are undergoing intensive care and have indwelling peripheral or central venous lines. Other causes should be sought in patients with normal immunity.

Dermatophyte infections (tinea) are caused by various species of trichophyton or epidermophyton and are usually transmitted by direct contact (e.g. from animals). Their culture and identification requires special mycological techniques, though these are not essential when the clinical picture is unequivocal. In inflammatory intertrigo, however, the distinction by culture between candida and a dermatophyte is important because griseofulvin and tolnaftate are ineffective against candida. Tinea may affect various superficial sites, but invasion of mucous membranes and deep tissues has not been described. An allergic response to the infecting dermatophyte can occasionally arise, with blisters developing on non-infected as well as infected areas of skin. The treatment of dermatophyte infections may be unsuccessful until the animal source has been removed or controlled.

Systemic treatment of severe infections: Most experience has been with griseofulvin, though treatment with this agent is not always successful. Griseofulvin in a single daily dose of 0.5–0.75 g or 10 mg/kg with a fatty meal is continued for 3–6 weeks or longer if necessary. Contra-indications are pregnancy and liver damage. An alternative systemic treatment is oral ketoconazole 200 mg daily, or fluconazole (p. 204), which is better tolerated.

Milder infections respond well to topical preparations. Infections of the scalp and hair require systemic therapy. Apart from a number of old benzoic acid derivatives such as compound benzoic acid (Whitfield's) ointment, tolnaftate is the preparation of choice for the topical treatment of dermatophyte infections. Newer preparations such as the imidazoles (clotrimazole, econazole, miconazole, sulconazole), naftifin and ciclopiroxolamine have the advantage of additional activity against Candida albicans. A longer course of topical treatment is advisable.

Fungal infections of the nails: Ringworm of the nails (tinea unguium) is caused by dermatophytes, although candida and some moulds (e.g. Scopulariopsis, Hendersonula, Aspergillus spp.) can give rise to clinically similar nail infections. Mixed infections with candida and dermatophytes are not uncommon, particularly in the toenails (as isolated lesions or accompanied by tinea pedis or tinea at other sites).

Severe cases should be *treated* with oral griseofulvin until the natural growth of the nail eliminates the inhibited (though still living) fungi, a process which may require several (4–8) months. An alternative antifungal is oral fluconazole. Systemic treatment should be supplemented by local antifungal agents (clotrimazole, miconazole, ciclopiroxolamine) and by mechanical measures (nail-filing). Fungal infections of the nail of the big toe are the most difficult to treat and may require surgical removal.

Microsporum infections affect the scalp, involve anthropophilic strains (Microsporum audouinii) and are very contagious, particularly among school children. The hair is fluorescent under Wood's light. The differential diagnosis in tinea capitis is trichophytosis. The *treatment of choice* is griseofulvin.

Pityriasis versicolor is caused by Pityrosporum (Malassezia) furfur. Its occurrence depends on host and environmental factors (heat, sweating, corticosteroids). Many local agents are effective. The *drug of choice* is selenium sulphide 2.5%, which should be carefully painted and left on the skin foci overnight on two occasions 8 days apart, or used as a shampoo. Topical clotrimazole and miconazole are also effective.

Seborrhoeic dermatitis due to Pityrosporum ovale (orbiculare) also responds both to selenium sulphide and to imidazoles. This condition is commoner in patients with AIDS. Opinions vary as to whether fungal infection is the cause of seborrhoeic dermatatis, and the name "seborrhoeic dermatitis" is also used for other, non-infectious, forms of dermatitis.

Candida infections (thrush) are usually caused by Candida albicans, occasionally by other species (e. g. C. tropicalis, C. pseudotropicalis). Though species of torulopsis can often be demonstrated, they rarely cause disease. Candida albicans is often part of the normal body flora (mouth, gut), and its growth can be selected by antibiotics, oral contraceptives, pregnancy, diabetes, iron deficiency, impaired host defences and AIDS. In many patients the precipitating cause of the candida infection is not known.

Candida infections may be localised at various sites:

Genital thrush occurs in women as vulvovaginitis with redness, itching, whitish plaques and a creamy discharge, and in men as balanitis. Topical *treatment* is with an imidazole such as clotrimazole, miconazole, econazole, or with ciclopiroxolamine or nystatin, for 1–2 weeks. Povidone iodine or amphotericin B may also be used locally. Both sexual partners should be treated. Relapse or reinfection are common, but are not usually due to drug resistance. In patients with recurrent genital thrush fluconazole orally 0.05 g once daily up to 3 months can be effective during treatment.

Oral thrush occurs particularly in the immunocompromised premature neonate or infant, in the child or adult during antibiotic therapy, and in AIDS, immunosuppression or in the severely ill elderly patient. The *treatment of choice* is topical nystatin as an oral suspension (100,000 units in 1 ml) instilled around the mouth every 3–6 hours. The suspension should then be swallowed, since the oesophagus is also often affected. Lozenges containing amphotericin B are also available. Oral candidosis in AIDS patients usually responds poorly to topical treatment and requires systemic fluconazole.

Candida oesophagitis is a serious complication that is often associated with oral thrush and particularly affects neutropenics and patients with severe T-cell deficiencies. Candida oesophagitis is very rare in other groups of patients. The diagnosis is not straightforward, and may require a barium swallow and possibly oesophagoscopy. Since candida oesophagitis can provide the initial focus for fungaemia, blind treatment is justifiable on clinical suspicion (pain on swallowing). The *drugs of choice* are oral nystatin or amphotericin B, given as a suspension. Severe cases or profoundly immunosuppressed patients should also be treated with systemic fluconazole.

Candida enteritis is rare. Yeasts found in the faeces are usually clinically insignificant. Candida albicans only causes inflammatory changes in the gut in oncological patients and the profoundly immunosuppressed. In recurrent genital candidiasis, however, the intestinal tract can act as a reservoir which should be controlled by oral nystatin or amphotericin B.

Candida pneumonia is also a rare complication of severe immunosuppression and usually arises as a result of candida septicaemia (e. g. from a colonised central venous line), but occasionally also by aspiration. The condition is difficult to recognise, because yeasts in expectorated sputum are usually oral contaminants. For confirmation of candida pneumonia, the organisms should be demonstrated in large numbers in specimens obtained by transtracheal aspiration or bronchoscopy. Yeasts (usually torulopsis) in material aspirated from the trachea in the absence of pneumonia are a frequent finding in patients treated with prolonged intubation and ventilation.

Confirmed cases of candida pneumonia should receive *systemic chemotherapy* with a combination (which is synergistic) of amphotericin B and flucytosine; in less severe cases, or where the isolate is resistant to flucytosine, i. v. or oral fluconazole may be considered. Because of the large particle size of candida, inhaled nystatin is of no value in the treatment of candida pneumonia.

Candida infections of the urinary tract: In normal urine, yeasts are absent or only present in very low numbers. Candida tropicalis and Torulopsis glabrata may be found as well as C. albicans, but are generally of little clinical significance. Yeasts in the urine usually originate not from the bladder but from genital thrush. Suprapubic aspiration to confirm the diagnosis of a fungal urinary infection is therefore always advisable before embarking on potentially risky antifungal therapy. Asymptomatic funguria with large numbers of yeasts can resolve spontaneously in a very short time. Diabetes mellitus, an indwelling urinary catheter and renal transplantation are all important predisposing factors for urinary tract infection with yeasts. Candida albicans may also be found in low numbers in the urine of patients with multiple renal foci from candida septicaemia, which can also give rise to foci in the mucosa of the bladder wall.

The *treatment of choice* is fluconazole, which is excreted in high concentrations in the urine. Amphotericin B i. v. should only be considered in cases of proven candida septicaemia, and renal function must be closely monitored during its use.

Candida septicaemia: The portal of entry is usually a long-standing intravenous line. A rare but very dangerous condition is postoperative candida endocarditis following the implantation of an artificial heart valve. Candida albicans sometimes invades the bloodstream in neutropenic patients, but septicaemia with this organism in other patients is most uncommon. The most important sign is fever; metastatic foci are occasionally found in the retina, brain and kidney. Candida may only be isolated from blood culture when there is massive fungaemia, though C. albicans is frequently found in the urine in this condition.

The *treatment of choice* is a combination of amphotericin B with flucytosine. Any colonised foreign body should if possible be removed; 10 days of systemic fluconazole should be given even after the removal of an infected venous catheter, and patients with less severe symptoms (transient fungaemia) may also be treated with oral fluconazole. Replacement of the infected heart valve in candida endocarditis is usually unavoidable.

Candida infections of the skin are a common inconvenience but are not usually dangerous. Intertrigo, perianal eczema, napkin dermatitis, balanitis, chronic paronychia, perlèche and otitis externa are all caused predominantly by Candida albicans. Local maceration of the skin with bacterial superinfection can contribute to the pathogenesis of these conditions. Congenital cutaneous candidosis is occurs seldomly. Redness, severe itching and peeling (hyperkeratosis) are all suggestive of cutaneous candidosis. Candida granulomas have been described, particularly in young children with congenital immunological deficiencies. They tend to affect the face and scalp, and the causative organisms are easily demonstrated.

Treatment is with topical antifungal agents. Polyenes (nystatin, amphotericin B) or imidazoles (clotrimazole, econazole, ketoconazole, miconazole, sulconazole) may be applied as creams, dusting powders, ointments, solutions or sprays. Alternatives are ciclopiroxolamine, natamycin or povidone iodine. Griseofulvin and tolnaftate are ineffective in yeast infections, and flucytosine should be avoided because of the risk of resistance. Systemic fluconazole should only be used in severe infections. Severe itching may be a sign of an associated allergic response, which is sometimes controllable by a short course of a topical corticosteroid. Precipitating factors such as macerated skin should be removed wherever possible.

Chronic mucocutaneous candidosis (candidosis granulomatosa) mainly occurs in children. The cause is always a primary or acquired immune defect, which may occur either singly or as a combined immunodeficiency (with T-cell deficiencies); the latter can often only be demonstrated by complex immunological methods.

The *treatment* of chronic mucocutaneous candidosis is difficult. Primary immunological disorders are not usually curable, and improvement is difficult to achieve. Long-term topical antifungal therapy is often ineffective. Oral ketoconazole for long periods seems to be the best option at present, though relapses and hepatotoxicity may occur. Fluconazole is better tolerated but evidence of its efficacy in this condition is not yet available. The combination of amphotericin B with flucytosine should be considered when the infecting organisms are resistant to other forms of treatment.

Aspergillus infections: Aspergillus fumigatus is the most important human pathogen, and other species (A. nidulans, A. glaucus) rarely cause disease. A. flavus is medically important on account of the production of aflatoxins in food but does not cause infections, A. fumigatus is widespread in the environment (earth, areas of dampness, flowerpots, dust, rotting wood), and its spores are frequently inhaled and expectorated without ill effect. The finding of one colony of A. fumigatus in sputum culture on a single occasion is not, therefore, indicative of disease; however, its presence repeatedly or in massive numbers in a patient with a compatible clinical picture is strong evidence of infection because A. fumigatus is not a component of the normal body flora. Culture is best achieved on fungal media incubated at 40–45° C; in addition, A. fumigatus antigen can be detected in serum by ELISA. A. fumigatus gives rise to several types of disease, namely:

1. **Bronchopulmonary aspergillosis:** In addition to a purely allergic disease which is expressed as asthma and arises through the inhalation of spores, an invasive infection can arise in which the bronchi are attacked and the bronchial wall destroyed. Chemotherapy can be used rationally only when aspergilli have been shown to be present. Purely allergic aspergillosis should be treated with corticosteroids.

2. **Aspergilloma** is a non-invasive infection of pre-existent cavities (lung cysts or old tuberculous cavities) and is often associated with haemoptysis. The chest X-ray is characteristic and shows a fungal mass containing crescents of air. Aspergilloma does not respond to local or systemic chemotherapy, and the only available treatment at present is surgical removal.

3. **Invasive pulmonary aspergillosis** presents in patients with severe immunosuppression (e.g. leukaemia) as a pneumonia that is resistant to antibacterial therapy. Cavitation and haemoptysis often occur.

4. **Aspergillus septicaemia** occurs in immunosuppressed patients. The portal of entry is sometimes a colonised indwelling venous line, but is often not recognised (lungs, intestinal tract, nasal sinuses). Haematogenous spread leads to infected infarcts and metastatic abscesses, principally in the brain, kidneys, myocardium or liver. Blood culture is usually negative.

5. **Rare forms** of aspergillosis include eye infections, otitis externa, sinusitis and the colonisation of chronic skin ulcers or burns.

Treatment: The chemotherapy of aspergillus infection is difficult, and the relatively toxic combination of amphotericin B with flucytosine at full dosage for a long course (see pp. 193 and 210) is still recommended. A new oral alternative is itraconazole, although there is little clinical experience with this agent in aspergillosis at the time of writing (see p. 202). Other imidazoles (miconazole i.v., ketoconazole orally) are less promising. Local treatment (e.g. inhalation of amphotericin B in bronchopulmonary aspergillosis) is rarely effective. The *prognosis* of invasive aspergillus infections in leukaemia is poor, even with optimal treatment.

Phycomycoses are caused by various phycomycetes, the commonest of which are Rhizopus and Mucor (mucormycoses). The portals of entry are the skin, mucous membranes and infected venous catheters. In immunosuppressed patients and ketoacidotic diabetics, these fungi can penetrate arterial walls and cause thrombosis and infarcts of the brain and other organs. Superficial infections of the skin, external ear and oesophageal and gastric mucosa can give rise to areas of purulent necrosis. The diagnosis of the cause of these is easier than that of pulmonary infection (infarcts), infections which spread to the brain (e. g. from the orbits) or disseminated disease. Amphotericin B is sometimes effective.

Histoplasmosis: see p. 386.

Cryptococcosis: see p. 541.

The **coccidioidomycoses** are caused by Coccidioides immitis and occur in North, Central and South America. They can occur in 3 forms, namely a primary pulmonary form, a primary extrapulmonary form and a disseminated form. The diagnosis is made microscopically, culturally, serologically and sometimes by means of a skin test. Amphotericin B, miconazole and ketoconazole are effective though not very reliable.

References

AMPEL, N. M. et al.: Coccidioidomycosis: Clinical update. Rev. Infect. Dis. *11:* 897 (1989).
DENNING, D. W. et al.: Treatment of invasive aspergillosis with itraconazole. Am. J. Med. *86:* 791 (1989).
EDWARDS, J. E., JR.: Candida Species. In: G. L. MANDELL, R. G. DOUGLAS, JR., and J. E. BENNETT (eds.), Principles and Practice of Infectious Diseases (3rd ed.). New York: Churchill Livingstone, 1990. P. 1943.
LEVITZ, S.: Aspergillosis. Infect. Dis. Clin. North Am. *3:* 1, 1989.
SAAG, M. S., W. E. DISMUKES: Azole antifungal agents: Emphasis on new triazoles. Antimicrob. Agents Chemother. *32:* 1 (1988).

35. Toxoplasmosis

The **diagnosis** of toxoplasmosis should always be properly confirmed before starting treatment with pyrimethamine and a sulphonamide because of the risk with this combination of damage to the bone marrow. The demonstration of specific antibodies at low titre is not in itself evidence of active disease because up to 60–80% of the population may have latent infection and a positive serological reaction is therefore a quite frequent finding.

The following may be regarded as **diagnostic criteria** of active toxoplasmosis:
1. In congenital toxoplasmosis and during the first few months of life, the presence of *toxoplasma trophozoites* shown microscopically in a stained CSF deposit. The

CSF has a high protein content and low cell count, including erythrocytes and occasional eosinophils. A marked eosiniphilia is sometimes found in the peripheral blood.
2. A significant (4-fold) *rise in serum antibody titre* in the Sabin-Feldman dye test, complement fixation test, indirect toxoplasma immunofluorescence reaction or ELISA, in the presence of clinical symptoms. A single high titre is suspicious but not diagnostic. On the other hand, the detection and subsequent disappearance of *toxoplasma-specific IgM* is proof of acute toxoplasmosis. If possible, a pair of sera should be taken from the patient, the first in the acute phase and the second about two weeks later, and tested in parallel on the same occasion. Serological results should always be interpreted with caution in view of the relative rarity of florid infection. Toxoplasma antibodies (other than complement-fixing ones) can persist for life after subclinical infections also.

The newborn baby can have maternal IgG antibodies which have crossed the placenta and whose titres gradually decline in the first few months of life. An increased total IgM in the presence of a positive Sabin-Feldman dye test and a compatible clinical picture in the neonate should arouse suspicion of active infection, which can be confirmed by demonstrating toxoplasma-specific IgM antibodies by immunofluorescence. The absence of specific IgM does not exclude the diagnosis, however, because a substantial number of neonates with acute toxoplasmosis have no detectable toxoplasma-specific IgM in the first few weeks of life. Toxoplasma-specific IgM may still be detectable during the early post-natal period in the mother, however. When the condition is suspected in the neonate despite the absence of specific IgM detectable by immunofluorescence, serum should be retested after 2–4 weeks by the double-sandwich ELISA technique, which is more sensitive. False positive reactions may be excluded by IgM-capture ELISA.

Toxoplasma-specific IgM in pregnancy is a sign that the mother has recently become infected, since IgM antibodies usually disappear within a few weeks, whereas IgG antibodies persist. Infections have, however, been described that were acquired before the start of pregnancy and in which specific IgM antibodies persisted for up to 10 months. In immunosuppressed (and particularly AIDS) patients with active toxoplasmosis, serological diagnosis is unreliable. In AIDS patients with isolated toxoplasma choroidoretinitis or cerebral abscess, serum titres are often strikingly low.
3. The *histological* demonstration of toxoplasmas or a typical histological picture in a biopsied lymph node in the lymphoglandular form of the disease or in the septicaemic form with lymphadenitis. The presence of trophozoites is evidence of active toxoplasmosis, whereas encapsulated forms (pseudocysts) are also found in latent toxoplasmosis. In immunosuppressed patients (e.g. with AIDS), a CT scan and brain biopsy may be needed to detect foci of cerebral toxoplasmosis or to establish another cause of the symptoms.

4. *Culture of the organisms* by inoculation into mice, guinea pigs or hamsters of material from CSF, blood, placenta or fresh organ biopsies. The test animals must be shown beforehand to be free of naturally acquired infection.

The **clinical symptoms** are varied and none is specific for toxoplasmosis. The features of congenital disease include encephalitis, intracerebral calcification, choroidoretinitis, hydrocephalus, microcephaly, hepatosplenomegaly and jaundice, all of which can also be found in congenital cytomegalovirus infection. Acquired toxoplasmosis is equally difficult to recognise clinically, because other infective agents can cause similar symptoms (septicaemia, encephalitis and lymphadenopathy). Patients who are receiving oncological treatment (particularly for lymphoma), immunosuppressive therapy, or who have AIDS, can succumb to disseminated toxoplasmosis with encephalitis, pneumonia, and myocarditis. This is either the reactivation of a chronic latent infection or the result of a severe primary infection. Toxoplasmosis has also been transmitted by organ transplantation from an infected donor when the recipient was seronegative.

Treatment: Pyrimethamine and sulphonamides inhibit parasitic folic acid synthesis by attacking at different points on the folate pathway. These drugs act synergistically on extracellular trophozoites, which are the actively proliferating forms of toxoplasma, but not on tissue pseudocysts. This treatment is therefore only effective in acute infection and at best converts active disease into an inactive stage in which spontaneous healing can occur. Despite effective treatment, antibody titres can remain high for a considerable time or even increase.

The principal **side-effects** of pyrimethamine are the depression of haemopoiesis (neutropenia, thrombocytopenia, anaemia), insomnia and rashes. In patients with cerebral involvement there is a risk of central nervous effects (e.g. convulsions), and the dose should be built up gradually. The side-effects of sulphonamides include neutropenia, haematuria, fever and transient rashes. At the first signs of bone marrow toxicity (for which white cell and platelet counts should be performed 2–3 times a week), a reduction in dose should first be tried. Folinic acid (leucovorin) may be given as an antidote in a dose in adults of 6 mg i.m. for 3 days. Folinic acid rescue does not counteract the antibacterial or antiprotozoal activity of folate acid antagonists. The blood picture often returns to normal, and treatment with pyrimethamine and sulphonamides may be resumed at lower dosage. In other cases, treatment may have to be interrupted, then continued after an interval for marrow recovery with spiramycin or clindamycin.

There are several therapeutic regimens and dosage recommendations. If the dosage is too low, treatment may be ineffective; if too high, the risk of blood dyscrasias is increased. There is still some controversy about the necessary duration of treatment, the choice of sulphonamide preparation and the best alternative drug to use in patients intolerant of the pyrimethamine/sulphonamide combination. Animal experiments suggest that roxithromycin (see p. 160) and azithromycin (see p. 164) are effective in toxoplasmosis. The treatment of toxoplasmosis is made more difficult by the fact that the range of available sulphonamides varies from country to country, and in some countries many sulphonamides are unobtainable. Sulphadiazine, which is recommended in the USA in a daily dose of 4 g, is relatively poorly tolerated. In Europe, the long-acting sulphonamides sulphamethoxydiazine, sulphamethoxazole or sulphalene, are generally preferred (for dosage, see Table 70). Dapsone may be substituted for the sulphonamide.

1. **Congenital toxoplasmosis:** In the first year of life, every child with demonstrable infection should be treated, regardless of whether symptoms are present or not. The dose of *pyrimethamine* is 1 mg/kg (or 15 mg/m^2) daily for the first 2 days, then every second or third day (pyrimethamine has a half-life of 4–5 days). In severe infections the same single dose may be given daily for 3 weeks. The child should always receive a *sulphonamide* as well (e.g. sulphamethoxydiazine 25 mg/kg daily). To reduce the risk of bone-marrow suppression, *folinic acid* (leucovorin) 1 mg is given with each dose of pyrimethamine. A 3-week course of pyrimethamine and sulphonamide may be followed by *spiramycin* 100 mg/kg daily in 3 divided oral doses for 6 weeks (see p. 166). The efficacy of this agent is still not clearly established, so it is not generally recommended. This initial treatment (pyrimethamine/sulphonamide for 3 weeks, then spiramycin for 6 weeks) is repeated 3–4 times during the first year of life in accordance with the clinical picture. In patients with active CNS infection or choroidoretinitis (which carries a risk of blindness), supplementary *prednisone* 1.5 mg/kg/day should be given for several months if necessary, until there is a clear improvement.

In asymptomatic neonates whose mothers had acute toxoplasmosis during pregnancy, a 3-week course of pyrimethamine and sulphonamide, possibly followed by 4–6 weeks of spiramycin, should be given for reasons of safety until after the time when congenital infection can be ruled out serologically. Some 70% of infected children are asymptomatic in the neonatal period and first develop symptoms months or years later. If toxoplasmosis is confirmed, treatment is continued in the usual way. Further treatment is not necessary after the first year of life.

2. **Toxoplasmosis in pregnancy:** An infection acquired in pregnancy should not be treated with pyrimethamine/sulphonamide in the first trimester because of the possible teratogenicity of this combination. Spiramycin 3 g daily by mouth is an alternative which should prevent fetal infection. If, nevertheless, the fetus does become infected, spiramycin has no further effect on the disease. An infection newly acquired in the second half of pregnancy may be treated with either pyrimethamine/sulphonamide or spiramycin.

Dosage recommendations:
a) 2-weekly cycles of pyrimethamine 25 mg every third day
  + a sulphonamide (for daily dose, see Table 70)

Table 70. Dosage of drugs in toxoplasmosis (see text for details).

Drug	Daily dose (in adults)
Pyrimethamine	25–50 mg (50–100 mg in AIDS)
Sulphadiazine *or* Sulphamethoxydiazine *or* Sulphamethoxazole *or* Sulphalene	4 g 1 g initially, then 0.5 g 2 g initially, then 1 g twice daily 2 g every 3–4 days
Spiramycin	3 g
Clindamycin	1.8–2.4 g
Fansidar prophylaxis against the relapse of cerebral toxoplasmosis in AIDS	2 tablets of Fansidar 0.525 g once a week (1 tablet contains pyrimethamine 25 mg and sulphadoxine 0.5 g)

+ folinic acid (leucovorin) 5 mg every 3rd day orally or i.v. are given throughout pregnancy, separated by intervals of four weeks during which no treatment is given.

b) 3-weekly cycles of spiramycin 3 g daily, separated by intervals of 2 weeks when no treatment is given, are continued throughout pregnancy. Spiramycin is well tolerated but its therapeutic efficacy is still in dispute.

3. **Acquired lymphoglandular toxoplasmosis** (in immunologically intact patients): pyrimethamine 50 mg on the first day, then 25 mg daily + a sulphonamide (e.g. sulphamethoxydiazine 1 g initially, then 0.5 g daily) for 2 weeks. Further courses of treatment should not be given even if serum antibody titres remain high.

4. **Reactivated toxoplasmosis:** In immunosuppressed and AIDS patients, severe encephalitis and other organ disease can arise as a result of the reactivation of old, latent toxoplasmosis. Severe primary infections can also occur in immunosuppressed patients. Such cases should be treated with pyrimethamine (25–50 mg daily and a sulphonamide (for daily dose, see Table 70) for a longer period until all signs of active infection have resolved (at least 2 months and usually 6 months or longer). Treatment for longer periods is usually necessary in patients with AIDS. This combination may also prevent pneumocystis pneumonia and thus replaces co-trimoxazole, which would otherwise be necessary. In very severe infections in AIDS patients, the individual dose of pyrimethamine may be increased to 100 mg. In patients with sulphonamide intolerance (a frequent problem in AIDS), pyrimethamine may be combined with clindamycin 2.4 g daily by mouth, or dapsone (see p. 274).

Relapse of cerebral toxoplasmosis in AIDS may be prevented by taking 2 tablets of Fansidar 0.525 g weekly for as long a period as necessary.

5. **Choroidoretinitis** can also arise through the reactivation of latent foci of toxoplasmosis in the eye and should be treated for at least 4 weeks with pyrimethamine 25 mg every second day + a sulphonamide (for dosage, see Table 70). For foci of toxoplasma near the macula, prednisone 60–100 mg daily should be given as well. About ⅔ of patients respond well to this regime and require no further treatment; the remainder will require repeated cycles of pyrimethamine and sulphonamide. Clindamycin is unreliable in ocular toxoplasmosis.

References

DANNEMANN, B. R., D. M. ISRAELSKI, J. S. REMINGTON: Treatment of toxoplasmic encephalitis with intravenous clindamycin. Arch. Intern. Med. *148:* 2477 (1988).
DESMONS, G., J. COUVREUR: Congenital toxoplasmosis. A prospective study of 378 pregnancies. New Engl. J. Med. *290:* 1110 (1974).
HOHLFELD, P., F. DAFFOS, P. THULLIEZ et al.: Fetal toxoplasmosis: outcome of pregnancy and infant follow-up after in-utero treatment. J. Pediatr. *115:* 765 (1989).
JEANNEL, D., D. COSTAGLIOLA, G. NIEL, B. HUBER, M. DANIS: What is known about the prevention of congenital toxoplasmosis? Lancet *336:* 359 (1990).
MCCABE, R. E., S. OSTER: Current recommendations and future prospects in the treatment of toxoplasmosis. Drugs *38:* 973–987 (1989).
MCCABE, R. E., J. S. REMINGTON: Toxoplasma gondii. In: G. L. MANDELL, R. G. DOUGLAS, JR., and J. E. BENNETT (eds.), Principles and Practice of Infectious Diseases (3rd ed.). New York: Churchill Livingstone, 1990.
WILSON, C. B.: Treatment of congenital toxoplasmosis during pregnancy. J. Pediatr. *116:* 1003 (1990).

36. Malaria

Incidence: Many cases of malaria are imported every year into Europe from areas where malaria is endemic, usually by travellers who have not taken adequate antimalarial prophylaxis. As in the endemic regions themselves, several *forms* of malaria caused by different *species* of the malaria parasite may be seen, namely:
1. *Tertian (benign) malaria* (Plasmodium vivax, occasionally P. ovale) with attacks of fever every 48 hours.
2. *Quartan malaria* (P. malariae) with bouts of fever every 72 hours.
3. *Falciparum (malignant) malaria* (P. falciparum) with irregular attacks. This is the most severe form of malaria and has the greatest variety of symptoms.
4. *Double infections.*

Malaria can develop at a variable time after the patient has left the endemic area, is often not immediately recognised and can, particularly in the case of falciparum malaria, be severe and sometimes fatal. A detailed travel history is therefore essential in any patient with an unexplained fever who presents in a temperate country after recent travel abroad, so that the diagnosis of malaria can, if suspected, be confirmed rapidly and treatment started. The laboratory diagnosis is best made by examination of a thick and a thin blood film taken either during or between attacks of fever and stained by the Giemsa method. Specific serum antibodies may be detectable by indirect immunofluorescence; this can be a useful technique when the blood film is temporarily negative, as is sometimes the case in falciparum malaria. Daily blood films are advisable to monitor the first few days of treatment.

Choice of drugs: *Chloroquine,* a 4-aminoquinoline, acts on the schizonts and trophozoites (ring forms) which are found in the erythrocytes and, when given alone, can achieve a **clinical cure** of chloroquine-sensitive falciparum malaria, in which secondary tissue forms are not found. In tertian and quartan malaria, *primaquine,* an 8-aminoquinoline, is used to eliminate the gametes and exoerythrocytic forms (but not the schizonts). To achieve a **radical cure** of tertian and quartan malaria, therefore, primaquine should be given for the 14–21 days which immediately follow the course of chloroquine. Since only primaquine eliminates the gametes to give a radical cure, even patients with chloroquine-sensitive falciparum malaria are best treated with primaquine immediately after their course of chloroquine.

Pyrimethamine, a diaminopyrimidine, acts primarily on exoerythrocytic forms and in antimalarial chemotherapy is used with a *sulphonamide,* sulphadoxine, as a fixed-dose combination (Fansidar) to treat chloroquine-resistant falciparum malaria. *Quinine* has once more become a valuable drug in the initial treatment of very severe cases of malaria, particularly when chloroquine-resistant. *Mefloquine* is also used to treat falciparum malaria, especially "breakthrough malaria" when chloroquine prophylaxis has failed. It is also important for the prophylaxis of travellers from non-endemic areas to parts of the world where there is chloroquine-resistant falciparum malaria. Halofantrine is a new agent for the treatment of chloroquine-resistant falciparum malaria. **Prophylaxis** of malaria in a strict sense (the prevention of infection) is not yet possible because no drug has been developed that kills the sporozoites at the time of their transmission from mosquito to man. The regular intake of chloroquine or other drugs as antimalarial prophylaxis (see Table 72) is used to inhibit the development of blood schizonts and thus to suppress the clinical disease.

Treatment of the malarial attack: Chloroquine is the drug of choice for the treatment of *benign malarias.* The adult dosage regimen for chloroquine for non-immune persons, which gives an approximate total cumulative dose of 25 mg/kg of chloroquine base, is:

Table 71. Antimalarial drugs and their dosages.

Indication	Drug	Dosage	
		Adults	Children
Uncomplicated malaria (except from areas with chloroquine-resistance); no previous prophylaxis	Chloroquine (diphosphate) orally	0.6 g base followed by 0.3 g base after 6, 24 and 48 h (1 tablet = 0.15 g base = 0.25 g salt)	10 mg/kg base (0.6 g maximum) followed by 5 mg/kg base after 6, 24 and 48 h
Uncomplicated falciparum malaria in areas with chloroquine resistance, particularly when chloroquine prophylaxis has failed	Oral quinine (sulphate), followed by pyrimethamine-sulphadoxine (Fansidar) orally	Quinine (sulphate) 0.65 g every 8 h for 3 days, then a single dose of Fansidar 3 tablets	Quinine (sulphate) 10 mg/kg every 8 h (maximum 0.65 g daily), followed by a single dose of Fansidar as follows: 2–11 mo: ¼ tab; 1–4 y: ½ tab; 5–6 y: 1 tab; 7–9 y: 1½ tabs; 10–14 y: 2 tabs; >14 y: 3 tabs.
	or Mefloquine orally (Note: no sequential agent required)	1.25–1.5 g base as 0.75 g (tabs. 3) initially, 0.5 g (tabs. 2) after 6 h, then 0.25 g (tabs. 1) after 12 h.	A single dose of 25 mg/kg base, i.e. 0.25 g (tabs. 1) per 10 kg, or tabs. ¼ per 2.5 kg
	or Tetracycline	0.25 g every 6 h for 7 d	Not recommended in children aged less than 8 years
Severe disease requiring parenteral therapy in areas with chloroquine resistance	Quinine (dihydrochloride) i.v. or, when unobtainable, quinidine i.v.	0.6 g of the salt in 300 ml of physiological saline as a 4-h infusion every 8 h (max. 1.8 g daily) for 7 d or until oral treatment can be resumed	8 mg/kg of the salt as a 4-h infusion every 8 h (maximum 1.8 g daily) for 7 d or until oral treatment can be resumed
Concurrent agent in chloroquine- and Fansidar-resistant falciparum malaria	Doxycycline + quinine (sulphate)	0.20 g every 24 h for 7 d, given with quinine 0.1 g every 12 h for 7 d	Caution in children
Sequential agent for prevention of relapse: P. vivax and P. ovale only	Primaquine (phosphate) orally	15 mg of base daily for 14 days	0.3 mg/kg of base daily (max. 15 mg) for 14 days

- an initial dose of 0.6 g of base (which corresponds to chloroquine diphosphate 1 g, or 4 tablets), then
- a single dose of 0.3 g of base after 6 to 8 h, then
- a single dose of 0.3 g daily for 2 days.

The dosage regimen for chloroquine for children depends on their age. Infants are given an initial dose of 100 mg of base, followed by 50 mg after 6, 24 and 48 h. The corresponding doses for pre-school children are 200 and 100 mg, and for schoolchildren (up to adult size) 300 and 150 mg.

This treatment alone may be adequate for P. malariae infections but, in the case of *P. vivax* and *P. ovale,* a radical cure (to destroy parasites in the liver and thus prevent relapses) is required. This is achieved with **primaquine** base 15 mg (adults) or 0.25 mg/kg (children), equivalent to primaquine diphosphate 26 mg (adults), up to a maximum of 15 mg daily for 14–21 days. A double dose (or twice the length of treatment) is recommended for Chesson-type strains of P. vivax from south-east Asia and the western Pacific. Primaquine can give rise to haemolysis in patients with glucose-6-phosphate dehydrogenase deficiency, and patients who may be deficient in this enzyme should be screened beforehand. If deficient, primaquine in a dose for adults of 30 mg once a week for 8 weeks has been found useful and without undue harmful effects; regular erythrocyte counts should be performed during treatment. Chloroquine and primaquine should be taken after meals to avoid gastric intolerance.

Because of the seriousness of the disease and the risk of fatal complications, every patient who has returned from an endemic area with suspected falciparum malaria should be managed in a hospital with appropriate intensive care facilities. Severe falciparum malaria, particularly from areas with chloroquine resistance, should be treated initially with an intravenous infusion of **quinine hydrochloride** (see Table 71) or with **quinidine** in the same dose as quinine (see below). Patients who are given parenteral quinine require continuous blood-pressure and ECG monitoring because of the danger of hypotension and cardiac arrhythmias; cardiotoxicity is more likely with quinidine. Incipient renal failure, which may herald the blackwater fever that results from massive intravascular haemolysis, should be carefully watched for. Complications are more common with severe parasitaemia (>10% of erythrocytes infected). Smaller doses of chloroquine may be sufficient to treat malaria in patients with partial immunity, such as adult inhabitants of endemic regions who take no drug prophylaxis.

Chloroquine resistance: Chloroquine-resistant falciparum malaria occurs particularly in central and eastern Africa, more recently in western Africa, as well as in south-east Asia, the Indian subcontinent, the islands of the Western Pacific and in South America. Chloroquine resistance must be assumed if falciparum malaria breaks through in a person who has taken regular chloroquine prophylaxis. It is recognised by the persistence of fever and of trophozoites (ring forms) in the blood after 1–2 days of chloroquine treatment or, in less severe attacks, by relapse. Chloroquine resistance is linked not infrequently with pyrimethamine resistance. Mefloquine or quinine may be given by mouth to patients with chloroquine-resistant malaria who can swallow tablets and have no serious manifestations (e. g. impaired consciousness).

The adult dosage regimen for *mefloquine* by mouth is 20 mg/kg (of mefloquine base) as a single dose, or (preferably) as 2 divided doses 6–8 hours apart. The dosage regimen for *quinine* (as the hydrochloride, dihydrochloride or sulphate salt) by mouth is:
– 0.6 g (adults) and 25 mg/kg (children) every 8 hours for 3–7 days or until the parasitaemia has disappeared. Quinine may be given alone or in combination with doxycycline, pyrimethamine-sulfadoxine (Fansidar) or clindamycin, depending on the sensitivity of local strains.

Oral quinine is well tolerated by children, although the salts are bitter.

Mefloquine, quinine and pyrimethamine-sulphadoxine are contraindicated in pregnancy. Halofantrine is a new agent for the treatment of Chloroquine-resistant malaria.

Malarial prophylaxis (suppression): The most important point to remember is that prophylaxis is relative, not absolute, and that breakthrough can occur with any of the drugs recommended anywhere in the world. Personal protection against mosquito bites (nets, insect repellents) is very important. When deciding which drugs to use for prophylaxis, the current malarial situation in the country to be visited should be considered. In countries where there is no chloroquine resistance, chloroquine base 0.3 g (equivalent to diphosphate 0.5 g = 2 tablets) should be taken regularly once a week; children should receive 50 mg (1st year of life), 50–100 mg (1–4 years), 100–150 mg (5–8 years), and 150–300 mg (9–15 years). This prophylaxis should be taken from one week before entry into the endemic region until 6 weeks after leaving it. When the risk is increased or the disease is suspected, a consecutive course of primaquine 15 mg daily for 2 weeks should be taken in order to avoid later disease with exoerythrocytic forms of P. vivax or ovale. Chloroquine is completely safe in pregnancy.

Mefloquine is the only drug that gives effective prophylaxis for short visits (up to 3 months) in areas where chloroquine-resistant malaria is endemic. Prophylaxis with 0.25 g base once weekly should be started 1 week before arrival in the endemic area and continued for 2 weeks after leaving. For longer visits (>3 weeks), 0.25 g of base every 2 weeks is sufficient. Resistance to mefloquine has been reported. An alternative to mefloquine is halofantrine which seems to be better tolerable. In areas with chloroquine-resistant falciparum malaria, the combination of chloroquine plus pyrimethamine-sulphadoxine (Fansidar) can also be used, but is not reliable in Africa on account of the frequent resistance there to pyrimethamine. Since sulphadoxine frequently gives rise to allergies (Lyell's

Table 72. Chemoprophylaxis of malaria (treat for up to 6 weeks after leaving the endemic area).

Name of drug	Dosage	
	Adults	Children
Chloroquine	300 mg base weekly or 75 mg base daily	<1 year: 37.5–50 mg base 1–3 years: 75 mg base 4–6 years: 100 mg base 7–10 years: 150 mg base 11–16 years: 200–300 mg base (once weekly)
Mefloquine	250 mg base weekly	15–19 kg: 62.5 mg 20–30 kg: 125 mg 31–45 kg: 187.5 mg (once weekly)
Pyrimethamine-sulphadoxine	Pyrimethamine 25 mg + sulphadoxine 0.5 g (= 1 tablet) weekly	<1 year: ⅛ tablet 1–4 years: ¼ tablet 5–8 years: ½ tablet 9–12 years: ¾ tablet (once weekly)
Proguanil	100 (–200) mg daily	1–2 years: 25–50 mg 3–6 years: 50–75 mg 7–10 years: 100 mg (daily)

syndrome; discontinue if itching or rashes occur) and pyrimethamine is teratogenic, this compound should be used with caution. Chloroquine plus proguanil (Paludrine) are also recommended (see Table 72). In areas with chloroquine resistance or multiple resistance, doxycycline 0.1 g daily alone (starting 1–2 days before exposure and continuing for 4 weeks afterwards) may be useful, but can give rise to photosensitivity.

References

BRASSEUR, P., J. KOUAMOUO, R. S. MOYOU, P. DRUILH: Emergence of mefloquine-resistant malaria in Africa without drug pressure. Lancet *336:* 59 (1990).
BRECKENRIDGE, A.: Risks and benefits of prophylactic antimalarial drugs. Brit. med. J. *299:* 1057 (1989).
COOK, G. C.: Prevention and treatment of malaria. Lancet *1:* 32–37 (1988).
Centers for Disease Control: Recommendations for the preventing of malaria among travelers. M.M.W.R. *39* (RR-3): 1–10 (1990).
Centers for Disease Control: Recommendations for the prevention of malaria among travelers. J. amer. med. Ass. *263:* 2739, 2734, 2737 (1990).
DE SOUZA, J. M., U. K. SHETH, R. M. G. DE OLIVEIRA et al.: An open, randomized, phase III clinical trial of mefloquine and of quinine plus sulfadoxine-pyrimethamine in the treatment of symptomatic falciparum malaria in Brazil. Bull. Wld. Hlth. Org. *63:* 603 (1985).

Gay, F., M. H. Binet, M. D. Bustos et al.: Mefloquine failure in a child contracting falciparum malaria in West Africa. Lancet *335:* 120 (1990).
Guinn, T. C., R. F. Jacobs, G. J. Mertz: Congenital malaria: a report of four cases and a review. J. Pediatr. *101:* 229 (1982).
Looareesuwan, S., R. E. Phillips, N. J. White et al.: Quinine and severe falciparum malaria in late pregnancy. Lancet *2:* 4 (1985).
Malin, A. S., A. P. Hall: Falciparum malaria resistant to quinine and pyrimethamine-sulfadoxine successfully treated with mefloquine. Brit. med. J. *300:* 1175 (1990).
Martin, S. K., A. M. J. Oduola, W. K. Milhous: Reversal of chloroquine resistance in Plasmodium falciparum by verapamil. Science *235:* 899–901 (1987).
Miller, K. D., H. O. Lobel, R. F. Satriale et al.: Severe cutaneous reactions among American travellers using pyrimethamine-sulfadoxine (Fansidar) for malaria prophylaxis. Am. J. Trop. Med. Hyg. *35:* 451 (1986).
Petersen, E., B. Hogh, I. C. Bygberg, F. T. Black: Malaria chemoprophylaxis: why mefloquine? Lancet *336:* 811 (1990).
Practical Chemotherapy of Malaria: WHO Publications, Geneva 1990.
Wernsdorfer, W. H., I. McGregor (eds.): Malaria. Churchill Livingstone, London 1989.

37. Helminth Infections

Helminths are parasitic worms. They often have a complex life-cycle with a period of development outside the definitive host, either in soil or in some intermediate host. Helminths of medical importance fall into three main groups: *cestodes (tapeworms), nematodes (roundworms),* and *trematodes (flukes).* Some are found worldwide, including the cestodes Echinococcus granulosus (dog tapeworm and cause of hydatid cysts), Hymenolepis nana (dwarf tapeworm), Taenia saginata (beef tapeworm) and T. solium (pork tapeworm), the nematodes Ascaris lumbricoides (giant roundworm), Enterobius vermicularis (oxyuris, threadworm, pinworm), Trichinella spiralis (a tissue roundworm and cause of trichinosis) and Trichuris trichiura (whipworm), and the trematode Fasciola hepatica (liver fluke). Diphyllobothrium latum (the fish tapeworm) is found chiefly in Finland. Others are distributed principally in parts of the tropics and subtropics, including the nematodes Ancylostoma duodenale (hookworm), Brugia malayi (the cause of Brugian or Malayan filariasis), Dracunculus medinensis (guinea worm), Loa loa (African eye worm; a filaria), Necator americanus (hookworm), Onchocerca volvulus (the cause of river blindness in West Africa; a filaria), Strongyloides stercoralis (the cause of strongyloidiasis) and Wucheria bancrofti (the cause of tropical elephantiasis; a filaria). They also include the trematodes Clonorchis sinensis (Chinese liver fluke), Fasciolopsis buski (intestinal fluke), Paragonimus westermani (lung fluke), Schistosoma haematobium, S. mansoni and S. japonicum (the blood flukes, which cause schistosomiasis, or bilharzia). Loa loa, onchocerca and wucheria are transmitted by biting insects and are of great economic importance in the populations affected because of the disabilities they cause.

The **diagnosis** of a helminth infection is based on the clinical picture and the demonstration of the parasite. The ova of helminths may be detected by microscopic examination of an unstained faecal smear prepared by mixing a loopful of faeces (avoiding large particles) with a drop of water on a slide and covering with a coverslip. The detection rate may be improved by saline enrichment (unsuitable for schistosomes and the fish tapeworm), which is achieved by mixing 1 part of faeces with 20 parts of a saturated solution of NaCl. After the suspension has stood for 20 min, a loop of diameter ½ cm and bent at a right angle is applied horizontally to the surface of the liquid, and 3 drops are put singly on to a slide which is then examined microscopically without a coverslip by focusing on the surface of the suspension. Alternatively, ova may be concentrated by centrifugation after ether extraction of an emulsion of sieved faeces in 10% formalin solution; a drop of unstained or iodine-stained centrifuged deposit on a slide is examined microscopically as above. Threadworm and tapeworm eggs are best obtained either with a sellotape slide, in which the sticky surface is applied to the anal skin, or from a moist cotton-wool swab applied to the anal margin; they are then examined unstained on a microscope slide.

Treatment: The treatment of infestations with **nematodes** (roundworms) is summarised in Table 73 and 4a.

Antihelminthics are not always immediately effective in *threadworm infections*, which are the commonest helminths of medical importance in temperate countries such as north-western Europe. Their use should be combined with hygienic measures (handwashing and nailbrushing after food and toilet, a bath immediately after rising in the morning) to break the cycle of auto-infection. All members of the patient's immediate family should be treated simultaneously. Mebendazole is

Table 73. Range of activity of the principal antihelminthic agents.

Parasite	Thiabend-azole	Pyrantel	Mebend-azole	Iver-mectin	Pyrvi-nium	Bephe-nium
Ascaris	++	+++	+++	+++	++	++
Enterobius	++	+++	+++	+++	+++	0
Trichuris	++	++	+++	+++	0	0
Hookworms	+++	+++	+++	+++	0	++
Strongy-loides	+++	+	++	+++	0	+
Trichinella	0	0	++	+++	0	0
Cutaneous larva migrans	+++	?	?	+++	0	0

Efficacy: +++ = good; ++ = moderate; + = slight; 0 = nil.

37. Helminth Infections

Table 74a. Treatment of infestations with nematodes (roundworms).

Infestation	Drug of choice and dosage	Remarks	Alternative treatments
Ankylostoma duodenale (hookworm)	Pyrantel 10 mg/kg as a single dose (maximum 1 g of base)	Side-effects: gastro-intestinal upset, fever, rashes. Avoid in liver impairment.	Mebendazole Bephenium Ivermectin
Ascaris	Pyrantel 10 mg/kg as a single dose (maximum 1 g of base)	Side-effects: diarrhoea, nausea, vomiting. Avoid in pregnancy.	Mebendazole Piperazine salts
Cutaneous larva migrans	Thiabendazole; apply suspension topically	Failure in forms not caused by hookworm larvae (sparganosis, myiasis)	Ivermectin
Dracunculus (guinea worm)	Niridazole 25 mg/kg daily in 3 divided doses for 10 days. Max. daily dose 1.5 g	Remove worms where possible	Mebendazole
Enterobius (Oxyuris)	Pyrantel 10 mg/kg as a single dose, repeated if necessary after 1 week	Treat the whole family (reinfections are common)	Mebendazole Pyrvinium
Filaria	Diethylcarbamazine 2 mg/kg 3 times a day for 3 weeks	Allergy due to lysis of parasites (fever, urticaria), possibly needing steroids	Ivermectin
Strongyloides (dwarf thread-worm)	Thiabendazole 25 mg/kg twice daily for 3 d. Maximum daily dose (adults): 3 g	Treat asymptomatic cases as well because of the risk of generalised infection	Mebendazole Albendazole
Toxocara	Diethylcarbamazine 0.5 mg/kg daily for 3 days, then slowly increased to 3 mg/kg daily for 3 weeks	Only in severe disease and unfavourable site (e.g. the eye), if necessary with prednisone (if hypoxia due to lung involvement)	Thiabendazole
Trichinella	Mebendazole 300 mg 3 times a day for three days, then 500 mg 3 times a day for 10 d	Give steroids in severe disease (myocarditis, cerebral involvement and for Herxheimer reaction)	Ivermectin
Trichuris (whipworm)	Mebendazole 100 mg twice daily for 3 days (for adults and children)	Side-effects: diarrhoea, abdominal pain. Avoid in pregnancy	Albendazole Ivermectin

Table 74b. Treatment of infestations with cestodes (tapeworms).

Infestation	Drug of choice and dosage	Remarks	Alternative treatments
Cysticercus (larval form of T. solium)	Praziquantel 17 mg/kg 3 times a day for 14 days, with steroids if cerebral involvement	Transient side-effects: headache, abdominal pain, confusion, urticaria	Albendazole
Diphyllobothrium latum (fish tapeworm)	Niclosamide 2 g as for taenia, with vitamin B_{12} supplements if necessary	see taenia	see taenia
Echinococcus granulosus	Albendazole 400 mg twice daily for 4 weeks (repeated if necessary)	Side-effects: diarrhoea, abdominal pain, rare leukopenia, alopecia	
Echinococcus multilocularis	Albendazole or mebendazole	Parasitolysis may occur with rupture of cysts, which may not all be eliminated	Surgical excision necessary
Hymenolepis nana (dwarf tapeworm)	Praziquantel 25 mg/kg as a single dose	Transient side-effects: headache, abdominal pain, confusion, urticaria	Niclosamide
Taenia saginata, T. solium	Niclosamide 2 g as a single dose (in children aged 2–8 y, 1 g; aged <2 y, 0.5 g)	Well tolerated, no laxative effect. Elimination of the scolex is necessary	Praziquantel

Table 74c. Treatment of infestations with trematodes (flukes).

Infestation	Drug of choice and dosage	Remarks	Alternative treatments
Clonorchis sinensis (Chinese liver fluke)	Praziquantel 25 mg/kg 3 times a day for one day	Transient side-effects: headache, abdominal pain, confusion, urticaria	
Fasciola hepatica	Bithionol 40 mg/kg every second day (10–15 doses in all)	Side-effects: malaise, diarrhoea, vomiting, photosensitisation (dermatitis), cardio-toxicity (bed-rest advisable)	
Paragonimus (lung fluke)	Praziquantel 25 mg/kg 3 times a day for 2 days	Transient side-effects: headache, abdominal pain, confusion, urticaria	Bithionol
Schistosoma (Bilharzia)	Praziquantel 40 mg/kg as a single dose	Transient side-effects: headache, abdominal pain, confusion, urticaria	Oxamniquine

the drug of choice for patients aged over 2 years, given as a single dose followed, if reinfection occurs, by a second dose after 1–2 weeks. Piperazine salts are best given daily for 7 days, with a further 7-day course if necessary after an interval of 1 week. Pyrantel is given as a single dose with 1 or 2 further doses if necessary at intervals of 2 weeks.

The results of treatment of *other roundworm infections* have improved dramatically since the introduction of pyrantel, mebendazole and, more recently, the new macrolide ivermectin. This compound is a derivative of avermectin B_1, one of a group of macrocyclic lactone antibiotics produced by Streptomyces avermitilis. Ivermectin has been extensively used by veterinarians and has already proved a major advance in the treatment of onchocerciasis, for which it is now the drug of choice, and possibly of other helminthic infections. The use of ivermectin seems not to be accompanied by the severe side-effects (Mazzotti reaction) to dead tissue filarial larvae associated with the piperazine derivative diethylcarbamazine (DEC), which was previously the only drug of proven value in filariasis. A particular advantage of all these new agents is their broad range of activity, since patients from countries with poor sanitation often have multiple infection with, for example, ascaris, hookworm and trichuris. A single dose of pyrantel and pyrvinium is often sufficient therapy. Mebendazole is better tolerated than thiabendazole, which can cause dizziness, fatigue, flatulence and headaches. Mebendazole, pyrantel and thiabendazole should be avoided in pregnancy.

Infections with the *intestinal nematodes* have traditionally been treated with a variety of compounds of variable efficacy, including bephenium, piperazine and tetrachloroethylene. More recently, levamisole and pyrantel pamoate have emerged as useful antihelminthics, and now the benzimidazoles (mebendazole, thiabendazole and the veterinary compound albendazole) have become the drugs of choice for many intestinal roundworm infections, although their expense limits their use in poorer countries. Infections with ascaris are usually eradicated by a single dose of pyrantel 10 mg/kg (maximum 1 g), which may occasionally produce mild nausea but is otherwise a very safe drug. Alternatives are mebendazole 100 mg twice daily for 3 days, and piperazine in a single dose equivalent to 4 g of piperazine hydrate.

Hookworms (Ancylostoma duodenale, Necator americanus) live in the upper small intestine and draw blood from the point of their attachment to their host, resulting in an iron-deficiency anaemia that requires treatment in addition to the expulsion of the worms. Pyrantel is very effective in a single dose of 10 mg/kg (max. 1 g), as is mebendazole 100 mg twice daily for 3 days. Although bephenium is still widely used as a single dose of 2.5 g repeated after 1–2 days, it is unpleasant to take and its activity against Necator americanus is unreliable.

The *tissue roundworms* of medical importance include the *filariae* and the *guinea worm* (Dracunculus medinensis). Diethylcarbamazine is effective against microfilariae and adults of Brugia malayi, Loa loa, and Wucheria bancrofti and must be given under close medical supervision to minimise reactions (Mazotti reaction) to dead tissue microfilariae. Treatment is commenced with a dose of 1 mg/kg, increased gradually over 3 days to 6 mg/kg daily in divided doses, and maintained for 21 days; this usually gives a radical cure. Since there is a risk of encephalopathy, this treatment must be stopped at the first sign of cerebral involvement. Ivermectin is now the drug of choice for *onchocerciasis;* a single oral dose of 200 µg/kg produces a prolonged reduction in microfilarial levels, and annual retreatment should be given until the adult worms die out. Reactions are usually slight and generally take the form of temporary aggravation of itching and rash.

The guinea worm, Dracunculus medinensis, may be killed and removed from tissues with the aid of a course of niridazole. The use of niridazole does not remove the need for sterile dressing of the ulcer caused by the guinea worm and for its extraction wherever possible under sterile conditions. Mebendazole at a dosage of 200 mg twice daily for 7 days has been reported from India as effective, as is metronidazole in a dose of 400 mg three times a day for 5 days.

The treatments of choice of **intestinal tapeworm infections** (see Table 74b) are niclosamide 2 g (4 tablets) and the hydroxyquinoline derivative praziquantel as a single adult dose of 10–20 mg/kg after a light breakfast. Constipated patients should be encouraged to empty their bowels before treatment. The cure rate is greater than 95%. The course may be repeated if further proglottids are passed. Hymenolepis nana is more resistant and requires an initial dose of niclosamide 2 g, then 1 g daily for 6 days; praziquantel in a single dose of 25 mg/kg is more effective. For hydatid disease caused by tapeworms, chemotherapy is not curative but only an adjunct to surgical removal. Cerebral cysticercosis, caused by autoinfection with the larval form of T. solium, may respond to praziquantel given together with steroids. Diphyllobothrium latum, the fish tapeworm, can cause a form of pernicious anaemia because of competition of the worm for vitamin B_{12}. The treatment is with niclosamide 2 g.

Praziquantel is also effective in most **trematode infections** (see Table 74c) and is the only agent to be highly active against all three species of schistosoma that commonly infect man. The dose is 40 mg/kg as a single oral dose (60 mg/kg in 3 divided doses on one day for infections with S. japonicum). No serious toxic effects have been reported. Of the currently available schistosomicides, praziquantel has the best combination of clinical efficacy, broad-range activity and low toxicity. Oxamniquine, an oral quinoline compound, is effective against S. mansoni infections only. The dosage ranges from 15 mg/kg as a single dose to a total of 60 mg/kg over 2–3 days, depending to the geographical region. This drug can occasionally cause epileptic fits. Metriphonate is an organophosphorus compound which is only effective against S. haematobium infections. It is given by mouth in 3 doses of 7.5 mg/kg at intervals of 2 weeks, and should be used with caution in patients likely to be frequently exposed to organophosphorus insecticides.

There is no entirely satisfactory treatment of infections with other trematodes of medical importance such as Fasciola hepatica (liver fluke), Clonorchis sinensis (Chinese liver fluke) and Parogonimus westermani (lung fluke), all of which are acquired by eating uncooked contaminated food. Bithionol, a halogenated phenol originally used as a skin antiseptic, probably offers the best chance of cure but is toxic. Praziquantel may be more effective and less toxic than bithionol, but there have been reports of failure in fascioliasis.

References

Drugs for parasitic infections. Med. Lett. Drugs. Ther.: *32:* 23–32 (1990).
JAMES, D. M., H. M. GILLES: Human antiparasitic drugs: pharmacology and usage. John Wiley & Sons Ltd., Chichester 1985.
KEITH, P. W., J. MCADAM (Eds.): New strategies in parasitology. Churchill Livingstone, London 1989.
KING, C. H., A. A. F. MAHMOUD: Drugs five years later: Praziquantel. Ann. Intern. Med. *110:* 290–296 (1989).
LEECH, J. H., M. A. SANDE, R. K. ROOT: Parasitic Infections. Churchill Livingstone, London 1988.
LEVIN, M. L.: Treatment of trichinosis with mebendazole. Am. J. Trop. Med. Hyg. *32:* 980 (1983).
LOSCHER, T., H.-D. NOTHDURFT, L. PRUFER, F. VON SONNENBURG, W. LANG: Praziquantel in chlonorchiasis and opisthorchiasis. Tropenmed. Parasitol. *32:* 234 (1981).
MCADAM, K. P. W. J.: New Strategies in Parasitology: Churchill Livingstone, London 1989.
OTTESEN, E. A.: Filariases and tropical eosinophilia. In: WARREN, K. S., A. A. F. MAHMOUD: Tropical and Geographical Medicine. S. 390. McGraw-Hill, New York 1984.
PACQUE, M., B. MUNOZ, B. M. GREENE: Community-Based Treatment of Onchocerciasis with Ivermectin: Safety, Efficacy, and Acceptability of Yearly Treatment. J. Inf. Dis. *163:* 381–385 (1991).
RICHARDS, F., P. M. SCHANTZ: Treatment of taenia solium infections. Lancet *1:* 1264 (1985).
SCHANTZ, P. M., H. VAN DEN BOSSCHE, J. ECKERT: Chemotherapy of larval echinococcosis in animals and humans: a review. Z. Parasitenk. *67:* 5 (1982).
SCHENONE, H.: Praziquantel in the treatment of hymenolepis nana infection in children. Am. J. Trop. Med. Hyg. *29:* 329 (1980).
SOTELO, J., F. ESCOBEDO, J. RODRIGUEZ-CARBAJAL: Therapy of parenchymal brain cysticercosis with praziquantel. N. Engl. J. Med. *310:* 1001 (1984).
SOTELO, J., B. TORRES, F. RUBIO-DONNADIEU: Praziquantel in the treatment of neurocysticercosis: Longerm follow-up. Neurology *35:* 752 (1985).
WHO Model Prescribing Information: Drugs Used in Parasitic Diseases. WHO Publications, Geneva 1990.

D. General Rules for Antimicrobial Therapy

1. Choice of Antibiotic

a) Preliminary Remarks

The choice of an antibiotic and the management of antibiotic therapy are governed by:
1. the clinical situation of the patient (e.g. florid acute pyelonephritis);
2. the pathogens isolated from or associated with the particular infection and their antibiotic susceptibilities ("culture and sensitivities");
3. the patient's underlying disease, including pre-existing illness, impaired renal function, age and history of allergy;
4. the properties of the antibiotic (active principle, toxicity, kinetics, presentation and possible side-effects).

These factors determine the choice, dosage and prospects of success of the antibiotic. The choice of antibiotic is, contrary to widely held belief, solely the decision of the clinician. The antibiotic susceptibility pattern tells him which antibiotics should *not* be given, and is *not* in itself a recommendation for the use of any particular antibiotic unless so indicated by a clinical microbiologist in full consultation with the clinician.

b) Forms of Therapy

Directed (or "targeted") **treatment** is the ideal. First, the causative organism is isolated and its antibiotic sensitivity pattern determined. The various possibilities for directed therapy are summarised in Table 77.

As a general rule, because of the low risk of biological side-effects, the most active, best tolerated antibiotic with the narrowest spectrum is chosen (e.g. benzylpenicillin for pneumococcal infections). Directed chemotherapy is often not possible because facilities for rapid bacteriological investigation are not readily available. Even under optimal conditions, directed chemotherapy may be the exception rather than the rule. Directed chemotherapy is important, however, in chronic infections due to resistant micro-organisms (e.g. pseudomonas or staphylococci).

Table 75. Clinical use of the more important antibiotics.

Bacterial species	Benzylpenicillin	Ampicillin, amoxycillin	Azlocillin	Mezlocillin	Piperacillin	Di-, flucloxacillin	Cefazolin, cefazedone	Cefuroxim, cefotiam	Cefoxitin	Cefotaxime	Cefaclor	Imipenem	Gentamicin, tobramycin	Amikacin	O-, ciprofloxacin	Doxycycline	Co-trimoxazole	Erythromycin	Clindamycin	Vancomycin
Group A and B streptococci	●	+	+	+	+	+	+	⊕	+	+	+	⊕	+	+	+	+	+	⊕	⊕	+
Pneumococci	●	+	+	+	+	+	+	⊕	+	+	⊕	⊕	○	○	+	+	+	⊕	⊕	⊕
Enterococci	+	●	⊕	●	⊕	○	○	○	○	○	○	⊕	○	○	+	⊕	+	⊕	○	⊕
Staphylococcus aureus	⊕	+	+	+	+	●	●	●	⊕	+	+	⊕	+	+	⊕	+	+	⊕	●	●
Staphylococcus epidermidis	○	○	○	○	○	⊕	⊕	⊕	+	+	+	⊕	+	+	⊕	○	○	+	●	●
Listeria	+	●	+	⊕	⊕	○	○	○	○	○	○	⊕	+	+	⊕	+	+	+	+	+
Meningococci	●	+	+	+	+	+	+	⊕	+	⊕	+	⊕	+	+	⊕	+	+	+	○	○
Gonococci	+	+	+	+	+	+	+	●	●	●	+	●	+	+	●	+	⊕	+	○	○
Branhamella	+	+	+	+	+	+	+	⊕	+	⊕	+	⊕	+	+	⊕	●	⊕	⊕	○	○
Haemophilus influenzae	○	⊕	⊕	⊕	⊕	○	+	⊕	+	●	⊕	⊕	+	+	⊕	●	⊕	+	○	○
Mycoplasma pneumoniae	○	○	○	○	○	○	○	○	○	○	○	○	○	○	+	●	○	⊕	○	○
Legionella pneumophila	○	○	○	○	○	○	○	○	○	+	○	+	○	○	+	+	○	●	○	○
E. coli	○	⊕	+	●	●	○	⊕	●	●	●	⊕	●	⊕	⊕	⊕	+	●	○	○	○
Klebsiella pneumoniae	○	○	○	+	⊕	○	+	⊕	●	●	+	●	●	●	●	⊕	●	○	○	○
Enterobacter aerogenes	○	○	○	○	+	○	+	⊕	⊕	●	+	●	●	●	●	+	⊕	○	○	○
Enterobacter cloacae	○	○	○	○	○	○	○	○	○	○	○	●	⊕	●	●	+	+	○	○	○
Proteus vulgaris	○	○	⊕	●	●	○	+	⊕	●	●	○	●	●	●	●	+	●	○	○	○
Proteus mirabilis	○	●	●	●	●	○	⊕	⊕	●	●	+	●	●	●	●	+	●	○	○	○
Pseudomonas aeruginosa	○	○	●	⊕	●	○	○	○	○	+	○	⊕	●	●	●	○	○	○	○	○
Serratia marcescens	○	○	○	+	+	○	○	○	+	●	○	●	⊕	●	⊕	○	+	○	○	○
Yersinia enterocolitica	○	○	○	○	○	○	+	+	+	+	○	⊕	+	+	●	⊕	●	○	○	○

Table 75. (continued)

Bacterial species	Benzylpenicillin	Ampicillin, amoxycillin	Azlocillin	Mezlocillin	Piperacillin	Di-, flucloxacillin	Cefazolin, cefazedone	Cefuroxim, cefotiam	Cefoxitin	Cefotaxime	Cefaclor	Imipenem	Gentamicin, tobramycin	Amikacin	O-, ciprofloxacin	Doxycycline	Co-trimoxazole	Erythromycin	Clindamycin	Vancomycin
Salmonella typhi	O	+	O	O	O	O	O	O	O	●	O	+	O	O	●	O	●	O	O	O
Salmonella typhimurium	O	⊕	+	+	+	O	+	+	+	⊕	+	⊕	O	O	●	+	●	O	O	O
Shigella	O	●	+	+	+	O	+	+	+	⊕	+	⊕	O	O	●	⊕	●	O	O	O
Bacteroides fragilis	O	O	⊕	+	⊕	O	O	O	⊕	O	O	●	O	O	+	+	+	+	●	O
Bacteroides melaninogenicus	●	+	+	+	+	O	O	+	⊕	+	O	●	O	O	+	⊕	+	+	●	O
Clostridia	●	+	+	+	+	+	+	+	+	+	⊕	●	O	O	+	⊕	O	⊕	+	⊕
Treponema pallidum	●	+	+	+	+	+	⊕	⊕	+	+	O	+	O	O	O	⊕	O	+	O	O
Chlamydia psittaci	O	O	O	O	O	O	O	O	O	O	O	O	O	O	+	●	O	+	O	O
Chlamydia trachomatis	O	O	O	O	O	O	O	O	O	O	O	O	O	O	+	●	⊕	●	O	O

● = very active, first choice for treatment, ⊕ = good activity, second line antibiotic, + = active but only recommended in special cases, or not at all, O = inactive.

Directed therapy unfortunately has several limitations:
1. At least 48 h are required before the results of culture and antibiotic sensitivities are available.
2. Clinical efficacy may be jeopardised by the presence of an unrecognised mixed infection.
3. Contaminants or superficial commensal flora are frequently mistaken for pathogens.
4. Bacteriological laboratory error may misdirect therapy.
5. In many infections (e.g. cholangitis and pneumonia) the causative organisms are often not demonstrable.
6. Directed therapy can only be satisfactorily managed when there is ready access to a diagnostic microbiological laboratory.

In everyday clinical practice, **calculated** (or "best guess") **treatment** is usually started. For this, an antibiotic is chosen which would be effective against the expected range of micro-organisms and which has the required pharmacokinetic

Table 76. Clinical use of the more important antibiotics against less common pathogens.

Bacterial species	Benzylpenicillin	Ampicillin	Cefazolin	Cefoxitin	Cefotaxime	Imipenem	Gentamicin	Doxycycline	Chloramphenicol	Erythromycin	Clindamycin	O-, Ciprofloxacin	Co-trimoxazole
Acinetobacter	∅	∅	∅	∅	±	+	+	±	∅	∅	∅	⊞	∅
Actinomyces israeli	⊞	+	+	+	+	+	∅	+	±	+	+	±	+
Aeromonas hydrophila	∅	∅	∅	+	+	+	+	+	+	∅	∅	+	+
Bacillus anthracis	⊞	+	+	+	+	+	+	+	+	+	+	+	+
Bordetella pertussis	∅	+	∅	∅	∅	?	∅	⊞	+	⊞	∅	+	+
Borrelia burgdorferi	⊞	+	+	+	+	+	?	+	+	+	∅	∅	∅
Borrelia recurrentis	+	+	+	+	+	+	?	⊞	+	+	∅	∅	∅
Brucella	∅	∅	∅	∅	∅	?	+	⊞	+	∅	∅	+	∅
Campylobacter jejuni	∅	+	∅	∅	±	+	+	+	+	⊞	∅	+	∅
Citrobacter	∅	∅	∅	∅	±	+	⊞	+	+	∅	∅	+	⊞
Corynebacterium diphtheriae	⊞	+	+	+	+	∅	+	+	+	+	+	+	+
Erysipelothrix rhusiopathiae	⊞	+	+	+	+	+	∅	+	+	+	+	+	+
Francisella tularensis	∅	∅	∅	∅	?	?	⊞	⊞	+	∅	∅	?	∅
Fusobacteria	⊞	+	+	+	+	+	∅	+	+	∅	⊞	+	+
Haemophilus ducreyi	∅	+	+	+	+	?	?	+	+	+	∅	+	⊞
Leptospira	⊞	+	+	+	+	?	?	⊞	+	?	?	?	∅
Nocardia asteroides	∅	∅	∅	∅	+	+	∅	+	∅	∅	+	?	⊞
Pasteurella multocida	⊞	+	+	+	+	+	+	+	+	?	+	+	+
Pseudomonas cepacia	∅	∅	∅	∅	∅	∅	∅	∅	+	∅	∅	±	+
Pseudomonas mallei	∅	∅	∅	∅	?	?	+	⊞	+	∅	∅	+	+
Xanthomonas maltophilia	∅	∅	∅	∅	∅	∅	∅	+	+	∅	∅	±	+
Pseudomonas pseudomallei	∅	∅	∅	∅	?	?	∅	+	+	∅	∅	?	+
Rickettsia	∅	∅	∅	∅	∅	∅	∅	⊞	⊞	+	∅	+	∅

⊞ = most active; + = moderately active; ± = doubtful activity; ∅ = inactive; ? = unknown.

properties. Thus wound infections, for example, which are usually caused by staphylococci or streptococci, are generally treated differently from urinary infections, which are generally caused by Enterobacteriaceae. The correct assessment of the clinical situation and a detailed knowledge of the possible causative micro-organisms are particularly important for calculated (or "best guess") chemotherapy.

In severe infections where a causative organism has not been isolated this calculated therapy should be given as **intervention therapy** following a set protocol. It is important here that the appropriate initial therapy can be complemented by further drugs if a response does not occur. As an example, a simplified treatment scheme for leukopenic patients with fever is quoted (based on proposals by the Paul Ehrlich Society, see Fig. 65, p. 607).

Table 77. Facultative pathogens, common infections and antibiotic therapy.

Name and synonyms	Usual site of occurrence	Typical infections	Effective antibiotics
Staphylococcus aureus	Skin, upper respiratory tract	Boils, infected wounds, mastitis, purulent parotitis, suppurative pneumonia, antibiotic-induced enterocolitis, food poisoning, infections associated with foreign bodies, osteomyelitis	Flucloxacillin, clindamycin, (when sensitive, benzylpenicillin), erythromycin, fusidic acid, cefazolin, vancomycin
Staphylococcus epidermidis	Always on the skin, nasal mucosa	Occasional cause of endocarditis, infections associated with foreign bodies (e.g. valve implants)	As Staphylococcus aureus (see above)
Streptococcus pyogenes	Throat	Erysipelas, scarlet fever, angina, rheumatic fever, puerperal sepsis, cellulitis, septicaemia	Benzylpenicillin, phenoxymethylpenicillin, in cases of allergy erythromycin, cefazolin, an oral cephalosporin
Streptococcus pneumoniae, pneumococci	Upper respiratory tract	Lobar pneumonia, bronchitis, sinusitis, corneal ulcer, meningitis, empyema, septicaemia, otitis media	As Streptococcus pyogenes (see above)
Group B streptococci, Streptococcus agalactiae	Genital tract, intestines, cause of animal infections	Neonatal septicaemia and meningitis, gynaecological infections, pyelonephritis	Benzylpenicillin (possibly with gentamicin), cefuroxime, cefotaxime
Enterococcus faecalis, Enterococcus faecium	Intestines, urethra	Urinary infections, mixed infections of intestinal origin, septicaemia, endocarditis	Ampicillin, erythromycin, doxycycline, vancomycin, mezlocillin
Other aerobic streptococci, viridans and non-haemolytic streptococci	Upper respiratory tract, intestines	Subacute bacterial endocarditis	Benzylpenicillin, cefazolin, clindamycin, vancomycin

Table 77 (continued).

Name and synonyms	Usual site of occurrence	Typical infections	Effective antibiotics
Anaerobic streptococci, peptostreptococci	Mouth, intestines, vagina	Mixed infections of intestinal or genital origin, dental infections, brain and lung abscess	Benzylpenicillin or clindamycin (in mixed infections with staphylococci)
Escherichia coli	Intestines, possibly also the mouth and vagina	Urinary infections, pyelonephritis, neonatal meningitis, cholangitis	Amoxicillin, mezlocillin, piperacillin, (where sensitive) co-trimoxazole, cephalosporins, gentamicin, amoxycillin/clavulanate, new quinolones
Organisms of the Kebsiella enterobacter group	Respiratory tract, intestines	As with E. coli, also Klebsiella pneumonia	Cefotaxime, gentamicin, amikacin, co-trimoxazole, doxycycline
Proteus species Pr. vulgaris, Pr. mirabilis, Pr. rettgeri	Intestines	Urinary infections, and occasionally in pyelonephritis, burns, wound infections, chronic otitis	Mezlocillin, cefoxitin, amikacin, gentamicin, co-trimoxazole
Pseudomonas aeruginosa	Not normally on skin or mucous membranes, but found in sewage and the environment, sometimes found in the intestines	Wound infections, particularly burns, chronic otitis, urinary infections, septicaemia, chronic bronchitis, ecthyma gangrenosum, umbilical infections	Tobramycin, gentamicin, amikacin, azlocillin, piperacillin, ceftazidime, cefsulodin, new quinolones, aztreonam
Haemophilus influenzae	Respiratory tract	Chronic bronchitis, bronchopneumonia, otitis media, sinusitis, conjunctivitis, meningitis, septicaemia, epiglottitis	Cefuroxime, cefotaxime, new quinolones, cefaclor, cefixime, doxycycline
Bacteroides melaninogenicus	Upper respiratory tract, rare in the intestines	Dental sepsis, lung abscess, empyema, brain abscess	Benzyl penicillin, metronidazole

Table 77 (continued).

Name and synonyms	Usual site of occurrence	Typical infections	Effective antibiotics
Bacteroides fragilis	Mouth, intestines	Mixed infections of intestinal origin, appendicitis, pylephlebitis, septic thrombophlebitis, genital infections, abscesses with fetid pus	Metronidazole, cefoxitin, clindamycin, imipenem, also mezlocillin or piperacillin (in large dosage)
Candida albicans	Skin, mouth, intestines	Candida stomatitis (thrush), vaginitis, balanitis, occasional pneumonia, oesophagitis, septicaemia. Common in skin infections, e.g. as intertrigo and nail infections	Clotrimazole, nystatin, miconazole, ketoconazole (topical) amphotericin B, flucytosine or fluconazole i.v. in systemic infection

Other severe infections, e.g. secondary infections in AIDS, pneumonia or peritonitis, can also be treated according to a protocol of intervention therapy.

The most comprehensive form of antibiotic treatment is **very broad-spectrum therapy** ("omnispectrum therapy"), which may have to be given on empirical grounds. Certain antibiotic combinations (e.g. cefotaxime + piperacillin + vancomycin) and some new agents, e.g. imipenem or ciprofloxacin, may encompass almost the entire range of pathogens for a given clinical infection. Such very broad-spectrum treatment, however, is indicated in only a very few clinical situations, e.g. bone-marrow insufficiency (as in leukaemia), rapidly changing infecting organisms (e.g. burns), mixed infections (e.g. peritonitis) and as the initial treatment of life-threatening infections (e.g. septic shock).

The fourth use of antibiotics is an **antibiotic prophylaxis.** This is intended to protect from new infection (e.g. treatment of siblings exposed to scarlet fever or meningococcal meningitis), from relapse of infection (e.g. in rheumatic fever), and from serious complications (e.g. as perioperative prophylaxis).

c) Chemotherapy in Practice

In severe illnesses, antibiotic therapy in hospital by the parenteral route is usually preferred. In general practice, simpler oral treatment is usually sufficient for the less severe illnesses encountered there.

α) Parenteral Therapy

In hospitals, severe, life-threatening infections are often encountered and require prompt, effective treatment. The most important of these are septicaemia, secondary pneumonias, severe wound infections, meningitis, peritonitis and biliary infections. There is in addition the large area of perioperative prophylaxis.

Stock antibiotics for hospital use include some or all of:
Benzylpenicillin
An acylamino penicillin (e.g. azlocillin, piperacillin)
A basic cephalosporin (e.g. cefazolin, cefuroxime)
A broad-spectrum cephalosporin (e.g. cefotaxime or ceftriaxone)
An aminoglycoside (e.g. gentamicin, tobramycin)
Metronizadole
Modern parenteral antibiotic therapy in hospitals is thus largely based on the *penicillins, cephalosporins* and *aminoglycosides*.

Antibiotics reserved for special indications in hospital would include:
1. New quinolones (intracellular or multiresistant organisms)
2. Imipenem (broad-spectrum antibiotic)
3. Aztreonam (cephalosporin allergy, enterobacteria, pseudomonas)
4. Ceftazidime (pseudomonas)
5. Flucloxacillin, dicloxacillin (staphylococci)
6. Ampicillin, amoxycillin (enterococci, listeria)
7. Ticarcillin/clavulanate (pseudomonas, enterobacteria)
8. Vancomycin (staphylococci)
9. Clindamycin (staphylococci, anaerobes)
10. Amikacin, netilmicin (resistant organisms)
11. Erythromycin (legionellosis, penicillin allergy)
12. Rifampicin (in combination with other agents to treat endocarditis with multiresistant organisms, legionellosis, tuberculosis and opportunistic mycobacterial infections)
13. Fusidic acid (severe or deep-seated staphylococcal infections)
14. Fosfomycin (β-lactam allergy, staphylococci)

Less severe infections can occur in hospital just as in general practice, and should be treated with oral antibiotics in the same way (see p. 583).

β) Oral Therapy

Infections treated by general medical practitioners in the community will usually be caused by a different range of organisms from those seen in hospital. Urinary infections, respiratory infections and mild wound infections can often be treated with oral antibiotics. Parenteral antibiotics are impractical in general practice.

Stock oral antibiotics for general practice include:
Antibiotic: *Alternatives:*
Phenoxymethylpenicillin   Propicillin
Amoxycillin   Bacampicillin
Doxycycline   Minocycline
Trimethoprim   Co-trimoxazole
Erythromycin   Clarithromycin, roxithromycin
Norfloxacin   Ciprofloxacin, ofloxacin
Cefaclor   Cefixime, cefpodoxime

Oral antibiotics reserved for special indications include:
Amoxycillin/clavulanate (co-amoxiclav)
Penicillinase-stable penicillins (flucloxacillin, dicloxacillin)
Clindamycin
Metronidazole
Ampicillin and tetracycline should now be replaced by better absorbed derivatives (e.g. amoxycillin, bacampicillin, doxycycline). Other oral antibiotics (e.g. fusidic acid and rifampicin) are rarely indicated.

2. Antibiotic Combinations

An infection caused by a single, known pathogen should in principle be treated with a single antibiotic. There is, however, an increasing tendency to treat with antibiotic combinations. Reasons for the use of combinations are
1. to achieve synergy,
2. to extend the spectrum of activity,
3. to delay the development of resistance.

Synergy can arise in various ways, such as
a) blockade of sequential enzymes in the bacterial metabolic pathway (e.g. co-trimoxazole),
b) blockade of enzymes produced by bacteria (e.g. by penicillinase inhibitors such as clavulanic acid),
c) enhancement of the penetration of one antibiotic (e.g. gentamicin) by another (e.g. penicillin),
d) effect on different binding proteins (with β-lactam antibiotics).

Synergy may be expected on theoretical grounds with certain antibiotic combinations, but it must be demonstrated scientifically *in vitro and in vivo* before it can be relied on in treatment. Antagonism found *in vitro* is not necessarily present in vivo.

Principal indications for treatment with antibiotic combinations
1. In *enterococcal infections*, penicillins alone do not have adequate bactericidal activity; high doses of penicillin can even impair bactericidal activity (the Eagle phenomenon). Reliable bactericidal activity can only be obtained by combining the penicillin with an aminoglycoside, and such a combination should always be used when treating enterococcal endocarditis.
2. The combination of an aminoglycoside (e. g. tobramycin) with an acylaminopenicillin (e. g. azlocillin) is superior to treatment with a single agent in severe *pseudomonas infections*, as shown in vitro, in animals and in patients. The combination of a cephalosporin with gentamicin is more effective than one or other as a single agent in the treatment of severe *klebsiella infections* (septicaemia, pneumonia).
3. Combined treatment inhibits or delays the development of resistance in *tuberculosis* and increases the activity of antituberculous drugs on strains of tubercle bacilli with reduced sensitivity.
4. In *severe candida infections*, the combination of amphotericin B and flucytosine achieves better clinical results than one or other alone. Amphotericin B is very toxic and can be given in a lower dose.
5. In *toxoplasmosis*, pyrimethamine and sulphonamides inhibit sequential stages of the metabolic pathway of the parasites.
6. *Infections associated with foreign bodies or implants* can only be eliminated by a bactericidal antibiotic combination, if at all.
7. *Endocarditis*. Infection is as difficult to eradicate from heart valves as it is from foreign bodies, and a bactericidal combination of antibiotics is almost always necessary.
8. *Severe impairment of host defences* (leukaemia, immunosuppression). Mixed infections often occur, which are difficult to treat. An antibiotic combination with a very broad spectrum (e. g. cefotaxime + azlocillin or gentamicin) is necessary because of the risk of rapid changes in infecting agent.
9. *Mixed infections*, e. g. in peritonitis or bronchiectasis, must be treated by antibiotic combinations if a single agent with activity against all the organisms involved is not available.
10. *Initial chemotherapy* given as a "best guess" in a life-threatening clinical situation before the results of culture are available. A combination of at least two antibiotics is usually required if all the likely infecting organisms are to be included.

Possible errors in therapy with antibiotic combinations:
1. *Underdosage* of one or both components because of reliance on presumed synergistic activity.
2. Combination of two antibiotics which are *not fully effective* at the site of infection because of their different pharmacological properties in the target organ (e. g. the brain).

3. *Cumulative toxicity* of two antibiotics in combination, each of which has related side-effects, e. g. vancomycin and gentamicin (both ototoxic).

Fixed combinations of antibiotics in commercial preparations are generally *undesirable* since individual dosage becomes more difficult and there is a risk of underdosage of individual components, as well as of stereotyping the antibiotic therapy. Differences in pharmacokinetic properties of the individual components may result in various ratios of the combination in the different compartments of the body. The frequent underdosage of fixed combinations means that antibacterial activity may not be achieved in the tissues. Fixed combinations of ampicillin with cloxacillin or flucloxacillin (co-fluampicil) are seldom indicated in the treatment of severe infections; many gram-negative bacilli (including Escherichia coli) are resistant to ampicillin, and cephalosporins have more reliable activity. Rational combinations which are clinically beneficial include combinations of trimethoprim with a sulphonamide, and of amoxycillin or ticarcillin with clavulanic acid.

3. Route of Administration

The decision of whether to give an antibiotic orally, parenterally or topically depends on the clinical picture, the condition of the patient and the general circumstances. Some antibiotics can only be given orally (e. g. phenoxymethylpenicillin, propicillin), while others (e. g. amikacin) are only given parenterally, because they are not absorbed in the intestine. Because of their toxicity, some antibiotics, e. g. neomycin, paromomycin, nystatin etc., are unsuitable for systemic use and are only used topically. Many antibiotics may be given both orally and parenterally.

The **parenteral route** generally gives more complete absorption than the oral. This is why antibiotic treatment of serious infections should be *started intravenously* as a slow injection or short infusion, to achieve rapid, high and, where possible, bactericidal blood and tissue concentrations. Once the patient's condition begins to improve, treatment is continued by mouth. *Continuous i. v. infusion* is only recommended with bacteriostatic drugs to obtain sustained high concentrations. High peaks of concentration, as after i. v. injection, give more favourable tissue concentrations of penicillins and cephalosporins than the longer and more sustained concentrations which result from constant i. v. infusion of the same daily dose. Tissue concentrations depend not only on the mode of action, however, but also on the rate of diffusion and other factors such as half-life, protein-binding, lipophilia, molecular size etc. Isotonic solutions are often better tolerated when given i. v. They are produced in volumes which vary with the individual preparation. Antibiotics should not be mixed with other drugs (vitamins, heparin etc.), with plasma concentrates or with amino acid infusions because of the possible risk of inactivation.

Intramuscular injection achieves a depot effect with poorly soluble antibiotics such as procaine penicillin. The absorption of the antibiotic can, however, be delayed in shock or dehydration. If the patient has poor veins, an antibiotic normally given i.v. may have to be injected i.m. (e.g. cefotaxime). I.m. injection is not advisable in patients with a bleeding tendency; certain antibiotics (e.g. cephalothin and erythromycin) cause marked local inflammation when given i.m., and increase the serum LDH and CK.

When an antibiotic powder is dissolved in the fluid in the ampoule, the resultant volume will be larger than that of the original solvent. The instructions for reconstitution should therefore be carefully followed, particularly when only part of the contents of the ampoule is to be used (e.g. in children).

Absorption after **oral administration** varies considerably with different antibiotics. While sulphonamides, chloramphenicol, minocycline etc. are almost completely absorbed by mouth, the absorption of phenoxymethylpenicillin, ampicillin, cloxacillin and tetracycline is only partial. The *rate of absorption* also depends on the galenic preparation, which can vary between preparations of the same antibiotic (e.g. phenoxymethylpenicillin and tetracycline). Antibiotics should not be given by mouth to patients who are unconscious, vomiting, or who have dysphagia or gastric diseases. Unreliable patients, especially when treated as outpatients, are not suitable for oral therapy. The oral absorption of certain antibiotics also depends on whether the stomach is empty or full. Phenoxymethylpenicillin, cloxacillin and lincomycin, for example, should be given fasting, whereas griseofulvin is best absorbed after a fatty meal.

Because absorption is unreliable, antibiotics should not generally be given **rectally** by suppository. An exception is metronidazole, which is well absorbed by this route.

The **dosage interval** required depends on the speed of absorption, metabolism and excretion. If the antibiotic is absorbed and eliminated rapidly, e.g. benzylpenicillin sodium injected i.v., the interval between doses must be shorter than for oral penicillins which are absorbed more slowly. The question of the optimal dosage interval (see Fig. 64) is somewhat controversial. Too long a dose interval, even when recommended as advantageous by the manufacturer, can give rise to risk of failure. On the other hand, persistently high concentrations are not necessary for bactericidal antibiotics. Questions of dosage are not appropriate to marketing strategy.

The **tolerance** of an antibiotic can vary with different routes of administration. Rapid i.v. injection (e.g. of tetracycline) often causes venous inflammation and unwanted systemic effects, while gastrointestinal upset is more frequent after

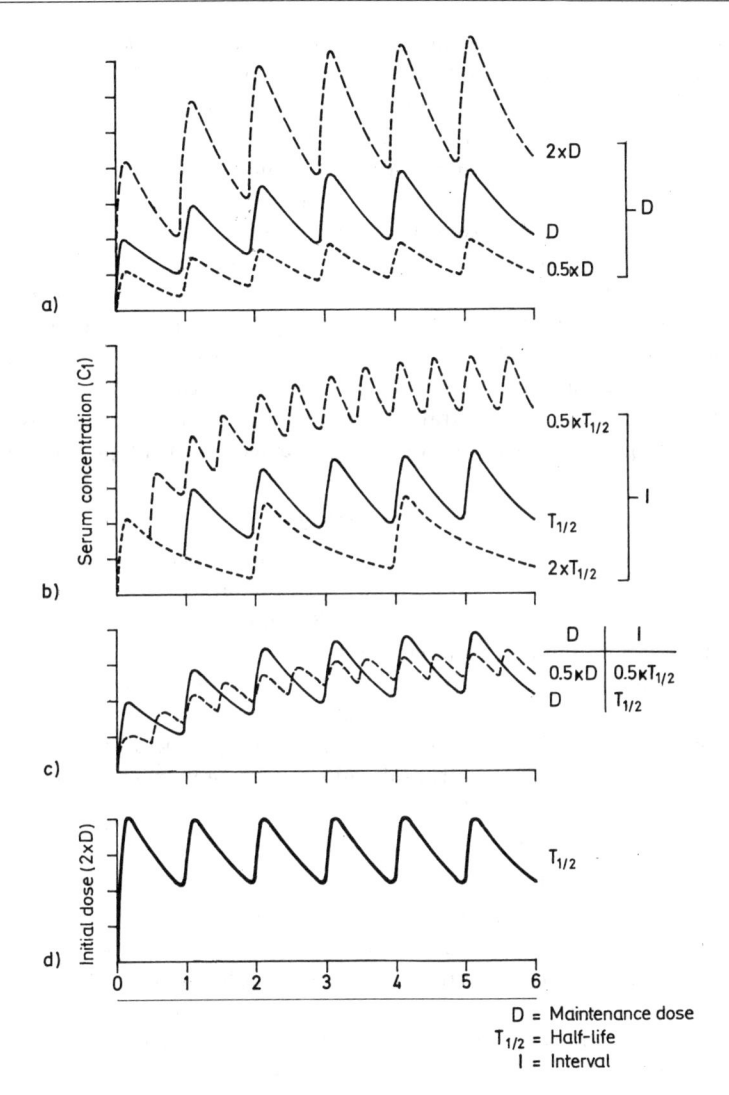

Fig. 64. Effect of dosage on accumulation of a drug on repeated administration at various intervals.

D = Maintenance dose
$T_{1/2}$ = Half-life
I = Interval

taking tetracycline by mouth. Local pain and inflammation are quite common after i.m. injection of almost all the cephalosporins, and should be avoided by mixing with a local anaesthetic or by giving i.v. Intolerance is sometimes attributed to additives or to the electrolyte content (Na).

Topical administration of an antibiotic is generally free of side-effects, although some absorption leading to side-effects is possible when antibiotics are applied topically to large wounds or instilled in large amounts into body cavities. Penicillins and cephalosporins should not be applied to the skin or mucous membranes because of the danger of allergy. Antibiotics which cannot be given systemically because of their toxicity are preferred for topical use because a systemic agent can still be given if resistant bacterial flora are selected. Topical antibiotics are only likely to be effective in very superficial skin infections, and a spray or solution is generally better for this purpose than a cream or ointment; an oil-in-water emulsion is also preferable to an ointment. Eye, nose or ear drops containing antibiotics should be given at concentrations which are tolerated by the tissues. The same applies to aerosols and the intrathecal, intra-articular, intra-pleural, intraperitoneal or intravesicular instillation of antibiotics. Repeated systemic dosage generally gives more prolonged activity than topical treatment.

4. Dosage

The principal objective in giving an antibiotic is to achieve a concentration at the site of infection which is sufficient to kill or inhibit the growth of the bacteria present. The dosage required to achieve this aim cannot always be predicted by fixed rules; it must often be adjusted to suit the individual case. Important factors are the sensitivity of the causative organisms, the pharmacokinetics and tolerance of the antibiotic in relation to the patient's age and illness, and the site of the infection. The dose recommendations made by the manufacturers are sometimes also influenced by commercial considerations, with preference for underdosage (less expensive) or twice-daily dosage (more convenient). Overdosage is less frequently recommended.

Tolerance of the antibiotic: If dose-related side-effects are to be avoided, the *maximum* daily and total dosage should *not as a rule be exceeded*. The penicillins and, to a lesser extent, the cephalosporins have such broad therapeutic ranges that dose-related side-effects are extremely uncommon. The practice in some countries is therefore to give higher doses of these substances than strictly necessary in order to effect a cure as rapidly as possible. With most other antibiotics, however, side-effects regularly occur when the maximum recommended dosage is exceeded.

A *moderate* dose is generally sufficient for less severe infections or when the causative organism is very sensitive, in which case the risk of dose-related side-effects is less. If the infection does not respond, the dose can be increased up to the maximum recommended. With some antibiotics such as the tetracyclines, however, increasing the oral dose does not result in proportionately higher blood concentrations because gastrointestinal absorption is already taking place at the maximal rate. Some compounds, e.g. amphotericin B, are given in gradually increasing doses up to their level of tolerance.

Sensitivity of the causative organism: The dosage of an antibiotic should be such that the minimal inhibitory concentration of that antibiotic against the organism concerned lies within the therapeutic range of that agent at the site of infection. Very sensitive bacteria such as Group A streptococci are adequately treated with quite low daily doses of an antibiotic such as benzylpenicillin. Less sensitive organisms such as pseudomonas may be better treated by a synergistic combination of antibiotics than by an excessive dosage of a single agent. Difficult infections such as endocarditis may require the antibiotic dosage to be adjusted in relation to the sensitivity of the patient's isolate.

Pharmacokinetics: Absorption, distribution, metabolism, conjugation and elimination differ depending on the antibiotic, underlying disease and age of the patient. The dose and dose interval of a given antibiotic are generally determined from the *blood concentration time curve* (absorption, half-life etc.) and the *urinary recovery*. Oral dosage must be higher than parenteral to achieve the same blood concentrations because oral absorption is often poor, with the exception of the sulphonamides and chloramphenicol. To produce therapeutically effective blood and tissue concentrations rapidly at the beginning of treatment, the initial dose may be given intravenously or at double the usual dose. A lower dosage may be sufficient in cardiac failure or renal impairment (see p. 598). Regular assays may be necessary in the treatment of difficult cases in order to avoid excessively high concentrations.

Site of infection: An important factor in successful treatment is the ability of the antibiotic to diffuse into the infected tissue. Infections in poorly accessible sites, such as bone, meninges, abscess cavities, may need to be treated by combining the maximum tolerated systemic dose with local instillation etc. The dose of penicillin or ampicillin necessary to treat bacterial meningitis may need to be 10–20 times higher than normal, particularly when meningeal inflammation subsides, since penicillins pass relatively poorly into the cerebrospinal fluid.

Paediatric dosage may be based on the *average body surface area of* children, from which the following rules have been derived:

Age (years)	Fraction of adult dosage
¼	⅙
½	⅕
1	¼
3	⅓
7	½
12	⅔

In clinical practice, antibiotics are usually dosed according to *body weight*. The usual daily doses for children given in Table 78 apply to infants and small children. Applying the rules of body weight to older children could result in excessive doses, higher even than those recommended for adults. For this reason, *surface area* should be the determining factor for children of school age. Children between 6 and 9 years thus receive one-half, and children between 10 and 12 years about two-thirds of the dosage recommended for adults.

Dosage in premature and full-term neonates and infants during the first month of life: At this age, the excretion of antibiotics whose main route of elimination is through the kidneys is *delayed* because of renal immaturity; the peak blood levels decline more slowly and the dose-intervals may need to be 2 to 3 times longer than with older children. Individual variations in the *degree of renal immaturity* between premature and full-term babies must, however, be taken into account. Special care is necessary in the first few days of life, whilst accumulation is less common after the first week. In particular, potentially toxic antibiotics should only be given in very low doses, or at extended dose-intervals. It may be helpful to assay the *serum concentration* immediately before the next dose (the trough or residual level). Commercial kits are now available for rapid radio-immunoassay and enzyme immunoassay of aminoglycosides and require only very small samples of blood. Largely non-toxic antibiotics, such as the penicillins, can be given without serious risk in the normal childhood dosage (Table 79).

Duration of treatment: The duration of treatment depends on the course of the disease and the species of causative organism and should be long enough to eradicate the infection. *Longer courses of treatment* are needed for chronic infections such as tuberculosis, fungal infections etc., and also in septicaemic illnesses with a tendency to relapse or recur (e. g. staphylococcal septicaemia, brucellosis, endocarditis). *Prophylaxis* against relapse is particularly recommended in rheumatic fever. Longer courses of antibiotic are often necessary in patients with impaired immunity (leukaemia, deficiencies etc.) who tend to relapse when treatment is discontinued.

Table 78. Daily dosage of important antimicrobial agents in adults and children.

Antibiotic	Route	Adults	Children (except neonates)
Benzylpenicillin	i. v., i. m.	0.6–30 (–12 g)	24–60 (–600) mg/kg
Phenoxymethylpenicillin	orally	1–2 g	30–60 mg/kg
Di-, flucloxacillin	orally, i. v.	2–4 (–10) g	100 (–200) mg/kg
Ampicillin	orally	3–4 g	100–150 (–200) mg/kg
	i. v.	1.5–6 (–20) g	100 (–200–400) mg/kg
Amoxycillin	orally	1–1.5 (–3) g	50 mg/kg
Azlo-, mezlo-, piperacillin	i. v.	6 (–15) g	100 (–200) mg/kg
Cefazolin, cefazedone, cefoxitin, cefotiam, cefamandole, cefotaxime, ceftazidime	i. v.	3–6 g	60 (–150) mg/kg
Cefuroxime	i. v.	2.25–4.5 g	60 (–150) mg/kg
Ceftriaxone	i. v.	2–4 g	30–60 mg/kg
Cefaclor, cefadroxil,	orally	1.5–3 g	50–100 mg/kg
Cefixime	orally	0.4 g	8 mg/kg
Imipenem	i. v.	1.5–2 (–4) g	30–60 mg/kg
Aztreonam	i. v.	3–6 (–8) g	45–90 (–120) mg/kg
Co-amoxiclav	orally	1.87 g	45 mg/kg
	i. v.	3.6 g	60 mg/kg
Genta-, tobramycin, netilmicin	i. m.	(0.16–) 0.24–0.32 g	3–5 mg/kg
Amikacin	i. m.	1 g	15 mg/kg
Spectinomycin	i. m.	2 g (once only)	–
Doxycycline	orally, i. v.	0.1–0.2 g	2–4 mg/kg
Tetracycline	orally	1–1.5 (–2) g	20–30 mg/kg
Rolitetracycline	i. v.	(0.25–) 0.5	10 mg/kg
Erythromycin	orally, i. v.	1–2 g	30–50 mg/kg
Fusidic acid	orally	1.5 (–3) g	20 mg/kg
Vancomycin	i. v.	2 g	20–40 mg/kg
Clindamycin	orally, i. v., i. m.	0.6–1.2 (–2.4) g	10–20 mg/kg
Metronidazole (anaerobes)	orally, i. v.	1–1.2 (–2) g	14–21 mg/kg
Rifampicin	orally, i. v.	0.6 g	10 mg/kg
Fosfomycin	i. v.	6–15 g	100–240 mg/kg
Chloramphenicol	orally, i. v.	2–3 g	50 (–80) mg/kg
Ofloxacin	orally	0.4 g	–
	i. v.	0.2 g	–
Ciprofloxacin	orally	0.5–1 (–1.5) g	–
	i. v.	0.2–0.4 g	–
Norfloxacin, enoxacin	orally	0.8 g	–
Co-trimoxazole*	orally	(0.9–) 1.9 (–2.8) g	20–30 mg/kg
Trimethoprim	orally	0.4 g	6 mg/kg

* Higher dosage required in pneumocystis pneumonia (see p. 387).

Table 79. Dosage in the first month of life.

Age Weight	1st–4th week <2000 g	Daily dose (mg/kg) 1st week >2000 g	2nd–4th week >2000 g
Benzylpenicillin*	60	90–120	90–120
Piperacillin*, mezlo-, azlocillin*, flucloxacillin*	100	100–200	100–200
Ampicillin*	100	100–200	100–200
Cefotaxime* Ceftazidime* Cefuroxime*	(60–)100	100	100(–150)
Gentamicin, tobramycin	2	2	3
Amikacin	10	15	15
Vancomycin	20	20	30
Metronidazole	10	10	20
Amphotericin B	0,5	0,5	0,5(–1)
Erythromycin	20	20	30
Cefaclor	50	50–100	50–100
Chloramphenicol*	25	25	25–50

* higher dosage in meningitis

5. Side-effects

Side-effects may be *toxic, allergic or biological*. **Acute** toxicity, as may occur after larger doses of colistin, should be distinguished from **chronic** toxicity (e. g. with chloramphenicol, which can cause anaemia and neutropenia after longer periods of treatment). Some antibiotics have little toxicity, such as penicillins, cephalosporins, fusidic acid etc., while others are potentially very toxic, such as polymyxin, aminoglycosides, amphotericin B etc., all of which can cause both reversible and irreversible damage when given in excessive dosage. Side-effects can also occur at normal dosage, however, particularly when the antibiotic accumulates as a result of inadequate detoxification by the liver or impaired excretion in cardiac and renal insufficiency. Potentially toxic antibiotics should therefore be used with care in patients with *metabolic, hepatic or renal disease, cardiac failure, pregnancy,* and in *premature and full term neonates.* Antibiotics which act at intracellular sites (e. g. rifampicin, co-trimoxazole, and isoniazid) are also often haemato- and hepatotoxic. Certain very toxic antibiotics such as neomycin, paromomycin, bacitracin, tyrothricin and nystatin are unsuitable for

5. Side-effects

systemic use and can only be safely given topically, although even then some absorption can occur and give rise to toxic effects. The recommended dose should not, therefore, be exceeded, and highly concentrated solutions which could irritate or inflame tissues should be avoided. A curare-like respiratory paralysis by neuromuscular blockade can occur after the intraperitoneal or intrapleural instillation of neomycin, gentamicin, tobramycin, streptomycin or amikacin.

Table 80 lists the possible side-effects of systemic antibiotic therapy. The **frequency** of their occurrence varies with different antibiotics. The only use nowadays for streptomycin, for example, is in the treatment of tuberculosis. Polymyxin B, colistin and kanamycin should only be used topically. Because of the very small risk of severe bone marrow suppression chloramphenicol should only be given in serious infections where other agents are less effective. Erythromycin estolate, but not the other forms of erythromycin, frequently causes allergic cholestatic hepatitis. During *pregnancy,* ototoxic and potentially cytotoxic antibiotics and tetracyclines are only justifiable in life-threatening infections. Newly developed drugs are not generally recommended during pregnancy for many years. Sulphonamides must not be given to pregnant women in the week before the estimated date of delivery, nor to newborn babies in the first few weeks of life, as this could cause hyperbilirubinaemia with the risk of kernicterus. Potentially toxic antibiotics (see Table 80) should be avoided in the *newborn* because of the immaturity of renal function and the risk of accumulation.

Allergic side-effects occur mainly with the *penicillins* and *cephalosporins* and are commoner when the drug has been given parenterally and topically than orally. The effects are variable and include different types of rash, urticaria, eosinophilia, oedema, fever, conjunctivitis, cutaneous photosensitivity reactions and immunological abnormalities in the blood. They can occur early in treatment when the patient is already allergic, or as a late reaction, usually after 9–11 days. Ampicillin and amoxycillin rashes are only partially allergic in nature (see p. 40). The most serious allergic response is *anaphylactic shock,* which can be fatal. Sulphonamides cause various hypersensitivity reactions such as rashes, Stevens-Johnson syndrome, exfoliative dermatitis and blood dyscrasias. Allergic reactions are not uncommon with cephalosporins, vancomycin, streptomycin and the nitrofurans, but are rarely associated with the systemic use of other antibiotics except for contact hypersensitivity after topical application.

Biological side-effects arise through the *influence of the antibiotic on the normal bacterial flora on the skin or mucous membranes.* They are commonly associated with broad-spectrum antibiotics such as the tetracyclines, ampicillin and amoxycillin, but can occasionally complicate treatment with narrow-spectrum antibiotics as well. The overgrowth of fungi such as Candida albicans can produce superinfections such as candida stomatitis (oral thrush), and occasionally oesophagitis, pneumonia, balanitis, proctitis and vaginitis. The diagnosis of superficial candida infections should be confirmed microscopically.

Table 80. Important side effects of antimicrobial agents.

Antimicrobial	Side-effects							Contra-indicated (except in life-threatening disease)		
	Allergy	Haematotoxicity	Nephrotoxicity	Hepatotoxicity	Neurotoxicity	Biological	Other	Pregnancy (1st trimester)	Neonatal period	Severe renal failure
Benzylpenicillin	++					+	±			
Methicillin	++	+	+							×
Flucloxacillin	++					±		1,2		
Ampicillin	⊞⊞		±			±	+	3		
Co-amoxiclav	⊞⊞		±			±	+	3	×	?
Azlo-, mezlocillin, piperacillin	++	+				±	+	2		
Cefazolin	+	±	±				±	1,2		
Cefoxitin	+	±					±	1		
Cefotaxime	+	±					±	1		
Latamoxef	+	±					±	1,7	?	?
Cefoperazone	+	±					±	1,3,7	?	?
Aztreonam	+	±					±	2,3,7	×	
Imipenem	+	±	±		+		±	2,3,7	×	?
Tetracyclines	±	±	±	+			+	2,3	×	×	×
Chloramphenicol	±	⊞				±	+	3	×	×	
Gentamicin	±		+		⊞⊞		±	4	×		
Amikacin	+		+		⊞⊞		±	4	×		
Erythromycin	±			+[1]			±	1,2,3			
Clindamycin	±			±			⊞	3			
Fusidic acid	±			+				1,3,5			
Vancomycin	++	±	±		+			1,2	×		
Isoniazid	±	±		+	⊞⊞			5			
Rifampicin	+	+	+	⊞⊞	+			3,5	×	×	
Ethambutol	±			±	⊞⊞			5			
Streptomycin	+	±	±		⊞⊞		±	4,5	×	×	×
Amphotericin B	±	±	⊞⊞	±	±			1,2			×
Flucytosine		⊞⊞		++				3,5			
Griseofulvin	+	±	±	±		±		3	×	×	
Miconazole	++	±		+		+		3	×	×	
Ketoconazole	+	±		⊞⊞		±		3	×	×	

Table 80 (continued).

Antimicrobial	Side-effects							Contra-indicated (except in life-threatening disease)		
	Allergy	Haematotoxicity	Nephrotoxicity	Hepatotoxicity	Neurotoxicity	Biological	Other	Pregnancy (1st trimester)	Neonatal period	Severe renal failure
Sulphonamides	++	±	±	±			3	×	×	×
Co-trimoxazole	++	+	+	+		+	3	×	×	×
Nitrofurantoin	⊞⊞	±		+	⊞⊞		3,6	×	×	×
Norfloxacin	s				+	s	2,3,5	×	×	
Ofloxacin	s				+	s	2,3,5	×	×	
Ciprofloxacin	s				s	s	2,3,5	×	×	
Metronidazole	s	+			+		2,3	×		

[1]) as estolate

Key to side effects: ++ = relatively frequent, + = occasional, ± = rare, ⊞⊞ = principal complication and often the limiting factor in therapy, 1 = local intolerance with i.m. or s.c. injection, 2 = venous irritation with i.v. injection, 3 = gastrointestinal intolerance, 4 = histamine release, 5 = development of secondary resistance, 6 = pneumonia or pulmonary fibrosis, 7 = bleeding tendency, × = contra-indicated

Superinfection with multiresistant bacteria such as MRSA (methicillin-resistant Staphylococcus aureus), Pseudomonas aeruginosa, klebsiella, serratia or acinetobacter) can cause stomatitis, pneumonia, wound infections, abscesses and occasionally septicaemia in immunosuppressed or severely debilitated patients.

Antibiotic-induced enterocolitis can follow treatment with ampicillin, tetracyclines, clindamycin and other broad-spectrum agents. It is a life-threatening condition with severe, bloody diarrhoea, dehydration, a pseudomembranous fibrinous exudate in the stool and shock, and is caused by the overgrowth of toxin-producing strains of Clostridium difficile. A clinically similar form of severe enterocolitis following antibiotic therapy is due to staphylococcal overgrowth and can be rapidly diagnosed by the demonstration of numerous clusters of gram-positive cocci in a gram-stained smear of the stool. The treatment of both conditions consists of rapid and intensive replacement of fluid and electrolyte losses, together with oral vancomycin (see p. 406). Other, less severe, forms of diarrhoea caused by disturbance of the intestinal flora regress rapidly when the antibiotic is discontinued and are also helped by dietary measures.

6. Cost of Treatment

The cost of antibiotic therapy can be considerable. Ideally, the choice of antibiotic should be based only on the best interests of the particular patient, with expense a secondary consideration. Inadequate treatment can in the long term cost more if an acute infection (e.g. sore throat) develops into a chronic process (e.g. endocarditis). On the other hand, once the decision to treat with antibiotics has been taken, there is no virtue in preferring a very expensive drug when a cheaper alternative is equally satisfactory, nor in giving excessive dosage or too long a course. Cost reductions are only acceptable when they are not made at the expense of quality or clinical judgement.

Different brands of the same antibiotic have been shown to vary considerably in their bioavailability and incidence of side-effects. Where preparations are otherwise similar, the drug with the optimal bioavailability should be chosen.

The price comparisons in Tables 81a and b are made on the basic costs of the preparations as quoted in the British National Formulary (1991). The costs of the dispensed medicines are always greater, particularly when dispensing costs are included. Bulk orders by large hospitals, hospital districts or regional pharmacies can benefit from considerable discounts.

Table 81a. Relative costs of oral antibiotics based on the basic net price of each preparation (British National Formulary, 1991, No. 22).

Antibiotic	Daily dose for adults	Daily cost in GB£
Phenoxymethylpenicillin	1.0 g	0.07
Ampicillin	2.0 g	0.28
Amoxycillin	1.5 g	0.84
Co-amoxiclav	1.5 g	1.93
Flucloxacillin	2.0 g	1.12
Cephalexin	1.5 g	0.96
Cephradine	2.0 g	1.40
Cefaclor	1.5 g	2.60
Cefixime	0.4 g	2.56
Cefuroxime axetil	0.5 g	1.80
Tetracycline	2.0 g	0.12
Doxycycline	0.1 g	0.42
Minocycline	0.2 g	1.19
Erythromycin	2.0 g	0.40
Clindamycin	0.6 g	1.81
Ciprofloxacin	1.5 g	4.50
Ofloxacin	0.4 g	1.47
Fusidic acid	1.5 g	4.17
Vancomycin	0.5 g	12.62
Nitrofurantoin	0.4 g	0.30
Co-trimoxazole	1.92 g	0.31
Trimethoprim	0.4 g	0.09

Table 81a (continued).

Antibiotic	Daily dose for adults	Daily cost in GB£
Chloramphenicol	1.5 g	0.49
Metronidazole	1.2 g	0.22
(suppository)	2.0 g	1.36
Rifampicin	0.6 g	0.76
Isoniazid	0.3 g	0.05
Ethambutol	15 mg/kg	0.67
Pyrazinamide	30 mg/kg	0.29
Amphotericin B	0.8 g	1.19
Flucytosine	200 mg/kg	13.20
Griseofulvin	1.0 g	0.24
Fluconazole	0.05 g	2.37
Ketoconazole	0.2 g	0.52
Nystatin	2×10^6 units	0.34

Table 81b. Relative costs of parenteral preparations based on the basic net price of each preparation (British National Formulary, 1991, No. 22).

Antibiotic	Daily dose for adults	Daily cost in GB£
Benzylpenicillin	6.0 g	1.20
Azlocillin	6.0 g	15.06
Flucloxacillin	2(–4) g	6.12 (–12.24)
Piperacillin	6(–12) g	18.24 (–36.03)
Co-amoxiclav	3(–4) g	8.10 (–10.80)
Ticarcillin/clavulanate	12(–18) g	21.16 (–31.74)
Cefazolin	2(–4) g	9.80 (–18.52)
Cephradine	2(–8) g	3.96 (–15.60)
Cefuroxime	2.25(–4.5) g	7.92 (–15.87)
Cefoxitin	3(–6) g	14.76 (–29.52)
Cefotaxime	2(–12) g	9.90 (–59.40)
Cefsulodin	1(–4) g	11.30 (–45.20)
Ceftazidime	3(–6) g	29.70 (–59.40)
Aztreonam	3(–6) g	26.85 (–53.70)
Imipenem	1.5(–3) g	45.00 (–90.00)
Gentamicin	0.24(–0.48) g	4.77 (– 9.54)
Tobramycin	0.24(–0.48) g	7.89 (–15.78)
Netilmicin	0.3 g	8.64
Amikacin	1.0 g	20.28
Tetracycline	1(–2) g	4.06 (– 8.12)
Teicoplanin	0.2(–0.4) g	26.72 (–53.44)
Vancomycin	2.0 g	53.44
Ciprofloxacin	0.2(–0.4) g	24.00 (–48.00)
Metronidazole	1.5 g	4.34

7. Antibiotic Therapy in Renal Insufficiency

Mode of excretion: Whereas antibiotics such as benzylpenicillin, cefazolin, gentamicin and vancomycin are almost entirely excreted in the urine, most other antibiotics are only partially eliminated through the kidneys, either in unchanged active form or as inactive metabolites, which the remainder passing out through the bile and intestinal tract.

The *urinary recovery* is an important basic parameter in chemotherapy. Only very small amounts of active minocycline, erythromycin, fusidic acid, oxacillin and cefoperazone appear in the urine; the bulk is metabolised in the body and excreted predominantly in the faeces. Accumulation and prolongation of the *elimination half-life* (Table 82) is seen in renal insufficiency and depends on the mode of excretion and rate of metabolism of the antibiotic given.

The degree of renal failure is most closely reflected in the reduction in *creatinine clearance* (and less well by serum urea and creatinine values). A creatinine clearance of >40 ml/min usually corresponds to a serum creatinine value of <2 mg/dl, a creatinine clearance of 20–40 ml/min to a serum creatinine of 2–4 mg/dl, and a creatinine clearance of 10–20 ml/min to a serum creatinine of 4–8 mg/dl. The risk of side-effects depends not only on the degree of accumulation, but also on the potential toxicity of the antibiotic. From this experience, certain rules can be drawn up for the dosage of antibiotics in renal failure, which are summarised in Table 82.

Table 82. Elimination half-lives of antibiotics that require the interval between average single doses to be modified in renal failure.

Antibiotic	Half-life (h)		Dose-interval (h) at a creatinine clearance (ml/min) of				Urinary recovery (%) (parenteral dose, normal renal function)
	Normal	Severe renal failure	>80	50–80	10–50	<10	
Amikacin	2.3	72–96	8	24	24–72	72–96	90
Ampi-, amoxicillin	1.0	8.5	6	8	12	12–24	60
Azlocillin	1.25	8–10	6	8	8	12–24	95
Aztreonam	1.7	6–9	6	8	12	24	70
Benzylpenicillin	0.65	7–10	6	8	8	12	90
Cefaclor	1.0	6–10	6	8	8	12	60
Cefadroxil	1.5	5–20	12	12	24	36	85
Cefazolin	1.5	5–20	6	8	12	24	90

7. Antibiotic Therapy in Renal Insufficiency

Table 82 (continued).

Antibiotic	Half-life (h)		Dose-interval (h) at a creatinine clearance (ml/min) of				Urinary recovery (%) (parenteral dose, normal renal function)
	Normal	Severe renal failure	>80	50–80	10–50	<10	
Cefoperazone	2.0	5–10	8	8	8	12	20
Cefotaxime	1.0	14	8	8	8	12	50
Cefoxitin	0.75	5–10	6	8	12	24	90
Ceftazidime	2	15–25	8	12	24	48	90
Ceftriaxone	7–8	12–15	12–24	24	24	24	50
Cefuroxime	1.2	5–20	6	8	12	24	90
Cephalexin	1.0	30	6	6	8	24–48	90
Cephalothin	0.65	3–18	4–6	6	6	8	65
Ciprofloxacin	3–4	10	12	12	12	24	40
Clindamycin	3	3–5	6	6	8	12	40
Flucloxacillin	0.75	8	6	8	8	12	35
Fluconazole	25	98	24	48	72	96	70
Flucytosine	3–4	70	6	8	12–24	Avoid	90
Gentamicin, tobramycin	2	60	8	12	18–24	48	90
Imipenem	1	3–4	6	8	12	12–24	20
Latamoxef	2.0	5–20	8	8	12	24	75
Lincomycin	5	10–13	8	8	12	12	40
Metronidazole	7	8–12	8	8	12	24	30
Mezlocillin	0.8	6–14	6	8	8	12–24	60
Oxacillin	0.4	2	4–6	6	6	8	25
Piperacillin	1.0	6–10	6	8	8	12–24	60
Tetracycline	8–9	30–128	6	12	48	72–96	60
Ticarcillin	1.1	16	6	8	12	24–48	95
Trimethoprim/ sulphamethoxazole	10 12	12–24 24–48	12	12	24	Avoid Avoid	60 80
Vancomycin	6	250	12	72	240	240	85

Potentially nephrotoxic antibiotics include *amphotericin B* (used for the treatment of generalised fungal infections and contra-indicated in severe renal failure), *bacitracin, neomycin* and *paromomycin*, which are still used as topical antibacterial therapy.

Cephaloridine, which is now obsolete, can cause acute tubular necrosis at high dosage (>4–6 g daily). *Cephalothin* and *cephradine* are also nephrotoxic in very high doses. The nephrotoxicity of the *newer cephalosporins*, on the other hand, is negligible.

Polymyxins can accumulate in renal insufficiency and cause a number of symptoms of neurotoxicity; they should therefore no longer be used systemically.

Streptomycin, kanamycin, amikacin, gentamicin, sisomicin, tobramycin, netilmicin and *capreomycin* are also potentially nephrotoxic and can also be neurotoxic if they accumulate. They should therefore only be given to patients with renal insufficiency who have severe infections, at reduced dosage and with careful monitoring of blood concentrations. The initial dose of gentamicin, tobramycin or netilmicin is 1.5–2 mg/kg. As maintenance dose, the usual daily dose x creatinine clearance/100 is recommended. The ototoxicity is increased by the simultaneous administration of certain diuretics, e.g. frusemide (see p. 138). Various rapid methods are now commercially available to laboratories which enable precise results of assays of concentrations of gentamicin, tobramycin, amikacin and netilmicin in small samples of blood (suitable for paediatric use) to be made available to the requesting clinician within less than an hour of receipt of the sample. The blood concentration immediately before a repeated dose (trough or valley level) is particularly useful and, if the dose-interval is correct, need not be significantly greater than the concentration in a patient with normal renal function dosed at standard intervals. Therapeutic levels 1 h after i.v. infusion over 20–30 min of gentamicin, tobramycin or netilmicin are 5–10 mg/l, of amikacin 20–40 mg/l.

Of the penicillins, only *methicillin* has been reported to cause renal damage; this agent was superceded some years ago by the more active, nontoxic isoxazolyl penicillins oxacillin, cloxacillin and flucloxacillin (see p. 36). In renal failure, apalcillin saturates the capacity of the liver for biliary excretion, leading to excessive blood concentrations.

Antibiotics whose dose should be reduced in renal impairment: The *tetracyclines* are 10–25% excreted by the kidneys when given orally and 50–70% when given i.v. They can accumulate in patients with renal insufficiency and cause toxic liver damage. *Demeclocycline* can cause a nephrogenic diabetes insipidus and should not be used in patients with pre-existing renal damage. *Doxycycline* and *minocycline* do not accumulate in renal failure, however, and should be always preferred.

β-lactam antibiotics should be carefully dosed in renal insufficiency and very high doses avoided. A combination with gentamicin or other potentially toxic antibiotics (see above) should be avoided when acute renal failure is imminent. *Lincomycin* and *clindamycin* are given at ¼ to ⅓ the normal dose in severe renal insufficiency. A dose reduction is also necessary for *flucytosine* (Table 82 and p. 210) and for *quinolones* (see pp. 240 and 244).

Most of the sulphonamides still in use are more water-soluble and less acetylated than earlier compounds, and so no longer cause renal damage under normal conditions of excretion. When renal function is impaired, however, they should be given at reduced dosage. This applies particularly to *sulphadiazine*, which should not be used in patients who are dehydrated, uraemic or who have pre-existing renal damage. The excretion of *sulphamethoxydiazine* and other *long-acting sulphonamides* is retarded when the creatinine clearance is less than 30 ml/min, and the daily dose should be halved below this value. Sulphonamides should not be given to patients whose creatinine clearance is less than 20 ml/min. *Co-trimoxazole* should not be used when the creatinine clearance is less than 15 ml/min, and at values of 15–30 ml/min the daily dose should be halved.

Nitrofurantoin in renal insufficiency leads to severe neurotoxic effects (polyneuritis etc.) and is best avoided even in low-grade renal impairment.

Antibiotics which require no dose reduction in renal insufficiency: *Benzylpenicillin* is so non-toxic that it can be given in the normal daily dose even though considerable accumulation occurs in renal insufficiency. The dose-interval may, however, be prolonged in severe renal impairment. Doses of benzylpenicillin above 6 g a day can give rise to convulsions in uraemic patients, so this upper limit should not be exceeded.

Ampicillin, azlocillin, cloxacillin, dicloxacillin, flucloxacillin, mezlocillin, oxacillin and *piperacillin* may all be used in moderate dosage in renal insufficiency.

In uraemia, the electrolyte content of the antibiotic must be taken into account, especially of the disodium salts *ceftriaxone, fosfomycin* and *ticarcillin*, and of *benzylpenicillin potassium*.

Of the *cephalosporins*, cefotaxime, cefoperazone, ceftriaxone and some others are about one-third metabolised in the body and therefore accumulate less than the other cephalosporins. In patients with severe renal insufficiency, therefore, the dose-interval has to be increased accordingly, although the standard unit doses may still safely be given. *β-Lactam antibiotics with substantial biliary elimination* (cefoperazone, mezlocillin), accumulate less than those with a predominantly renal excretion pathway, although saturation of the capacity for biliary elimination may occur (apalcillin).

Erythromycin, fusidic acid, rifampicin and *metronidazole* are well tolerated in renal insufficiency provided that liver function is unimpaired. *Doxycycline* may also be used without restriction in renal failure. The daily dose of *chloramphenicol*, which is predominantly excreted in the urine, does not have to be reduced in patients with poor renal function because accumulation of the antibacterially inactive metabolites does not apparently give rise to side-effects. When liver function is also impaired, however, and detoxification by glucuronidation is reduced, chloramphenicol should be avoided. *Ketoconazole, itraconazole* and *miconazole* may also be given at normal dosage in renal failure, but fluconazole may accumulate.

Antibiotic therapy in anuria: In acute anuria, antibiotics that require no dose reduction in renal impairment may be given at full dosage. These are chloramphenicol, doxycycline, erythromycin, fusidic acid, the penicillins (except apalcillin and ticarcillin), and rifampicin. In patients on intermittent *haemodialysis* or *peritoneal dialysis*, antibiotics are often necessary (e. g. because of an arteriovenous shunt infection). If drugs that do not accumulate are inappropriate for the infection present, other antibiotics that have to be given at extended intervals may have to be considered. The dosage depends on the residual diuresis, the possibility of extra-renal elimination, the frequency of dialysis, and whether the antibiotic is dialysable. Plasma urea and creatinine values are unsuitable criteria for deciding the dosage regime of antibiotics in patients on dialysis. Highly toxic antibiotics such as amphotericin B and vancomycin should generally only be given as a single dose to dialysis patients. Since they are not dialysable and have virtually no extra-renal pathway of elimination, therapeutic concentrations persist in the blood for weeks. A further dose is only permissible after a long interval and after the results of an assay have been obtained.

Antibiotics are generally given to uraemic patients by the parenteral route, since the absorption and tolerance of oral doses can be affected by uraemic gastritis. The normal dose should be given at the end of each dialysis session since most antibiotics are dialysable (with the exception of amphotericin B, clindamycin, doxycycline, erythromycin, teicoplanin, fusidic acid, lincomycin and probably also rifampicin). Benzylpenicillin and the penicillinase-stable penicillins such as flucloxacillin are only partially removed by dialysis. Published data about the elimination half-lives of antibiotics during dialysis are sometimes contradictory, possibly as a result of variation in the properties of different dialysis membranes and in the dialysis period. The addition of antibiotics to the dialysis fluid should be considered as a possible route of administration, since most antibiotics diffuse into the blood during dialysis.

Peritoneal dialysis is less effective and certain haemodialysable antibiotics (e. g. cefazolin) are not, or only partially, removed. Most antibiotics behave similarly in both peritoneal and haemodialysis. If an antibiotic is added to the fluid during peritoneal dialysis, it can diffuse into the blood and cause side-effects. Ampicillin, mezlocillin, cephalothin, cefotaxime and oxacillin may all be added with relative safety to dialysis fluid to give concentrations of 50 mg/l in patients with peritonitis; this causes an initial increase in the serum concentration, which then decreases through metabolism and extra-renal excretion. Aminoglycosides should not be given intraperitoneally because of the risk of neuromuscular blockade, but clindamycin and teicoplanin may be used for instillation. Fungal peritonitis following peritoneal dialysis may be treated by the instillation of amphotericin B or miconazole. For the treatment of peritonitis in CAPD, see p. 412.

References

GILBERT, D. N., W. M. BENNETT: Use of antimicrobial agents in renal failure. Infect. Dis. Clin. North Am. *3:* 517 (1989).

8. Antibiotic Therapy and Abnormal Liver Function

Contra-indications: The liver plays an important part in the metabolism and detoxification of drugs. Antibiotics which cannot be detoxified in patients with hepatic insufficiency can give rise to serious side-effects. Chloramphenicol, nalidixic acid, norfloxacin and the sulphonamides are conjugated with glucuronic acid in the liver and excreted in this form in the urine. These antibiotics may be contra-indicated in severe liver disease and particularly in hepatorenal failure, since the blood concentrations of the free antibiotics are then markedly raised.

Use with caution: Antibiotics that are excreted through the liver into the intestine (e.g. ciprofloxacin, cefoperazone, ceftriaxone, erythromycin, fusidic acid, mezlocillin, nafcillin) should be used with caution in patients with *hepatitis* and *cirrhosis;* β-lactams that are predominantly excreted in the bile (apalcillin, cefoperazone, ceftriaxone) are best avoided altogether in patients with any liver disease. Clindamycin is also metabolised in the liver and accumulates when liver function is impaired.

Because *clotting disorders* often accompany severe liver disease, antibiotics which themselves give rise to a bleeding tendency (cefoperazone, latamoxef, ticarcillin) are best avoided in patients with liver disorders.

Antibiotics that are mainly eliminated unchanged through the kidneys (e.g. benzylpenicillin, cefoxitin, cefuroxime, cephalexin, gentamicin) may safely be used even in patients with severe liver damage. Slight elevation of serum transaminases (e.g. from 10 to 25 i. u./ml) have been reported for all β-lactam antibiotics. These aetiologically obscure increases in transaminase are harmless, and are not due to any detectable disturbance of liver function.

Potentially hepatotoxic drugs: Certain antibiotics (see below) can, however, be hepatotoxic when overdosed or when there is pre-existing liver damage. The combination with other potentially hepatotoxic drugs should be avoided. There is also a danger from drug interactions.

Tetracyclines given parenterally in large doses (2–4 g i. v. daily) can cause toxic liver damage (hepatic dystrophy and fatty degeneration), which can be fatal. The relative frequency of such toxicity in pregnancy suggests that hepatopathy of pregnancy can be triggered by tetracycline therapy; the extent to which pre-existing renal impairment or liver damage is responsible remains unclear. In patients with normal liver function given the correct dosage (1–2 g by mouth or 0.5–0.75 g parenterally), tetracyclines would not be expected to cause liver damage *per se*. They should, however, be avoided in patients with cirrhosis, hepatic coma and hepatitis.

Rifampicin often induces liver enzymes and gives rise to raised transaminases and other liver disorders (sometimes accompanied by jaundice) which have proved fatal in a few cases. Rifampicin is contraindicated in acute liver disease, particularly acute hepatitis. *Isoniazid* (INH), *prothionamide* and *pyrazinamide* can also be hepatotoxic, and caution is advised in the use of these drugs.

Griseofulvin can be hepatotoxic in patients with pre-existing liver damage and should never be used for the long-term treatment of fungal infections in patients with liver disease. Ketoconazole and rarely fluconazole can also cause liver damage (see p. 199 and p. 204).

Jaundice and abnormal liver function tests are occasionally seen during *clindamycin* therapy. *Nitrofurantoin* and *sulphonamides* should only be used with caution in hepatic impairment and should be stopped immediately if liver function is severely reduced.

Potentially hepatotoxic antimicrobials should not be given to patients with viral hepatitis; thus, urinary-tract infections in such patients should not be treated with *co-trimoxazole*. The behaviour of the quinolones is not yet fully understood; they are, however, extensively metabolised in the liver.

Intrahepatic cholestasis: *Erythromycin estolate* (erythromycin lauryl sulphate) and *triacetyl oleandomycin* can give rise to cholestatic hepatosis of clearly allergic origin when given for periods of more than 10 days or in repeated courses. Features of obstructive jaundice appear, with an increase in serum alkaline phosphatase, fever and eosinophilia. These changes are benign and rapidly disappear after treatment has stopped, but are the reasons for which erythromycin ethyl succinate and stearate are now preferred.

In **hepatic coma,** oral aminoglycoside treatment (e. g. with neomycin) may be given to reduce the intestinal production of ammonia. This has led to an improvement in many patients, the basis for which is not entirely clear. Oral aminoglycosides cannot sterilise the contents of the intestine, but they can reduce the enteric bacterial counts considerably. Prolonged oral treatment with aminoglycosides may lead to small-intestinal villous atrophy and is therefore not recommended.

References

Lebel, M. H.: Pharmacology of antimicrobial agents in children with hepatic dysfunction. Pediatr. Infect. Dis. 5: 686 (1986).

9. Antibiotic Therapy in Granulocytopenic Patients

When the bone marrow fails, as occurs in the advanced stages of leukaemia, agranulocytosis or pancytopenia (peripheral granulocyte count below 700/µl), the body's resistance is lowered to such an extent that the further course of the disease becomes dominated by severe infections of the skin, mucous membranes or internal organs. Resistance to infection is also markedly reduced by the immunosuppressive properties of most cytotoxic agents.

Causative organisms: The most important causative organisms (Table 83) are bacteroides, Escherichia coli, klebsiella, pseudomonas and staphylococci. The entire range of facultative pathogens must, however, be considered. The main reservoir of organisms is the colonic and oral flora. Infections with exogenous pathogens, including Clostridium perfringens, legionella, listeria, meningococci, and salmonellae can progress with great rapidity in the granulocytopenic patient. The incidence of tuberculosis in granulocytopenics is also increased, usually as an exacerbation of an earlier infection. Infections with fungi (e.g. aspergillus, candida, cryptococcus) often arise as, though less frequently, do infections with protozoa (e.g. pneumocystis, toxoplasma). When viral infections (e.g. cytomegalovirus, herpes, varicella) occur, they tend to be particularly severe.

Treatment: There are many potential causes of fever in the granulocytopenic patient, and antibiotic therapy often cannot be directed against a particular pathogen. Even when an organism has been isolated, a broad range of facultative pathogens should be covered by the antibiotic combination used. Narrow-

Table 83. Common causes of fever in granulocytopenic patients.

Common situations	Blood transfusion Drug fever Enteritis Infected venous catheters (with thrombophlebitis) Oesophagitis, oral necrosis Pneumonia Septicaemia or bacteraemia Skin infections (e.g. abscesses, ecthyma) Underlying disease (e.g. necrosis of tumor, lymphoma))
Common causes	Bacterial infection (e.g. anaerobes, enterobacteria, listeria, mycobacteria, pseudomonas, staphylococci, legionella, salmonellae)
	Fungal infections (e.g. aspergillus, candida)
	Parasitic infections (e.g. amoebae, Pneumocystis carinii, Toxoplasma gondii)
	Viral infections (e.g. cytomegalovirus, hepatitis, herpes simplex, papovaviruses, parotitis, varicella zoster)

spectrum chemotherapy in the granulocytopenic patient often merely brings about a rapid change to another infecting micro-organism. Previous antibiotic treatment should be taken into account when choosing antibiotics and, where possible, an antibiotic combination should be selected that has not been used in the recent past. It is important in granulocytopenic patients that antibiotic therapy be started promptly. Once specimens for microbiological investigation have been obtained, a **bactericidal combination of drugs** should be started as soon as possible, although it may require subsequent modification in the light of results. Combinations that are active against a wide range of facultative bacterial pathogens, such as cefotaxime + azlocillin, can have their bactericidal activity enhanced by the addition of an aminoglycoside (e.g. gentamicin). The aminoglycosides appear to be less active in the absence of functioning granulocytes, however, and in granulocytopenic patients should only be used in a bactericidal combination as above.

A suggested scheme of **intervention therapy** in the granulocytopenic patient with a fever is shown in Fig. 65, in which the crucial factor is the response to the intervention. Problems arise with those patients in whom the elevated temperature persists despite apparently appropriate treatment; in these patients the chemotherapy should be supplemented as guided by the clinical features, for which there are certain rules.

Intervention therapy in patients with granulocytopenia is also made much more difficult when signs of an allergic reaction occur whilst the patient is receiving a β-lactam combination. Unless there is absolutely no alternative, antibiotics should not be continued in the presence of a drug rash.

The most important **index of effective therapy** is defervescence. The response to antibiotics is often difficult to assess. A prolonged fever usually suggests the presence of resistant organisms. Non-bacterial infections may be present, for example, Aspergillus fumigatus, cytomegalovirus or Pneumocystis carinii. In some cases, treatment may have to be based on clinical suspicion alone because the hazards of confirming the diagnosis in a thrombocytopenic patient from a tissue biopsy would be too great. Every effort should, nevertheless, be made to identify the causative organism of a pneumonia (Table 84) or gastroenteritis (Table 85). Treatment is almost always blind. If antibacterially active antibiotics have failed, a trial of antifungal therapy should be started with fluconazole, itraconazole, and possibly also amphotericin B + flucytosine.

Fungal infections: *Superficial candida infections* in granulocytopenic patients respond poorly to nystatin treatment; most need treatment with ketoconazole, fluconazole or itraconazole. If a *systemic fungal infection* is suspected, flucytosine (6–10 g daily by mouth) may be given in combination with amphotericin B. Oral ketoconazole is not very reliable but may be tried. *Aspergillus infection* leads mainly to fever and resistant pneumonia; the fungus is difficult to demonstrate and is sometimes not found until autopsy. Treatment with amphotericin B +

```
                    Granulocytopenia
                    Signs of infection
                    Temperature >38.5°C  ──→ Blood culture
                              │
                              ▼
              Immediate broad-spectrum intervention
                   therapy for at least 4 days
```

| Acylaminopenicillin + aminoglycoside e.g. piperacillin + tobramycin | or | Modern cephalosporin + aminoglycoside e.g. ceftazidime + tobramycin | or | Acylaminopenicillin + aminoglycoside e.g. piperacillin + cefotaxime |

Defervescence = responder

Continue initial therapy for a further 2–4 (8) days

Non-responder
Further investigations

Supplement therapy according to clinical situation (e.g. with vancomycin, rifampicin)

Continue supplemented therapy for 4 days

Non-responder
Suspect fungal infection

Supplementary antifungal therapy

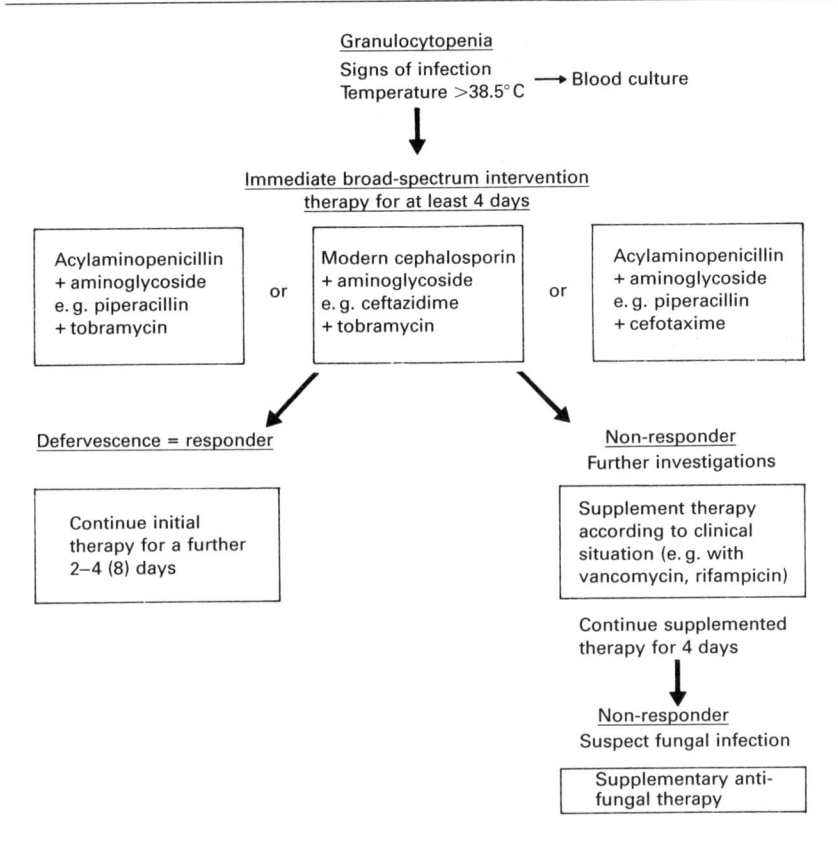

Fig. 65. Scheme of intervention therapy in granulocytopenic patients.

flucytosine or with itraconazole must therefore be begun on clinical suspicion. Other fungal species such as Cryptococcus neoformans and Mucor can also cause infections in these patients.

In *herpes simplex* and *varicella zoster* infections, acyclovir is effective. High doses of co-trimoxazole are indicated if there are clinical signs or radiological evidence of *Pneumocystis carinii* infection. *Toxoplasmosis* may be treated with pyrimethamine + a sulphonamide, and intestinal *giardiasis* with metronidazole.

Overt infections in granulocytopenic patients carry a poor **prognosis,** often progressing to septicaemia and shock, or to the development of extensive areas of non-reactive necrosis. The absence of functioning granulocytes cannot be fully compensated for by antibiotic therapy. Where a granulocyte transfusion is possible, its use should be carefully considered, particularly in reversible forms of granulocytopenia.

Table 84. Causes of pneumonia in granulocytopenic patients.

Cause of pneumonia	Detection
Pneumococci Haemophilus	Culture (sputum, blood), microscopy (sputum), latex agglutination (serum)
Staphylococci	Culture (sputum, possibly blood)
Mycobacterium tuberculosis	Culture, microscopy (sputum, tracheal aspirate)
Enterobacteria Pseudomonas Anaerobes	Culture (tracheal aspirate)
Cytomegalovirus, measles and varicella zoster viruses	Tissue culture, microscopy (immunofluorescence), antigen detection, possibly serology
Candida albicans Cryptococcus neoformans	Culture (tracheal aspirate), latex agglutination (serum)
Pneumocystis carinii Toxoplasma gondii	Microscopy (bronchoscopy with lavage), lung biopsy, possibly serological (fluorescent antibodies)

Table 85. Causes of gastroenteritis in granulocytopenic patients.

Cause of gastroenteritis	Detection
Salmonellae Shigellae Yersinia Pseudomonas Campylobacter jejuni	Culture
Clostridium difficile	Culture, toxin detection
Rotavirus	ELISA or latex test
Candida	Microscopy, culture
Cryptosporidium	Microscopy
Giardia lamblia	Microscopy, antigen detection
Strongyloides	Antibodies (EIA)

Prophylaxis: The poor prognosis of established infection is the basis for prophylaxis in patients during the phase of granulocytopenia. The most sophisticated procedure is protective isolation in an isolation unit with decontamination. There are various systems of isolation unit (e.g. incubators, "life island", a controlled-environment ward, laminar airflow systems). The aim of these systems is to prevent contact with exogenous organisms. All such isolation systems are expensive and require intensive staffing, and so are not available for most patients. They can, moreover, give rise to considerable psychological problems.

It is also still not clear whether exogenous or endogenous infections are more important in such patients, but there is no doubt that endogenous infections play a major role. Isolation units *per se* are therefore of no value unless they are used in conjunction with bacterial decontamination of the patient, by which is meant a marked reduction and, if possible, elimination of the body's own bacterial flora.

Decontamination consists essentially of a reduction in the mouth and intestinal flora and the almost complete elimination of the skin flora. There is no optimal method for achieving intestinal decontamination (sometimes mis-named sterilisation), but one combination used for this purpose is neomycin (2–4 g daily), polymyxin B (0.4–0.6 g daily) and nystatin (1.5–3 million units), all given by mouth. Bacteroides species are unaffected by this combination. The large number of tablets required (ca. 20/day) can also cause difficulty, which may be overcome by giving the drugs as a powder. Oral gentamicin, vancomycin and other antibiotics are used in the USA. The mouth flora may by reduced by various local antibiotics and disinfectants, but complete suppression of bacterial growth is seldom achieved. Well-tolerated antibacterial disinfectants should be used for skin decontamination, paying special attention to certain skin areas (axillae, anal region). Decontamination carries the risk of selection of resistant organisms, and regular bacteriological surveillance is advisable.

Selective decontamination, in which facultative pathogens are eliminated but non-pathogenic flora (e. g. lactobacilli) remain unaffected, is theoretically a better method because it should preserve the natural colonisation resistance of the colon. The chemotherapeutic agents currently available hardly meet this requirement. The greatest experience has been gained with co-trimoxazole and the polymyxins. Norfloxacin and ciprofloxacin have also been considered. The importance of blood levels in prophylaxis with co-trimoxazole or quinolones is not clear. Their use is *de facto* a case of selective gut decontamination with simultaneous prophylaxis against often fulminating streptococcal and enterobacterial infections.

In several studies, prophylactic intestinal decontamination with or without the systemic use of antibiotics to reduce the frequency of bacterial superinfection has proved of value in reducing the frequency of bacterial superinfection in myelosuppression. Immunoglobulins are only justifiable where specific deficiencies have been demonstrated. To prevent *cytomegalovirus* infection (e. g. in bone marrow transplantation), cytomegalovirus immunoglobulin may be used. Prophylactic co-trimoxazole (p. 223) may be used to prevent *Pneumocystis carinii pneumonia* (PCP).

References

ARMSTRONG, D.: Infection in the Patient with Neoplastic Disease. In: R. E. WITTES (ed.). Manual of Oncologic Therapeutics. Philadelphia: Lippincott, 1989.

BODEY, G.: Antimicrobial Prophylaxis for Infection in Neutropenic Patients. In: J. S. REMINGTON, M. N. SWARTZ (eds.). Current Clinical Topics in Infectious Diseases. New York: McGraw-Hill, 1988, pp. 1–43.

EORTC International Antimicrobial Therapy Cooperative Group: Gram-positive bacteraemia in granulocytopenic cancer patients. Eu. J. Cancer. *26:* 569–574 (1990).
HAUER, C., C. URBAN, I. SLAVC: Imipenem-antibiotic monotherapy in juvenile cancer patients with neutropenia. Pediatr. Hematol. ONCOL. *7:* 229–241 (1990).
HOLLERAN, W. M., J. R. WILBUR, M. W. DE GREGORIO: Empiric amphotericin B therapy in patients with acute leukemia. Rev. Infect. Dis. *7:* 619 (1985).
HUGHES, W. T., et al.: Guidelines for the use of antimicrobial agents in neutropenic patients with unexplained fever. J. Infect. Dis. *161:* 381 (1990).
KOVATCH, A. L., E. R. WALD, V. C. ALBO et al.: Oral trimethoprim/sulfamethoxazole for prevention of bacterial infection during the induction phase of cancer chemotherapy in children. Pediatrics *76:* 754 (1985).
LUNDGREN, G., H. WILCZEK, B. LÖNNQVIST et al.: Acyclovir prophylaxis in bone marrow transplant recipients. Scand. J. Infect. Dis. *Suppl. 47:* 137 (1985).
RUBIN, M., et al.: Gram-positive infections and the use of vancomycin in 550 episodes of fever and neutropenia. Ann. Intern. Med. *108:* 30 (1988).

10. Antibiotics in Pregnancy

Antibiotics have not been shown to be particularly teratogenic in man, but have also not been studied particularly for that effect. **In the first trimester,** therefore, it is advisable to avoid antimicrobials which may have cytotoxic activity, such as amphotericin B, chloramphenicol, co-trimoxazole, flucytosine, griseofulvin, nitrofurantoin, nitroimidazoles, pyrimethamine, rifampicin and the quinolones (see Table 86).

Between months 4 and 10, tetracyclines should only be given when alternative antibiotics have failed, because of the risk of impairment of skeletal growth and of yellow discoloration of the child's teeth. Ototoxic antibiotics (aminoglycosides) have caused damage to the fetal inner ear during pregnancy and should therefore be avoided except in life-threatening infections. Quinolones are contraindicated in pregnancy (see p. 235). Flucytosine can damage fetal blood cells and is contraindicated throughout pregnancy, as is amphotericin B. New antibiotics should in general only be given with great caution during pregnancy.

In the last week before the estimated date of delivery, sulphonamides and co-trimoxazole should be avoided because of the increased risk of neonatal jaundice by displacement of bilirubin from its binding sites on plasma proteins, which can lead to bilirubin encephalopathy (kernicterus). Nitrofurantoin shortly before birth can result in neonatal haemolytic anaemia as a result of immaturity of enzyme systems.

Well tolerated in pregnancy are penicillins, cephalosporins, erythromycin and fusidic acid which should always be considered first. The penicillins azlocillin, mezlocillin and piperacillin, the established cephalosporins (cefuroxime, cefotaxime and ceftazidime), imipenem and the monobactams (e. g aztreonam) have all greatly extended the spectrum of activity of the β-lactam antibiotics, so that

10. Antibiotics in Pregnancy

Table 86. Use of important antimicrobials in pregnancy.

Period	Generally safe	Safety not established	Avoid because of side-effects	Potentially teratogenic or cytotoxic
Months 1–4	Amoxycillin, ampicillin, azlocillin, benzylpenicillin, cefazolin, cefotaxime, cefoxitin, ceftazidime, cefuroxime, erythromycin, flucloxacillin, fusidic acid, mezlocillin, oral cephalosporins, phenoxymethylpenicillin	New penicillins and new cephalosporins, imipenem, aztreonam, clavulanate (risk clearly very low), other new substances	Aminoglycosides, amphotericin B, clindamycin, flucytosine, tetracyclines, ketoconazole, fluconazole, itraconazole	Chloramphenicol, ethionamide, flucytosine, griseofulvin, nitroimidazoles, nitrofurantoin, pyrimethamine, quinolones, rifampicin, sulphonamides, trimethoprim
Months 5–10	see months 1–4	–	see months 1–4	–
Last week before delivery	see months 1–4	–	as for months 1–4, plus co-trimoxazole, nitrofurantoin, sulphonamides	–

Substances not mentioned in this table should be assumed to be unsuitable for use in pregnancy.

aminoglycosides and other potentially toxic antibiotics can now generally be avoided even in severe infections.

Placental transfer: Penicillins and cephalosporins are found to different extents in the fetal circulation after being taken by the mother. The concentrations of benzylpenicillin, the acylaminopenicillins and cephalosporins in the umbilical cord blood are known to be about 50% of those in the mother's serum. Aminoglycosides, erythromycin and clindamycin only cross the placenta to a very limited extent. As a result of fetal renal excretion, the penicillins and cephalosporins are concentrated in the amniotic fluid which is then swallowed by the fetus, allowing partial reabsorption of these antibiotics through the fetal gastrointestinal tract. When given continuously in sufficient dosage, therefore, this recirculation means that these antibiotics can be present in considerably higher concentrations in amniotic fluid than in the maternal blood, allowing therapeutically effective concentrations to be achieved in the fetal blood.

References

Chow, A. W., P. J. Jewesson: Pharmacokinetics and safety of antimicrobial agents during pregnancy. Rev. Infect. Dis. 7: 287 (1985).
Gibbs, R. S.: Severe infections in pregnancy. Med. Clin. North. Am. 73: 713–721 (1989).
Medical Letter. Nitrofurantoin in pregnancy. Med. Lett. Drugs Ther. 28: 32 (1986).
Medical Letter. Safety of antimicrobial drugs in pregnancy. Med. Lett. Drugs Ther. 29: 61 (1987).

11. Antibiotic Therapy in the Neonatal Period

Tolerance of antibiotics: The newborn baby, particularly when premature, does not detoxify and metabolise certain antimicrobials in the same way as adults, because of hepatic immaturity. Chloramphenicol in the standard dose of 80 mg/kg will cause the grey baby syndrome in the newborn (see p. 128), so that only 25 mg/kg should be given in the first two weeks of life, and 50 mg/kg in the third and fourth weeks. Sulphonamides, co-trimoxazole, nitrofurantoin and tetracyclines are unsuitable for the treatment of infections in the neonatal period on account of their poor tolerance. Although not licensed for use in the newborn, imipenem and metronidazole may be given for severe infections in individual cases.

Because of renal immaturity, the mean *half-life* of almost all antibiotics varies in the newborn according to the week of life; for carbenicillin (now obsolete), for example, it is 5 h in the first week, 3 h in the second week and 2.5 h in the third and fourth weeks, after which it converges on the adult value of about 1 h. Erythromycin, which is incompletely absorbed, almost completely metabolised, and mainly eliminated in the bile, is the only antibiotic with a constant half-life in this age-group. The variation in antibiotic half-life according to age in weeks of the baby is of little practical importance for the penicillins and cephalosporins, which are well tolerated, although unexplained convulsions in a newborn baby receiving large doses of penicillin, especially if they occur in the first few days of life, should be considered as a possible side-effect of the antibiotic.

Dosage: The daily doses for neonates (see Table 79, p. 592) are generally similar to those recommended for infants, and are based on body weight. These doses are calculated from empirical data such as the sensitivity of the causative organism, the tolerance and pharmacokinetics of the antibiotic and the site of the infection. The doses of penicillins and cephalosporins may be increased several-fold without harm. Thus an average daily dose is recommended for infections with organisms of normal sensitivity, and a higher dose for bacteria with moderate or only slight sensitivity. The normal dose-interval in the newborn may be doubled in view of the renal immaturity.

Published reports often suggest a higher dose (5–6 mg/kg) of gentamicin than that given in Table 79 because the blood concentrations of gentamicin in newborn babies given adequate doses are generally less than those found in adults. The reason for this observation is not completely clear, but could be because gentamicin is deposited to a greater extent in the neonatal than in the adult kidney. The renal accumulation of gentamicin would explain the prolonged urinary excretion of the antibiotic, which may continue for weeks after cessation of therapy.

Antibiotics in breast milk: Whenever a lactating mother is given chemotherapeutic agents, their transfer into the breast milk is to be expected. Sulphonamides, tetracyclines, chloramphenicol and isoniazid achieve high concentrations in breast milk. No drugs that are contraindicated in the newborn should therefore be given to the breastfeeding mother. Penicillins, cephalosporins and aminoglycosides are only present in small quantities in the milk and are therefore generally harmless unless the baby is already allergic to them.

References

GREENOUGH, A., J. OSBORNE, S. SUTHERLAND (eds.): Congenital, perinatal and neonatal infections. Churchill Livingstone, London 1992.
ISAACS, D., E. R. MOXON (eds.): Neonatal infection. Butterworth-Heinemann, Oxford 1991.
MCCRACKEN, G. H., JR., J. D. NELSON: Antimicrobial Therapy for Newborns. Grune and Stratton, New York 1977.
MCCRACKEN, G. H., B. J. FREIJ: Clinical pharmacology of antimicrobial agents. In: REMINGTON, J. S., J. O. KLEIN (eds.): Infectious Diseases of the Fetus and the Newborn Infant. pp. 1020–1078, Saunders, Philadelphia 1990.
REMINGTON, J. S., J. KLEIN (eds.): Infectious Diseases of the Foetus and Newborn Infant. WB Saunders, Philadelphia 1990.
SEVER, J. L., J. W. LARSEN, J. H. GROSSMAN: Handbook of perinatal infections. 2nd ed. 1989.
SPRITZER, R., H. J. VAN DE KAMP, G. DZOLJIC, P. J. SAUER: Five years of cefotaxime use in a neonatal intensive care unit. Pediatr. infect. Dis. J. *9:* 92 (1990).

12. Prophylaxis

In clinical practice, the distinction between prophylaxis and early treatment is often blurred. The indiscriminate use of antibiotics for prophylaxis is clearly as misguided as their total avoidance. There are now several generally agreed conventions which apply to the following sets of circumstances:
1. Prophylaxis of infection, i.e. the suppression after exposure of an infectious agent during its incubation period (e.g. malaria);
2. Prophylaxis of relapse of infections that have already occurred in the patient (e.g. rheumatic fever);
3. Prophylaxis of complications, i.e. the prevention of frequent complications by the early treatment of an unavoidable infection (e.g. in prolonged open heart operations, operations on the opened bowel, contaminated wounds, compound fractures).

1. **Prophylaxis of infection:** During the *incubation period* of bacterial infections, specific, correctly dosed chemosuppression given for a sufficient time can prevent, attenuate or delay the onset of that infection.

After exposure to *whooping cough*, infants and children with severe underlying disease (e. g. leukaemia, renal disease) should be given erythromycin in normal dosage for 1–2 weeks, or longer for more prolonged exposure.

Conversion in the tuberculin test in non-immunised children with no clinical signs of tuberculosis is an indication for isoniazid treatment for at least 6 months (see p. 522).

Exposure of *syphilis* warrants prophylaxis with a penicillin, e. g. a single i. m. injection of benzathine penicillin 1.44 g or i. m. benethamine, procaine and benzylpenicillins ("Triplopen") 1 vial. If treatment is given with penicillin at too low a dose, syphilis can be masked.

For post-exposure prophylaxis of *scarlet fever*, phenoxymethylpenicillin should be given for 5–10 days in a daily dose of 250 mg (infants), 500 mg (older children) and 1 g (adults).

Close contacts of cases of *meningococcal infection*, i. e. contacts (usually family members) who sleep in the same household or dormitory, contacts who have had saliva exchange (kissing, mouth-to-mouth resuscitation) or in an outbreak (particularly of group C disease) who attend the same class, school or play group may be given prophylaxis with rifampicin for 2 days in a twice-daily dose of 10 mg/kg (children up to 12 years) and 600 mg (patients older than 12 years). Ofloxacin, ciprofloxacin and minocycline may also be used. If the index strain is already known to be sensitive, a twice-daily dose of sulphadiazine 250 mg (infants), 500 mg (children aged 1–12 years) and 1 g (adults) for 2 days may be used; however, prophylaxis should not be delayed until sensitivities of the index strain become known.

Rifampicin 20 mg/kg/day (maximum 600 mg daily) for four days should be offered to the following groups of contacts of invasive *Haemophilus influenzae type b infection* (meningitis, epiglottitis, septic arthritis or septicaemia): household members in households where there is an index case of any age, and another child aged under 3 years; classroom contacts (teachers and children) where 2 or more cases of disease have occurred within 120 days; and index cases before discharge from hospital. Pregnant or breastfeeding women, children aged less than 3 months, and persons with severe hepatic dysfunction should be excluded from this recommendation.

2. **Prophylaxis of relapse:** The risk of relapse of *rheumatic fever* through a fresh streptococcal infection can be reduced by the regular administration of phenoxymethylpenicillin. If the patient will comply, an oral dose of 250–500 mg daily is sufficient. A more reliable method is to give benzathine penicillin 0.75 g i. m. once a month, unless there is any suspicion of penicillin allergy, when erythromycin, cephalexin or a sulphonamide should be used.

Prophylaxis of *endocarditis* is important in patients with abnormal or damaged heart valves, after an earlier attack of bacterial endocarditis, in congenital heart disease or after an earlier cardiac operation, or whenever the patient requires a surgical procedure which may give rise to transient bacteraemia (e. g. dental extraction, urological or gynaecological operation). A penicillin, erythromycin or vancomycin are used and detailed regimens are described on p. 347.

Prevention of *recurrent ascending urinary-tract infection:* Young women not infrequently suffer from recurrent cystitis, often related to sexual activity ("honeymoon cystitis") but sometimes due to anatomical or physiological abnormalities such as too short a urethra or infrequent micturition. The frequency of recurrence can be reduced by regular small doses of an antimicrobial such as co-trimoxazole 240 mg or cephalexin 250 mg post-coitally or regularly every evening over a period of time. Such prophylaxis of recurrence of ascending urinary-tract infection should not be confused with suppressive therapy in full dosage as is given, for example, to patients with infected renal stones.

Patients with *recurrent erysipelas* may be protected by long-term phenoxymethylpenicillin or an i. m. injection of one ampoule of benzathine penicillin once a month.

3. **Prophylaxis of complications:** In unavoidable infections (e. g. from contaminated wounds, colonic operations), antibiotics are justifiable to avoid potentially dangerous complications. Since bacterial colonisation can only be reduced temporarily by this means, this type of prophylaxis carries the risk of superinfection or of changes in the infecting organism and should therefore by given for short periods only.

Patients who have *aspirated* material (unconsciousness, drowning, poisoning etc.) require antibiotics to reduce the risk of secondary pneumonia. Since anaerobes of the bacteroides group are the principal causes of aspiration pneumonia, an antibiotic active against anaerobes such as metronidazole or clindamycin should be included.

Patients with a history of tuberculosis who require *high-dose prednisone therapy* should be given prophylactic isoniazid (5 mg/kg/day) to prevent reactivation of old tuberculosis.

Patients with *bone-marrow suppression* should be given parenteral antibiotics when they are severely granulocytopenic (see p. 605). The full range of facultatively pathogenic organisms should be covered. This prophylaxis can be extended by intestinal decontamination with, for example, neomycin, polymyxin B and nystatin. Even so, some gaps in the antibiotic spectrum will remain and infection with resistant organisms can still occur.

The most important indication for prophylactic antibiotics, including perioperative prophylaxis (p. 431) is to *prevent the infective complications of surgery.* The principal indications are:

operations in heavily colonised areas (particularly the colon and uterus),
sternotomy,
neurosurgical operations,
implantation of intravascular devices,
bites, penetrating and crush injuries, including stab and bullet wounds,
trauma involving the paranasal sinuses or joints,
fracture of the base of the skull,
lower limb amputation for ischaemia,
gas-gangrene prophylaxis.

Prophylaxis in surgery can be derived from two different indications, namely:
a) a high frequency of mostly mild secondary infections, and
b) the risk of rare but catastrophic postoperative complications.

Various antibiotics may be given parenterally for these indications (see p. 432). The choice is governed by the possible range of organisms and by the results of relevant studies. In many operations, staphylococci, streptococci and gram-negative bacilli pose the greatest threat, against which basic or intermediate cephalosporins are active. *Anaerobes*, particularly Bacteroides fragilis, are of greatest importance in abdominal surgery and gynaecology, and clindamycin and metronidazole are the most effective agents. To prevent gas gangrene after lower limb amputation for ischaemia, moderate doses of penicillin are sufficient.

Staphylococci are important causes of infection after sternotomy, intravascular implantation of foreign bodies and in neurosurgery, and prophylaxis must be effective against penicillin-resistant strains. Either flucloxacillin or cefazolin are particularly suitable. Newly developed antibiotics should not be used for prophylaxis.

In the past, antibiotic prophylaxis in surgery was often started too late and continued for too long. It is important that antibiotics are not started until just before, or even during the operation. If during an operation an unexpected situation arises that needs antibiotic cover (e. g. the opening of a viscus), they should be given without delay by the anaesthetist. Controlled studies have shown that prophylaxis given for too long is of no value and may even lead to serious complications (superinfection by resistant organisms). Views on the optimal duration of perioperative prophylaxis vary from one dose to 3 days, and it is here that prophylaxis and early treatment may overlap. Prophylaxis of the infective complications of surgery should not be confused with prolonged perioperative therapy in septic surgery.

References

Conte, J. E., Jr.: Antibiotic Prophylaxis: Non-Abdominal Surgery. In: Remington J. S., M. N. Swartz (eds.), Current Clinical Topics in Infectious Diseases. Boston: Blackwell Scientific (Vol. 10), 1989, pp. 254–305.

Medical Letter. Antimicrobial prophylaxis in surgery. Med. Lett. Drugs Ther. *31:* 105 (1989).

Index

Abortion, febrile 448
-, septic 332
Abscess 479
- and cellulitis, eyelid 459
-, cerebral 365
-, circumorbital 464
-, lung 390
-, retropharyngeal 369
-, sweat gland 479
Absorption rate 13
Acne 482
Acrosoxacin (rosoxacin) 233
Actinomycosis 481, 512
Acyclovir 278
Adenine arabinoside 292
Administration 585
-, topical 588
Adnexitis 447
AIDS 290, 530
Allergy to penicillin 29
Amantadine 297
Amikacin 145
Aminocyclitol 267
Aminoglycosides 5, 134
Amoxycillin 43, 110
Amphotericin B 191
Ampicillin 39, 114
Anaerobic infections 321
Angina, Ludwig's 369
Antagonism 583
Anthrax 499
-, cutaneous 479
Antibiotic, choice of 575
-, combinations 583
-, prophylaxis 581
Antibiotics, breast milk 613
-, glycopeptide 176
-, pregnancy 610
-, topical 185
Antiviral agents 278
Apalcillin 59
Appendicitis 410
ARC (AIDS related complex) 290

Arthritis, purulent, acute 440
Aspergilloma 553
Aspergillosis, bronchopulmonary 553
-, invasive pulmonary 553
Aspergillus infections 552
- -, AIDS 542
Azidamphenicol 126
Azidocillin 33
Azidothymidine 288
Azithromycin 164
Azlocillin 53
Azoles 196
AZT 288
Aztreonam 107

Bacampicillin 45
Bacitracin 186
Bacterial infections, acute 478
Bartholinitis 441
β-lactam antibiotics 3, 19
β-lactamase inhibitors 110
Bifonazole 208
Biliary infections 414
Blennorrhoea 462
Blepharitis 458
Body fluids 14
Borreliosis 361, 480
Botulism 407
Bronchiectasis 375
Bronchiolitis 375
Bronchitis, acute 372
-, chronic 373
Brucellosis 506

Candida infections, AIDS 540
- -, skin 552
Candidosis, chronic mucocutaneous 552
- granulomatosa 552
CAPD 412
Capreomycin 273
Carbenicillin 48
- esters 48
Carfecillin 48

Carindacillin 48
Cefaclor 92
Cefadroxil 92
Cefamandole 66
Cefazedone 63
Cefazolin 63
Cefetamet 98
Cefixime 95
Cefmenoxime 80
Cefmetazole 75
Cefoperazone 89
Ceforanide 90
Cefotaxime 80
Cefotetan 74
Cefotiam 66
– hexetil 102
Cefoxitin 71
Cefpirome 91
Cefpodoxime proxetil 100
Cefsulodin 88
Ceftazidime 80
Ceftizoxime 80
Ceftriaxone 80
Cefuroxime 66
– axetil 99
Cellulitis 479
–, orbital 460
Cephalexin 92
Cephalosporins 62
–, aminothiazole 80
–, oral 92
Cephamycins 71
Cephradine 92
Chalazion 459
Chemoprophylaxis in surgery 432
Chloramphenicol 126
Cholera 402
Choroidoretinitis 559
Ciclopiroxolamine 213, 483
Cilastatin 103
Cinoxacin 233
Ciprofloxacin 242
Clarithromycin 161
Clavulanic acid 110, 113
Clindamycin 171
Clofazimine 276
Clostridium difficile 169, 173, 399
Clotrimazole 205
CMV, lungs 388
CNS infections 351
Co-amoxiclav 110

Coccidial infections 409
Coccidioidomycoses 554
Colistin 186
Colitis, ulcerative 410
Colpitis, amine 444
Combinations, fixed 585
Conjunctival infections 460
Conjunctivitis, adenovirus 463
–, bacterial, acute 461
–, –, chronic 463
–, inclusion 462
–, neonatal 461
Corneal infections 463
Co-tetroxazine 225
Co-trimazine 225
Co-trimetrole 225
Co-trimoxazole 220
Crohn's disease 410
Cryptosporidial infections 539
Cystic fibrosis 376
Cystitis 426
Cytomegalovirus, AIDS 545

Dacryoadenitis 459
Dacryocystitis 460
Dapsone 274
Daptomycin 182
Decontamination 609
–, selective 609
Demeclocycline 118, 123
Dermatitis, exfoliative 478
–, seborrhoeic 550
Dermatophyte infections 548
Dialysis, peritoneal 602
–, –, ambulatory, continous 412
Diaminopyrimidine-sulphonamide
  combinations 225
Diarrhoea, Traveller's 403
Dicloxacillin 36
Diphtheria 370
–, conjunctival 461
–, cutaneous 480
Dosage 588
– in neonates 590
–, paediatric 589
Doxycycline 118
Dysentery, amoebic 407
–, balantidial 408
–, shigella 400

Econazole 206
Ecthyma gangrenosum 479

Empyema 391, 415
–, subdural 366
Endocarditis 342
–, campylobacter 346
–, fungal 346
–, prevention of 347
–, Q-fever 346
Endometritis 447
Endophthalmitis, bacterial 465
Enoxacin 246
Enteritis 395
–, campylobacter 401
–, candida 550
–, salmonella 400
–, vibrio parahaemolyticus 407
Enterobacter aerogenes 310
– cloacae 310
Enterobacteriaceae 307
Enterococci 320
Enterocolitis, antibiotic-associated 406
–, antibiotic-induced 595
–, necrotising 405
Epididymitis 428
Epiglottitis 372
Erysipelas 479
–, auricle 471
–, eyelid 459
Erysipeloid 479, 499
Erythrasma 480
Erythromycin 150
Escherichia coli 310
Ethambutol 265
Ethionamide 270
Eye infections 453

Fever, glandular 370
–, granulocytopenic patients 605
–, pontiac 389
–, rheumatic 493
–, scarlet 495
Fleroxacin 248
Flomoxef 78
Flucloxacillin 36
Fluconazole 204
Flucytosine 209
Fluoquinolones 236
Food poisoning 399
Formophthalylsulphacarbamide 215
Fosfomycin 183
Fungal infections 548
– –, granulocytopenic patients 606

Fungal infections, nails 549
– –, skin 482
Furuncle 479
–, ear 471
–, eyelid 459
–, nose and lip 469
Fusafungin 191
Fusidic acid 174

Gall bladder 415
Ganciclovir 286
Gangrene 479
–, gas 340, 497 f
Gastritis 393
Gastroenteritis, Escherichia coli 402
–, granulocytopenic patients 608
–, viral 405
Gastrointestinal infections 393
Gentamicin 135
Giardiasis 408
Gingivitis, necrotising, acute 371
Gonorrhoea 428
Granuloma, swimming pool 480
Grey syndrome 128
Griseofulvin 211
Group B streptococci 319
Gynaecological infections 441

Haemophilus influenzae infections 314
Hand infections 434
Helicobacter pylori 393
Helminth infections 565
Herpes, AIDS 545
– simplex 459
Herxheimer reaction 31
Histoplasmosis 386
HIV infection 290
Hordeolum, external 458
–, internal 458
Hpersensitivity to penicillin 29
Hypopyon 463

Idoxuridine 295
Imipenem 103
Immunoglobulins 302
Infected burns 433
– gangrene 436
Infections, corneal margin 464
–, ear, nose, throat 467
Influenza 529
– pneumonia 530

Infusion bacteraemia 334
INH 258
Interferon α 298
- β 298
- γ 299
Interferons 298
Isoconazole 208
Isoniazid 258
Itraconazole 202

Josamycin 159

Kanamycin 188
Keratitis, herpetic 464
-, parenchymatous 465
Keratoconjunctivitis, allergic 465
Keratomycosis 465
Ketoconazole 199
Klebsiella pneumoniae 310

Laryngitis 372
Latamoxef 76
Legionellosis 388
Leprosy 526
Leptospirosis 510
Lid infections 458
Lincomycin 168
Lincosamides 168
Listeriosis 500
Liver abscess 413
- -, amoebic 408
- function, abnormal 603
Lomefloxacin 251
Loracarbef 102
Lyme disease 361, 480
Lymphadenitis, cervical 474

Macrolides 150
Malaria 559
- prophylaxis 563
Mastitis 450
Mastoiditis 473
Mecillinam 60
Melioidosis 341
Meningitis 351
-, campylobacter 361
-, cryptococcal, AIDS 541
-, fungal 362
-, listeria 359
-, tuberculous 524
Meningo-encephalitis, amoebic 362

Meningo-encephalitis, herpes 362
Methicillin 36
Metronidazole 252
Mezlocillin 55
Miconazole 197
Microsporum infections 549
Minocycline 118
Mononucleosis, infectious 370
Mucoviscidosis 376
Mupirocin 190
Mycobacterial infections, AIDS 543
Mycosis, skin of the eyelid 459
Myositis, clostridial 497

Nafcillin 36
Naftifin 214
Nalidixic acid 233
Natamycin 196
Nematodes 566
Neomycin 188
Netilmicin 144
Nimorazole 252
Nitrofurans 227
Nitrofurantoin 227
Nitrofurazone 231
Nitroimidazoles 252
Norfloxacin 236
Nystatin 195

Oesophagitis, candida 550
Ofloxacin 239
Ophthalmia, gonococcal 462
Opportunistic infections 533
Orchitis 428
Ornidazole 252
Osteomyelitis 437
-, upper and lower jaws 469
Otitis externa 471
- -, malignant 471
- media 471
- -, chronic 473
Oxacillin 36
Oxiconazole 208
Oxytetracycline 118

Pancreatitis 413
Papovavirus 546
Parametritis 447
Paromomycin 190
Paronychia 434
Parotitis, suppurative 470

Pefloxacin 250
Pelvic inflammatory disease 447
Pelvo-peritonitis 447
Penicillin 23
–, benzyl 26
–, combinations 62
– G (benzyl) 26
–, phenoxy 33
–, phenoxymethyl 33
Penicillins, acylamino 53
–, amino 39
–, carboxy 48
–, isoxazolyl 36
Pericarditis 349
–, rheumatic 350
–, tuberculous 350
–, viral 351
Perichondritis, auricular 470
Peritonitis 411
Peritonsillar 369
Perlèche 470
Pertussis 509
Pharmacokinetics 12
Pharyngitis 368
Phenethicillin 33
Phycomycoses 554
Pimaricin 196
Pipemidic acid 233
Piperacillin 57, 117
Pityriasis versicolor 549
Pivampicillin 44
Pivmecillinam 60
Pleurisy, exudative 524
Pneumocystis carinii pneumonia 387, 536
Pneumonia 376
–, aspiration 383
–, candida 551
–, granulocytopenic patients 608
–, influenza 383
–, interstitial 381, 387
–, newborn 383
–, postoperative 436
–, RSV 388
–, varicella 388
Polyenes 191
Polymyxin B 186
Polymyxins 186
Prophylaxis 613
–, perioperative, cardiac operations 348
Propicillin 33
Prostatitis 428

Protein binding 14
Proteus species 311
Prothionamide 270
Pseudomonas infections 313
Puerperal fever 449
Pyelonephritis 424
–, pregnancy 425, 451
Pyoderma 478
Pyrazinamide 272
Pyrexia during labour 451

Quinolones 231

Resistance, bacterial 8
–, cross 12
Respiratory infections 367
Retrobulbar injection 455
Rhinitis 368
Ribavirin 293
Rickettsial infections 511
Rifabutin 277
Rifampicin 261
Rolitetracycline 118
Rosacea 482
Roxithromycin 160

Salmonella excretors 505
– infections 502
Salmonellosis, gastrointestinal 504
Sepsis, puerperal 332
Septic shock 338
Septicaemia 325
–, aspergillus 553
–, biliary 330
–, candida 551
–, clostridial 498
–, foreign body 333
–, neonatal 334
–, postoperative 331, 435
–, salmonella, AIDS 544
–, staphylococcus 335
–, – epidermidis 335
Serratia marcescens infections 312
Sexually transmitted diseases 484
Side-effects 592
–, biological 593
Sinusitis, maxillary 469
–, –, ethmoidal, frontal, sphenoidal 468
Sisomicin 142
Skin infections 475
Spectinomycin 149

Spiramycin 166
Staphylococcal infections 316
Staphylococcus aureus 316
– epidermidis 318
– saprophyticus 318
Stomatitis 470
–, angular 470
–, candida 371
Streptococcal infections 319
Streptococcus pyogenes infections 319
Streptomycin 267
Strongyloides infections 409
Subconjunctival injection 455
Sulbactam 114
Sulphadiazine 215, 225
Sulphaguanidine 215
Sulphalene 215
Sulphamethoxazole 215, 220
Sulphamethoxydiazine 215
Sulphametopyrazine 215
Sulphametrole 225
Sulphamoxole 215
Sulphaurea 215
Sulphonamides 215
Surgical infections 430
Synergy 583
Syphilis 484
–, congenital 487
–, pregnancy 487

Talampicillin 47
Tapeworm infections 570
Tazobactam 117
Teicoplanin 180
Temafloxacin 251
Temocillin 52
Tenovaginitis 434
Tetanus 496
Tetracyclines 118
Tetroxoprim 225
Therapy, antibiotic, granulocytopenic patients 605
–, –, haemodialysis 602
–, –, neonatal period 612
–, –, renal insufficiency 598
–, intervention 578
–, –, AIDS 535
–, –, granulocytopenic patients 607
Thiamphenicol 131
Thioamides 270
Thrush 550

Thrush, genital 550
–, oral 371, 550
Ticarcillin 50, 113
Tinea 548
Tinidazole 252
Tissue penetration 13
Tobramycin 141
Tolnaftate 214
Tonsillitis 368
Toxic shock syndrome 451
Toxoplasmosis 538, 554
–, acquired lymphoglandular 558
–, AIDS 538
–, congenital 557
–, pregnancy 557
–, reactivated 558
Trachoma 462
Transfer, placental 610
Treatment, cost of 596
Trematode infections 570
Tribavirin 293
Trifluridine 296
Trimethoprim 220, 226
Triplopen 33
Trometamol 183
Tuberculosis 513
–, cervical lymph nodes 524
–, cutaneous 480, 525
–, mesenteric lymph nodes 524
–, miliary 524
– of bone and joint 525
–, urogenital 525
Tularaemia 480, 508
Typhoid, paratyphoid fevers 502
Tyrothricin 186

Ulcer, buruli 480
–, corneal 463
–, peptic 393
Urethritis 426
–, candida 428
–, chlamydial 428
–, trichomonas 428
Urinary infections, acute 421
– –, candida 551
Urogenital infections 417

Vaginitis in adults 443
–, candida 444
Vaginosis, bacterial 444
Vancomycin 176

Vidarabine 292
Vulvitis 442
Vulvovaginitis in children 442

Waterhouse-Friderichsen syndrome 337
Whipworm infections 409
Whitlow 479

Wound infections 430
– –, prophylaxis 431

Yersiniosis 401

Zidovudine 288
Zoster, ophthalmic 465
–, varicella, AIDS 545